AGING, PLACE, and HEALTH

A GLOBAL PERSPECTIVE

William A. Satariano , PhD, MPH
Professor, Epidemiology and Community Health Sciences
School of Public Health University of California, Berkeley

Marlon Maus, MD, DrPH, FACS
Adjunct Professor, Community Health Sciences
School of Public Health University of California, Berkeley

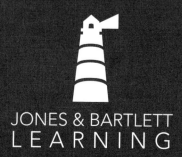

JONES & BARTLETT
LEARNING

World Headquarters
Jones & Bartlett Learning
5 Wall Street
Burlington, MA 01803
978-443-5000
info@jblearning.com
www.jblearning.com

Jones & Bartlett Learning books and products are available through most bookstores and online booksellers. To contact Jones & Bartlett Learning directly, call 800-832-0034, fax 978-443-8000, or visit our website, www.jblearning.com.

Substantial discounts on bulk quantities of Jones & Bartlett Learning publications are available to corporations, professional associations, and other qualified organizations. For details and specific discount information, contact the special sales department at Jones & Bartlett Learning via the above contact information or send an email to specialsales@jblearning.com.

Production Credits

VP, Executive Publisher: David D. Cella
Publisher: Michael Brown
Associate Editor: Lindsey Mawhiney Sousa
Associate Editor: Danielle Bessette
Production Manager: Carolyn Rogers Pershouse
Senior Production Editor: Nancy Hitchcock
Senior Marketing Manager: Sophie Fleck Teague
Production Services Manager: Colleen Lamy
Manufacturing and Inventory Control Supervisor:
   Amy Bacus

Product Fulfillment Manager: Wendy Kilborn
Composition: Integra Software Services Pvt. Ltd.
Director of Rights & Media: Joanna Gallant
Rights & Media Specialist: Merideth Tumasz
Media Development Editor: Shannon Sheehan
Cover Image (Title Page, Part Opener, Chapter Opener):
   Hands: © Shutterstock, Inc./Dewald Kirsten;
   Buildings: © Shutterstock, Inc./Bariskina
Printing and Binding: Edwards Brothers Malloy
Cover Printing: Edwards Brothers Malloy

Library of Congress Cataloging-in-Publication Data
Names: Satariano, William, author. | Maus, Marlon, author.
Title: Aging, place, and health : a global perspective / William Satariano, Marlon Maus.
Description: Burlington, Massachusetts : Jones & Bartlett Learning, [2018] | Includes bibliographical references and index.
Identifiers: LCCN 2016056018 | ISBN 9781284069389
Subjects: | MESH: Aged | Geography, Medical | Geriatrics | Health Policy | Internationality
Classification: LCC RA418 | NLM WT 100 | DDC 362.1--dc23
LC record available at https://lccn.loc.gov/2016056018

6048

Printed in the United States of America
21 20 19 18 17   10 9 8 7 6 5 4 3 2 1

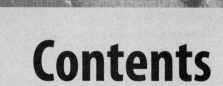

Image: Hands © Shutterstock, Inc./Dewald Kirsten; Buildings © Shutterstock, Inc./Bariskina.

Contents

Preface

William A. Satariano and **Marlon Maus**

An older Dutch couple, out for an evening stroll in Amsterdam in 1995, turn a corner and are startled by the sight of advancing German soldiers marching down the street, as they had marched each night on patrol in 1944.

This unsettling sight is the centerpiece of the 1995 installation "The Neighbor Next Door" by artist Shimon Attie, which presents a visceral multimedia interpretation of the experiences of those driven into hiding by the Nazi regime that reflects on the relationships among place, memory, and identity (Shainman, 2014).

Attie's art, in his own words, is designed to "unlock the memory of place" by projecting, with an elaborate system of lasers, documentary film footage of where the events took place so many years before. By projecting the film from 1944 onto the street in Amsterdam, he unlocked the memory of that place through

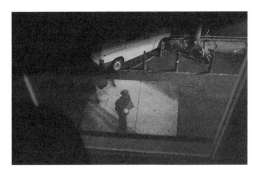

Shimon Attie. Scene from *Prinsengracht*. On-location film projection, from the project *The Neighbor Next Door*, Amsterdam, 1995.

Courtesy of the artist and Jack Shainman Gallery, New York.

the image of life-size German soldiers. Some of the other people walking that night stop, turn, and avoid the exhibition; others walk among the figures, directly confronting the images of the German soldiers who had occupied their country during World War II.

"Unlocking the memory of place" is central to the thesis of this book. We argue that to understand the epidemiology of aging and health, it is important to incorporate information about place across the life course. As Robert Bevan (2007) writes, a place represents a "touchstone for collective memory."

In 2006, one of us published a book titled *Epidemiology of Aging: An Ecological Approach* (Satariano, 2006). That book sought to provide an overview of research and practice in the epidemiology of aging. An ecological model was employed to provide coherence to the consideration of aging: "Patterns of health and well-being are due to a dynamic interplay of biological, behavioral, social, and environmental factors that play out over the life course of individuals, families, neighborhoods, and communities." Each chapter of the book addressed an important topic in aging from survival to function, depression, and health conditions. At the end of the book, the translation of the aging research into practice and policy was considered. While the current text builds on the 2006 book and a general, ecological model, a number of important differences and enhancements exist.

First, and most important, this text represents a collaboration among experts in the field of aging and public health. What was a challenging endeavor barely a decade ago became a Sisyphean task given the truly exponential growth of information in research, teaching, and policy related to the area of aging studies, and in particular the epidemiology of aging. What a single author could have hoped to review and summarize back then, now requires proficiency in multiple areas of expertise.

We came to the field of aging and public health along different paths. While one of us (Satariano) entered the field from the social sciences, the other (Maus) approached aging and public health from clinical medicine and ophthalmology. We invited the authors whose work is presented in this text to join the project based on their expertise in particular areas of aging research, practice, and policy. Each set of authors kindly agreed to prepare a chapter, treating their topic (e.g., cognitive function) as an outcome in epidemiological research. In addition to addressing the significance of the topic, each author reviewed conceptual and measurement issues, implications for practice and policy, and future directions for research. We asked the authors to look broadly and identify key research throughout the world.

Second, this text is written from a global perspective. As noted previously, each author was asked to adhere to that perspective and identify work from countries throughout the world, not just the United States. Our purpose, then, is to provide a comprehensive examination of aging research by topic, and not by country. Therefore, this text does not provide a compendium of aging research from each country, as has been done by other authors. For example, Robinson and colleagues (2007) developed an excellent book on global aging, which uses that approach.

Third, an ecological model, in many ways, captures the intersection of time and place. While the 2006 book addressed the topics of life course and place, it did so very briefly and did not reflect at all the state of outstanding research today. The current text has been expanded to capture the nuances of these important topics.

Fourth, in addition to key topics in the epidemiology of aging, this text includes two important chapters on the translation of research into practice and policy. These chapters are written from different perspectives—one focusing on social and behavioral programs and the other emphasizing more place-based programs.

Fifth, we have included a chapter on the conduct of international studies on aging, with a particular focus on research from developing countries.

Sixth, we address key statistical issues as a roadmap for future research in aging.

Finally, we conclude with a chapter on final directions. As noted previously, we asked each author to discuss future research: which research is anticipated? Which research should be conducted? In the final chapter, we attempted to look across the chapters and provide a summary of key areas for future research. Each of the authors collaborated in the preparation of the final chapter.

This edition is intended for a wide audience that includes not only other experts in the field and academics, but also students, practitioners, and interested researchers from other disciplines. We hope that our text will help inspire further progress in the global effort toward a "state of complete physical, mental, and social well-being, not merely the absence of disease or infirmity" (World Health Organization, 1946) of our older population.

Note that the words "epidemiologic" and "epidemiological" are used interchangeably throughout the book.

▶ References

Bevan, R. (2007). *The destruction of memory: Architecture at war.* London, UK: Reaktion Books.

Robinson, M., Novelli, W., Pearson, C., & Norris, L. (2007). *Global health and global aging.* San Francisco, CA: Jossey-Bass.

Satariano, W. (2006). *Epidemiology of aging: An ecological approach.* Sudbury, MA: Jones and Bartlett.

Shainman, J. (2014). Shimon Attie: Artist page: Jack Shainman Gallery. *YouTube.* Available at https://www.youtube.com/watch?v=wUkWcfyx8hk

World Health Organization. (1946). Preamble to the Constitution of the World Health Organization as adopted by the International Health Conference, New York, 19–22 June, 1946. *Official Records of the World Health Organization, 2,* 100; entered into force on 7 April 1948.

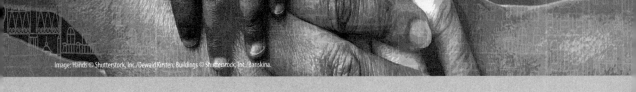

Acknowledgments

We and several of the authors of this volume (Ory, Prohaska, Smith, Snowden, and Steinman) were very fortunate to be members of the Centers for Disease Control and Prevention (CDC) Healthy Aging Research Network (HAN). HAN comprises a network of research institutions and scholars conducting research practice in healthy aging. For its members, it represents a welcoming forum for the exchange of ideas on this important topic. Leaders of HAN include Lynda Anderson and Basia Belza. In addition to these colleagues, we would like to thank our colleagues and associates for their steadfast support in the task of preparing this book, including, but not limited to, Brenda Eskenazi, Meredith Minkler, S. Leonard Syme, John Swartzberg, Debbie Jan, Dion M. Shimatusu-Ong, and Susan Ivey.

And, of course, we wish to express our love and gratitude to our families and friends:

- William: My wife, Enid Satariano; my daughter, Erin Schwass, and her family Kenneth, George, and Nate; and my son, Adam Satariano, and his family Nickie, Leo, and Kai
- Marlon: My partner, Alan Selsor; my mother, Josele Cesarman; my father, Teodoro Maus; and my sister, Tamara, and her family Marcos, Alexis, Jose, and Ivan

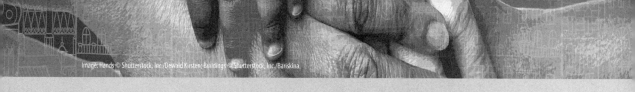

About the Authors

William A. Satariano obtained a BA degree from Santa Clara University (1968), a PhD in sociology from Purdue University (1973), as well as an MPH (1978) and an MS in epidemiology (1979) from University of California, Berkeley. Prior to returning to Berkeley in 1989 as a faculty member, he served as Deputy Director of Epidemiology at the Michigan Cancer Foundation (now the Karmanos Cancer Institute) (1980–1989). He is the recipient of grants and contracts from the National Cancer Institute, the National Institute of Aging, the Centers for Disease Control and Prevention, and the Robert Wood Johnson Foundation. He held the Berkeley Endowed Chair in Geriatrics from 2012–2015. He is the author of *The Epidemiology of Aging: An Ecological Approach* (Jones & Bartlett, 2006). His research interests include aging, health, and function; cancer survival; the effects of the built environment on health behavior and health status in older populations; and technology and aging. Most recently, he and Marlon Maus and other colleagues have been collaborating on the development and evaluation of an iPad-based app ("WordWalk") to encourage walking and brain health among older adults.

Marlon Maus was born and raised in Mexico. He received a BA degree from Brown University (1981) and a medical degree from Jefferson Medical College (1985). His ophthalmology residency at Wills Eye Hospital (1989) was followed by an orbital surgery and neuro-ophthalmology fellowship (1990) and an oculoplastic fellowship at Massachusetts Eye and Ear Infirmary through Harvard University (1991). He then became director of the residency and emergency services at Wills Eye Hospital, where he did research and published extensively on surgical techniques and oculoplastics. He then joined the School of Public Health at University of California, Berkeley, receiving an MPH degree and a doctorate in public health (2011). His present research centers on the relationship between the built environment and public health, including visual disabilities, with a focus on aging. He is collaborating with William Satariano and other colleagues on various projects.

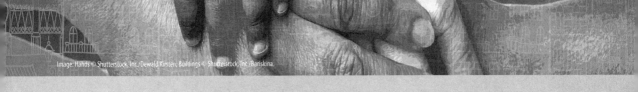

Contributors

Jose Almirall
Adjunct Professor
Université de Sherbrooke
Québec, Canada

Karen Bandeen-Roche, PhD
Hurley-Dorrien Professor and Chair of
  Biostatistics
John Hopkins Bloomberg School of Public
  Health
Baltimore, Maryland

Cynthia Boyd, MD, MPH
Associate Professor of Medicine
Division of Geriatric Medicine and
  Gerontology
Johns Hopkins University School of
  Medicine
Baltimore, Maryland

W. Thomas Boyce
Lisa and John Pritzker Distinguished
  Professor of Development and Behavioral
  Health
Departments of Pediatrics and Psychiatry
University of California, San Francisco
San Francisco, California

Paul Brewster, PhD
Institute on Aging and Lifelong Health
University of Victoria
Victoria, British Columbia, Canada

Brian Buta, MHS
Program Manager
Center on Aging and Health
Division of Geriatric Medicine & Gerontology
Johns Hopkins University School of Medicine
Baltimore, Maryland

Ralph Catalano, PhD
Professor of the Graduate School, Public
  Health
University of California, Berkeley
Berkeley, California

Paulo Chaves, MD, PhD
Leon Medical Centers Chair in Geriatrics in
  the Herbert Wertheim College of Medicine
Director of the Benjamin Leon Center for
  Geriatric Research and Education
Florida International University
Miama, Florida

April M. Falconi, PhD
Postdoctoral Research Scholar
Stanford University
Stanford, California

Martin Fortin, MD, MSc
Professor
Department of Family Medicine and
  Emergency Medicine
Université de Sherbrooke
Quebec, Canada

Lori A. Goehring, BA
Research Assistant
Health and Disability Research Institute
Boston University School of Public Health
Boston, Massachusetts

Emily A. Greenfield, PhD
Associate Professor
School of Social Work
Affiliate of the Institute for Health, Health
  Care Policy, & Aging Research
Rutgers, The State University of New Jersey
New Brunswick, New Jersey

Alan E. Hubbard
Professor of Biostatistics
School of Public Health, University of
  California, Berkeley
Berkeley, California

Alan M. Jette, PhD
Director, Health and Disability Research
  Institute
Boston University School of Public Health
Boston, Massachusetts

Julene K. Johnson, PhD
Professor, Institute for Health & Aging
  and Center for Aging in Diverse
  Communities
University of California, San Francisco
San Francisco, California

Wenjun Li, PhD
Associate Professor of Medicine
University of Massachusetts Medical
  School
Worcester, Massachusetts

Molly E. Marino, MPH
Health and Disability Research Institute
Boston University School of Public Health
Boston, Massachusetts

Richard Marottoli, MD, MPH
Professor of Medicine
Yale University School of Medicine
New Haven, Connecticut

María J. Marquine, PhD
Assistant Professor
University of California, San Diego
San Diego, California

Christine M. McDonaugh, PhD, PT, MS
Research Assistant Professor, Health and
  Disability Research Institute
Department of Health Law, Policy, and
  Management
Boston University School of
  Public Health
Boston, Massachusetts

Nadia Minicuci, PhD
Biostatistician
National Research Council, Neuroscience
  Institute
Padova, Italy

Keith Diaz Moore, PhD, AIA
Dean, College of Architecture + Planning
University of Utah
Salt Lake City, Utah

Dan M. Mungas, PhD
Adjunct Professor
Associate Director, University of California,
  Davis Alzheimer's Disease Research Center
Sacramento, California

Anna Napoles, PhD, MPH
Professor, Department of Medicine
University of California San Francisco
San Francisco, California

Desmond O'Neill, MD, FRCPI
Professor of Medical Gerontology
Trinity College Dublin
Dublin, Ireland

Marcia G. Ory, PhD, MPH
Health Promotion and Community Health
  Sciences
School of Public Health, Texas A&M
  University,
College Station, Texas

Thomas R. Prohaska
Dean
College of Health and Human Services
George Mason University
Fairfax, Virginia

Aline Ramond, MD, PhD
Postdoctoral Fellow
University of Sherbrooke
Quebec, Canada

Taina Rantanen
Professor of Gerontology and Public Health
University of Jyväskylä
Jyväskylä, Finland

Bruce Reed, PhD
Director, Division of Neuroscience,
    Development, and Aging
Center for Scientific Review, National
    Institutes of Health
Bethesda, Maryland

Andrew Scharlach, PhD
Kleiner Professor of Aging
School of Social Welfare
University of California, Berkeley
Berkeley, California

Matthew Smith, PhD, MPH, CHES, FAAHB
Associate Professor
Institute of Gerontology, Department of
    Health Promotion and Behavior, College of
    Public Health
The University of Georgia
Athens, Georgia

Mark Snowden, MD, MPH
Associate Professor
Department of Psychiatry and Behavioral
    Sciences
University of Washington, School of Medicine
Seattle, Washington

Leslie Steinman, MSW, MPH
Research Scientist, Health Promotion
    Research Center
University of Washington, School of Public
    Health
Seattle, Washington

Sarah L. Szanton, PhD, ANP, FAAN
Professor and PhD Program Director
Associate Director for Policy, Center on
    Innovative Care in Aging,
Joint Appointment with the Department of
    Health Policy and Management,
Johns Hopkins School of Nursing and
    Bloomberg School of Public Health
Baltimore, Maryland

Afshin Vafaei, MD, PhD
Post-Doctoral Fellow
Centre for Addiction and Mental Health
Toronto, Ontario, Canada

Ravi Varadhan, PhD
Associate Professor
Division of Biostatistics and Bioinformatics,
    Department of Oncology
John Hopkins University
Baltimore, Maryland

Jeremy D. Walston, MD
Raymond & Anna Lublin Professor of
    Geriatric Medicine
Johns Hopkins University School of
    Medicine
Baltimore, Maryland

Qian-Li Xue, PhD
Associate Professor of Medicine, Biostatistics,
    Epidemiology
Johns Hopkins School of Medicine,
    Department of Medicine Division of
    Geriatric Medicine and Gerontology,
    and Johns Hopkins Center on Aging and
    Health
Baltimore, Maryland

Maria Victoria Zunzunegui
Honorary Professor
School of Public Health, University of
    Montreal
Montreal, Canada

SECTION I

Background

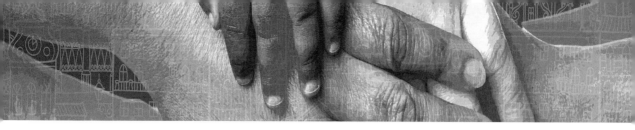

CHAPTER 1

Global Aging of the Population: The Significance of an Epidemiological Perspective

William A. Satariano and **Marlon Maus**

ABSTRACT

The purpose of this chapter is to provide an overview of **global aging** through the prism of the Epidemiologic Transition Theory. While the human population is aging, the extent and nature of that aging process vary by geographic location. There are more older adults living in the industrialized developed world, but growth in the aging population is occurring more rapidly in the developing world. Despite its overall utility, the Epidemiologic Transition Theory is a work in progress. This chapter reviews suggested ways to improve the effectiveness of the Epidemiologic Transition Theory so as to provide an evidence base for the development of programs and policies to enhance healthy aging. Finally, we consider the development of the epidemiology of aging as a field of study to foster future global studies in aging.

KEYWORDS

aged	healthy aging	climate change
epidemiology	global aging	

▶ Introduction

Today, older people constitute a larger segment of the world's population than at any other time in history. In 2010, an estimated 524 million people were **aged** 65 or older—8% of the world's population. By 2050, this number is expected to nearly triple to approximately 1.5 billion, representing

16% of the world's population (National Institute on Aging, 2011). The aging of the population is not limited to any one part of the world or segment of the population; rather, it is a global phenomenon.

TABLE 1-1 displays the current size and future projections for the size of the older population by region of the world between

TABLE 1-1 Percentage of the Total Population Accounted for by Elderly Persons, by Age and Region, 2000–2050

Region	Year	65 Years and Older (%)	75 Years and Older (%)	80 Years and Older (%)
Europe	2000	14.0	5.6	2.8
	2015	16.3	7.7	4.3
	2030	23.1	10.8	6.3
	2050	28.6	15.7	10.2
North America	2000	12.6	6.0	3.3
	2015	14.8	6.3	3.8
	2030	20.3	9.4	5.4
	2050	20.7	11.6	8.0
Oceania	2000	10.2	4.5	2.4
	2015	12.7	5.4	3.2
	2030	16.3	7.5	4.4
	2050	20.0	10.6	6.6
Asia	2000	5.9	1.9	0.8
	2015	7.7	2.7	1.3

(continues)

Region	Year	65 Years and Older (%)	75 Years and Older (%)	80 Years and Older (%)
	2030	11.9	4.5	2.2
	2050	18.0	8.5	4.9
Latin America/ Caribbean	2000	5.5	1.9	0.9
	2015	7.4	2.8	1.5
	2030	11.6	4.5	2.4
	2050	18.1	8.4	4.9
Near East/North Africa	2000	2.9	0.8	0.3
	2015	3.1	1.0	0.4
	2030	3.7	1.3	0.6
	2050	5.3	1.8	0.9

TABLE 1-1 Percentage of the Total Population Accounted for by Elderly Persons, *(continued)* by Age and Region, 2000–2050

Reprinted with permission from NRC. PREPARING FOR AN AGING WORLD: THE CASE FOR CROSS-NATIONAL RESEARCH. In N. A. O. Sciences (Ed.), 2001 by the National Academy of Sciences, Courtesy of the National Academies Press, Washington, D.C. Data from U.S. Bureau of the Census 2000.

2000 and 2050 (Sciences National Research Council, 2001). Two points are clear from these data. First, there is considerable variation among regions. In 2000, the percentage of the population aged 65 and older ranged from 14% in Europe to 2.9% in sub-Saharan Africa. Second, as illustrated in **FIGURE 1-1**, in 2050, although Europe is expected to continue to lead the world in the percentage of older people (nearly 30%), older adults in a number of other regions—most notably, Asia, Latin America, and the Caribbean, the Near (or Middle) East, and North Africa—are expected to account for a much higher percentage of the total populations of those areas than they do today. In some cases, the percentages in the latter regions will even approximate the percentages that are expected for North America and Oceania. These data indicate that there is a difference in the percentage of people aged 65 and older between the so-called developed and developing world (or, stated differently, between high-, middle-, and low-income countries).

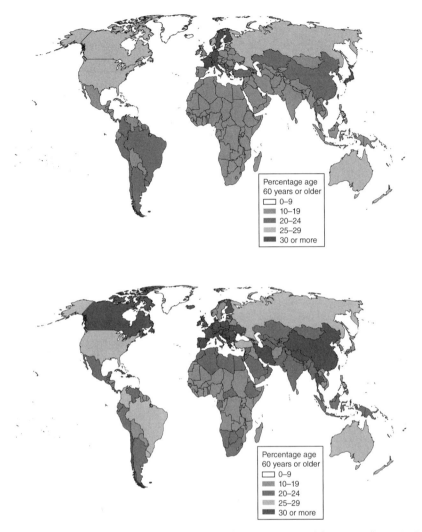

FIGURE 1-1 Proportion of population aged 60 years or older, by country, 2015 (above, top illustration) and 2050 projection (above, bottom illustration).

Reproduced from: WHO. World report on ageing and health. 2015. Luxembourg, Luxembourg. 2015:1-260.

Between 1950 and 2050 (and even more markedly in the 2100 projection), we can see a transformation from a population pyramid to what is, in effect, a population dome (**FIGURE 1-2**). In this case, the greater absolute size of the population in the developing world contributes significantly to the shape of the dome. Thus, it is quite clear that it is not possible to picture the aging of the population without appreciating the significance of place.

▶ Healthy Aging and Place

Background

Why are these demographic trends so important? Put succinctly, the aging of the population represents one of the most significant public policy issues facing society today. Not only has the

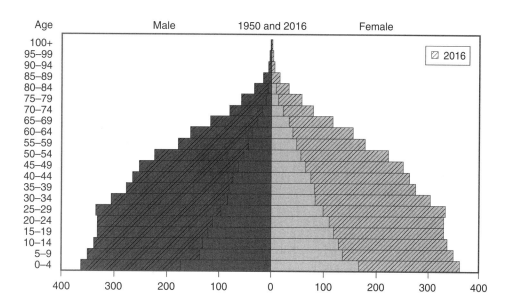

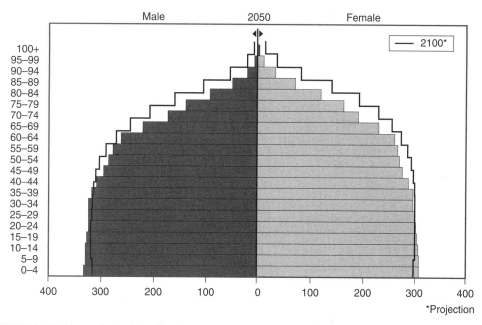

FIGURE 1-2 World population (in millions), 1950–2050 (2100 projection).

Data from: U.S. Census Bureau, 2000a; "The World in 2100" 2011, *The Economist* online; The United Nations 2013; *CIA World Factbook* 2016.

increase in the sheer number of older individuals focused the public's attention on this change in demographics, but the current and future levels of that population's health and vitality are also of widespread concern. The aging of the population is associated with an increase in the incidence and prevalence of chronic diseases and disability. In addition to representing an increase in pain and suffering, it is associated with increased costs for health care and long-term services. In 2014, the World Health Assembly asked the Director-General to develop a comprehensive global strategy and action plan on aging and health. The resulting World Health Organization (WHO, 2015) strategy was designed to enhance and maintain the health and function of an aging population by focusing on the intersection of population and places. This strategy to foster "healthy aging" is also reflected in a statement prepared by the Centers for Disease Control and Prevention's (CDC) Healthy Research Network:

> Healthy aging is the development and maintenance of optimal physical, mental, and social well-being and function in older adults. It is most likely to be achieved when physical environments and communities are safe, and support the adoption and maintenance by individuals of attitudes and behaviors known to promote health and well-being; and by the effective use of health services and community programs to prevent or minimize the impact of acute and chronic disease on function (CDC, 2015).

In short, to understand and promote **healthy aging**, it is necessary to understand the significance of place.

Epidemiological Transitions and Changes in Life Expectancy

What accounts for differences in the age distribution of populations around the world? The Epidemiologic Transition Theory, as first published

by Omran in 1971, was originally presented as an attempt to both describe and explain these global patterns. The basic proposition of this theory is that the increases in life expectancy (a key health outcome) have been caused primarily by changes in the age distribution of the population and associated primary causes of death—that is, by a substitution of early-onset infectious and parasitic diseases, occurring largely among infants, children, and young adult women, for late-onset degenerative causes of death, such as heart disease and cancer, occurring largely among older adults (Omran, 1971). This epidemiological transition is attributable to a variety of factors that are associated primarily with the forces of modernization. Key factors include improvements in public hygiene, sanitation, and housing; improvements in nutrition, food production, and processing; and later, immunization and other medical innovations. Likewise, improved access to formal education by females has been identified as an important factor (Aviles, 2001). Because infants and children of both genders and adolescent and young adult women are at greatest risk of early death from infectious and parasitic conditions, reduction in the incidence of these diseases led to improvements in life expectancy. The initial improvements in life expectancy, therefore, were due to early reduction of infant and maternal mortality. People, then, typically survive their early years to develop degenerative, chronic conditions later in life.

This epidemiological transition, as originally proposed, has evolved in three stages:

1. The age of pestilence and famine
2. The age of receding pandemics
3. The age of degenerative and human-made diseases

High fertility and high mortality characterized the age of pestilence and famine in primarily agrarian societies. Although mortality rates were high in this era, periodic fluctuations occurred in those rates due to epidemics that regularly affected the population. Influenza, pneumonia, diarrhea, smallpox, and tuberculosis, as well as trauma and infections associated with childbirth, were conditions that most commonly affected the population during this period.

During the time of receding pandemics, basic improvements in living standards, public sanitation, housing, and nutrition reduced the incidence of pandemics and parasitic disease, especially among infants, children, and young mothers. The development and dissemination of medical and public health measures, such as new immunization and community screening programs, sustained this transition. Following a reduction in mortality rates, a reduction in birth rates occurred. As the risk of early death from infectious and parasitic diseases declined, more people survived to their later years. A larger cohort reached the age of employability, resulting in an increase in the labor supply and an enhancement of economic productivity and associated goods and services. This outcome is described as the "first dividend" of the epidemiological transition. With the growing size of the aging population, there is an accumulation of capital and further economic development—the "second dividend" of the epidemiological transition.

When the primary cause of death is no longer infectious and parasitic diseases, but rather degenerative and so-called human-made diseases, such as heart disease, cancer, and stroke, society enters into the third period: the age of degenerative and human-made diseases. Relatively low and stable birth and death rates characterize this period. Overall, then, the transition from the first stage to the third stage results in a progressive aging of the population.

Different regions of the world are currently in different stages of development along this trajectory. Some regions of the world are presently in the third stage of development; others are not. As noted previously, the age distribution of the world population is quite variable. Indeed, Omran (1971) proposed that the nature and timing of the transition depend on the time period, country, the stage of modernization, and, it may be hypothesized, the degree of contact that a country has with other regions in different stages of transition.

According to Omran, while each region may proceed through a similar demographic and epidemiological transition, each region is characterized by a different pattern, pace, determinants, and consequences of that evolution.

Omran (1971) identified three models of epidemiological transition as part of his theory. The Classic or Western Model is characterized by a gradual, progressive transition from high mortality and high fertility to low mortality and low fertility. This transition, as experienced by Western Europe and the United States, was stimulated in large part by socioeconomic factors. Specific factors included the sanitary revolution of the late 1800s, coupled with the development and dissemination of medical and public health innovations during the early period of the 1900s. In the second and third decades of the 1900s, chronic and degenerative disease replaced infectious diseases as the primary causes of death.

In contrast, the second model, the Accelerated Epidemiologic Transition Model, was evident in countries such as Japan. Although the factors that stimulated the transition in these countries were similar to the factors that affected the transition in the Classic Model, Omran (1971) contends that the process occurred more quickly. The epidemiological transition that occurred at this time and in these regions of the world was affected by interaction with other regions— the United States and Western Europe—that had made the same transition decades before. Interaction among countries may take different forms, including contact made through global systems of communication and trade.

Finally, the Contemporary (or Delayed) Epidemiologic Transition Model, the third model, characterizes the ongoing transition that is taking place today in many developing nations. Mortality rates in a number of these countries began to decline at the end of the 1800s, but accelerated after World War II. At the same time, many of these countries are still characterized by high fertility rates. Although socioeconomic factors contributed significantly to this transition, as was the case with the first two models, public health and medical interventions played, and continue to play, a more significant role in their epidemiological transition.

Some evidence has been found that supports the premise that the aging of the population in the developing countries is occurring more rapidly than it did in developed countries. One measure used by the U.S. Census Bureau is the time it takes for the percentage of people aged 65 and older in a country's population to increase from 7% to 14% of its total population. For example, in the developed world, it took more than 115 years (from 1865 to 1980) for the senior population in France to increase from 7% to 14%, compared to only 26 years (from 1970 to 1996) for this same change to occur in Japan (Kinsella & He, 2009) (**FIGURE 1-3**). In contrast, in developing countries, it is estimated that this time will range from 30 years for Chile (from 2000 to 2030) to only 15 years for Tunisia (from 2020 to 2035) (Sciences National Research Council, 2001).

Epidemiologic Transition Theory and Economic Outcomes

The epidemiological transition has important implications for economic outcomes. The population age structure is associated with issues of employment, productivity, retirement and long-term care (Mason & Lee, 2011). The epidemiological transition, as noted previously, affects the age distribution of the population and, in turn, the proportion of employed and retired people in the country. As Mason and Lee (2011, p. 2) write:

> In many countries, the boom in the working-age population is drawing to a close and the future will be dominated by growth in the 60+ population. For the world as a whole, those in the working ages currently outnumber those 60+ by 4 to 1. By 2050 the ratio is projected to drop to 2 to 1. The third phase of the global age transition is without precedent. Populations in the future will be much older than ever before in human experience.

One of the major issues is to understand the effects of this epidemiological transition on the "generational economy"—that is, the intergenerational distribution and flow of economic resources. While the Epidemiologic Transition Theory outlines this process in broad strokes, one of the challenges will be to specify the economic outcomes within and between developed and developing countries over time.

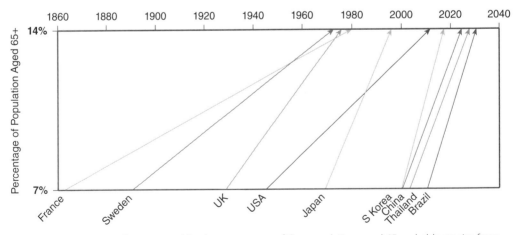

FIGURE 1-3 Time required or expected for the percentage of the population aged 65 and older to rise from 7% to 14% of the total population

One basic measure to characterize this process is the elderly support ratio. This ratio represents the number of people aged 65 and older per 100 persons aged 20 to 64. In the United States, the elderly support ratio is anticipated to increase from 21 in 2000 to 37 in 2030. While this increase is noteworthy, it is even more dramatic in other developing nations. For example, the elderly support ratio in Italy is expected to increase from 29 to 49 between 2000 and 2030; in Japan, it will increase from 27 to 52 over the same time period. Although less pronounced, the elderly support ratio is also expected to increase among developing nations. For example, in Asia the ratio is expected to increase from 12 to 26 in China between 2000 in 2030, from 9 to 15 in India, and from 11 to 27 in Thailand. In Latin America and the Caribbean, the elderly support ratio will range from 13 to 28 in Chile and from 8 to 11 in Guatemala (Kinsella & He, 2009).

In addition to summarizing the age distribution of the population, the elderly support ratio is useful for estimating the proportion of the population (those aged 20 to 64 years) theoretically available to contribute to the overall economic productivity of the country in general and to the economic support for older adults aged 65 and older in particular. (In the United States, this support comes in the form of such transfer programs as Social Security and Medicare.) The significance of the ratio will vary with the scope of each country's economic transfer programs and the perceived need demonstrated by the country's elderly, as reflected by their level of health and functioning. Given the recent attempts to reduce trade and immigration barriers among countries, developed countries have incentives to reduce their elderly support ratios by encouraging migration of younger workers from other countries, most notably developing countries. While immigration of younger workers to countries with high support ratio is a reasonable policy, especially for the European Union, it has been a source of intense debate. Opponents of immigration cite the social and economic costs of facilitating the assimilation of immigrants. In recent years, concerns have arisen that the migrant population, especially from the Middle East, may include terrorists or people who are supportive of terrorism. No doubt that opposition to immigration contributed to the results of the 2016 referendum in the United Kingdom, in which the country's voters chose to leave the European Union ("Brexit"). Attempts to reduce costs by modifying the timing and amount of pensions have also led to intense debate and unrest, including riots in the streets of Greece and France.

The Epidemiologic Transition Theory, as originally presented, provides a parsimonious framework for considering the interrelationship of life expectancy, morbidity, and mortality within a global-historical context. It also underscores the significance of socioeconomic and environmental factors in this transition. It represents a synthesis of demographic and epidemiological principles. Despite its utility as a general framework, the theory remains incomplete—it is very much a work in progress. It is important to note that Omran (1971) concluded his original paper by acknowledging that there are inherent difficulties in attempting to formulate such a comprehensive theory, especially when it seeks to incorporate such a vast array of social, economic, demographic, and epidemiological factors. To his credit, Omran called on other researchers to assist in expanding the theory.

Epidemiologic Transition Theory: Reflections and Revisions
Age of Delayed Degenerative Diseases: A Fourth Stage

A range of issues have been raised since the publication of Omran's original paper in 1971. Fifteen years after the publication of this seminal paper, Olshansky and Ault (1986) proposed that the final stage of the theory (the age of human-made diseases) no longer accurately characterized many of the developed nations. Instead, they suggested, many of these countries were better characterized by a fourth stage—the age of delayed degenerative diseases.

PEARL 1-1 The Elderly Support Ratio and the Prospects of a "Third Demographic Dividend"

The elderly support ratio is a simple summary measure that indicates the number of people aged 65 and older for every 100 adults aged 20 to 64. In general, this ratio is designed to identify and monitor the older, "dependent" segment of the population as compared to the adult "productive" segment of the population. The elderly support ratio has been increasing in both the developed and developing worlds. While not a perfect measure, it suggests that an increasingly large older population may emerge that is more dependent on a shrinking productive, working population.

Linda Fried (2016), however, indicates that the future need not be so dire. She argues that if we investigate in strategies and programs to enhance the health and well-being of people across the life course, there is an increased likelihood that we will be able to produce a healthier older population—in effect, compressing multiple health and disability to the last years of life. More important, Fried contends that we can invest in programs and policies to encourage this healthier older population to continue to contribute to the well-being of society, through either paid employment or volunteerism.

Following from the Epidemiologic Transition Theory, if the first and second demographic dividends are derived from an expanding employed population and associated economic savings, then a third dividend may be obtained from the societal benefits and contributions derived from a healthy elderly population. The aging population should be thought of as a natural, renewable resource, rather than exclusively a societal challenge and problem. This means, then, that the elderly support ratio does not necessarily have to indicate "dependency," but rather "opportunity."

When Omran's original paper was published in 1971, Olshansky and Ault (1986) argued that Omran and others did not fully appreciate the long-term significance of the decline in coronary heart disease that began in 1967 and 1968. The general consensus at the time was that life expectancy, approximately 70 years at that time, had reached its biologic limit and it was very unlikely that there would be any meaningful improvement in life expectancy beyond that point. This proved not to be the case. While the death rates declined initially among middle-aged people, later declines occurred among older age groups. The development of new drugs and antibiotics and improved methods of diagnosing and treating degenerative diseases and their complications served to postpone deaths from these diseases by slowing the rate of chronic disease progression and by reducing case-fatality rates. In addition to advances in medical technology, lifestyle changes occurred, such as reductions in smoking and improved exercise and dietary behavior. In the United States, access to health services for the elderly was improved through the introduction of the Medicare program in the 1960s. In contrast to improvements in life expectancy that were driven by reductions in infant and maternal mortality at the turn of the century, current and future gains in life expectancy are attributable to reductions in mortality among older age groups. Just as the initial epidemiological transitions resulted in infectious and parasitic diseases being replaced by chronic diseases, as argued by the authors, the most recent transition has resulted in the age at death changing from the young old to the oldest old.

Olshansky and Ault (1986) argued that this period of increased age at onset of degenerative conditions is important for two reasons: (1) the size, age, and gender distribution of the older population, and (2) the health and vitality of the older population. Indeed, the relationship between the increased age at onset of chronic diseases and associated levels of health and vitality continues to be a topic of some debate, especially in the United States. It is generally acknowledged today, including by Omran (1983), that the

Epidemiologic Transition Theory consists of the four stages outlined in this section. Other points are being considered in more detail.

Multiple Epidemiological Transitions

Progressive and sustained improvements in life expectancy and the resultant aging of the population are fundamental propositions of the Epidemiologic Transition Theory, as originally proposed. It is assumed that all societies and regions of the world will experience improvements in life expectancy, albeit in their own time and in their own way. Although the timing of the Epidemiologic Transition Theory may vary, as represented by the three models of epidemiological transition (Classic or Western Model, Accelerated Epidemiologic Transition Model, and Contemporary (or Delayed) Epidemiologic Transition Model), it is assumed that all societies will eventually proceed through a similar process, whether it be the United States, Japan, or Tunisia. To date, however, there is only limited evidence of that common transition for a subset of developed nations.

Events in Russia and other states in the former Soviet Union after 1990 indicate that life expectancy can be quite fragile, with any gains being lost in a relatively short period of time (Notzon et al., 1998; Shkolnikov, McKee, & Leon, 2001). Specifically, between 1990 and 1994, life expectancy for Russian men and women declined dramatically from 63.8 and 74.4 years, respectively, to 57.7 and 71.2 years. Over the same period in the United States, life expectancy increased for both men and women from 71.8 to 78.8 years, respectively, to 72.4 and 79.0 years. Closer inspection reveals that more than 75% of the decline in Russian life expectancy was due to increased mortality rates for people ages 25 to 64 years. Leading causes of death included cardiovascular diseases, injuries, pneumonia, influenza, chronic liver diseases and cirrhosis, and other alcohol-related causes. Researchers concluded that the dramatic decline in life expectancy was

due to a variety of factors, including economic and social instability, high rates of tobacco and alcohol consumption, poor nutrition, depression, and deterioration of the healthcare system (Leon et al., 1997).

The presumption that the Epidemiologic Transition Model is uniform within countries has also been criticized (Gaylin & Kates, 1997; Heuveline, Guillot, & Gwatkin, 2002; Mackenbach, 1994). For example, the United States is included with other developed nations in the third or fourth stage of transition. According to some critics, this presumption neglects the heterogeneity (or health disparities) that exists with both developed and developing countries. The epidemiological profile of some residents of developed countries may actually be more akin to that posited for stage 2 than the profile associated with stage 3 or 4. This difference is reflected, in turn, in the health disparities that exist in countries such as the United States and other developed countries—disparities that are often associated with differences in race, ethnicity, and socioeconomic status. Rather than one epidemiological transition, multiple transitions may occur within single countries, with this diversity then being reflected in the heterogeneity of multiple health conditions within a country. Developed and developing countries are characterized by a variety of conditions, including both chronic and infectious diseases.

Robine and Michel (2004) argue that a general theory of population aging must take these multiple patterns into account. In a commentary that accompanied the Robine-Michel paper, Guralnik (2004) summarizes their position as follows:

> There may be a circulating back, where, first, sicker people survive into older age and disability rises, then the number of years lived with disability decreases as new cohorts of healthier people enter old age, but, finally, the number of years lived with disability rises again when the average age of death goes so high that many people spend their last

years at advanced old age burdened by multiple chronic diseases and frailty. And as if all of this were not complex enough, Robine and Michel proposed that it is happening at different times in different countries and perhaps seen at different times in the same country within different population subgroups. Particularly provocative and worthy of serious consideration is their proposal that all these changes, both expansion and compression of morbidity, are part of a single unifying process, a "general theory on population aging," and are simply different stages of a single transition. (p. 606)

Primary and Multiple Causes of Death

There is also concern that the proposed transition from infectious and parasitic causes of death in stage 1 (age of pestilence and famine) to chronic disease in stage 3 (age of degenerative

and human-made diseases) is overly simplistic (**FIGURE 1-4**). While a general transition from infectious diseases to chronic diseases as the major health concerns might occur, the presence of other co-occurring diseases and disability is not given sufficient attention. For example, while chronic diseases may be leading causes of death during stage 3, other diseases, such as acquired immunodeficiency syndrome (AIDS) or other infectious diseases, may make significant contributions to the disease burden of a population. This is an example of syndemics, defined as "the concentration and deleterious interaction of two or more diseases or other health conditions in a population, especially as a consequence of social inequity and the unjust exercise of power" (Singer, 2009, p. xv). Syndemics may be a particular problem in developing countries. In these areas, not only do we find infectious diseases, but also the emergence of chronic conditions, such as diabetes and depression, co-occurring at the same time and among the same populations. Given the limited health and medical resources of many developing

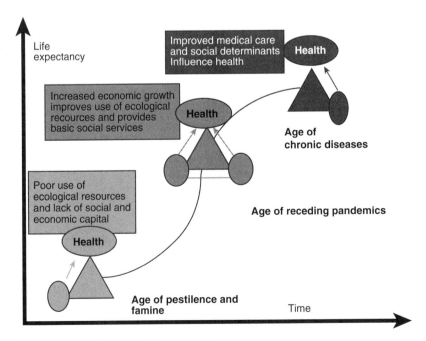

FIGURE 1-4 Epidemiologic Transition Model.
Reproduced from: Manju, Pilania. Epidemiological transition. Available at: http://www.slideshare.net/ManjuPilania/epidemiological-transition-43609219, slide 10.

countries, their healthcare systems are not sufficiently comprehensive to deal with a range of conditions. Most importantly, the presence and severity of multiple morbidities of this kind may affect the timing and nature of the epidemiological transition and the aging of the population. It is recommended that the Epidemiologic Transition Theory be expanded to include an appreciation of health disparities within countries.

Life Changes and Epidemiological Transitions

There is a growing appreciation that aging is not confined to the last part of life, but represents a process that covers the full course of human development. Put differently, patterns of aging and the risk of disease and disability in the middle and later years are affected by events occurring earlier in life, including events prior to birth. As Kuh and colleagues (2014, p. 238) write, "A life course approach in **epidemiology** investigates the biological, behavioral, and social pathways that link physical and social exposures and experiences during gestation, childhood, adolescence, and adult life, and across generations, to changes in health and disease risk later in life." By expanding gerontology to include elements of demography, epidemiology, and human development, it becomes possible to identify periods of vulnerability and resiliency across the life course. Moreover, one can address the temporal interaction of individual and environmental factors (both natural and built) as they influence multiple outcomes of health and well-being.

It is recommended, therefore, that a more complete consideration of the Epidemiologic Transition Theory incorporate a life course perspective—namely, information about individual and environmental factors over the life course from the early years to the middle and later years.

Climate Change

There is scientific consensus that the global climate is becoming progressively warmer, as indicated by increasing trends in both air and ocean temperatures (Intergovernmental Panel on Climate Change, 2014). **Climate change**, in turn, is associated with severe weather events, such as heatwaves, droughts, wild fires, hurricanes, and floods (HelpAge International, 2004). Other evidence indicates that climate change negatively affects agriculture and livestock, especially among subsistence farmers. Finally, climate change may elevate the risk of water- and food-borne diseases and respiratory conditions associated with a rise in increasing heat and reduction in overall air quality.

While the general population is adversely affected by conditions and events associated with climate change, the effects are especially severe among older adults (Gamble et al., 2013). Older adults are more likely than younger people to suffer from chronic conditions and disabilities, experience poorer immune function, and have less adaptive capacity. They are less likely to be mobile, whether "mobility" is defined as being able to walk for extended distances or drive a car safely during stressful and difficult circumstances (Satariano et al., 2012). They are less likely, therefore, to escape and survive major climatic events, such as floods, heatwaves, and hurricanes (Klinenberg, 2015).

It is a perfect storm. At precisely the time that we are entering a period of major climatic events and great storms, more people are reaching an age at which they are least able to deal with the environmental chaos—a stage of significant vulnerability—than at any other time in history. To date, however, these environmental data have not been included in a consideration of epidemiological transition.

Other Environmental Factors

Recent work suggests that other environmental factors may also affect the epidemiological transition. For example, Jared Diamond's book *Guns, Germs, and Steel* (1999, p. 16) is based on a question that is very similar to the basic questions that led to development of the Epidemiologic Transition Theory: "Why did human development proceed at such different rates on different continents?" Diamond contends that differences in human development and demography, such as the aging of populations, may have been affected by differences in land topography and natural resources. Specifically, differences in topography may have affected the opportunities for the production and accumulation of food through the availability and domestication of wild plant and animal species as well as the likelihood of contacts among populations and resultant opportunities for the diffusion of technology and social, political, and economic organization.

According to Diamond (1999), Eurasia had a greater variety of wild plant and animal species available for domestication. Moreover, sustained contact with animal species led to the establishment of immunities to particular types of infectious and bacterial diseases. In addition, contact and diffusion of innovations among populations were more likely in Eurasia, because of its east-west major axis and the relative absence of such geographic barriers as major north-south mountain ranges. In contrast, interhemispheric diffusion made no contribution to Native America's complex societies, which were isolated from Eurasia at low latitudes by broad oceans, and at high latitudes by geographic barriers and a climate suitable only for hunting and gathering. Together, these factors helped to support the development of a larger, more diverse, and more organized population in Eurasia. Work similar to Diamond's can serve as a model to broaden the scope of the Epidemiologic Transition Theory.

Epidemiologic Transition Theory: Final Thoughts

The Epidemiologic Transition Theory has contributed to our understanding of the global patterns of aging and longevity among developed and developing nations. The strengths of this theory can be summarized as follows:

■   The theory casts the study of aging, health, and longevity into a broad historical and global context. The causes and consequences of aging and longevity are not restricted to one country, in one period of history.

■   The theory emphasizes the effects of social, economic, and political forces on changes in patterns of longevity and the age profile of nations.

Together, these characteristics set the stage for the development of global and regional strategies to understand and enhance the health and functioning of older populations.

While the Epidemiologic Transition Theory provides a broad and useful template, combining principles of demography and epidemiology, it is very much a work in progress (Omran, 1971). As noted here, it is necessary to expand the set of individual and environmental factors to better capture the global heterogeneity among and within nations. The causes and consequences of aging and health disparities should be a centerpiece of the epidemiological transition. Environmental factors must be expanded to include both the built and natural environments, as is the case with climate change. It is necessary to look beyond single causes of death to better capture the rich tapestry of health and well-being that exists in populations as part of everyday life. Moreover, the life course approach—a growing focus of researchers' attention—should be central to work in this area. Expanding our understanding in this way will require innovative strategies to obtain rich sources of data from countries throughout the world. Epidemiology will play a key role in enriching scientific research in the epidemiological transition.

▶ Toward an Epidemiology of Aging

From a historical perspective, chronological age has been a key variable in epidemiological studies of disease and disability. Indeed, age is so closely aligned with the incidence of disease and disability that it has been necessary to adjust or "hold constant" the effects of age, so that the significance of other variables could be noted. It is ironic, then, that while chronological age has figured so prominently in the study of epidemiology, the epidemiology of aging, as a separate field, is of relatively recent origin.

In 1972, the National Institutes of Health (NIH) convened the first conference on the epidemiology of aging in Washington, D.C. The epidemiology of aging was presented (in many ways, introduced) at this conference as a field that should address the underlying physiological factors that characterized aging—in fact, the factors that served as markers of aging. These markers were considered to be distinct from individual chronic conditions, but perhaps represented the physiological foundation that affected relative host susceptibility to all health conditions and disabilities. As Adrian Ostfeld, chairperson of the NIH conference, indicated in his opening remarks:

> The epidemiologic method has been traditionally used in the study of specific diseases, first the communicable and later the chronic disorders. Some of us think that the time has come to apply these fruitful methods to a phenomenon broader and more complex than any illness, the condition of aging itself. (*Epidemiology of Aging*, 1975, p. 1)

Ostfeld went on to describe the challenges faced by researchers in this new field:

> But the challenge of applying epidemiologic methods to the study of aging is far more difficult one than applying them to a disease. A clear, valid, and reliable definition of aging remains to be formulated. The units of aging capable of study range from intracellular enzyme activity to overall mortality rates, with subcellular particles, cells, hormones, immune processes, tissues, organs, and neural and endocrine biofeedback mechanism[s] in between. This conference represents a small beginning in considering how we may use epidemiologic methods in partnership with other disciplines in attempting to improve our understanding of aging at all levels of living organism. (*Epidemiology of Aging*, 1975, p. 1)

In 1977, a second conference was convened, in part to take stock of the progress that had been made in the intervening five years (Haynes & Feinleib, 1980). The consensus was that some progress had been made, but more governmental support was required to support the methods and sources of longitudinal data that were necessary to develop this field.

In 1974, the National Institute on Aging (NIA) was established, as part of the Research on Aging Act, as one of the institutes of the NIH. One branch of this new institute was dedicated to epidemiology, demography, and biometry. Among the primary objectives of this branch was the description and explanation of patterns of aging, health, and functioning in human populations.

The establishment of the NIA helped, of course, to draw additional attention to the emerging field of the epidemiology of aging. The epidemiology, demography, and biometry branch stimulated the development of new national population surveys on aging, such as the National Health and Nutrition Examination Survey I. This survey, together with other collaborative studies, provided a picture of the aging population. The NIA also fostered the development of epidemiological studies of aging from established population-based studies as the original cohorts of those studies aged. Exemplars for this type of study include the Framingham Heart Study, the Honolulu Heart Study, and the Alameda County Study. This was exactly the type of study called for by Ostfeld and others at the first NIH meeting on the epidemiology of aging—aging studies that reflected an efficient and effective use of current resources. The advantage of this type of study is that information has been collected for extended periods of time, often following the cohort from the middle to senior years.

More recent NIA-funded studies have used longitudinal designs that were developed specifically for the purpose of conducting research on aging. Reflecting the global significance of aging, a variety of studies of this kind have been undertaken. The NIA initiated a collaborative study in 1984 that serves as an exemplar for many of these studies. The Established Populations for Epidemiologic Studies of the Elderly (EPESE) was the first collaborative, community-based study devoted specifically to the study of the epidemiology of aging, health, and functioning (Huntley et al., 1993). It was based on three population-based samples: East Boston, Massachusetts; New Haven, Connecticut; and selected counties in Iowa. Later, the collaboration was expanded to include selected counties in North Carolina. EPESE is important for a variety of reasons:

- Although not representative of the nation, the collaboration was perhaps the largest and most representative study of aging undertaken in the United States. The samples from New Haven and North Carolina also included valuable information about African Americans.
- The study protocol consisted of a home interview that included the respondents' reports of health and functioning as well as direct assessments of physical performance. Respondents were asked to perform specific tasks that were designed to assess upper- and lower-body function, walking speed, balance, and fine dexterity. The inclusion of these items was a major innovation in population-based studies and supported an observation made by Robert Wallace that many of the research methods used in community studies were first developed in laboratory and clinical settings.

- The EPESE protocol arguably has become the standard protocol for epidemiological studies of this kind, providing the bases for comparisons of aging populations throughout the world. For example, the protocol or key components of the protocol have been used as part of longitudinal studies in Amsterdam, Berlin, and Beijing.

Global Studies in the Epidemiology of Aging

An increased number of studies have addressed the epidemiology of aging worldwide—most notably, longitudinal studies that provide an opportunity to examine health, functioning, and longevity in aging populations. The World Health Organization has contributed significantly to the development of these global studies on aging. WHO-sponsored studies have provided useful, comparative information, which will be critical for the refinement of the Epidemiologic Transition Theory. One major contribution to the global epidemiology of aging includes the use of global measures, such as the global burden of disease (GBD). GBD was developed originally in a 1990 study by the WHO to assess the burden of disease consistently across diseases, risk factors, and geographic regions (Lopez A &, Murray, 1996).

Global Burden of Disease

Assessment of the global burden of disease entails a systematic, scientific effort to quantify the comparative magnitude of health loss due to diseases, injuries, and risk factors by age, sex, and geography for specific points in time. It measures burden of disease using the disability-adjusted life-year (DALY). This time-based measure combines the years of life lost due to premature mortality and the years of life lost due to time lived in states of less than full health. By looking specifically at health loss, rather than income or productivity loss, the GBD approach provides an opportunity to see the big picture; to compare diseases, injuries, and risk factors; and to understand in a given place, time, and age-sex group what are the most important contributors to health loss (Murray et al., 2012).

In its latest iteration, GBD 2010 has dramatically expanded the scope of the 1990 GBD exercise originally commissioned by the World Bank, which assessed 107 diseases and injuries, together with 10 risk factors. The GBD 2010 assessed 235 causes of death and 67 risk factors (Horton, 2012).

By providing a "level playing field," the GBD approach encourages a better understanding of the priorities for comparisons across countries independent of other considerations such as political or economic status. In addition, it highlights the importance of disability caused by conditions such as mental health disorders, substance use, musculoskeletal disease, diabetes, chronic respiratory disease, anemia, and loss of vision and hearing. Particularly in an aging population, disability from disease and injury becomes an increasingly important issue for all health systems. Although current and future aging populations may be healthier than their counterparts in previous generations, more people will be spending more years of their lives with more illnesses. Women are hit especially hard by disability: Women aged 15 to 65 years lose more healthy life to disability than men (WHO, 2000).

The latest GBD measures show that 52.8 million deaths occurred in 2010 compared to 46.5 million deaths in 1990. Population health continues to improve, with life expectancies for men and women increasing, which in turn results in a greater proportion of deaths taking place among people older than 70 years. There has also been substantial progress in preventing premature deaths from heart disease and cancer in several areas around the world.

Some other measures remain subjects of concern. One in four deaths in 2010 was from heart disease or stroke, and 1.3 million deaths were due to diabetes. Deaths from road traffic injuries increased by almost half. Blood pressure is the biggest global risk factor for disease,

followed by tobacco, alcohol, and poor diet. Moreover, young adults are emerging as a new and neglected priority in global health: GBD 2010 found that young adults, especially men, are dying in far higher numbers than previously (Horton, 2012).

The findings from the GBD 2010 study will improve our understanding of the priority of health challenges, as will new multi-county studies on disease epidemiology. This study should provide the essential health intelligence to help guide policy debates about the most urgent global health challenges, and how well we are addressing them (Murray et al., 2012).

The World Health Organization and other international organizations have called for

PEARL 1-2 Global Studies on Aging and Team Science

The development of a new generation of global studies on aging will require good ideas and good organization. The World Health Organization, among other national and international scientific bodies, has contributed significantly to the development of global studies in aging. These studies are critical for establishing evidence-based programs and policies to foster the health and well-being of a growing and increasingly diverse aging population. Daniel Stokols and colleagues (2008) have argued that scientific enterprises, especially those involving multidisciplinary collaboration, require effective systems of organization. Ideas do not advance in a vacuum. As we move forward to study and enhance the health and well-being of populations across the life course, we need to study, in turn, the most effective organizational strategies to achieve that end. What is the best way to bring together and sustain scientists, practitioners, policy makers, and other stakeholders to advance the study of healthy aging? Following the path suggested by Stokols and colleagues, we need to invest in the "science of team science" as it pertains to global aging.

more global studies on aging and more training programs in aging research (WHO, 2000, 2015). One of the concerns expressed about global studies on aging is the lack of a comprehensive and uniform evidence base. Detailed research is available for some countries, typically upper-income or developed nations, but very little has been done for developing countries. Notably, research is lacking that would support the development of a uniform evidence base for the hypotheses generated from the Epidemiologic Transition Theory. To bridge this gap, a growing set of global studies are addressing aging, including Healthy Ageing across the Life Course (HALCyon) (Kuh et al., 2014). Other studies include the Study on Global AGEing and Adult Health (SAGE), the Survey of Health, Ageing, and Retirement in Europe (SHARE), 10/66 Dementia Research Group, and the International Mobility in Aging Study (IMIAS). With a well-developed set of global studies, including those from developing countries, it will be possible to establish a better understanding of the epidemiology of aging. This evidence base, in turn, will serve as the foundation for practices and policies to foster healthy aging.

Epidemiology of Aging: The Core Questions

Epidemiology, both as a perspective and as a set of analytic methods, is especially well suited to examine patterns of health and functioning in an aging population. Epidemiology is based on the premise that health outcomes are not distributed randomly in the population; rather, the incidence and prevalence of health outcomes, as well as the duration and quality of life, follow specific patterns. The purpose of epidemiology is to describe and explain those patterns in the population. This information, in turn, establishes the foundation for future public health interventions. The important questions are how best to prevent and postpone disease and disability and to maintain

and even enhance the health, independence, and mobility of an aging population:

- What is the overall distribution of the health outcome in the population, such as the number and types of subclinical conditions, diseases, levels of functioning, limitations, disability, and survival? How does the health outcome vary among age groups? How does it change as people age? To what extent does the health outcome vary within age groups?
- To what extent do differences among and within age groups vary by gender, race, ethnicity, socioeconomic status, and geographic region? One example is the difference among groups in the age of the onset of a particular condition.
- To what extent do differences among and within age groups vary by other factors associated with health, functioning, behavior, social factors, and the physical environment? Although these factors are important in their own right, they also serve to explain the associations between health outcomes and age, gender, race, ethnicity, socioeconomic status, and geographic region.
- To what extent are differences among and within age groups associated with age differences in the following:
  - The prevalence of the same risk factors
  - The salience or strength of the same risk factors
  - The frequency and timing of exposure over the life course to the same risk factors
  - Exposure to a different set of risk factors
- How does the timing of these factors across the life course, coupled with developmental physiological factors, affect the subsequent risk of disease, disability, and death in the middle and senior years?
- What are the biologic, behavioral, social, and environmental factors associated with the maintenance of health and functioning among older people, or so-called healthy aging? Special attention should be

given to those older people who maintain their health and functioning despite having a risk-factor profile that should elevate their risk for disease, disability, and death. The study of aging and resiliency is central to a consideration of healthy aging.

▶ Conclusion and Future Directions

The aging of the population is a global issue. This issue encompasses not just the sheer number of older people in the population, but also the implications of that aging population for patterns of health, functioning, and longevity, as well as the number and types of resources that will be needed to address the needs of that aging population. The Epidemiologic Transition Theory is one common framework that may be used to describe and explain the patterns of health and functioning in the population. While this theory is a work in progress, it can serve as a roadmap that will pay additional dividends for our society today and in the future.

The Epidemiologic Transition Theory highlights the dividends derived from an aging population, including the expansion of the increased workforce and later an accumulation of economic assets. Linda Fried (2016) argues that we should look to the future and the potential of deriving a third dividend from the aging population. That is, as we focus on strategies to maintain health and well-being in the aging population (i.e., healthy aging), we may be able to develop strategies that will create the opportunities for older adults to contribute to the overall quality of life of the society at large. To accomplish that task and realize this third dividend, we will need to develop a global evidence base to understand more clearly why some older people are at elevated risk of health problems and functional disabilities, while others are able to maintain their health and well-being and adapt to the demands of a changing society. That information, in turn, will serve as the foundation for the practices and policies to enable a growing and increasingly diverse population to age healthfully and potentially contribute to the well-being of the society at large (third dividend). Finally, as noted by many of the authors in this volume, individual- and place-based programs and policies to enhance health and well-being must focus on people across the life course from gestation to old age.

References

Aviles, L. (2001). Epidemiology as discourse: The politics of development institutions in the epidemiological profile of El Salvador. *Journal of Epidemiology and Community Health, 66*, 164-171.

Centers for Disease Control and Prevention (CDC). (2015). *Healthy aging: Helping older Americans achieve healthy and high-quality lives.* Atlanta, GA: Author. Available at: https://www.cdc.gov/chronicdisease/resources/publications/aag/pdf/2015/healthy-aging-aag.pdf

Diamond, J. (1999). *Guns, germs, and steel: The fates of human societies.* New York City, NY: W. W. Norton & Company.

Epidemiology of aging: Summary report and selected paper from a research conference on epidemiology of aging. (1975). Bethesda, MD: National Institutes of Health.

Fried, L. P. (2016). Investing in health to create a third demographic dividend. *Gerontologist, 56*, S167-S177.

Gamble, J. L., Hurley, B. J., Schultz, P. A., Jaglom, W. S., Krishnan, N., & Harris, M. (2013). Climate change and older Americans: State of the science. *Environmental Health Perspectives, 121*, 15.

Gaylin, D. S., & Kates, J. (1997). Refocusing the lens: Epidemiologic transition theory, mortality differentials, and the AIDS pandemic. *Social Science & Medicine, 44*, 609-621.

Guralnik, J. M. (2004). Population aging across time and cultures: Can we move from theory to evidence. *Journals of Gerontology Series A, Biological Sciences and Medical Sciences, 59*, M606-M608.

Haynes, S. G., & Feinleib, M. (1980). Second conference on the epidemiology of aging: Proceedings of the second conference March 28-29, 1977. Bethesda, MD: National Institutes of Health.

HelpAge International. (2004 [cited 2015]). Global ageing statistics. Available at: http://www.helpage.org/resources/ageing-data/global-ageing-statistics/

Heuveline, P., Guillot, M., & Gwatkin, D. R. (2002). The uneven tides of the health transition. *Social Science & Medicine, 55*, 313-322.

Horton, R. (2012). GBD 2010: Understanding disease, injury, and risk. *Lancet, 380,* 2053-2054.

Huntley, J., Ostfeld, A. M., Taylor, J. O., Wallace, R. B., Blazer, D., Berkman, L. F.,... Scherr, P. A. (1993). Established populations for epidemiologic studies of the elderly: Study design and methodology. *Aging Clinical and Experimental Research, 5,* 27-37.

Intergovernmental Panel on Climate Change. (2014). *Climate change 2014: Impacts, adaptation, and vulnerability: Regional aspects.* Cambridge, UK: Cambridge University Press.

Kinsella, K., & He, W. (2009). *An aging world: 2008: International population reports.* Washington, DC: U.S. Government Printing Office.

Klinenberg, E. (2015). *Heat wave: A social autopsy of disaster in Chicago.* Chicago, IL: University of Chicago Press.

Kuh, D., Karunananthan, S., Bergman, H., & Cooper, R. (2014). A life-course approach to healthy ageing: Maintaining physical capability. *Proceedings of the Nutrition Society, 73,* 237-248.

Leon, D. A., Chenet, L., Shkolnikov, V. M., Zakharov, S., Shapiro, J., Rakhmanova, G., Vassin, S., McKee, M. (1997). Huge variation in Russian mortality rates 1984–94: Artefact, alcohol, or what? *Lancet, 350,* 383-388.

Lopez, A. D., & Murray, C. J. (1996). *The global burden of disease: A comprehensive assessment of mortality and disability from diseases, injuries, and risk factors in 1990 and projected to 2020.* Boston, MA: Harvard School of Public Health.

Mackenbach, J. (1994). The Epidemiologic Transition Theory. *Journal of Epidemiology and Community Health, 48,* 329-331.

Mason, A., & Lee, R. (2011). Population aging and the generational economy: Key findings. *Population Aging and the Generational Economy: A Global Perspective,* 3-31.

Murray, C. J. L., Ezzati, M., Flaxman, A. D., Lim, S., Lozano, R., Michaud, C.,... Lopez, A. D. (2012). GBD 2010: Design, definitions, and metrics. *Lancet, 380,* 2063-2066.

National Institute on Aging. (2011). *Global health and aging: 2011.* Contract No.: # 11-7737. Bethesda, MD: National Institutes of Health.

Notzon, F. C., Komarov, Y. M., Ermakov, S. P., Sempos, C. T., Marks, J. S., & Sempos, E. V. (1998). Causes of declining life expectancy in Russia. *Journal of the American Medical Association, 279,* 793-800.

Olshansky, S. J., & Ault, A. B. (1986). The fourth stage of the epidemiologic transition: The age of delayed degenerative diseases. *Milbank Quarterly,* 355-391.

Omran, A. R. (1971). The epidemiologic transition: A theory of the epidemiology of population change. *Milbank Memorial Fund Quarterly, 49,* 509-538.

Omran, A. R. (1983). The Epidemiologic Transition Theory: A preliminary update. *Journal of Tropical Pediatrics, 29,* 305-316.

Robine, J.-M., & Michel, J.-P. (2004). Looking forward to a general theory on population aging. *Journals of Gerontology Series A: Biological Sciences and Medical Sciences, 59,* M590-M597.

Satariano, W. A., Guralnik, J. M., Jackson, R. J., Marottoli, R. A., Phelan, E. A., & Prohaska, T. R. (2012). Mobility and aging: New directions for public health action. *American Journal of Public Health, 102,* 1508-1515.

Sciences National Research Council (Ed.). (2001). *Preparing for an aging world: The case for cross-national research.* Washington, DC: National Academy Press.

Shkolnikov, V., McKee, M., & Leon, D. A. (2001). Changes in life expectancy in Russia in the mid-1990s. *Lancet, 357,* 917-921.

Singer, M. (2009). *Introduction to syndemics: A critical systems approach to public and community health.* San Francisco, CA: Jossey-Bass/John Wiley & Sons.

Stokols, D., Hall, K. L., Taylor, B. K., & Moser, R. P. (2008). The science of team science: Overview of the field and introduction to the supplement. *American Journal of Preventive Medicine, 35,* S77-S89.

World Health Organization (WHO). (2000). *The implications for training of embracing a life course approach to health.* Geneva, Switzerland: WHO & International Longevity Centre-United Kingdom.

World Health Organization (WHO). (2015). *World report on ageing and health.* Luxembourg, Luxembourg: Author.

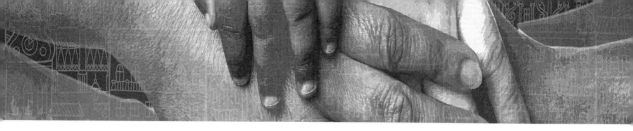

CHAPTER 2

Aging, Health, and the Environment: An Ecological Model

Marlon Maus and **William A. Satariano**

ABSTRACT

Research into the epidemiology of aging is an increasingly complex discipline in the face of a growing older population and the exponential growth of information in the field. To study, measure, describe, and test the multiple factors and hypotheses that make up the study of aging in the 21st century requires a conceptual framework that takes into account these numerous components. The ecological model is exceptionally well suited to consider the various determinants of health at multiple levels. In the framework used in this text, the model is essentially integrated into a life course perspective, as it is now generally accepted that factors occurring early in life have an important effect on how people age. The concept of "place," which suggests that where people age, including the built environment, is an essential contextual element that must also be incorporated when exploring the field of aging.

KEYWORDS

ecological model	epidemiology of aging	aging research
life course perspective	resilience	

▸ Introduction: Why Use an Ecological Model and a Life Course Perspective in the Epidemiology of Aging?

Epidemiology has been defined as the study and analysis of the patterns, causes, and effects of health and disease conditions in defined populations. It is one of the main pillars of public health, as it helps design the studies and interventions that support evidence-based practices and that shape the policy decisions that are ultimately responsible for how contemporary health care is typically provided. When epidemiology targets the fast-growing aging population, it must address various topics that are related to health, functioning, and longevity. Some of the leading areas of research include the effects of age and aging on survival and mortality and the causes of death; physical functioning, disability, and activities of everyday life; cognitive functioning; depression and other psychosocial disorders; falls and injuries; frailty and geriatric syndromes; and, of course, disease and comorbidities.

Ample evidence shows that no single factor can explain why some people—and, indeed, some populations—are able to do well as they age, whereas others do not (Violence Prevention Alliance, 2016). Rather, it is the interactions among the many factors, at many levels and over the life course, that determine the health outcomes we are considering.

The Institute of Medicine (IOM) has defined the **ecological model** as "a model of health that emphasizes the linkages and relationships among multiple factors (or determinants) affecting health" (Gebbie, Rosenstock, & Hernandez, 2003, p. 1). In the first edition of this text, the ecological model was used as a conceptual framework that focuses on the age-associated patterns of health, functioning,

and longevity by considering the determinants of health at various levels from the individual and the interpersonal to the community and policy levels over the life course. The original IOM model is adapted here to illustrate the determinants and ecological nature of health across the life course and includes elements such as biological factors, personal relationships, community contexts, and wider societal factors, as well as traditional demographics such as place, gender, race, ethnicity, and socioeconomic status (Committee on Assuring the Health of the Public in the 21st Century, 2002). In addition, we incorporate more recent work that has been done to enhance our understanding of "life course" and "place"—two key components of the ecological model. We advocate that an ecological framework with a **life course perspective** is the ideal lens that can treat the interaction between factors at different levels with equal importance to the factors within a single level (Violence Prevention Alliance, 2016).

Many appeals have been made to move modern epidemiology from the study of proximate, individual-level risks to the social-ecological perspective that would allow greater insights into the complex social and environmental systems that are the context for health and disease; thinking about population health; and using life course models of disease risk acquisition (McMichael, 1999). This approach is particularly important in view of how the growing world population and economic activity are affecting the environment and its relationship with the health of an aging population.

The ecological approach is contextual in nature and requires an awareness of the multifaceted nature of the conditions and motivations for the expression of behavior across environmental conditions (Kelly, 2006). The ecological approach both to research and practice has been described as having four constituent facets: (1) It takes into account the interrelationships of persons and settings,

(2) It is based on ecological knowledge, (3) It uses a collaborative style, and (4) It is based on social processes (Kelly, 2006).

The ecological model provides a sense of "the big picture" by enabling epidemiological research in aging to combine knowledge from a wide range of scientific disciplines, including the biologic, behavioral, social, and environmental health sciences. Whereas the ecological model focuses on a static picture of an individual or a population, the addition of a life course perspective provides a temporal progression that connects the various elements of an ecological model to the health outcomes at the various stages of life. As an example, studies show that in utero exposure to the 1918 flu pandemic had long-lasting negative health consequences much later in life, including a higher probability of developing coronary heart disease, diabetes, kidney disorders, or generally poor health (Garthwaite, 2008). Other evidence shows that a cohort with fetal exposure to a pandemic performs significantly worse in terms of educational attainment and has a lower chance of marriage than its contemporaries without such exposure (Neelsen & Stratmann, 2012). This concept is explored in greater detail in the chapter on early-life predictors of late-life health.

It is not just the events very early in life that manifest themselves as changes in health late in life. In fact, events occurring at every stage in life affect subsequent stages of life. The cumulative progression that occurs over the life course can include both events with negative effects and events with positive effects. In addition, these events can, and do, take place at every level of the ecological model throughout the life course. Community and societal events, such as an economic recession or a war, may have as powerful effects on health outcomes later in life as those occurring at the individual biological level.

Finally, for a universal and comprehensive understanding of the **epidemiology of aging**, the "global perspective" approach mentioned in this text's title becomes indispensable. The study and research of health in the 21st century must take place in a vastly more interconnected world. In such a world of networks, mathematical models show that even though most nodes are not neighbors of one another, most nodes can be reached from every other node by a small number of hops or steps (Telesford, Joyce, Hayasaka, Burdette, & Laurienti, 2011). These nodes, representing individuals, their peer groups, families, communities, schools, and workplaces, are embedded in the broad economic, cultural, social, and physical environmental conditions at the local, national, and global levels, and are now intimately interconnected by technology, such as social media or ubiquitous transportation. Moreover, all of these interactions are taking place in the context of potentially cataclysmic events that know no geographic borders, such as climate change and massive population migrations resulting from political, economic, and environmental events.

▶ **The Ecological Model**

In this section, we present an ecological model with a life course perspective that serves as the framework for the other chapters in this text, and is intended to be used as a guide for what is being done and an agenda for what should be done in the field of the epidemiology of aging. By looking at key topic areas in this field as outcomes rather than as distinct areas of research, we suggest that the following areas are intimately interrelated: survival and mortality; physical functioning and activities of everyday life; crashes; cognitive functioning; depression; falls and injuries; and disease and comorbidities. In addition, we attempt to integrate the conclusions from these discussions into a blueprint for future directions that may help researchers, students, and practitioners plan for potential activities and allocate resources.

An Overview

As the fraction of older adults in the world population continues to increase, the need to fulfill the World Health Organization's (WHO, 1946) definition of health—"a state of complete physical, mental, and social well-being and not merely the absence of disease or infirmity"— takes on a new level of urgency. The medical model that has dominated the U.S. healthcare system since the 19th century and for much of the 20th century is an untenable approach to preventing disease, improving health, and maintaining a state of well-being in older adults. No longer is it sufficient to look at only disease and injury and their outcomes; instead, it is necessary to recognize the importance of the social and physical environments

that shape patterns of health and of disease as well as our responses to them over the entire life cycle (Fielding, Teutsch, & Breslow, 2010). Some of the determinants of health in the ecological model are listed in **TABLE 2-1**. For communities to be healthy, meaning that they have the capacity to allow each individual to be healthy, they must address all of these factors.

The idea of a social ecological perspective has its origins in the writings of Kurt Lewin, starting in the 1930s. Lewin (1935) sought to understand how individuals and their social environments mutually affect each other across the lifespan. While originating in the field of social psychology, the ecological perspective has actually been used in various disciplines for more than a century (Green, Richard, &

TABLE 2-1 Examples of Determinants of Health Within an Ecological Model

Biological Factors	Living and Working Conditions
Genetic characteristics Lipid levels	Employment/living wage Income Educational attainment Healthy homes Walkable communities Transportation systems
Individual Behaviors	**Broad Social, Economic, Cultural, Health, and Environmental Conditions and Policies at the Global, National, State, and Local Levels**
Physical activity Diet Tobacco use	Climate change Medical care system Air pollution Discrimination and stigma War, terrorism, natural disaster Agricultural policy
Social, Family, and Community Networks	
Social support/social capital Intact families Schools	

Reproduced from: Fielding JE, Steven Teutsch MD M, Breslow L. A framework for public health in the United States. Public Health Reviews. 2010; 32:174., Table 1.

Potvin, 1996). Barker (1968; writing in the field of "ecological psychology"), Bronfenbrenner, and others began to extend the ecological perspective to account for the complexity of individuals developing within embedded systems. Bronfenbrenner (1979), in particular, specified micro-, meso-, exo-, and macro-subsystems as constituting the settings and life space within which an individual develops. These levels correspond to the concentric circle levels depicted in **FIGURE 2-1**. In this model, each of the subsystems influences the individual and the other subsystems and helps us understand behavior in the context of the interplay between the individual and the environment. McLeroy further defined these concentric circles as a comprehensive social ecological model for health promotion that depicts interrelated systems at the intrapersonal, interpersonal, organizational, community, and policy levels (McLeroy,

Bibeau, Steckler, & Glanz, 1988) (Ferraro & Morton, 2016).

In the 1980s, the approach led to the development of variations of the ecological model that have been widely used in health promotion, health psychology, epidemiology, and maternal and child health. Today, these variations continue to expand and replace limited behavioral change models as means to investigate the relationship between global environmental change and human health (Stokols, 1992). For example, there is currently a considerable enthusiasm for using an ecological approach in public health and epidemiology. The ecological model has become an integral component of public health training and competencies, such as those developed by the Association of Schools and Programs of Public Health (ASPPH) and by the Council on Linkages Between Academia

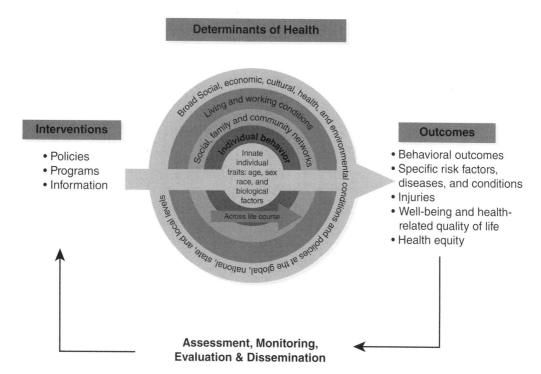

FIGURE 2-1 Action model to achieve the *Healthy People 2020* overarching goals.

and Public Health Practice (Public Health Foundation [PHF]).

The ecological model also serves as the basis for various position documents by leading national and international organizations, including *Healthy People 2010*, which outlines the U.S. public health agenda for the first part of the 21st century (U.S. Department of Health and Human Services, 2000); the IOM (2001) reports on health behaviors; and the model proposed for the National Institutes of Health (NIH) population disparities centers (Warnecke et al., 2008). Its usefulness and applicability to various populations and settings make the ecological framework ideal for use in the international public health arena, such as WHO's (2004) Global Strategy on Diet and Physical Activity and Health, WHO's (2003b) Framework Convention on Tobacco Control, the Bangkok Charter on Health Promotion in a Globalized World (2006), and the Ottawa Charter on Health Promotion (WHO, 1996).

Finally, the ecological model is able to take into account various determinants of health in a broader context, making it especially relevant in view of the need to address social inequalities in health such as socioeconomic, cultural, racial, and ethnic factors, as well as the built environment and access to health care (Krieger, 2001; Marmot, Friel, Bell, Houweling, & Taylor, 2008; Marmot & Wilkinson, 2005; Wilkinson & Marmot, 2003).

What Is It?

An ecological model is predicated on the idea that health and health behaviors are determined by influences at multiple levels, including personal (i.e., biological, psychological), behavioral, organizational/institutional, environmental (i.e., social and physical), and policy levels. It assumes that the dynamic interrelationships among these health determinants throughout the life course result in patterns of health and well-being for individuals, families, and communities (Smedley & Syme, 2001).

This model is useful to the researcher, for whom it provides a framework for the study of

the epidemiology of aging. For the practitioner, use of the ecological models makes it more likely that interventions will be more effective by addressing determinants at all levels.

A practical example of the application of the ecological model is in tobacco control, where multilevel interventions, including environmental and policy components, have been effective in creating long-term, population-wide improvements in health behavior and health outcomes (*Healthy People 2020*, 2010). The ecological model suggests that the need for supportive social and physical environments, together with motivation and instruction, is necessary to produce widespread and long-lasting change.

In this text, topics are considered as health outcomes of an aging population. For each topic, we must keep in mind the ecological model where the determinants of health act at multiple levels, and recognize that the determinants and ecological nature of health act across the life course. This model also serves to connect possible interventions in public health with their health outcomes by identifying multiple points of possible intervention—from the microbiologic to the environmental levels—to postpone the risks of disease, disability, and death, and to enhance the chances for health, mobility, and longevity.

Historically, the visual metaphor for the ecological model is based on Bronfenbrenner's theory of development and seeks to capture the multilevel, integrated quality of this model (McLaren & Hawe, 2005). This depiction consists of a series of concentric circles, each of which represents a level of influence on behavior exerted by the overall physical environment, which in turn contains societies and populations (the epidemiological terrain), public policy, community, organizations, interpersonal processes, single individuals, intrapersonal factors, and individual physiological systems, tissues, and cells, and finally (in biology) molecules. There is an explicit assumption of interactions and reciprocal influences among the various levels.

In the original version of the model, there was no overt consideration of the effect of a life course perspective. Indeed, it was not until relatively recently that the importance of devoting explicit attention to human development across the life course became evident, as researchers realized that exposures in early life can be linked to outcomes in later life (*Healthy People 2020*, 2010). The perinatal and adult periods can be connected by studying how early-life factors, together with later-life factors, contribute to health outcomes (Lynch & Davey Smith, 2005). The implication is that the different factors that operate within the nested genetic, biological, behavioral, social, and economic contexts change as a person develops (*Healthy People 2020*, 2010).

▶ The Life Course Perspective

One of the essential features of the ecological model used in this text is that it integrates a life course perspective in its application to the epidemiology of aging. This approach is consistent with the current trends in public health practice and research, as noted by the *Healthy People 2020* (2010) report. One of the overarching goals in this report is the application of an ecological model that promotes "healthy development and healthy behaviors at every stage of life." The rationale underlying this application stems from the fact that the various determinants of health and the context in which they interact, including genetic, biological, behavioral, social, and economic factors, change as a person develops. Thus, a life course perspective is critical as we look to improve the health and quality of life of older adults and aging populations.

An Overview

A life course perspective examines the biological and behavioral pathways that link physical and social exposures during gestation, childhood, adolescence, and adult life to changes in health and disease risk later in life (Kuh, Richards, Cooper, Hardy, & Ben-Shlomo, 2013). Such a multidisciplinary framework helps us understand the importance of time and timing in associations between exposures and outcomes at the individual and population levels (Lynch & Davey Smith, 2005). This approach aims to consider the way that time and timing of various factors, such as physical growth, reproduction, infection, social mobility, and behavioral transitions, influence health and disease in older adults, and how these temporal processes are interconnected and manifested in population-level disease trends (Lynch & Davey Smith, 2005).

Historically, as research experience with a life course approach increased, particularly in the epidemiology of chronic diseases, various models were proposed. These models distinguished between critical or sensitive period models (with or without later-life modifiers) and risk accumulation models, attempting to identify both the timing and the type of exposures and to determine when in the life course these exposures "get under the skin" and leave biological imprints that later may manifest as adult chronic conditions (Kuh & Ben-Shlomo, 2016).

Essentially, these models represent the mechanisms by which exposures are believed to influence the development of health and disease over the life course (*Healthy People 2020*, 2010). In the critical periods model, the biological or behavioral systems are "programmed" during periods of high sensitivity. It is hypothesized that specific exposures (such as low birth weight) during times of rapid growth and development affect the risk of disease later in life by adjusting the structure or function of organs, tissues, and body systems (Kuh & Ben-Shlomo, 2016). Later risk factors may or may not modify these biological imprints.

The risk accumulation model proposes that the exposures and their effects accumulate over the life course, like weathering of the landscape over time. Such a model suggests that adverse exposures at any stage in life cause biological system damage, which then manifests as chronic disease later in life. An alternative explanation is that a sequence of these exposures ("chain of risk") accumulates, but it is the final event that causes damage to health (Kuh & Ben-Shlomo, 2016).

A third important mechanism influencing these models is the concept that there is a pathway process whereby factors in the social and physical environment reinforce other influences (*Healthy People 2020*, 2010).

What Is It?

The *Healthy People 2020* (2010) report states that an important aim of studying social and physical environmental factors is to increase health equity. To do so, it is necessary to recognize the substantial, often cumulative effects of socioeconomic status and related factors on health, functioning, and well-being from birth throughout the life course. These effects occur across all ecological levels (individual, social and physical environmental, societal).

There are two distinct approaches to studying human development over the life course: the "life stages" approach and "developmental stages" approach. These approaches are complementary and overlapping. Life stages are used to divide the life course into discrete blocks (e.g., infancy, childhood) to facilitate monitoring. Thus, the life stages approach is cross sectional, and it offers a way to break up the life course into easily measured stages (*Healthy People 2020*, 2010). In contrast, the developmental stages approach is longitudinal, and offers a way to examine the impact of early life experiences and exposures on health status later in life.

An important development in the epidemiology of aging is the idea that there is much to be learned by studying the whole spectrum of health and aging, from those individuals who are aging well and have the best health (i.e., the highest-functioning individuals) to those who have the worst health or are experiencing accelerated aging (Kuh et al., 2013). This notion introduces two concepts based on the fact that any research or studies performed on older populations are done on the survivors who have lived long enough to get old: (1) Individuals may have an intrinsic functional or structural reserve, and (2) There may be a compensatory reserve based on the resilience of the individual.

FIGURE 2-2 illustrates the notion of a functional or structural reserve by showing the functional trajectories of body functions and

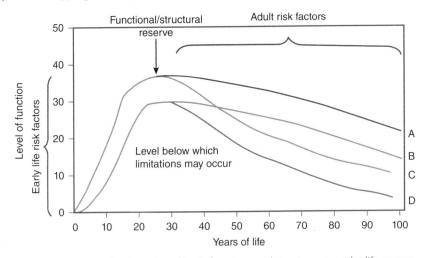

FIGURE 2-2 Functional trajectories of body functions and structures over the life course.

structures over the life course. Line A denotes the rapid growth and development during the prenatal, prepubertal, and pubertal periods, which reaches a peak or plateau at maturity. Line B shows how exposures and epigenetic mechanisms in early life, particularly during a critical developmental window, may leave imprints and have an effect on the structure or function of body systems. However, they may not have any appreciable effects on the rate of decline. Line C, in contrast, shows the accelerated aging processes leading to a more rapid functional decline. Finally, line D shows how various adverse exposures across the lifespan may affect the reserve and accelerate functional decline (Kuh et al., 2013).

An important question in the epidemiology of aging is why some people age better than others. One concept that complements a life course perspective and ecological model is the idea of **resilience**. We must consider the following questions when pondering the effects of resilience:

- To what extent is resilience determined by the ecological level—that is, by community, individual, and biological characteristics?
- How can resilience be developed, maintained, and enhanced to reduce health and social inequalities and achieve healthy aging across the life course?
- Can resilience be defined and measured so it informs research, policy, and practice?
- How do life course experiences influence health and resilience?

▶ The Importance of Place

While the ecological model stresses the importance of considering all levels affecting an individual, and a life course perspective tells us that these levels must be taken into account at all stages in life, most studies looking at healthy aging have traditionally focused on the role of individual factors in encouraging or preventing outdoor mobility such as functional status, self-efficacy, and outcome expectations (Kerr, Rosenberg, & Frank, 2012). Until relatively recently, research focusing on enabling older adults to age in place did not consider the importance of "place," especially the built environment.

This was not always the case. The public health profession originated in tandem with the city and land use planning profession; indeed, for much of the late 19th and early 20th centuries, they were almost united and were closely allied with the social welfare movement. The seven founders of the American Public Health Association in 1872 included an architect and a housing specialist (Jackson, Dannenberg, & Frumkin, 2013). Gains in life expectancy were to a great extent due to improvements in the built environment, including better and healthier housing, street design, and access to clean water, food, and air. With the advent of clinical medicine, the focus for much of public health shifted to interventions targeting individual diseases—both infectious and (later in the century) chronic. For the planning profession, the focus shifted to community design practices that were based on facilitating automobile travel (Kerr et al., 2012). This urban design strategy prioritized developing communities with lower residential densities and disconnected street networks with the purpose of preventing cars from traveling through neighborhoods. As a consequence, residential areas lost access to areas of employment, retail, and entertainment, making walking to these venues difficult for residents, especially older adults.

Nearly a century later, as the effects of these earlier decisions have become manifest, the idea that neighborhoods affect health has become widely accepted among researchers and policy makers (Yen, Michael, & Perdue, 2009). Community design that was supposed to promote public health, safety, and welfare has resulted in declining levels of physical activity and active transportation at a time when chronic diseases such as obesity and cardiovascular disease (CVD) are on the rise.

PEARL 2-1 Transdisciplinary Approach to Collaboration

A transdisciplinary approach to research and health interventions has become a requirement for obtaining funding from many governmental and grant funding organizations. These organizations realize that complex problems require an approach that encourages close collaboration between people in professions who do not necessarily share common academic homes (departments), language, concepts, and methods (Sallis et al., 2006). The partners must strive to understand and solve complex problems in the life-world, and view the complexities of the whole project, rather than one part of it. By transcending their own disciplines to inform one another's work, capture complexity, and create new intellectual spaces, the members of such transdisciplinary teams can potentially stimulate innovation in a broad range of disciplines (Roux, 2007; Sallis et al., 2006; Wiesmann et al., 2008).

With this realization has come a growing collaboration between the planning professions and public health professionals. This requires increased integration of public policy, architectural, and environmental leadership to create age-friendly urban environments and social institutions and roles for older adults that promote health through continued engagement (Fried, 2016). In addition, advocacy may be an effective strategy to encourage cities' adoption of innovations that affect the mobility and quality of life of older adults by emphasizing potential financial benefits to the city, and focusing on cities whose aging residents are particularly vulnerable to disease and disability (Lehning, 2012; Scharlach & Lehning, 2013).

The research examining the connection between the neighborhood environment and older adults' health and functioning is still very limited. A comprehensive literature review suggested the need for additional hypothesis-driven research based on models linking specific neighborhood exposure to health outcomes in older adults, new methods that define and measure "activity spaces" that are relevant to older adults, and integration of direct measurements of these spaces into research (Yen et al., 2009).

Why is this important in the study of epidemiology of aging, and specifically to the area of healthy aging? A landmark WHO (2015) report, *World Report on Ageing and Health*, assembled nearly 200 experts to outline a public health framework for action on healthy aging that is built around the concept of functional ability. In the report, this framework is defined as "the health-related attributes that enable people to be and to do what they have reason to value." This ability is, in turn, determined by both the intrinsic capacities of individuals and the influence of the environments they inhabit (Beard, Officer, & Cassels, 2016). Living longer cannot be the ultimate goal of public health if the extra longevity does not result in added years that are lived in good health and an aging population that becomes a growing human resource that can contribute to society in many ways, such as through a longer working life and the generative social capital of older adults, the "third demographic dividend" (Fried, 2016). This combination would contribute to stronger and wealthier societies, which in turn would benefit the young and increase society's ability to provide the humane supports needed at the end of life (Fried, 2016). Diminishing limitations in capacity for older adults to age in place while achieving their best possible health outcomes makes both societal and economic sense by diminishing demands for health care and social care and increasing the contributions that older adults can make.

When authors of other chapters in this text consider outcomes such as falls or mobility limitations and barriers, the notion of place is implicit in the entire narrative. As an example, it has been shown that when older adults have poor lower-body function, those who have less proximity to goods and services and report more barriers to walking experience more mobility disability compared to other older adults (Satariano et al., 2014).

In conclusion, the built environment influences the mobility of older adults, especially their physical activity. Addressing only intrapersonal ecological factors such as self-efficacy or social support without considering built environment factors such as walkability and access to recreation and services is much less likely to result in a physically active, mobile, and cognitively healthy older population (Carlson, Sallis, & Conway, 2012; Yen et al., 2009). It is hypothesized that built environment factors such as land-use patterns, esthetics, the accessibility and connectivity of urban design, housing quality and population density, pedestrian-friendly environments, and parks are all variables that may greatly affect the physical activity and patterns of mobility among older people (WHO, 2015). As yet, this area has not been studied with the significant attention it deserves.

▶ Resilience Later in Life

The concept of resilience is largely based on the general systems theories elaborated by von Bertalanffy (1968) and others. It was later developed and applied independently in the fields of ecology and psychology as a way of looking at systems of many kinds at many interacting levels, both living and nonliving, such as microorganisms, economies, children or families, a forest, or the global climate (Garmezy, 1971; Holling, 1973; Masten, 2014). Resilience is defined broadly as the capacity of a dynamic ecosystem to respond to a perturbation or disturbance by resisting damage and recovering quickly. In ecology, examples include the ecosystem's stability and capability of tolerating disturbances and restoring itself after fires, floods, deforestation, or fracking, for example. In psychology, particularly child development, the concept has deep roots in the aftermath of World War II, an event that exposed children and youth to severe traumatic experiences (Masten, 2014). Early

research in resilience and public health looked at protective factors in the area of developmental psychology (Garmezy, 1973; Werner, 1989; Werner, Bierman, & French, 1971). As the concept was applied to other populations, it became important to define resilience as a process that can be learned and developed, rather than an individual trait.

An ecological model and a life course process are suggested by the fact that the resilience response process unfolds over time and is embedded within the context. Indeed, it has been explicitly proposed that resilience should be placed in an ecological model that applies to individuals and their communities in later life (Aldwin & Igarashi, 2012). The study of resilience has been influenced by Bronfenbrenner's (1979) ecological model, which considers development "a person's evolving conception of the ecological environment, and his relation to it, as well as the person's growing capacity to discover, sustain, or alter its properties" (p. 9).

Resilience results from the ability of individuals facing stress or adversity to effectively use coping mechanisms in a process that promotes well-being. This method of adaptation may be particularly important in the face of the accumulation of risk factors over the course of a lifetime—that is, within the risk accumulation model, in which the cumulative risk factors result in chronic disease. With roots in the Latin verb *resilire* ("to rebound"), the concept of resilience has been adopted by social scientists to understand how some people escape the harmful effects of severe adversity, cope well, bounce back, or even thrive (Masten, 2014). The study of resilience focuses on one particular subset of processes associated with human development: those that enhance the experience of well-being among individuals who face significant adversity (Ungar, Ghazinour, & Richter, 2013). Thus the importance of the idea of resilience in the study of healthy aging that is explored in other chapters of this text.

Resilience later in life has been equated by Hochhalter, Smith, and Ory (2011) with successful or optimal aging that "leaves one ideally positioned to reach his or her goals." Adaptation occurs throughout the lifespan and has been described as active aging, defined by WHO as "the process of optimizing opportunities for health, participation, and security in order to enhance quality of life as people age" (Mutangadura, 2004, p. 12). While the concept of successful aging, as originally adopted by Rowe and Kahn (1997), helped focus on the idea that some people were better than others at progressing through the aging process, there has been some criticism that this perspective may stigmatize people with chronic disease as being "unsuccessful" in aging.

As we discuss in the next section, the epidemiology of aging, health, functioning, and longevity should be based on a perspective that considers the influences at multiple levels and that reflects the significant and dynamic interrelationships of those different levels of health determinants. This must be embedded in a life course perspective because the outcomes in later life can be linked to exposures in earlier life of individuals and populations.

▶ Epidemiology of Aging

In this section, we examine in greater detail some components of the various levels of the ecological model. Some of the most powerful determinants of health, which include genetic, behavioral, social, and environmental factors, are closely interconnected. **FIGURE 2-3** depicts the range of variables from the ecological model as being divided into three sections (circles). It is important to stress that these variables are interrelated; in other words, each variable affects and, in turn, is affected by each other variable. The model does not, however, imply specific, hypothesized causal relationships or causal links across independent, intermediary, and dependent variables. It is intended to serve as a graphic representation that can help guide our consideration of research in the epidemiology of aging.

In the first part (top circle) of Figure 2-3, we consider some of the more traditional components of epidemiology, while paying special attention to aging individuals and populations. These components include demographics such as age, gender, race and ethnicity, and socioeconomic status (SES). We then look at some of the social determinants of health such as social capital; the built environment (BE), physical environment, and living arrangements; social networks; and social support, which constitute a broader level of the ecological model. In the second part (middle circle) of Figure 2-3, we focus on more specific health behaviors known to exert major health effects on individuals and populations, such as tobacco exposure, alcohol consumption, physical activity (PA), diet and nutrition, and cognitive activity. Over the life course, the outcomes that are displayed in the second circle also may affect the variables listed in the first circle. The third circle represents vital status (alive or dead).

Epidemiology of Aging Research

In 1984, the WHO report *The Uses of Epidemiology in the Study of the Elderly* pointed out the existence of major gaps in knowledge about the state of health of elderly populations, even in the richest countries, and noted that these gaps were due in part to the problems of conceptualization and definition of health and to the difficulties of measuring it. Given that the purpose of health and social services directed toward this population is to improve the health and promote the well-being of the elderly, WHO suggested that health and well-being should be operationally defined, with the factors that affect these outcomes being ascertained and measured.

This conclusion was the direct result of the surprising lack of epidemiological research focusing on aging until the early 1980s (Davies, 1985). Although it was clear that the complex and intertwined causes and consequences of aging of populations demand an interdisciplinary approach, including input from the field of

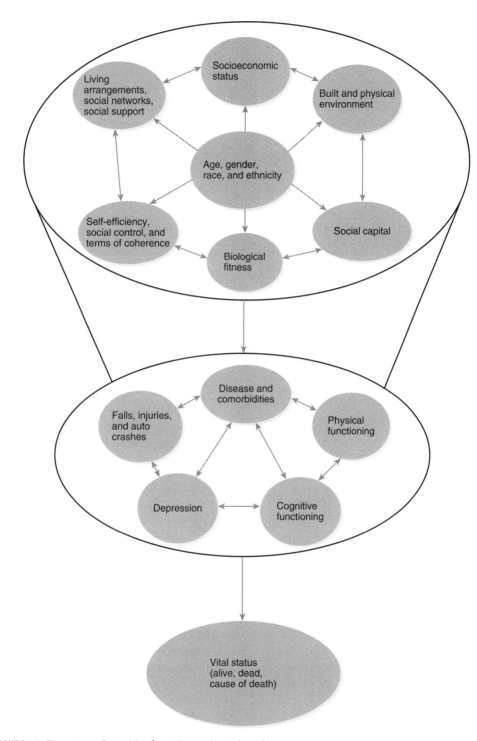

FIGURE 2-3 The range of variables from the ecological model.

epidemiology, most of the advances in **aging research** were made in separate scientific disciplines, such as cellular aging, sociology of aging, demography, and physiological, psychological, or economic areas; only few attempts at integrated or holistic approaches were made (Brenner & Arndt, 2004; Davies, 1985).

It is through the application of epidemiological methods to research related to aging individuals and populations that understanding of the need for, and some proposals of, appropriate definitions for this evolving field emerged. Epidemiology must play a major role in elucidating the determinants of health necessary for the elderly to remain healthy and independent so that they can continue to play an active role in society. Measures of health are difficult to obtain at any age; however, they become especially complicated with advancing age. It has been proposed that the maintenance or restoration of autonomy and independence are the ultimate measurable goals in this population. Thus, autonomy can be used as a reasonable proxy for health, albeit attended by further difficulties in attempting to define the concept operationally.

As defined by the Centers for Disease Control and Prevention (CDC), epidemiology is the study of the distribution and determinants of health-related states or events in specified populations, and the application of this study to the control of health problems (Dicker, Coronado, Koo, & Parrish, 2006). Who is affected and which specific factors put individuals at risk are key questions that researchers must address. Studies are usually distinguished as consisting either of descriptive epidemiology or analytical epidemiology. Descriptive epidemiology is concerned with the observational study of the occurrence of disease and other health-related characteristics in human populations. It deals with general descriptions concerning the relationship of disease to basic characteristics such as age, gender, race, occupation, social class, and geographic location (Porta, 2008). In the case of older adults, the incidence of functional impairments is a particularly important measure, in addition to

other measures such as mortality and prevalence of diseases or impairments.

For many chronic diseases and functional impairments, their incidence, mortality, and prevalence increase with age, and they often vary by sex even within the same age groups. Given this reality, it is important that measures be reported by age and sex (Brenner & Arndt, 2004). It is critical to avoid possible biases from changes in the age structure of populations over time or from the various populations being compared. To accomplish this goal, age-standardized measures of incidence, mortality, and prevalence may be used that assume a common fixed age structure of some "standard population," such as the world population, or some regional or national population.

While descriptive epidemiology can be used to generate hypotheses, testing those hypotheses requires the application of analytic epidemiology. Analytical epidemiology is used to identify the quality and the amount of influence that determinants have on the occurrence of disease or functional impairment. The usual way to gain this knowledge is by group comparisons using either case-control studies or cohort (longitudinal) studies.

Cohort studies are of particular importance in the area of the epidemiology of aging because they allow for the assessment of etiologic factors of multiple health outcomes that are encountered very frequently in the settings of comorbidity and multimorbidity common in older adults. It is also suggested that the quality of data on risk factors or protective factors is often superior in cohort studies, since this information is collected prospectively, rather than retrospectively as in case-control studies (Brenner & Arndt, 2004). In addition, the cohort approach is more effective in suggesting causal effects by providing stronger evidence regarding the temporal relationship between the occurrence of presumed risk and/ or preventive factors and the health outcome.

Observational studies are prone to the bias associated with confounding, which occurs when all or part of the apparent association between the exposure and the outcome is actually accounted for by other variables that affect the outcome and are not themselves affected by exposure (Porta, 2008). For example, various lifestyle factors, such as dietary habits, physical activity, smoking, and alcohol consumption, which are clearly related to a variety of health outcomes at old age, are often interrelated with each other (Brenner & Arndt, 2004). To address this possible bias, the other factors, as well as additional relevant factors such as age or gender, are carefully measured and controlled for in the analysis. Control for confounding is typically done by means of analytic methods such as multivariate analysis or other statistical models.

Health Behaviors

As we have previously argued, an integrated ecological life course model of aging considers that social and biological factors across life affect the probability of healthy aging. The demographic transition to greater life expectancy and the resultant older population is the result of many factors including better childhood nutrition, education, improvements in the environment, advances in medical science, public health, and lifestyle and behavior change. Health behaviors, such as physical activity, dietary practices and nutrition, tobacco exposure, and alcohol consumption, are especially associated with health, functioning, and longevity across the life course (Emmons, 2000). Such modifiable health behaviors could potentially be linked to as many as two thirds of all cancer deaths (Colditz et al., 2000).

Health behaviors play a central role in the life course model, acting in both the risk accumulation model and the "chain of risk" model that links exposures to impaired function. In short, the way we live (in terms of diet, physical activity, and area characteristics) has a direct effect on the likelihood of healthy aging, and life course influences determine the way we live (Kuh et al., 2013).

While very significant differences in life expectancy are apparent across the United States, studies show that the gap in lifespan between the rich and the poor has increased significantly in recent years. For poor Americans, where they live in the United States plays a key role in determining how long they live, while higher income is associated with greater longevity (Chetty et al., 2016). The differences in life expectancy have remarkably increased across income groups over time. Even so, the association between life expectancy and income varies substantially across areas; differences in longevity across income groups have decreased in some areas and increased in others. We now realize that life expectancy is correlated not only with health behaviors, as was traditionally the focus of public health interventions, but also with local area characteristics. The importance of place—of residential areas and the built environment in general—is an essential characteristic of the ecological model and life course perspective because "place" clearly possesses both physical and social attributes that can affect the health of individuals.

To investigate multiple different health outcomes, including chronic disease, morbidity and mortality, mental health, infant health, and birth outcomes, analytical techniques such as multilevel analysis are employed to study neighborhoods and the individuals who live in them (Pickett & Pearl, 2001). In accordance with the framework used in this text, this approach seeks to reconcile two divergent epidemiological paradigms—individual risk factor epidemiology and an ecological approach (Roux, 2007).

In the past, most studies looked at the association of place and specific diseases such as cancer, hypertension, or cardiovascular disease (Cubbin & Winkleby, 2005; Roux et al., 2001). More recently, other indicators have emerged, especially in the area of healthy aging, focusing on physical and cognitive capability (Murray & Stafford, 2014). One important aspect of studying the built environment is the measures used to describe it. These can be subjective, based on the perception of the environment by either the inhabitants or outside observers, or it can be objective, as when research relies on census data or observational measures of the actual buildings and streets and land-use records. An example of a self-reported function in older adults and their environment is an Alameda County study that looked at older adults experiencing severe difficulty with physical tasks (e.g., climbing stairs or lifting 10 pounds) (Balfour & Kaplan, 2002). As with all self-reported data, there is a risk of bias in studies that collect such data because the subjects may consistently over- or under-estimate the objective measures of the environment. One exception has been research of crime rates, where perceptions of safety and actual reported crime statistics have had a significant correlation with disability ("going-outside-the-home disability") (Beard et al., 2009).

Most studies looking at the association between cognitive functioning of older adults and the environment have primarily examined the socioeconomic characteristics of the environment (Murray & Stafford, 2014). Very few studies have looked at cross-sectional links between census-derived data and different tests of cognitive functioning. These links may include differences in cognition between individuals of high and low educational attainment as related to individual and environmental conditions. Showing that cognition varies across urban neighborhoods suggests that social context is an important factor in determining cognitive function among older adults (Wight et al., 2006).

The association between the residential area inhabited in childhood or early adulthood and healthy aging in later life is a major component of a life course approach and one that affects how communities are designed. Various international reports have stressed the importance of healthy and active aging and its relationship to external factors including the built environment (WHO, 2002, 2003a). The effects of human-made and natural environments (and the interactions between the two) on the development of chronic diseases are increasingly being recognized. Ideally, we would design communities specifically for active aging,

PEARL 2-2 Tobacco Control and Behavior Modification

Smoking is an important modifiable risk behavior that affects all other health outcomes in an older population. Although older people are less likely to smoke than younger people, in 2010 fewer than 10% of older people smoked, compared to almost 20% of younger people. Older adults who smoke face an elevated risk of health problems compared with those who do not smoke (West, Cole, Goodkind, & He, 2014) because older people typically have a longer history of tobacco use, are heavier smokers, are already suffering from smoking-related health conditions upon entering older ages, and have other comorbidities (Burns, 2000). Smoking remains a strong risk factor for premature mortality at older age, and smoking cessation is beneficial at any age (Gellert, Schöttker, & Brenner, 2012).

Studies show that residents living in resource-poor areas, such as those characterized by substandard housing conditions, differential access to health services, and lack of social organization, have a higher prevalence of smoking independent of individual social class and educational level (Shohaimi et al., 2000). The ecological model has become a key feature in the planning of interventions for tobacco control (Sallis et al., 2006; Warner, 2000.)

so that the community-based effects would take place throughout the life course. Furthermore, there is a need to understand how human-made environments affect us physically, and how these structural factors can help promote healthy active aging in populations with increased longevity.

Probably one of the most important modifiable health behaviors affecting healthy aging over the life course is physical activity—or more correctly, as WHO (2016) has indicated, physical *in*activity. WHO attributes approximately 3.2 million deaths each year to insufficient physical activity, with many developed and developing countries having populations in which as much as 50% of the adults are insufficiently active. In terms of both human and economic costs, the public health burden of inactivity is very significant, as mortality and chronic conditions tend to negatively impact quality of life as well as life expectancy for inactive individuals. Unfortunately, the growing levels of both inactivity and obesity pose (independent) major health problems in Western society (Colditz, 1999).

To understand how older adults are involved in physical activity, it must be realized that certain trends are associated with aging. Physical activity levels decline by age in adulthood and, in general, men are more active than women across all age groups (Ekelund, 2014). Most of these observations appear generalizable across cultures and ethnic groups, regardless of whether physical activity has been assessed by self-report or objective measurement.

In a comprehensive review of the available time-trend data from the United States, the following trends were observed with greater age, according to the type of physical activity:

- Relatively stable or slightly increasing levels of leisure-time physical activity
- Declining work-related activity
- Declining transportation activity
- Declining activity in the home
- Increasing sedentary activity

Collectively, these trends result in an overall trend of declining total physical activity (Brownson, Boehmer, & Luke, 2005). Causes of these trends may include changes in the built environment, such as urbanization, and an increasing proportion of the overall population being sedentary.

Cognitive ability in older adults reflects the interplay of various factors, including the baseline physical fitness from which adults progress and the level of activity they perform during the life course. Better fitness at baseline is associated with better cognitive function in healthy older adults, particularly on measures of global function and attention/executive function (Barnes, Yaffe, Satariano, & Tager, 2002).

Maintaining cognitive ability as a way to promote healthy aging may depend on a combination of various approaches. An increasing body of evidence suggests that physical exercise has beneficial effects on cognition by enhancing neuroplasticity, thereby preventing cognitive decline and pathological aging (Bamidis et al., 2014; Williams & Kemper, 2010). Combining physical activity with cognitive training might result in a mutual enhancement of both interventions and increased maintenance of cognitive ability due to the increased cardiovascular fitness level. The underlying mechanism might be the enhancement of an individual's capacity to respond to new demands with behavioral adaptations (Hötting & Röder, 2013).

A very exciting area of research is the use of technology to encourage physical activity in combination with cognitive training. Various reports suggest that simultaneous physical and cognitive exercise induce more beneficial cognitive effects than purely cognitive and physical interventions provided separately (Bamidis et al., 2014; Konstantinidis et al., 2012). An adaptation of so-called exergame training, which combines cognitive and physical activities in a game format, might be an effective way to promote physical and cognitive improvements among older adults (Maillot, Perrot, & Hartley, 2012). Using mobile technology to promote walking outdoors in a safe environment (such as parks or safe streets) and combining it with a cognitive intensive activity (such as a word game) in a group setting that also stimulates social interaction is another approach to increasing the physical activity of older adults (Satariano & Maus, 2016). Making physical activity accessible, fun, and safe by taking advantage of the rapidly advancing mobile technology may turn out to be one of the great success stories of the technological revolution of the 21st century.

WHO (2003a) has recognized that chronic disease must be seen in the context of the life course in the same way that both under- and over-nutrition, in addition to other factors mentioned previously, play a role in the development of chronic disease. The global epidemic of increasing obesity, diabetes, and other chronic noncommunicable diseases, for example, is affecting all economies—developing and transitional economies, less affluent segments within these regions, and developed countries. At the same time, an increasing number of communities and households have coincident under- and over-nutrition. Although genetic predisposition and fetal life programming do play roles in these phenomena, the most readily apparent association with the obesity/diabetes/chronic disease epidemic is a lifetime of exposures and influences (Darnton-Hill, Nishida, & James, 2004). A life course approach to research into dietary habits, particularly if focused on the period of life when food preferences are formed and in which families have constrained access to nutritionally adequate diets, has clear implications for designing nutrition interventions and educational programs (Wethington, 2005).

In conclusion, two of the most significant risk factors for poor health outcomes in older adults in terms of the life course are diet and physical activity. Their relationship to the human-driven changes in the physical environment and the aging of the world's population require that the modifiable social and environmental factors be addressed in both the study of the epidemiology of aging and the planning of public health interventions.

Measures

Global Burden of Disease. The global burden of disease (GBD) is an important measure used in international epidemiology, as it allows us to compare diseases, injuries, and risk factors, and to understand in a given place, time, and age–sex group which factors might make the most important contributions to health loss (Murray et al., 2012). GBD

has particularly useful applications in studies of aging populations, given that 23% of the total global burden of disease is attributable to disorders in people aged 60 years and older, especially in the high-income regions (Prince et al., 2015). Nevertheless, it has also been reported that per-capita disability-adjusted life-years (DALYs) are 40% higher in low-income and middle-income regions (Waddington, 2012).

Health, Functioning, and Longevity: Healthy Aging. The remaining components of the ecological model include measures of health, functioning, and longevity. With the exception of longevity and vital status, each of the measures of health and functioning serve both as outcomes and predictors. Other chapters of this text examine specific health outcomes, including mortality and causes of death.

▶ Conclusion and Future Directions

The ecological model assumes that patterns of health and well-being in human populations are associated with a dynamic interplay of biologic, behavioral, social, and physical environmental factors—an interaction that unfolds over the life course of individuals, families, and communities. Using this model enables us to represent a very complex set of factors and problems. We have come to realize that complex problems require an interdisciplinary approach and even a transdisciplinary approach. This kind of multifaceted approach, rather than just relying on increased innovation in the methods used within a single type of study, will be essential if we are to continue to advance our understanding of, and find solutions to, these problems. Given the high prevalence of multimorbidity during old age, a clinical approach that considers a single diagnosis

An exciting field that is developing due to the advances in genomics is "epigenetic epidemiology." The term *epigenetics* is described in a landmark article by Conrad Waddington (2012), in which he postulated that "between genotype and phenotype, and connecting them to each other, there lies a whole complex of developmental processes," the so-called epigenotype. This field offers the promise of "prediction, prevention, and treatment of a wide spectrum of common complex diseases" (Relton & Davey Smith, 2012).

Since epidemiology is concerned with group-level analysis, it can provide the much-needed methodology to identify the major determinants of epigenetic variation and their suggested contributions to health and disease. To accomplish this, it has been suggested that traditional epidemiology methods—such as population-based studies, twin studies, family-based studies, cross-sectional studies, and especially longitudinal cohort studies—will be applied to this new interdisciplinary field (Ng et al., 2012; Relton & Davey Smith, 2012).

in the epidemiology of aging would be too restrictive and would most likely fail to produce the desired studies and applications. Health outcomes cannot be simply considered separately, but rather development of new methods is required to adequately deal with multiple, complexly interrelated health outcomes (Brenner & Arndt, 2004).

Other suggestions for future directions in the epidemiology of aging include increased use of birth cohorts and other cohort studies under a life course perspective, the emergence of the field of epigenetic epidemiology, and the design of studies specifically for older populations rather than extrapolating based on younger populations.

Finally, by using the principles of epidemiological aging research, we can help create the solid scientific base necessary both to address the burden of disease in older populations and to promote healthy aging. We hope that this model will serve as the map that guides researchers, practitioners, and students in reviewing and evaluating the concepts, methods, and research in the epidemiology of aging.

References

Aldwin, C., & Igarashi, H. (2012). An ecological model of resilience in late life. *Annual Review of Gerontology and Geriatrics, 32,* 115-130.

Balfour, J. L., & Kaplan, G. A. (2002). Neighborhood environment and loss of physical function in older adults: Evidence from the Alameda County Study. *American Journal of Epidemiology, 155,* 507-515.

Bamidis, P. D., Vivas, A. B., Styliadis, C., Frantzidis, C., Klados M., Schlee. W.,… Papageorgiou, S. G. (2014). A review of physical and cognitive interventions in aging. *Neuroscience & Biobehavioral Reviews, 44,* 206-220.

The Bangkok charter for health promotion in a globalized world. (2006). *An Official Journal of the International Union for Health Promotion and Education* (Vol. 21, p. 10). Bangkok. Contract No.: S1.

Barker, R. G. (1968). *Ecological psychology: Concepts and methods for studying the environment of human behavior.* Stanford, CA: Stanford University Press.

Barnes, D., Yaffe, K., Satariano, W., & Tager, I. (2002). A longitudinal study of aerobic fitness and cognitive function in healthy older adults. *Neurobiology of Aging, 23,* S450.

Beard, J. R., Blaney, S., Cerda, M., Frye, V., Lovasi, G. S., Ompad, D.,… Vlahov, D. (2009). Neighborhood characteristics and disability in older adults. *Journals of Gerontology Series B: Psychological Sciences and Social Sciences, 64B,* 252-257.

Beard, J. R., Officer, A. M., & Cassels, A. K. (2016). The world report on ageing and health. *Gerontologist, 56,* S163-S166.

Brenner, H., & Arndt, V. (2004). Epidemiology in aging research. *Experimental Gerontology, 39,* 679-686.

Bronfenbrenner, U. (1979). *The ecology of human development: Experiments by design and nature.* Cambridge, MA: Harvard University Press.

Brownson, R. C., Boehmer, T. K., & Luke, D. A. (2005). Declining rates of physical activity in the United States: What are the contributors? *Annual Review of Public Health, 26,* 421-443.

Burns, D. M. (2000). Cigarette smoking among the elderly: Disease consequences and the benefits of cessation. *American Journal of Health Promotion, 14,* 357-361.

Carlson, J. A., Sallis, J. F., & Conway, T. L. (2012). Interactions between psychosocial and built environment factors in explaining older adults' physical activity. *Preventive Medicine, 54*, 68–73.

Chetty, R., Stepner, M., Abraham, S., Lin, S., Scuderi, B., Turner, N.,… Cutler, D. (2016). The association between income and life expectancy in the United States, 2001–2014. *Journal of the American Medical Association, 315*, 1750–1766.

Colditz, G. A. (1999). Economic costs of obesity and inactivity. *Medicine & Science in Sports & Exercise, 31*, S663–S667.

Colditz, G. A., Atwood, K. A., Emmons, K., Monson, R. R., Willett, W. C., Trichopoulos, D.,… Hunter, D. J. (2000). Harvard report on cancer prevention volume 4: Harvard cancer risk index. *Cancer Causes & Control, 11*, 477–488.

Committee on Assuring the Health of the Public in the 21st Century. (2002). *The future of the public's health in the 21st century.* Washington, DC: Institute of Medicine.

Cubbin, C., & Winkleby, M. A. (2005). Protective and harmful effects of neighborhood-level deprivation on individual-level health knowledge, behavior changes, and risk of coronary heart disease. *American Journal of Epidemiology, 162*, 559–568.

Darnton-Hill, I., Nishida, C., & James, W. (2004). A life course approach to diet, nutrition, and the prevention of chronic diseases. *Public Health Nutrition, 7*, 101–121.

Davies, A. M. (1985). Epidemiology and the challenge of ageing. *International Journal of Epidemiology, 14*, 9–19.

Dicker, R., Coronado, F., Koo, D., & Parrish, R. G. (2006). *Principles of epidemiology in public health practice.* Atlanta, GA: U.S. Department of Health and Human Services.

Ekelund, U. (2014). Lifetime lifestyles II: Physical activity, the life course, and ageing. *Life Course Approach to Healthy Ageing, 1*, 229–245.

Emmons, K. M. (2000). Health behaviors in a social context. In L. F. Berkman & I. Kawachi (Eds.), *Social epidemiology* (pp. 242–266).

Ferraro, K. F., & Morton, P. M. (2016). What do we mean by accumulation? Advancing conceptual precision for a core idea in gerontology. *Journals of Gerontology Series B: Psychological and Social Sciences.* doi: 10.1093/geronb/gbvo94, February 16, 2016.

Fielding, J. E., Teutsch, S., & Breslow, L. A framework for public health in the United States. *Public Health Reviews, 32*, 174.

Fried, L. P. (2016). Investing in health to create a third demographic dividend. *Gerontologist, 56*, S167–S177.

Garmezy, N. (1971). Vulnerability research and the issue of primary prevention. *American Journal of Orthopsychiatry, 41*, 101.

Garmezy, N. (1973). Competence and adaptation in adult schizophrenic patients and children at risk. *Schizophrenia: The First Ten Dean Award Lectures*, 163–204.

Garthwaite, C. (2008). *The effect of in-utero conditions on long-term health: Evidence from the 1918 Spanish flu pandemic.* Working paper, University of Maryland, Department of Economics.

Gebbie, K., Rosenstock, L., & Hernandez, L. M. (2003). *Who will keep the public healthy? Educating public health professionals for the 21st century.* (No. 030908542X). Washington, DC: Institute of Medicine of the National Academies. National Academies Press.

Gellert, C., Schöttker, B., & Brenner, H. (2012). Smoking and all-cause mortality in older people: Systematic review and meta-analysis. *Archives of Internal Medicine, 172*, 837–844.

Green, L. W., Richard, L., & Potvin, L. (1996). Ecological foundations of health promotion. *American Journal of Health Promotion, 10*, 270–281.

Healthy People 2020. (2010). *Secretary's Advisory Committee on Health Promotion and Disease Prevention Objectives for 2020.* Washington, DC: U.S. Government Printing Office.

Hochhalter, A. K., Smith, M. L., & Ory, M. G. (2011). Successful aging and resilience: Applications for public health and health care. In *Resilience in aging* (pp. 15–29). In B. Resnick, L. P. Gwyther & K. A. Roberto (Eds.), *Resilience in Aging* (pp. 15-29). New York: Springer.

Holling, C. S. (1973). Resilience and stability of ecological systems. *Annual Review of Ecology and Systematics*, Vol. 4, pp. 1–23.

Hötting, K., & Röder, B. (2013). Beneficial effects of physical exercise on neuroplasticity and cognition. *Neuroscience & Biobehavioral Reviews, 37*, 2243–2257.

Institute of Medicine (IOM). (2001). *Health and behavior: The interplay of biological, behavioral, and societal influences.* Report No.: 0309070309. Washington, DC: Author.

Jackson, R. J., Dannenberg, A. L., & Frumkin, H. (2013). Health and the built environment: 10 years after. *American Journal of Public Health, 103*, 1542–1544.

Kelly, J. (2006). *Becoming ecological: An expedition into community psychology.* New York, NY: Oxford University Press.

Kerr, J., Rosenberg, D., & Frank, L. (2012). The role of the built environment in healthy aging: Community design, physical activity, and health among older adults. *Journal of Planning Literature, 27*, 43–60.

Konstantinidis, E. I., Billis, A., Grigoriadou, E., Sidiropoulos, S., Fasnaki, S., & Bamidis, P. D. (Eds.). (2012). *Affective computing on elderly physical and cognitive training within live social networks.* Paper presented at the 7th Hellenic conference on Artificial Intelligence: Theories and applications. Springer, Berlin, Heidelberg.

Krieger, N. (2001). Theories for social epidemiology in the 21st century: An ecosocial perspective. *International Journal of Epidemiology, 30*, 668–677.

Kuh, D., & Ben-Shlomo, Y. (2016). Early life origins of adult health and aging. In: K. F. Ferraro (Ed.), *Handbook of aging and the social sciences* (8th ed., pp. 101-122). San Diego, CA: Academic Press.

Kuh, D., Richards, M., Cooper, R., Hardy, R., & Ben-Shlomo, Y. (2013). Life course epidemiology, ageing research and maturing cohort studies: A dynamic combination for understanding healthy ageing. In D. Kuh, R. Cooper, R. Hardy, M. Richards, & Y. Ben-Shlomo (Eds.), *A life course approach to healthy ageing: Life course approach to adult health series* (pp. 3-15). Oxford, UK: Oxford University Press.

Lehning, A. J. (2012). City governments and aging in place: Community design, transportation, and housing innovation adoption. *gerontologist*, *52*, 345–356.

Lewin, K. (1935). *A dynamic theory of personality: Selected papers*. D. K. Adams & K. E. Zener (Trans.). New York, NY: McGraw.

Lynch, J., & Davey Smith, G. (2005). A life course approach to chronic disease epidemiology. *Annual Review of Public Health*, *26*, 1–35.

Maillot, P., Perrot, A., & Hartley, A. (2012). Effects of interactive physical activity video-game training on physical and cognitive function in older adults. *Psychology and Aging*, *27*, 589.

Marmot, M., Friel, S., Bell, R., Houweling, T. A. J., & Taylor, S. (2008). Closing the gap in a generation: Health equity through action on the social determinants of health. *Lancet*, *372*, 1661–1669.

Marmot, M., & Wilkinson, R. (2005). *Social determinants of health*. Oxford, UK: Oxford University Press.

Masten, A. S. (2014). Global perspectives on resilience in children and youth. *Child Development*, *85*, 6–20.

McLaren, L., & Hawe, P. (2005). Ecological perspectives in health research. *Journal of Epidemiology and Community Health*, *59*, 6–14.

McLeroy, K., Bibeau, D., Steckler, A., & Glanz, K. (1988). An ecological perspective on health promotion programs. *Health Education and Behavior*, *15*, 351–377.

McMichael, A. J. (1999). Prisoners of the proximate: Loosening the constraints on epidemiology in an age of change. *American Journal of Epidemiology*, *149*, 887–897.

Murray, C. J. L., Ezzati, M., Flaxman, A. D., Lim, S., Lozano, R., Michaud, C.,… Lopez, A. D. (2012). GBD 2010: Design, definitions, and metrics. *Lancet*, *380*, 2063–2066.

Murray, E. T., & Stafford, M. (2014). Lifetime lifestyles III: Where we live, the life course, and ageing. In D. Kuh, R. Cooper, R. Hardy, M. Richards, & Y. Ben-Shlomo (Eds.). *A Life Course Approach to Healthy Ageing* (pp. 246–260). Oxford, UK: Oxford University Press.

Mutangadura, G. B. (2004). World health report 2002: Reducing risks, promoting healthy life. *Agricultural Economics*, *30*, 170–172.

Neelsen, S., & Stratmann, T. (2012). Long-run effects of fetal influenza exposure: Evidence from Switzerland. *Social Science & Medicine*, *74*, 58–66.

Ng, J. W., Barrett, L. M., Wong, A., Kuh, D., Smith, G. D., & Relton, C. L. (2012). The role of longitudinal cohort studies in epigenetic epidemiology: Challenges and opportunities. *Genome Biology*, *13*, 1.

Pickett, K. E., & Pearl, M. (2001). Multilevel analyses of neighbourhood socioeconomic context and health outcomes: A critical review. *Journal of Epidemiology and Community Health*, *55*, 111–122.

Porta, M. (2008). *A dictionary of epidemiology*. Oxford, UK: Oxford University Press.

Prince, M. J., Wu, F., Guo, Y., Gutierrez Robledo, L. M., O'Donnell, M., Sullivan, R.,… Yusuf, S. (2015). The burden of disease in older people and implications for health policy and practice. *Lancet*, *385*, 549–562.

Relton, C. L., & Davey Smith, G. (2012). Is epidemiology ready for epigenetics? *International Journal of Epidemiology*, *41*, 5–9.

Roux, A.-V. D. (2007). Neighborhoods and health: Where are we and where do we go from here? *Revue d'epidemiologie et de sante publique*, *55*, 13–21.

Roux, A. V. D., Merkin, S. S., Arnett, D., Chambless, L., Massing, M., Nieto, F. J.,… Watson, R. L. (2001). Neighborhood of residence and incidence of coronary heart disease. *New England Journal of Medicine*, *345*, 99–106.

Rowe, J. W., & Kahn, R. L. (1997). Successful aging. *Gerontologist*, *37*, 433–440.

Sallis, J. F., Cervero, R. B., Ascher, W., Henderson, K. A., Kraft, M. K., & Kerr, J. (2006). An ecological approach to creating active living communities. *Annual Review of Public Health*, *27*, 297–322.

Satariano, W. A., Kealey, M., Hubbard, A., Kurtovich, E., Ivey, S. L., Bayles, C. M.,… Prohaska, T. R. Mobility disability in older adults: At the intersection of people and places. *Gerontologist*. 2014. Vol. *00*, pp. 1–11.

Satariano, W., & Maus, M. (2016). *WordWalk: An application to promote physical and cognitive activity for older adults*.

Scharlach, A. E., & Lehning, A. J. (2013). Ageing-friendly communities and social inclusion in the United States of America. *Ageing & Society*, *33*, 110–136.

Shohaimi, S., Luben, R., Wareham, N., Day, N., Bingham, S., Welch, A.,… Khaw, KT. (2003). Residential area deprivation predicts smoking habit independently of individual educational level and occupational social class: A cross-sectional study in the Norfolk cohort of the European Investigation into Cancer (EPIC-Norfolk). *Journal of Epidemiology and Community Health*, *57*, 270–276.

Smedley, B. D., & Syme, S. L. (2001). Promoting health: Intervention strategies from social and behavioral research. *American Journal of Health Promotion*, *15*, 149–166.

Stokols, D. (1992). Establishing and maintaining healthy environments: Toward a social ecology of health promotion. *American Psychologist*, *47*, 6.

Telesford, Q. K., Joyce, K. E., Hayasaka, S., Burdette, J. H., & Laurienti, P. J. (2011). The ubiquity of small-world networks. *Brain Connectivity*, *1*, 367–375.

Ungar, M., Ghazinour, M., & Richter, J. (2013). Annual research review: What is resilience within the social ecology of human development? *Journal of Child Psychology and Psychiatry, 54,* 348–366.

U.S. Department of Health and Human Services. (2000). *Healthy People 2010: Understanding and improving health* (2nd ed.). Washington, DC: U.S. Government Printing Office.

Violence Prevention Alliance. (2016). *Ecological framework.* Geneva, Switzerland: Author. Available at: http://www.who.int/violenceprevention/approach/ecology/en/

Von Bertalanffy, L. (1968). *General systems theory: Foundations, development, applications.* New York, NY: Braziller.

Waddington, C. H. (2012). The epigenotype. *International Journal of Epidemiology, 41,* 10–13.

Warnecke, R. B., Oh, A., Breen, N., Gehlert, S., Paskett, E., Tucker, K. L.,... Flack, J. (2008). Approaching health disparities from a population perspective: The National Institutes of Health Centers for Population Health and Health Disparities. *American Journal of Public Health, 98,* 1608–1615.

Warner, K. E. (2000). The need for, and value of, a multi-level approach to disease prevention: The case of tobacco control. In B. D. Smedley and S. L. Syme (Eds.) *Promoting health: Intervention strategies from social and behavioral research* (pp. 417–449). Washington, DC: National Academies Press.

Werner, E. E. (1989). High-risk children in young adulthood: A longitudinal study from birth to 32 years. *American Journal of Orthopsychiatry, 59,* 72.

Werner, E. E., Bierman, J. M., & French, F. E. (1971). *The children of Kauai: A longitudinal study from the prenatal period to age ten.* Honolulu, HI: University of Hawaii Press.

West, L., Cole, S., Goodkind, D., & He, W. (2014). *65+ in the United States: 2010.* Washington, DC: U.S. Government Printing Office.

Wethington, E. (2005). An overview of the life course perspective: Implications for health and nutrition. *Journal of Nutrition Education and Behavior, 37,* 115–120.

Wiesmann, U., Biber-Klemm, S., Grossenbacher-Mansuy, W., Hadorn, G. H., Hoffmann-Riem, H., Joye, D.,... Zemp, E. (2008). Enhancing transdisciplinary research: A synthesis in fifteen propositions. In G. H. Hadorn, H. Hoffmann-Riem, S. Biber-Klemm, W. Grossenbacher-Mansuy, D. Joye, C. Pohl, U. Wiesmann, & E. Zemp (Eds.), *Handbook of Transdisciplinary Research* (pp. 433–441). New York: Springer.

Wight, R. G., Aneshensel, C. S., Miller-Martinez, D., Botticello, A. L., Cummings, J. R., Karlamangla, A. S.,... Seeman, T. E. (2006). Urban neighborhood context, educational attainment, and cognitive function among older adults. *American Journal of Epidemiology, 163,* 1071–1078.

Wilkinson, R. G., & Marmot, M. G. (2003). *Social determinants of health: The solid facts.* Geneva, Switzerland: World Health Organization.

Williams, K., & Kemper, S. (2010). Exploring interventions to reduce cognitive decline in aging. *Journal of Psychosocial Nursing and Mental Health Services, 48,* 42–51.

World Health Organization (WHO). (1946). Preamble to the Constitution of the World Health Organization as adopted by the International Health Conference, New York, 19–22 June, 1946. Official Records of the World Health Organization, no. 2, p. 100; entered into force on 7 April 1948. New York, NY: Author.

World Health Organization (WHO). (1984). *The uses of epidemiology in the study of the elderly: Report of a WHO Scientific Group on the Epidemiology of Aging.* WHO Technical Report Series 706.

World Health Organization (WHO). (1986). Ottawa charter for health promotion. *Canadian Journal of Public Health, 77,* 425–430.

World Health Organization (WHO). (2002). *Active ageing: A policy framework: A contribution of the World Health Organization to the Second United Nations World Assembly on Ageing.* Madrid, Spain: Author.

World Health Organization (WHO). (2002). *Diet, nutrition, and the prevention of chronic diseases: Report of a joint WHO/FAO expert consultation.* (No. 924120916X). Geneva, Switzerland.

World Health Organization (WHO). (2003b). *WHO framework convention on tobacco control.* Geneva, Switzerland: Author.

World Health Organization (WHO). (2004). *Global strategy on diet, physical activity, and health.* Geneva, Switzerland: Author.

World Health Organization (WHO). (2015). *World report on ageing and health.* Luxembourg, Luxembourg: Author.

World Health Organization (WHO). (2016). Physical inactivity: A global public health problem. Available at: http://www.who.int/dietphysicalactivity/factsheet_inactivity/en/

Yen, I. H., Michael, Y. L., & Perdue, L. (2009). Neighborhood environment in studies of health of older adults: A systematic review. *American Journal of Preventive Medicine, 37,* 455–463.

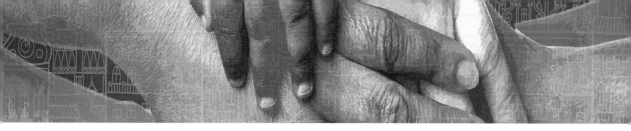

CHAPTER 3

Early-Life Predictors of Late-Life Health

April M. Falconi, Ralph Catalano, and **W. Thomas Boyce**

ABSTRACT

Although health in late life depends on an individual's environment and lifestyle during old age, conditions over the life course appear to "program" or influence the health trajectories that contribute to well-being in old age. This chapter reviews the literature that examines the linkages between conditions in early life and health in late life. Health conditions of adulthood associated with early-life exposures are described from two methodologically different, albeit similar disciplines. The first perspective, developmental epidemiology, studies how individually experienced, perhaps idiosyncratic risk factors or exposures to suspected pathogens influence individual health in late life. Examples of developmental influences on long-term health status are cited from the literature on both humans and animals. The second perspective, developmental demography, reviews work on how population cohorts exposed to aggregate stressors exhibit elevated morbidity and mortality in late life. The research cited draws from studies of both specific threats (e.g., famine, war, disease) and nonspecific threats to cohort health and survival. The measures used to draw linkages between early-life influences and late-life health—and the methodological issues associated with both developmental epidemiology and developmental demography—are assessed, elucidating areas of caution in the interpretation of study findings.

KEYWORDS

developmental epidemiology   critical periods
developmental demography   epigenetic

▶ Introduction

Why is epidemiology so interested in early-life predictors of later-life health? We suspect this interest reflects the longstanding strategy of public health reformers to target programming at infants and children. Doing so makes sense for two reasons. First, the public at large—whose support on the political front empowers reform—responds more to the pain of children than to that of other populations (Rogers, 2005; Shapiro, 2013). Second, such targeting not only improves the health of the young but also provides an opportunity for reformers to improve the lives of others for whom the general public has tended to show less concern—low-income mothers, for example.

Reformers have argued that improving the health of children reduces future dependence on tax-supported public programs and increases the productivity of the workforce (Belli, Bustreo, & Preker, 2005). This argument has been cited to intentionally frame much of public health programming, and the epidemiology that informs it, as investments in the young and productive, rather than as palliative measures for the old and needy.

The growing political and institutional influence of the elderly cohort suggests that public health practitioners' strategy of targeting the most politically advantageous group might cause the field to shift programming from the young to the old. Two circumstances, however, impede such a shift and continue to encourage work that we review here. First, more epidemiologists and public health professionals have focused on the health of the young than on the health of the old, thereby making such a strategic shift slow and fitful. Second, and more important for this chapter, such a shift would seem to be a palliative effort for the old—and, therefore, a violation of the manifest, intuitively compelling, and a widely accepted argument that investing in children returns dividends in the form of adult financial independence and a healthy, productive workforce.

Following intuition and the division of labor among disciplines and researchers, we have separated the work reviewed in this chapter into two perspectives. The first perspective, **developmental epidemiology**, asks whether individual exposure to suspected pathogens early in life increases the odds of poor health status late in life. The second perspective, **developmental demography**, asks whether historically observed conception or birth cohorts exposed to known or suspected stressors (e.g., famines) at **critical periods** in development exhibit unexpectedly high death rates late in life or live, on average, shorter lives than unexposed cohorts. This question should attract attention from readers of this volume because public health interventions to improve late-life health typically target "communities" or populations of functionally connected individuals (e.g., residents of a political jurisdiction that provides public health programs, members of an employment-based health plan, participants in a labor market or regional economy) in discreet time, rather than samples spread over too much time or a real space to engage in communal adaptations (**FIGURE 3-1**).

Studies of health over the life course in entire historical birth cohorts have increased in recent times for reasons other than growing curiosity about the association between early-life stressors and late-life health. In marked contrast to earlier times when researchers had little access to dependable life table data describing societies over many decades, almost any researcher with an Internet connection can now acquire precisely such data (University of California, Berkeley, & Max Planck Institute for Demographic Research, 2016). Methods for analyzing such data have also become increasingly available and understood (Coglan, 2016).

The literature introduced in this chapter has inspired its set of controversies: Which developmental periods (e.g., gestation, infancy, adolescence) leave young persons

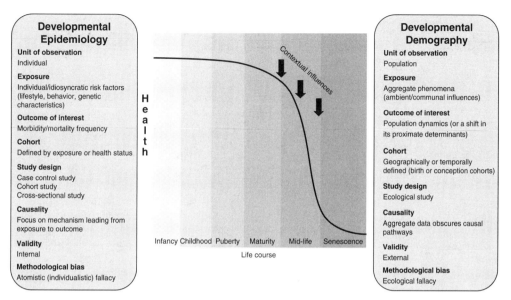

FIGURE 3-1 Developmental epidemiology and demography.
Contributed by Falconi, Catalano, and Boyce.

most vulnerable to which stressors, and why? How great a role does cognition play in inducing the vulnerability of critical periods, given that it must play a small role in utero or in infancy? Is the variation over birth cohorts in health measured, for example, in longevity, due to plasticity or selection in utero? How should we resolve differences between the interest of the collective and the preferences of parents in sheltering vulnerable children during critical periods? We do not offer answers to these questions here, but instead review work that we hope brings them to the reader's attention.

▶ Developmental Epidemiology

Developmental epidemiological research examines trajectories of risk biomarkers or surrogate endpoints to appraise the evidence indicating that early, pathogenic exposures inflate the odds of poor health status later in life. Although deep cultural traditions affirm the special sensibilities

of children and the echoing of childhood difficulties and stress into adult life, such views are now becoming more powerfully grounded in a new science describing the biological embedding of early social adversity (Boivin & Hertzman, 2012; Boyce, Sokolowski, & Robinson, 2012; Hertzman & Boyce, 2010). The formative observations of David Barker and his colleagues (Barker, 1990; Barker, Winter, Osmond, Margetts, & Simmonds, 1989), which indicate that adult coronary heart disease might be traceable to early life—especially prenatal, nutritional deficiencies—propelled such "developmental origins" research into the mainstream of contemporary epidemiological investigation. The Barker hypothesis and research enterprise began with an epidemiological comparison of the geographical distribution of infant mortality between 1921 and 1925 in England and Wales and the death rates from heart disease in adults, five decades later, between 1968 and 1978 (Barker & Osmond, 1986). Based on visible homologies in the geo-patterning of these measures, Barker proposed that fetal under-nutrition, resulting in intrauterine

PEARL 3-1   Developmental Origins of Health Outcomes in Older Adults

Barker's developmental origins work focused at the outset upon the role of intrauterine nutritional exposures or deficiencies in the "fetal programming" of vulnerability to ischemic heart disease, stroke, and hypertension. More recent research has broadened these observations to include exposures to psychosocial adversity and trauma, the origination of risk in both the preconceptual and early postnatal (roughly the first 1000 days of life) periods, the possible transmission of risk across generations, and an extension beyond cardiovascular outcomes to include obesity and metabolic syndrome, depression, and intelligence (Davey Smith, 2012).

  Work by Wadhwa and colleagues (Dunkel-Schetter, Gurung, Lobel, & Wadhwa, in press; Entringer & Wadhwa, 2013) has pointed out how psychological adversity, like nutritional insults, constitutes an important aspect of the intrauterine environment and may affect the structural and functional integrity of the developing organism. Their findings suggest that, among young adults who are exposed to significant adversities in intrauterine life, multiple forms of physiological dysregulation place them at substantial risk for developing complex, chronic diseases, including higher body mass index, insulin resistance, lipid dysregulation, and altered immune function. Psychological stressors occurring even during the preconception period or during the production of gametes appear capable of influencing developmental and health outcomes into the later periods of the human lifespan (Grandjean et al., 2015). Thus, social environmental exposures can become "embedded" within disease- and disorder-relevant biological processes, producing long-term liabilities to health and developmental achievements (Hertzman, 2012; Hertzman & Boyce, 2010).

growth retardation and low birth weight, might be causally implicated in the pathogenesis of ischemic heart disease, though that outcome emerged only decades later in the life course.

This broader assertion—namely, that what happens in very early life is substantively linked to the disorders and afflictions of later life—is a conviction that has crossed the boundaries of discipline, geography, and historical time. Ethologist Konrad Lorenz observed an instinctive parental "imprinting" of young goslings on the first perceived, moving objects within the hours immediately following hatching. Biologist René Dubos invoked "biological Freudianism" to argue that adverse exposures in childhood can produce lasting neurobiological risks that persist even when such exposures are later abated or removed (Dubos, Savage, & Schaedler, 1966). Further, three major reports—in the United States (Shonkoff & Phillips, 2000), the United Kingdom (Marmot, 2010), and Canada (Boivin & Hertzman, 2012)—have catalyzed strong consensus that the experiences of early life, as dramatically partitioned by aspects of socioeconomic status (SES) and social position, result in societies with widely divergent developmental and health outcomes.

Developmental Origins: Core Issues in the Epidemiological Science

Central to the promise of developmental origins research has been a set of converging insights from life course epidemiology and stress neurobiology that address critical issues identified by Kuh and Ben-Schlomo (2004) in their seminal life course approach to chronic disease epidemiology:

- The need to further elucidate the pathogenic mechanisms that could lead to socioeconomic partitioning of health outcomes across the lifespan
- The critical importance of understanding variation in susceptibility to adverse experiences

- The need for measures of biobehavioral indicators of stress and adversity effects that are valid and reliable short-term markers of increased risk for long-term impairments

Together, these three areas of investigation offer a wealth of evolving knowledge that could be used to close the gap between what we know about the predictors of health trajectories and what we do to enhance well-being over the life course.

The now broad evidence for profound, lifelong health effects of early socioeconomic disadvantage (see, e.g., Odgers, 2015) is rendered even more compelling by research examining how a mismatch between fetal expectations of the postnatal environment and actual postnatal conditions, along with the inherent plasticity of early developmental paths, can contribute to later-adult disease risk (Gluckman et al., 2009; Gluckman, Hanson, & Pinal, 2005). Such "developmental plasticity" employs the concept of conditional adaptation—that is, the idea that a genetically based program can be modified in response to changing environmental conditions to shape the unique characteristics of each individual.

Less well investigated is the often striking variation in individual susceptibility to maladaptive outcomes among those persons sustaining early developmental exposures. Sex differences in the developmental effects of low birth weight and gestational under-nutrition, for example, have been frequently noted but rarely studied as a phenomenon of interest within developmental origins research. As reviewed by Dasinger and Alexander (2016), researchers have repeatedly observed sex differences in blood pressure and other cardiovascular risk factors following an early developmental insult. These findings, moreover, are commensurate with several epidemiological studies revealing greater programming of hypertension among male fetuses that sustained compromised prenatal nutrition.

More broadly, such differential susceptibility to social and physical environments appears to operate bidirectionally, in both adverse and beneficial contexts, and results in a minority subpopulation with remarkably poor or unusually positive trajectories of health and development, contingent upon the character of environmental conditions (Boyce, 2016). Differences in contextual susceptibility appear to emerge in early development, as the interactive, adaptive products of genetic and environmental attributes, and can be detected at the levels of temperament and behavior, peripheral physiological systems, brain circuitry and neuronal function, and genetic and **epigenetic** variation.

Beyond these issues of socioeconomic disparities in health, variations in exposure susceptibility, and biobehavioral markers of adverse experience are other salient scientific dilemmas with which the developmental origins field has also had to come to terms. As recently reviewed by Gage and colleagues (2016), most developmental origins research has taken place using observational study designs, which are inherently incapable of generating strong causal inferences. Given the impossibility (and immorality) of conducting many of the randomized human experiments that could explicitly test causal hypotheses, such interpretations must be weighed against the possibilities of confounding, reverse causation, and the operation of various biases. Unfortunately, statistical attempts to adjust for measured and unmeasured confounding, selection bias, and other methodological flaws have serious limitations.

Another scientific dilemma is the reality that the effects of developmental experiences can change dynamically across the lifespan, especially in the early years, as critical and sensitive periods open and close. As Kuzawa and Thayer (2011) noted, human adaptation to environmental conditions takes place on numerous time scales, ranging from homeostatic changes that can occur over a period of seconds or minutes, to developmental plasticity that emerges over months or years, to conserved genetic changes that operate on a time scale of millennia. Within a person's development trajectory, the critical periods are those in which the presence or absence of important experiences or exposures results in irreversible changes in the brain circuitry that supports developmental advancement, while the sensitive periods are intervals in which the brain is especially responsive to such experience (Fox, Levitt, & Nelson, 2010). Both time-linked processes involve experience-dependent plasticity during defined, temporal windows of early life (Takesian & Hensch, 2013).

Wright and Christiani (2010) point out that the critical periodicity of growth and development occurs as a consequence of the timing and sequencing of important neurodevelopmental processes, such as cell migration, synaptic proliferation and pruning, changes in receptor density, and axonal myelination. For example, evidence shows that the brain is especially vulnerable to the deleterious effects of chemical exposures during early developmental periods, rendering children (as compared to adults) more vulnerable to toxic injury during critical periods of neurodevelopment. Such vulnerability also arises because of unique, early susceptibility to positive social environmental exposures. For example, in a random-assignment trial of foster-care placements for children in Romanian orphanages, Nelson (2014) has shown how neurobiological and developmental outcomes are dramatically improved when placements occur prior to age 2 years, but are unaffected when these interventions are delivered beyond that age (Zeanah, Gunnar, McCall, Kreppner, & Fox, 2011). The molecular substrates that underlie the occurrence of such critical periods—their openings and closings across developmental time—are being elucidated within animal models involving experimental manipulations at the neuronal and molecular levels (Takesian & Hensch, 2013).

Developmental Origins: Biological Mechanisms

Evidence for such biological mediation of developmental origins has emerged even within human samples, from a broad, diverse set of epidemiological observations. A variety of studies, for example, have documented associations between maternal and offspring cortisol levels within the setting of mothers' prenatal exposures to adversity and stress (Bowers & Yehuda, 2016). Only 10% to 20% of maternal cortisol passes through to the fetus, due to the placenta's protective conversion of cortisol to inactive metabolites. Thus, the placenta—an organ of fetal origin—plays a key role in the modulation of maternal glucocorticoid effects on the developing fetus. The placenta also produces a large output of the central corticotropin-releasing hormone (CRH), which has profound effects on both maternal and fetal immune function and may play a role in the onset of parturition (Wadhwa, 2005).

Beyond such directly shared neuroendocrine exposures, the transmission of disease risk from parent to child could occur through shared genetic risk, maternal exposures during intrauterine life, newborn experiences in early postnatal life, or direct transfer of parental exposure effects via gametes (Bowers & Yehuda, 2016). Epigenetic regulation of gene expression—through DNA methylation and post-translational histone modifications of the histone proteins around which DNA is wound—has become the focus of intensive study as a mechanism (and perhaps *the* mechanism) of developmental influences on long-term health status in both human and animal models (Boyce & Kobor, 2015).

Epigenetics has been defined as "the structural adaptation of chromosomal regions so as to register, signal, or perpetuate altered [gene] activity states" (Bird, 2007). Epigenetic mechanisms change gene activity or expression by altering chromatin organization, without modifying the genetic code of the DNA itself (Meaney, 2010). Throughout the course of life, epigenetic "marks" are placed and excised in response to environmental conditions and exposures. Because long-term changes in disease susceptibility and resistance can occur through these mechanisms, it is now presumed that epigenetic regulation of gene expression is a principal means by which early environmental exposures—to maternal nutrition, smoking, irradiation, and trauma, for example—exert health effects over the life course, even into old age.

In support of this view, a growing body of literature has offered evidence of associations between early-life perturbations and patterns of epigenetic marks and modifications. Essex et al. (2013), for example, found a pattern of DNA hyper- and hypo-methylation among 170 epigenetic sites within the inside lining of cheek cells from 15-year-old youth in the Wisconsin Study of Families and Work. This pattern of DNA methylation was significantly related, after correction for potential false discovery, to parental reports of adversity, such as parenting difficulties, role strains, and financial stressors, that occurred 10 to 15 years earlier in their children's infancy and preschool periods of development. Romens et al. (2015) studied methylation of the promoter region in the NR3C1 glucocorticoid receptor (GR) gene, whose expression is a key regulator of stress reactivity within the human adrenocortical system. Compared to their counterparts without abuse histories, maltreated children showed heightened methylation—an epigenetic mark that would result in diminished expression of GR and an upregulation in activation of the cortisol response system. Similarly, another study found a positive association between exposure to intimate-partner violence during pregnancy with the methylation status of the NR3C1 promoter of the child at 10 to 19 years of age (Radtke et al., 2011). Other work has implicated the methylation status and allelic variants of the serotonin transporter gene (*SLC6A4*)—which moderates linkages between environmental stressors and risk for psychopathology—as an additional molecular bridge across generations (Grabe et al., 2009; Taylor et al., 2006).

As summarized by Lester et al. (2016) in an introduction to an epigenetics-focused special issue of *Child Development*, differences in DNA methylation and other epigenetic marks have now been related to prenatal exposures to poor nutrition, maternal depression, post-traumatic stress disorder, and smoking, as well as postnatal factors such as environmental adversity, child maltreatment, and parental psychopathology. Further, within the physicochemical environment, prenatal alcohol and bisphenol-A exposures are known to impair fetal well-being through specific changes in the epigenome. When environmental perturbations such as these disrupt early developmental processes, they often engender epigenetic changes that drive differences in cellular gene expression, cell numbers, or cell location, which may collectively result in increased susceptibility to disease and disorder later in life (Grandjean et al., 2015). Downstream, the neurodevelopmental sequelae of such differences have been shown to include alterations in the size and integrity of brain structures such as the limbic circuitry, prefrontal cortex, and hippocampus.

What is less clear is whether epigenetic mechanisms also include the transmission of exposure-related epigenetic marks from one generation to another. All epigenetic marks are mitotically stable, allowing differences in gene expression to maintain specific cellular structures and functions over the life course; what is in question is whether such marks are also meiotically stable, surviving gamete production and embryogenesis. Mammalian development involves two early, distinctive phases of DNA methylation reprogramming—in germ cell development and in post-fertilization blastocyst formation—during which replication of parental epigenetic marks could theoretically occur (Santos & Dean, 2004). These processes appear to involve erasure of parentally acquired epigenetic marks, thereby preventing the transmission of experience-related chromatin modifications to the next generation.

Recent animal experiments have suggested that some of these modifications might not be completely erased, providing a possible means of transgenerational inheritance (van Otterdijk & Michels, 2016). What remains unclear is whether the same or similar processes occur during human embryogenesis, independent of the epigenetic influences of fetal, intrauterine experience. Epidemiological evidence from human populations has documented the transgenerational influences of parental and grandparental exposures (e.g., nutrition, smoking, irradiation) on disease risk in their progeny, along with evidence of shared epigenetic profiles implicated in such risk. Given that the ova from which such progeny are derived were formed during their maternal grandmother's pregnancy (i.e., during their mother's fetal life), gestational exposures could still potentially account for any epigenetic homologies across three sequential generations. Thus, evidence of epigenetic transmission into a fourth, unexposed generation is needed to confirm that true transgenerational, meiotic inheritance accounts for such homologies (van Otterdijk & Michels, 2016). Moreover, since the reproductive cells that give rise to an individual conceptus were formed during its grandmothers' pregnancies, exposures occurring two generations past can exert developmental influences on a current fetus in the F2 generation (van Otterdijk & Michels, 2016). Despite the methodologically challenging nature of such studies, at least one long-term, multigenerational project has documented stress exposure effects, in the form of ambivalent attachment behavior and poorer evaluative judgment, into the third generation beyond that of Holocaust survivors (Scharf, 2007).

Finally, events and exposures within developmental time, rather than historical time, also create constraints and opportunities for healthy development and the avoidance of disorder. The function of neuronal circuits in the brain is guided by experiences in postnatal life that regulate the maturation of inhibitory connections and interneurons (Hensch, 2005). Critical periods exist, for example, for the acquisition of language and discrimination of speech sounds in human infants (Weikum, Oberlander, Hensch, & Werker, 2012), and exposure to music can change auditory preferences in young mice by promoting changes in the anterior brain regions during an early critical period (Yang, Lin, & Hensch, 2012). Adult brain plasticity appears to become restricted by structural and functional developmental "brakes" that inhibit neurite growth and the balance between excitatory and inhibitory circuitry (Bavelier, Levi, Li, Dan, & Hensch, 2010). Genetic, pharmacologic, and environmental influences can all alter such plasticity, suggesting future opportunities for reopening closed critical periods, such as those for language acquisition or vision, or enhancing recovery from traumatic or cerebrovascular brain injury.

Developmental Origins: Animal Models

The seminal work of Meaney and colleagues (Szyf, McGowan, & Meaney, 2008; Weaver, 2009; Weaver et al., 2004; Zhang & Meaney, 2010) in a rat model of developmental plasticity demonstrated how naturally occurring and experimentally induced variations in maternal behavior during the immediate postnatal period can produce lifelong changes in neural, hormonal, cognitive, and behavioral responses to stress in pups. Specifically, maternal licking and grooming in the first several days of life downregulate pups' longterm hypothalamic–pituitary–adrenal (HPA) stress reactivity through changes in the neural system. Relatively high licking and grooming results in a downregulation of corticotro-pin-releasing hormone and diminished activation of the HPA axis (Hackman, Farah, & Meaney, 2010).

Other work in rat models of early infant maltreatment has demonstrated enduring methylation of the gene coding for brain-derived neurotrophic factor (BDNF), reduced BDNF expression, and extension of both epigenetic marks and maltreatment of young into a subsequent generation (Roth, Lubin, Funk, & Sweatt, 2009). Because BDNF is a key mediator of neural plasticity in brain regions such as the prefrontal cortex and hippocampus, such findings might present a legitimate model of the neurocognitive sequelae of transgenerational neglect and abuse of human children. Champagne and colleagues (2006) have also shown, in the same model, that the increased estrogen receptor-α (ER-α) expression that occurs in the medial preoptic area of the brain among high-licking and -grooming mothers is associated with cytosine methylation of the ER-α gene promoter. Others have shown how paternal stress can influence pup development through effects on sperm or on early paternal care (Dias & Ressler, 2014; Franklin et al., 2010).

Rodent models of cardiovascular risk following an early insult have shown, in parallel to observations in human populations, that male pups are more likely to develop blood pressure elevations following subjection to an early-life stressor, such as maternal separation (Loria, Pollock, & Pollock, 2010). Experimental work further shows that gestational dexamethasone exposure results in greater reductions in nephron numbers and glomerular filtration rates—both factors predisposing the later-age animal to the development of hypertension—among male rat pups (Dasinger & Alexander, 2016; Morton, Cooke, & Davidge, 2016).

Such animal models have the potential for exploring, through truly experimental designs, the effects of ancestral experience on behavioral and biological characteristics and the increased mental health risks among generations substantially removed from those

in which the original exposure occurred (McMullen & Mostyn, 2009). The translational implications of such experiments are legion, as they could potentially elucidate, or even ameliorate, the long-term sequelae of human tragedies such as the Holocaust, historical and present-day genocides, traumatic exposures to natural or created calamities, and the forced internment of indigenous children in boarding school environments.

Methodological Shortfalls and Their Remedies

Because epigenetic marks are likely to occur during critical periods of development, the systemic versus tissue-specific character of such marks should be taken into account when designing epidemiological studies to test developmental origins hypotheses. Investigations of epigenetic marks thought to generate generalized, cross-tissue alterations should focus on periconceptual exposures, while tissue-specific effects should be examined in relation to late gestational and postnatal exposures (Waterland & Michels, 2007).

The tissue-specific character of epigenetic processes also heightens the importance of careful biosample selection in epidemiological studies of developmental origins. While single-tissue sampling has been the technique most commonly employed to date, a more defensible and potentially more informative approach, especially in studies of early developmental influences, would be to sample multiple tissues that are representative of the different embryologic germ layers (i.e., endoderm, ectoderm, and mesoderm).

Moreover, while epigenetic studies in human populations have typically focused on DNA methylation within promoter regions of select, candidate genes with known linkages to the outcome of interest, the capacity for examining a far broader array of variably methylated sites, covering a wider sample of the entire epigenome, has grown exponentially in recent years. Opportunities for interrogating other epigenetic marks more directly relevant to gene expression, such as histone deacetylation, will surely become more available in coming years.

Another major interpretive difficulty in studies of intergenerational transmission is assessing whether offspring outcomes of stress exposure are due to the variable severity of the exposure or to its consequent behavioral or physical effects on the mother (Bowers & Yehuda, 2016). Because of this, studies of such transmission must be attentive to both the intensity of the maternal exposure and the mothers' symptoms of stress-induced biological change. Disentangling the confounding effects of shared environmental circumstances, such as poverty, and parental psychopathology that can induce experiences of adversity is also methodologically important.

Summary

Beginning in the early 1990s, a wealth of reports addressed the long-term biological, behavioral, and psychosocial processes that associate the chronic health conditions of adulthood with exposures to physical or social risk factors in early life. This linkage should come as no great surprise, given enduring cultural convictions—crossing geography and time—that the special sensibilities of young children, when exposed to psychological and physical adversities, can produce forms of morbidity extending well beyond the exposure itself and into the domains of adult life.

In continuing this line of developmental origins research, it will be important not only to further document intergenerational transmission, but also to study factors capable of interrupting the perpetuation of exposure effects and to clarify whether transmission plays an adaptive role among the progeny of affected individuals. With respect to the former issue, for example, Sharp and colleagues (2012) found that the frequency of human mothers' stroking of their infants at 5 to 9 weeks of age

moderated the association between prenatal depression and infants' negative emotionality and withdrawal of vagal tone in response to a stressor. With respect to the latter issue, more illuminating insights are needed into phenomena such as the higher obesity rates found among the children of mothers who were malnourished during pregnancy and the children of severe adversity survivors (e.g., Holocaust survivors) having biological response patterns directly opposing those of their parents (e.g., methylation of the *FKBP5* gene that co-regulates HPA reactivity). As reviewed by Entringer and Wadhwa (2013), both nutritional and traumatic intrauterine exposures are key environmental conditions determining natural selection and developmental plasticity, and the perturbation of stress response pathways may constitute an underlying mechanism for the nutritional effects on development with which the developmental origins hypothesis began. Finally, the developmental effects of nutritional and adversity-related insults in early life could help elucidate socioeconomic and racial disparities in disease risks that are among the most powerful determinants of health over the life course (Wise, 2016).

▶ Developmental Demography

Developmental research at the population level estimates the relative importance of early-life stressors for later-life health across populations in time or place (Kuh & Hardy, 2002). The "developmental origins hypothesis" implied by much of this work posits that stressors encountered early in life induce adaptive responses that promote survival in the short term, but come at a cost of adverse health outcomes later in life (Gluckman, Hanson, & Beedle, 2007). This work often focuses on conception or birth cohorts exposed to exogenous and virulent population stressors such as famine, war, or disease epidemics.

Famine

Researchers have estimated the effects of early-life exposure to famine on adult health using historical cohort data from the Finnish crop failure famine of 1866–1868, the Dutch Hunger Winter of 1944–1945, the Siege of Leningrad in 1944, seasonal famines in the Gambia between 1949 and 1994, and the Chinese Great Leap Forward famine of 1959–1961. Outcomes studied in this work include adult height and weight, glucose metabolism, blood pressure, lipid profile, metabolic syndrome, cardiovascular outcomes, self-reported health, mental performance and cognition, mental disorders, and adult mortality (Lumey, Stein, & Susser, 2011).

Consistent associations appear between famine exposure early in life and adult mental and metabolic health (Gluckman et al., 2007). Adult men and women in the Netherlands and in China exposed to famine in early life reportedly exhibited, for example, twice the risk for schizophrenia (Hoek, Brown, & Susser, 1998; St Clair et al., 2005). Offspring of mothers subjected to the Dutch Hunger Winter and the Chinese famine also exhibited an increased risk of obesity as adults (Luo, Mu, & Zhang, 2006; Roseboom et al., 2001), though some research claims the risk of obesity increased only among those exposed during the first half of the pregnancy (Gluckman et al., 2007; Hoek et al., 1998). Research suggests that the birth cohorts exposed to the Dutch and Chinese famines experienced a greater risk for impaired glucose tolerance as well (Lumey et al., 2011). Evidence, however, does not support an association between nutritional stress in early life and later-life mortality (Kannisto, Christensen, & Vaupel, 1997; Painter et al., 2005; Saxton, Falconi, Goldman-Mellor, & Catalano, 2013).

Several methodological artifacts may bias these findings toward the null hypothesis (Saxton et al., 2013). First, comparison groups (i.e., those categorized as "unexposed") typically include cohorts born closely before or after those exposed to famine, or from populations close in geographic proximity that presumably did not experience famine. Comparison groups in studies of the Dutch famine, for example, have included children born immediately before or after the famine; thus, these children experienced the stressors of either war and German occupation or post-war economic and civil disorganization. In short, the comparison cohorts also suffered exposure to stressors that could induce outcomes like those following from nutritional deficits (Saxton et al., 2013). As another example, Sweden's population has been used as a comparison group for the cohort exposed to the Finnish famine, yet the Swedish population similarly experienced the Spanish flu pandemic of 1918 and repeated crop failures (though with lesser effects on mortality) (Doblhammer, van den Berg, & Lumey, 2011).

Second, other stressors (e.g., war, extreme weather conditions, epidemic) often occur with—indeed, cause—famine, which complicates the process of teasing out the independent contribution of under-nutrition. The Dutch famine, for example, occurred during a particularly cold winter when German forces had occupied the Netherlands near the end of World War II (Lumey et al., 2011). The Chinese famine occurred against a backdrop of political coercion, terror, and systematic violence; and Finland suffered the Spanish influenza pandemic at the same time its people experienced famine (Doblhammer, van den Berg, & Lumey, 2013). Any or all of such factors acting independently or interactively could have contributed to the "programming" of adult health.

Third, selection bias may have distorted earlier study findings, given that the social and biological characteristics of women who conceive and give birth during famines may differ from those of women who conceive during other times (Doblhammer et al., 2013). Incidence of spontaneous abortions or early postnatal deaths may vary depending on the severity of the famine (or other coinciding stressors), resulting in a more or less robust population structure from which frailer individuals have been selected. Even so, results consistent across famines provide support for the contribution of population starvation or under-nutrition as the relevant exposure, and provide evidence for the pathways in which famine affects health in later life (Lumey et al., 2011).

Disease

Much research on the associations between disease exposure in early life and later-life morbidity and mortality has followed from the debate over the fetal origins hypothesis— that is, the idea that health effects can remain latent for many years and reflect some type of biological programming (Skogen & Overland, 2012). This association is also discussed in this text in the context of survival and mortality as they relate to a life course approach. Such research has tested whether the prenatal or postnatal period is most influential for adult disease (Power, Kuh, & Morton, 2013), but has predominantly focused on how exposure to infectious diseases in early life influences adult mortality.

One historical cohort study of 18th-century Sweden showed that the effects of disease load experienced during the first year of birth, as measured by the period infant mortality rate for that year, were strongly associated with old-age mortality. This association was driven mostly from outbreaks of infectious diseases, such as smallpox and whooping cough. The disease load on the mother during pregnancy did not appear significantly associated with old-age mortality (Bengtsson & Lindstrom, 2003).

In contrast, some studies of the long-term effects of influenza in pregnancy have found positive associations with later-life morbidities. Several ecological studies, for example, have shown correlations between prenatal exposure to influenza and schizophrenia. This relation has been found across different populations and cohorts, including Denmark, England and Wales, England alone, Scotland, Japan, and Australia (McGrath, Castle, & Murray, 1995).

One cohort study in the United States also has found an association between prenatal exposure to the 1918 influenza pandemic and adult disability. Children of infected mothers (who were born in early 1919) were approximately 20% more likely to be disabled compared with those born in early 1918 (who had virtually zero prenatal exposure to the 1918 pandemic) (Almond, 2006).

Findings from other ecological studies indicating associations between diseases experienced early in life and later-life morbidity include respiratory infections (e.g., pneumonia) in early life that are linked to later-life impairments in lung or respiratory function (Bengtsson & Lindstrom, 2003; Shaheen et al., 1994) and diarrhea and enteritis that are linked to cardiovascular conditions in both men and women and to respiratory cancer in men only (Buck & Simpson, 1982). Declining rates of tuberculosis (a disease that is typically acquired during childhood) in the 1800s and 1900s have been estimated to account for significant declines (between 30% and 40% in England and Wales) in adult mortality as well (Elo & Preston, 1992).

Establishing causality between disease exposure in childhood and adult morbidity and mortality remains difficult due to similar methodological challenges as those associated with studies on famine. First, aggregate data can obscure causal pathways. Other variables— such as the cold weather that occurred simultaneously with prior influenza epidemics—may explain the connection between early-life exposure and later-life health. It is also unknown whether study findings are reflective of mothers who actually had influenza; all that is known is that mothers were pregnant during a documented flu epidemic (McGrath et al., 1995).

Second, whether and when an infection in utero or in childhood manifests itself in disease or premature mortality later in life often reflects various environmental and personal characteristics (Elo & Preston, 1992) that aggregate historical data cannot measure. Ecological research testing the fetal origins of later life health can only establish that cohorts exposed to disease during infancy or prenatally may be more susceptible to higher morbidity or mortality rates in old age as an effect of this exposure (Bengtsson & Lindstrom, 2003). These associations provide little insight into the biological mechanisms that may, in part, produce them.

Third, many studies have not accounted for confounding factors that could have increased disease susceptibility in childhood and subsequent morbidity or mortality in adulthood. Disease exposure, therefore, may represent an intermediate risk factor in the overall causal chain between geographical or socioeconomic inequalities and later life health (Elford, Shaper, & Whincup, 1992).

War

Comparatively less research has investigated the effect of early-life exposure to war on later-life health, relative to studies on famine or disease. Most of the research that has been conducted in this area tests the association between exposure to war in utero or in infancy and elevated mortality at adult ages. Study findings consistently report that males and females born during wartime experience elevated mortality as adults. These results apply to cohorts of males and females born in Italy and in France during World War I (Casselli, 1990; Casselli & Capocaccia, 1989; Wilmoth, 1990) as well as to cohorts of male and females born during World War II in the Soviet Union (Anderson & Silver, 1989). Such literature supports the idea that adverse perinatal environments "scar" rather than "cull" members of exposed cohorts (Barker, 2007; Ben-Shlomo & Kuh, 2002; Gluckman, Hanson, Beedle, & Raubenheimer, 2008).

A few studies also report that cohorts of males and females who were adolescents during wartime experienced elevated mortality at older ages (Elo & Preston, 1992). The mechanisms explaining this phenomenon remain less explored relative to research on perinatal health. Some research suggests, however, that puberty represents another critical period in health, whose onset results in a cascade of physical, emotional, cognitive, and social changes. The underlying theory does not exclude women; however, the implications as they apply to female longevity remain less explored (Falconi, Gemmill, Dahl, & Catalano, 2014).

Study findings appear to support this theory, with research showing that cohorts of males, but not females, who were adolescents during World War I in Germany (Horiuchi, 1983) and during World War II in Japan experienced elevated mortality as older adults (Okubo, 1981). Males who were adolescents during both world wars in Italy experienced higher mortality at older ages (Casselli & Capocaccia, 1989). Only among cohorts of females who were adolescents in France during World War I has elevated mortality been observed at older ages (Wilmoth, 1990).

Methodological challenges that potentially threaten the validity or significance of research in this area include that other factors occurred simultaneously with war that may have confounded the effect between exposure and outcome. In England, for example, many lifestyle changes (especially related to diet) occurred during the course of World War II that also could have influenced the health and well-being of cohorts born in this era (Barker & Osmond, 1986). As another example, Italy experienced significant political, social, and economic unrest during both world wars, which undoubtedly had profound effects on the health of the Italian population through the rise and fall of fascism, mass unemployment, and food shortages (Harrison, 1998).

Nonspecific Threats to Cohort Health and Longevity

The preceding discussion implies that most contributors to the developmental demography literature infer from historic data that cohorts exposed in utero to the maternal stress response will adapt in ways that manifest with excess somatic or psychological morbidity late in life. An alternative argument posits that the apparent consensus arises as much from confirmation bias as from the data. This alternative view arises from two undisputed facts. First, fewer than half and as few as one fourth of human conceptions end spontaneously without a live birth (Boklage, 1990). Second, those fetuses surviving to birth include fewer twins, weigh more after adjusting for gestational age, exhibit fewer genetic and chromosomal abnormalities, and include fewer small-for-gestational-age males than fetuses spontaneously aborted (Simpson & Carson, 2013).

The literature that attempts to explain these facts argue that this "selection in utero" arises from mechanisms, conserved by natural selection, that reduce the likelihood that mothers will invest in offspring with relatively low prospects of yielding grandchildren (Catalano, Saxton, et al., 2012). The literature also suggests that spontaneous abortion becomes more common and selects on relatively smaller impediments to Darwinian fitness when environmental threats to infant survival increase and maternal energy to invest in infants decreases (Bruckner, Catalano, & Mortensen, 2016; Catalano, Goodman, et al., 2012).

These facts and their interpretation lead to conflicting predictions concerning the health during old age of survivors from cohorts subjected to relatively great selection in utero. The first prediction, consistent with the damage hypothesis offered by the literature, suggests that the survivors will suffer relatively great morbidity and shorter lifespans. This prediction assumes that normal fetuses suffer damaging hormonal abnormalities when the maternal stress response "dysregulates" gestation. The yield of spontaneous abortion rises in stressed cohorts because there is an increase in the rate of fetuses damaged seriously enough to fall below the fitness criterion needed to continue gestation. The surviving

fetuses may have made less damaging adaptations that leave them above the constant criterion for spontaneous abortion, but even relatively small damage to their "soma" (i.e., nonreproductive biology) renders them likely to suffer earlier death than cohorts in gestation during more benign times. The second, contrasting prediction of longer lifespan for birth cohorts in utero during stressful times assumes that the maternal stress response does not damage otherwise normal fetuses, but rather raises the level of fetal fitness needed for gestation to continue, leaving fewer but fitter fetuses in utero.

Empirical research supports the selection argument. Studies of longevity in countries with historical data of sufficient quality to warrant inclusion in the Human Mortality Database (i.e., Denmark, England and Wales, Finland, Iceland, Norway, and Sweden) report an inverse association, controlling for autocorrelation, over annual birth cohorts between male longevity and the ratio of male to female births (i.e., secondary sex ratio), a "signal" of relatively deep selection against frail males in utero (Catalano, 2011; Catalano & Bruckner, 2006a, 2006b). Other research reports that males from low secondary sex ratio cohorts in preindustrial Finland were less likely to die as infants and had more offspring than other males (Bruckner, Helle, Bolund, & Lummaa, 2015). The positive relationship between cohort secondary sex ratios and infant mortality has also appeared in contemporary data (Bruckner & Catalano, 2007).

Other outcomes than longevity and fitness appear associated with selection in utero. Studies of cohorts in utero at the time of the September 2001 terrorist attacks in the United States appear to have yielded fewer males than expected based on the number of females and based on other cohorts born earlier and later (Catalano, Bruckner, Marks, & Eskenazi, 2006). Germaine to argument here, males in those cohorts exhibited higher scores on cognitive ability tests than did other males (Bruckner & Nobles, 2013).

PEARL 3-2 Death Rates and Secondary Sex Ratios

In a direct test of the argument that selection in utero affects later-life health, Bruckner and Catalano (2007) hypothesized a positive association between the degree to which the secondary sex ratio of historical annual birth cohorts differed from values expected from trends and cycles (i.e., autocorrelation) and the degree to which death rates among males aged 55 through 79 differed from values expected from autocorrelation. The test used data from Denmark (1835–1913), England and Wales (1841–1913), and Sweden (1751–1913)—the countries with the longest available life-table data of dependable quality. The series all ended with cohorts born in 1913 because too many members of younger cohorts remained alive at the time of the test to estimate cohort lifespan. Results in all three societies showed, consistent with selection in utero, that males from birth cohorts with relatively low sex ratios lived relatively long lives.

A relatively small body of literature argues that puberty represents another critical or sensitive window, during which threatening environments may affect developmental trajectories and health later in life (Crone & Dahl, 2012; Kuh & Ben-Shlomo, 2004). A life history theory would suggest that environmental threats occurring during puberty result in a tradeoff of longevity (or adult health, more generally) for reproductive success (Ellis, Boyce, Belsky, Bakermans-Kranenburg, & van Ijzendoom, 2011; Selevan, Kimmel, & Mendola, 2000). A perceived threat occurring near or during puberty could, therefore, trigger a physiological response, such as earlier onset of puberty or accelerated growth. Such rapid and dramatic changes and growth, which are characteristic of critical periods, would lead to enhanced vulnerability to disease risk or otherwise pernicious effects on health (Hoyt & Falconi, 2015).

Historical data from three countries— England/Wales, France, and Sweden—support this theory (Falconi et al., 2014). Empirical findings show that life-threatening population stressors, as measured by nonspecific, elevated cohort mortality rates during puberty (ages 10 to 14), are inversely associated with cohort life expectancy at age 20. Significant findings have applied only to pubertal males, however, even though the underlying theory does not exclude effects on women. Nevertheless, no significant associations for females were found in any of the three societies (Falconi et al., 2014).

We infer from the developmental demography literature that ambient and communal stressors that affect whole populations affect the later-life health of cohorts that are in critical periods of early-life development when those stressors occur. There appears little controversy over the argument that infancy, and perhaps adolescence, "fits" the intuitive notion of a critical period, in that cohorts stressed at those times in the development arc exhibit worse health at old age compared to other cohorts.

More controversy greets the claim that gestation fits the intuitive narrative of a critical period in which pregnant women in stressed populations yield offspring who exhibit relatively bad health at old age. In fact, the work to date, although limited, suggests just the opposite outcome: Selection in utero may lead stressed populations to yield fewer but, on average, hardier birth cohorts, particularly males, who live longer than otherwise expected.

▶ Conclusion and Future Directions

We began this chapter with an explanation of why a volume concerned with health and well-being in late life would include a chapter describing the experiences of early life. Public health has a long tradition of focusing on the effects of environmental circumstances on the young. This focus likely arose from the assumption that making the environment safe for children would make it safe for other, less vulnerable members of the population and from the fact that public, and therefore political, support for the protection of children historically exceeded that for other groups (Rogers, 2005). The global increase in the absolute and relative sizes of the older population implies, however, that we should shift our focus to the opposite end of the lifespan. The elderly, after all, also appear vulnerable to environmental influences, and their political power grows with their number. This chapter argued that how we treat fetuses, infants, and children determines, in part, their health at old age.

Two arms of the literature can be cited to buttress our argument. The first, developmental epidemiology, suggests that circumstances in early life—indeed, perhaps in gestation—start men and women on trajectories that determine their physical and psychological well-being in old age. This work, at its best, strives for internal validity via prospective documentation of early life experiences and lifelong monitoring of respondent health. It sacrifices external validity, however, in that sampling and attrition may introduce bias and because the research effort, let alone the original researchers, is unlikely to survive to measure the health of respondents at old age.

In contrast, developmental demography offers increased historical external validity by retrospectively studying geographically defined cohorts from birth to death. The work compares the longevity of entire birth cohorts known to have suffered stressful circumstances in early life to that of cohorts born at other times or places. Findings from this line of research suggest that infancy and adolescence represent "critical periods" during which ambient stressors may reduce longevity among those surviving exposure. While this approach may increase historical external validity, it relies on gross categorization of exposed

cohorts and has not observed outcomes other than longevity. Moreover, its contemporary external validity remains unknown because it must, by axiom, study populations exposed seven or more decades earlier.

We note two important caveats for readers to consider. First, the strong and continuing connections among epidemiology, the public health profession, and the social reform movement imply that we exhibit confirmation bias when assessing work like that reviewed here (Ioannidis, 2005; Nickerson, 1998). We want to believe that the way we collectively treat pregnant women, infants, and children affects well-being throughout the remainder of life. Indeed, most readers of this volume probably exhibit this bias as well. Others whom we encounter, however, exhibit greater, and well-founded, skepticism about this relationship (Woolston, 2016).

Second, we do not imply that the "cohort effects" we inferred from the literature exceed, or even approach, the influence of "period effects" on the health and well-being of older persons (Barbi & Camarda, 2011; Catalano, 2002). As argued in the other chapters of this volume, the circumstances encountered in the day-to-day life of people surviving to old age dramatically affect the quality of their life. The work reviewed in this chapter does not support the argument that what occurred seven or more decades ago solely determined the health of our elderly population, leaving us no strategies by which we can improve their well-being.

Health in late life reflects not only contemporaneous conditions but also the biological forces and lifestyle factors that shape human ontogeny. Even so, empirical studies are needed that explain variation in vulnerability to exposures over the life course and their associated health outcomes. While research indicates sex differences exist in the body's regulatory systems, little is known about how sexual dimorphism contributes to differences in contextual susceptibility to stressors or their differential health effects at the population level. Differences in social standing or economic status may at least partially account for apparent gender differences in exposures and health outcomes. Future research may consider, therefore, the socioeconomic partitioning of health outcomes across the life course.

The effects of early-life exposures can change dynamically across the lifespan and vary not only by sex but also by age. Continued research on age-specific changes in gene expression, epigenetic changes over the life course, and the potential for either reversibility of epigenetic changes or the transmission of epigenetic marks to future generations will be important for understanding the determinants of aging and trajectories of age-related morbidities.

Lastly, while demographers typically focus on elements of population change (e.g., fertility, mortality, and migration), a growing number study disability. These biodemography studies characterize functionality over the life course and will, we expect, examine age and/or sex-specific processes critical to our understanding of how morbidity emerges and evolves in a population as it ages.

References

Almond, D. (2006). Is the 1918 influenza pandemic over? Long-term effects of in-utero influenza exposure in the post-1940 U.S. population. *Journal of Political Economy, 114*(4), 672-712.

Anderson, B. A., & Silver, B. D. (1989). Patterns of cohort mortality in the Soviet population. *Population and Development Review, 15*(3), 471-501.

Barbi, E., & Camarda, C. (2011). Period and cohort effects on elderly mortality: A new relational model for smoothing mortality surfaces. *Statistica, 71*(1), 51-69. doi: http://dx.doi.org/10.6092/issn.1973-2201/3604

Barker, D. J. (1990). The fetal and infant origins of adult disease. *British Medical Journal, 301*(6761), 1111.

Barker, D. J. (2007). The origins of the developmental origins theory. *Journal of Internal Medicine, 261*, 412-417.

Barker, D. J., & Osmond, C. (1986). Infant mortality, childhood nutrition, and ischemic heart disease in England and Wales. *Lancet, 1*(8489), 1077-1081.

Barker, D. J., Winter, P. D., Osmond, C., Margetts, B., & Simmonds, S.J. (1989). Weight in infancy and death from ischaemic heart disease. *Lancet, 2*(8663), 577-580.

Bavelier, D., Levi, D. M., Li, R. W., Dan, Y., & Hensch, T. K. (2010). Removing brakes on adult brain plasticity: From molecular to behavioral interventions. *Journal of Neuroscience, 30*(45), 14964-14971.

Belli, P., Bustreo, F., & Preker, A. (2005). Investing in children's health: What are the economic benefits? *Bulletin of the World Health Organization, 83*, 777-784.

Bengtsson, T., & Lindstrom, M. (2003). Airborne infectious diseases during infancy and mortality in later life in southern Sweden, 1766-1894. *International Journal of Epidemiology, 32*, 286-294.

Ben-Shlomo, Y., & Kuh, D. (2002). A life course approach to chronic disease epidemiology: Conceptual models, empirical challenges, and interdisciplinary perspectives. *International Journal of Epidemiology, 31*, 285-293.

Bird, A. (2007). Perceptions of epigenetics. *Nature, 44*(7143), 396-398.

Boivin, M., & Hertzman, C. (2012). *Early childhood development: adverse experiences and development.* Ottawa, ON: Royal Society of Canada, Canadian Academy of Health Sciences Expert Panel.

Boklage, C. E. (1990). The survival probability of human conceptions from fertilization to term. *International Journal of Fertility, 35*, 75-94.

Bowers, M. E., & Yehuda, R. (2016). Intergenerational transmission of stress in humans. *Neuropsychopharmacology, 41*(1), 232-244. doi: 10.1038/npp.2015.247

Boyce, T., Sokolowski, M. B., & Robinson, G. E. (2012). Toward a new biology of social adversity. *Proceedings of the National Academy of Sciences USA, 109*(suppl 2), 17143-17148. doi: 10.1073/pnas.1121264109

Boyce, W. T. (2016). Differential susceptibility of the developing brain to contextual adversity and stress. *Neuropsychopharmacology Reviews, 41*, 142-162.

Boyce, W. T., & Kobor, M.S. (2015). Development and the epigenome: The "synapse" of gene-environment interplay. *Developmental Science, 18*(1), 1-23.

Bruckner, T., & Catalano, R. (2007). The sex ratio and age-specific male mortality: Evidence for culling in utero. *American Journal of Human Biology, 19*(6), 763-773. doi: 10.1002/ajhb.20636

Bruckner, T., Catalano, R., & Mortensen, L. (2016). Spontaneous pregnancy loss in Denmark following economic downturns. *American Journal of Epidemiology.* doi: doi:10.1093/aje/kww003

Bruckner, T. A., Helle, S., Bolund, E., & Lummaa, V. (2015). Culled males, infant mortality, and reproductive success in a pre-industrial Finnish population. *Proceedings of the Royal Society B, 282*(1799), 20140835.

Bruckner, T., & Nobles, J. (2013). Intrauterine stress and male cohort quality: The case of September 11, 2001. *Social Science & Medicine, 76*, 107-114. doi: 10.1016/j.socscimed.2012.10.012

Buck, C., & Simpson, H. (1982). Infant diarrhoea and subsequent mortality from heart disease and cancer. *Journal of Epidemiology and Community Health, 36,* 27-30.

Casselli, G. (1990). The influence of cohort effects on differentials and trends in mortality. In J. S. Vallin, S. D'Souza, & A. Palloni (Eds.), *Measurement and analysis of mortality: New approaches* (pp. 229-249). Oxford, UK: Clarendon Press.

Casselli, G., & Capocaccia, R. (1989). Age, period, cohort, and early mortality: An analysis of adult mortality in Italy. *Population Studies, 43*(1), 133-153. doi: 10.1080/0032472031000143886

Catalano, R. (2002). Economic antecedents of mortality among the very old. *Epidemiology, 13,* 133-137.

Catalano, R. (2011). Selection in utero contributes to the male longevity deficit. *Social Science & Medicine, 72,* 999-1003.

Catalano, R., & Bruckner, T. (2006a). Male lifespan and the secondary sex ratio. *American Journal of Human Biology, 18,* 783-790.

Catalano, R., & Bruckner, T. (2006b). Secondary sex ratios and male lifespan: Damaged or culled cohorts. *Proceedings of the National Academy of Sciences USA, 103,* 1639-1643.

Catalano, R., Bruckner, T., Marks, A., & Eskenazi, B. (2006). Exogenous shocks to the human sex ratio: The case of September 11th in New York City. *Human Reproduction, 21,* 3127-3131.

Catalano, R., Goodman, J., Margerison-Zilko, C., Saxton, K., Anderson, B. A., & Epstein, M. (2012). Selection against small males in utero: A test of the Wells hypothesis. *Human Reproduction, 27,* 1202-1208.

Catalano, R., Saxton, K., Bruckner, T., Pearl, M., Anderson, B.A., Goldman-Mellor, S.,… Kharrazi, M. (2012). Hormonal evidence supports the theory of selection in utero. *American Journal of Human Biology, 24,* 526-532.

Champagne, F. A., Weaver, I. C., Diorio, J., Dymov, S., Szyf, M., & Meaney, M. J. (2006). Maternal care associated with methylation of the estrogen receptor-alpha 1β promoter and estrogen receptor-alpha expression in the medial preoptic area of female offspring. *Endocrinology, 147*(6), 2909-2915.

Coglan, A. (2016). *Little book of R for time series!* Cambridge, UK: Parasite Genomics Group, Wellcome Trust Sanger Institute.

Crone, E. A., & Dahl, R. E. (2012). Understanding adolescence as a period of social–affective engagement and goal flexibility. *Nature Reviews Neuroscience, 13,* 636-650.

Dasinger, J. H., & Alexander, B. T. (2016). Gender differences in developmental programming of cardiovascular diseases. *Clinical Science (London), 130*(5), 337-348. doi: 10.1042/CS20150611

Davey Smith, G. (2012). Epigenesis for epidemiologists: Does evo-devo have implications for population health research and practice? *International Journal of Epidemiology, 41*(1), 236-247.

Dias, B. G., & Ressler, K. J. (2014). Parental olfactory experience influences behavior and neural structure in subsequent generations. *Nature Neuroscience, 17*(1), 89-96. doi: 10.1038/nn.3594.

Doblhammer, G., van den Berg, G. J., & Lumey, L. H. (2011). *Long-term effects of famine on life expectancy: A re-analysis of the Great Finnish Famine of 1866–1868.* IZA Discussion Paper No. 5534.

Doblhammer, G., van den Berg, G. J., & Lumey, L. H. (2013). A re-analysis of the long-term effects on life expectancy of the Great Finnish Famine of 1866-68. *Population Studies, 67*(3), 309-322.

Dubos, R., Savage, D., & Schaedler, R. (1966). Biological Freudianism. *Pediatrics, 38*(5), 789-800.

Dunkel-Schetter, C., Gurung, R. A. R., Lobel, M., & Wadhwa, P. D. (In press). Stress processes in pregnancy and birth: Psychological, biological, and sociocultural influences. In A. Baum, T. Revenson, & J. Singer (Eds.), *Handbook of health psychology.* Hillsdale, NJ: Erlbaum.

Elford, J., Shaper, A. G., & Whincup, P. (1992). Early life experiences and cardiovascular disease: Ecological studies. *Journal of Epidemiology and Community Health, 46,* 1-11.

Ellis, B. J., Boyce, W. T., Belsky, J., Bakermans-Kranenburg, M. J., & van Ijzendoom, M. H. (2011). Differential susceptibility to the environment: An evolutionary-neurodevelopmental theory. *Developmental Psychopathology, 23,* 7-12.

Elo, I. T., & Preston, S. H. (1992). Effects of early-life conditions on adult mortality: A review. *Population Index, 58*(2), 186-212.

Entringer, S., & Wadhwa, P. D. (2013). Developmental programming of obesity and metabolic dysfunction: Role of prenatal stress and stress biology. *Nestlé Nutrition Institute Workshop Series, 74,* 107-120. doi: 10.1159/000348454.

Essex, M. J., Boyce, W. T., Hertzman, C., Lam, L. L., Armstrong, J. M., Neumann, S. M., & Kobor, M. S. (2013). Epigenetic vestiges of early developmental adversity: Childhood stress exposure and DNA methylation in adolescence. *Child Development, 84*(1), 58-75.

Falconi, A., Gemmill, A., Dahl, R., & Catalano, R. (2014). Adolescent experience predicts longevity: Evidence from historical epidemiology. *Journal of Developmental Origins of Health and Disease, 5*(3), 171-177. doi: 10.1017/S2040174414000105.

Fox, S. E., Levitt, P., & Nelson, C. A. (2010). How the timing and quality of early experiences influence the development of brain architecture. *Child Development, 81*(1), 28-40. doi: CDEV1380 [pii] 10.1111/j.1467-8624.2009.01380.x.

Franklin, T. B., Russig, H., Weiss, I. C., Graff, J., Linder, N., Michalon, A., ... Mansuy, I. M. (2010). Epigenetic transmission of the impact of early stress across generations. *Biological Psychiatry, 68*(5), 408-415. doi: S0006-3223(10)00576-7 [pii] 10.1016/j.biopsych.2010.05.036.

Gage, S. H., Munafo, M. R., & Smith, G. D. (2016). Causal inference in developmental origins of health and disease (DOHaD) research. *Annual Review of Psychology, 67*, 567-585.

Gluckman, P. D., Hanson, M. A., Bateson, P., Beedle, A. S., Law, C. M., Bhutta, Z. A., ... West-Eberhard, M. J. (2009). Towards a new developmental synthesis: Adaptive inflammatory exposure and human disease. *Lancet, 373*(9675), 1654-1657. doi: S0140-6736(09)60234-8 [pii] 10.1016/S0140-6736(09)60234-8.

Gluckman, P. D., Hanson, M. A., & Beedle, A. S. (2007). Early life events and their consequences for later disease: A life history and evolutionary perspective. *American Journal of Human Biology, 19*, 1-19.

Gluckman, P. D., Hanson, M. A., Beedle, A. S., & Raubenheimer, D. (2008). Fetal and neonatal pathways to obesity. *Frontiers of Hormone Research, 36*, 61-72.

Gluckman, P. D., Hanson, M. A., & Pinal, C. (2005). The developmental origins of adult disease. *Maternal and Child Nutrition, 1*(3), 130-141.

Grabe, H. J., Spitzer, C., Schwahn, C., Marcinek, A., Frahnow, A., Barnow, S., ... Rosskopf, D. (2009). Serotonin transporter gene (*SLC6A4*) promoter polymorphisms and the susceptibility to posttraumatic stress disorder in the general population. *American Journal of Psychiatry, 166*(8), 926-933. doi: 10.1176/appi.ajp.2009.08101542.

Grandjean, P., Barouki, R., Bellinger, D. C., Casteleyn, L., Chadwick, L. H., Cordier, S., ... Heindel, J. J. (2015). Life-long implications of developmental exposure to environmental stressors: New perspectives. *Endocrinology, 156*(10), 3408-3415. doi: 10.1210/EN.2015-1350.

Hackman, D. A., Farah, M. J., & Meaney, M. J. (2010). Socioeconomic status and the brain: Mechanistic insights from human and animal research. *Nature Reviews Neuroscience, 11*(9), 651-659. doi: nrn2897 [pii] 10.1038/nrn2897.

Harrison, M. (1998). The economics of World War II: An overview. In M. Harrison (Ed.), *The economics of World War II: Six great powers in international comparison* (pp. 1-42). Cambridge, UK: Cambridge University Press.

Hensch, T. K. (2005). Critical period plasticity in local cortical circuits. *Nature Reviews Neuroscience, 6*(11), 877-888. doi: nrn1787 [pii] 10.1038/nrn1787.

Hertzman, C. (2012). Putting the concept of biological embedding in historical perspective. *Proceedings of the National Academy of Sciences USA, 109*(suppl 2), 17160-17167.

Hertzman, C., & Boyce, T. (2010). How experience gets under the skin to create gradients in developmental health. *Annual Review of Public Health, 31*, 329-347.

Hoek, H. W., Brown, A. S., & Susser, E. (1998). The Dutch famine and schizophrenia spectrum disorders. *Social Psychiatry and Psychiatric Epidemiology, 33*(8), 373-379.

Horiuchi, S. (1983). The long-term impact of war on mortality: Old age mortality of the first World War survivors in the Federal Republic of Germany. *Population Bulletin of the United Nations, 15*, 80-92.

Hoyt, L. T., & Falconi, A. M. (2015). Puberty and perimenopause: Reproductive transitions and their implications for women's health. *Social Science & Medicine, 132*, 103-112. doi: 10.1016/j.socscimed.2015.03.031.

Ioannidis, J. (2005). Why most published research findings are false. *PloS Medicine, 2*(8), e124. doi: doi:10.1371/journal.pmed.0020124.

Kannisto, V., Christensen, K., & Vaupel, J. W. (1997). No increased mortality in later life for cohorts born during famine. *American Journal of Epidemiology, 145*(11), 987-994.

Kuh, D., & Ben-Shlomo, Y. (2004). *A life course approach to chronic disease epidemiology*. Oxford, UK: Oxford University Press.

Kuh, D., & Hardy, R. (2002). A life course approach to women's health: Linking the past, present, and future. In D. Kuh & R. Hardy (Eds.), *A life course approach to women's health* (pp. 397-412). London, UK: Oxford University Press.

Kuzawa, C. W., & Thayer, Z. M. (2011). Timescales of human adaptation: The role of epigenetic processes. *Epigenomics, 3*(2), 221-234. doi: 10.2217/epi.11.11.

Lester, B. M., Conradt, E., & Marsit, C. (2016). Introduction to the special section on epigenetics. *Child Development, 87*(1), 29-37.

Loria, A. S., Pollock, D. M., & Pollock, J. S. (2010). Early life stress sensitizes rats to angiotensin II-induced hypertension and vascular inflammation in adult life. *Hypertension, 55*(2), 494-499.

Lumey, L. H., Stein, A. D., & Susser, E. (2011). Prenatal famine and adult health. *Annual Review of Public Health, 32*, 237-262. doi: 10.1146/annurev-publhealth-031210-101230.

Luo, Z., Mu, R., & Zhang, X. (2006). Famine and overweight in China. *Review of Agricultural Economics, 28*(3), 296-304.

Marmot, M. (Ed.). (2010). *Fair society, health lives: Strategic review of health inequalities in England post-2010*. London, UK: Institute of Health Equity.

McGrath, J., Castle, D., & Murray, R. (1995). How can we judge whether or not prenatal exposure to influenza causes schizophrenia? In S. A. Mednick & J. M. Hollister (Eds.), *Neural development and schizophrenia* (pp. 203-214). New York, NY: Plenum Press.

McMullen, S., & Mostyn, A. (2009). Animal models for the study of the developmental origins of health and disease. *Proceedings of the Nutrition Society, 68*(3), 306-320.

Meaney, M. J. (2010). Epigenetics and the biological definition of gene × environmental interactions. *Child Development, 81*(1), 41-79.

Morton, J. S., Cooke, C. L., & Davidge, S. T. (2016). In-utero origins of hypertension: Mechanisms and targets for therapy. *Physiological Reviews, 96*(2), 549-603. doi: 10.1152/physrev.00015.2015.

Nelson, C. A. (2014). *Romania's abandoned children.* Cambridge, MA: Harvard University Press.

Nickerson, R. (1998). Confirmation bias: A ubiquitous phenomenon in many guises. *Review of General Psychology, 2*, 175-220.

Odgers, C. L. (2015). Income inequality and the developing child: Is it all relative? *American Psychologist, 70*(8), 722-731.

Okubo, M. (1981). *Increase in mortality of middle-aged males in Japan.* NUPRI research paper series No. 3. Tokyo, Japan: Nihon University Population Research Institute.

Painter, R. C., Roseboom, T. J., Bossuyt, P. M. M., Osmond, C., Barker, D. J., & Bleker, O.P. (2005). Adult mortality at age 57 after prenatal exposure to the Dutch Famine. *European Journal of Epidemiology, 20*, 673-676.

Power, C., Kuh, D., & Morton, S. (2013). From developmental origins of adult disease to life course research on adult disease and aging: Insights from birth cohort studies. *Annual Review of Public Health, 34*, 7-28. doi: 10.1146/annurcv-publhealth-031912-114423.

Radtke, K. M., Ruf, M., Gunter, H. M., Dohman, K., Schauer, M., Meyer, A., & Elbert, T. (2011). Transgenerational impact of intimate partner violence on methylation in the promoter of the glucocorticoid receptor. *Translational Psychiatry, 1*, e21.

Rogers, N. (2005). Vegetables on parade. In K. Warsh & V. Strong-Boag (Eds.), *Children's health issues in historical perspective* (pp. 23-72). Ontario, Canada: Wilford Laurier University Press.

Romens, S. E., McDonald, J., Svaren, J., & Pollak, S. D. (2015). Associations between early life stress and gene methylation in children. *Child Development, 86*(1), 303-309.

Roseboom, T. J., van der Meulen, J. H., Osmond, C., Barker, D. J., Ravelli, A. C., & Bleker, O. P. (2001). Adult survival after prenatal exposure to the Dutch famine. *Paediatric and Perinatal Epidemiology, 15*(3), 220-225.

Roth, T. L., Lubin, F. D., Funk, A. J., & Sweatt, J. D. (2009). Lasting epigenetic influence of early-life adversity on the *BDNF* gene. *Biological Psychiatry, 65*(9), 760-769. doi: S0006-3223(08)01530-8 [pii] 10.1016/j.biopsych.2008.11.028.

Santos, F., & Dean, W. (2004). Epigenetic reprogramming during early development in mammals. *Reproduction, 127*(6), 643-651.

Saxton, K., Falconi, A., Goldman-Mellor, S., & Catalano, R. (2013). No evidence of programmed late-life mortality in the Finnish famine cohort. *Journal of Developmental Origins of Health and Disease, 4*(1), 30-34.

Scharf, M. (2007). Long-term effects of trauma: Psychosocial functioning of the second and third generation of Holocaust survivors. *Developmental Psychopathology, 19*(2), 603-622.

Selevan, S. G., Kimmel, C. A., & Mendola, P. (2000). Identifying critical windows of exposure for children's health. *Environmental Health Perspectives, 108*, 451-455.

Shaheen, S. O., Barker, D. J., Shiell, A. W., Crocker, F. J., Wield, G. A., & Holgate, S. T. (1994). The relationship between pneumonia in early childhood and impaired lung function in late adult life. *American Journal of Respiratory and Critical Care Medicine, 149*, 616.

Shapiro, A. (2013, April 8). Why politicians want children to be seen and heard. National Public Radio, *Morning Edition*. Available at: http://www.npr.org/sections/itsallpolitics/2013/04/08/176339793/why-politicians-want-children-to-be-seen-and-heard

Sharp, H., Pickles, A., Meaney, M. J., Marshall, K., Tibu, F., & Hill, J. (2012). Frequency of infant stroking reported by mothers moderates the effect of prenatal depression on infant behavioral and psychological outcomes. *PLoS One, 7*(10), e45446.

Shonkoff, J. P., & Phillips, D. A. (Eds.). (2000). *From neurons to neighborhoods: The science of early childhood development.* Washington, DC: Committee on Integrating the Science of Early Childhood Development.

Simpson, J., & Carson, S. (2013). Genetic and nongenetic causes of pregnancy loss. *Glob Libr Women's Med, 3*(30), 4.

Skogen, J. C., & Overland, S. (2012). The fetal origins of adult disease: A narrative review of the epidemiological literature. *JRSM Short Reports, 3*(8), 59. doi: 10.1258/shorts.2012.012048.

St Clair, D., Xu, M., Wang, P., Yu, Y., Fang, Y., Zhang, F., … He, L. (2005). Rates of adult schizophrenia following prenatal exposure to the Chinese famine of 1959-1961. *Journal of the American Medical Association, 294*(5), 557-562.

Szyf, M., McGowan, P., & Meaney, M. J. (2008). The social environment and the epigenome. *Environmental and Molecular Mutagenesis, 49*(1), 46-60. doi: 10.1002/em.20357.

Takesian, A. E., & Hensch, T. K. (2013). Balancing plasticity/stability across brain development. *Progress in Brain Research, 207*, 3-34. doi: 10.1016/B978-0-444-63327-9.00001-1.

Taylor, S. E., Way, B. M., Welch, W. T., Hilmert, C. J., Lehman, B. J., & Eisenberger, N. I. (2006). Early family environment, current adversity, the serotonin transporter polymorphism, and depressive symptomatology. *Biological Psychiatry, 60*, 671-676.

University of California, Berkeley, & Max Planck Institute for Demographic Research. (2016). Human Mortality Database. Available at: http://www.mortality.org

van Otterdijk, S. D., & Michels, K. B. (2016). Transgenerational epigenetic inheritance in mammals: How good is the evidence? *The FASEB Journal, 30*(7), 2457-2465.

Wadhwa, P. D. (2005). Psychoneuroendocrine processes in human pregnancy influence fetal development and health. *Psychoneuroendocrinology, 30*(8), 724-743.

Waterland, R. A., & Michels, K. B. (2007). Epigenetic epidemiology of the developmental origins hypothesis. *Annual Review of Nutrition, 27*, 363-388.

Weaver, I. C. (2009). Epigenetic effects of glucocorticoids. *Seminars in Fetal and Neonatal Medicine, 14*(3), 143-150. doi: S1744-165X(08)00148-0 [pii] 10.1016/j.siny.2008.12.002.

Weaver, I. C., Cervoni, N., Champagne, F. A., D'Alessio, A. C., Sharma, S., Seckl, J. R., ... Meaney, M. J. (2004). Epigenetic programming by maternal behavior. *Nature Neuroscience, 7*(8), 847-854.

Weikum, W., Oberlander, T. F., Hensch, T., & Werker, J. (2012). Prenatal exposure to antidepressants and depressed maternal mood alter trajectory of infant speech perception. *Proceedings of the National Academy of Sciences, 109*(Supplement 2), 17221-17227.

Wilmoth, J. R. (1990). Variation in vital rates by age, period, and cohort. *Sociological Methodology, 20*, 295-335.

Wise, P. H. (2016). Child poverty and the promise of human capacity: Childhood as a foundation for healthy aging. *Academy of Pediatrics, 16*(3 suppl), S37-S45.

Woolston, C. (2016). Researcher under fire for *New Yorker* epigenetics article. *Nature, 533*(7603), 295. doi: 10.1038/533295f0.

Wright, R. O., & Christiani, D. (2010). Gene-environmental interaction and children's health and development. *Current Opinion in Pediatrics, 22*(2), 197-201.

Yang, E.-J., Lin, E. W., & Hensch, T. K. (2012). A critical period for acoustic preference in mice. *Proceedings of the National Academy of Sciences, 109*(Supplement 2), 17213-17220.

Zeanah, C. H., Gunnar, M. R., McCall, R. B., Kreppner, J. M., & Fox, N. A. (2011). VI. Sensitive periods. *Monographs of the Society for Research in Child Development, 76*(4), 147-162.

Zhang, T. Y., & Meaney, M. J. (2010). Epigenetics and the environmental regulation of the genome and its function. *Annual Review of Psychology, 61*, 439-466, C431_C433. doi: 10.1146/annurev.psych.60.110707.163625.

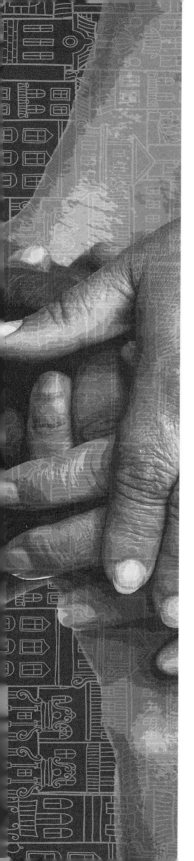

SECTION II

Aging, Health, and Function

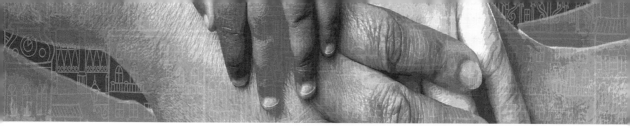

CHAPTER 4

Survival, Mortality, and Cause of Death

Taina Rantanen

ABSTRACT

This chapter gives an overview of predictors of mortality and changing patterns of mortality and longevity in the world. Mortality is an important component of population dynamics, in addition to birth rate and migration. A good indicator of population health, it is typically used in international comparisons to guide health policies. Even though mortality has decreased, which has led to aging of the overall population, the socioeconomic disparities in mortality have not vanished. Poorer countries have higher mortality rates than richer countries, and within countries those populations in lower socioeconomic positions have higher mortality rates than those in higher positions. Instead of systematically going through all factors predicting mortality, this chapter addresses some aspects of studies on aging, mortality, and longevity that have been debated recently, including socioeconomic disparities, biomarkers of aging, functional capacity, life course influences, the male–female survival paradox, and genetic versus environmental factors underlying mortality and longevity. Finally, compression of morbidity and the last years of life are discussed before presenting some ideas for future studies.

KEYWORDS

mortality	biomarkers	compression of
socioeconomic disparities	functional capacity	morbidity

Image: Hands © Shutterstock, Inc./Dewald Kirsten; Buildings © Shutterstock, Inc./Bariskina.

▶ Introduction

Long life is universally valued, and premature death is a tragedy. Research on **mortality** and survival helps us understand how societies and individuals can promote long and productive lives for all. Gerontologists are interested in the length of the lifespan because—in principle—the longer the life, the slower the aging process is. Length of life also informs public health. The shorter the lifespan, the more common are diseases and injuries underlying death. Especially in international comparisons and studies over long time periods, mortality data are typically more valid and extensive than data on other indicators of living conditions or population health.

Causes of death and predictors of mortality are distinct concepts. Causes of death refer to those factors that are the immediate contributors to death. The underlying cause of death is the factor that initiated the chain of events that led to death. Predictors of mortality refer to factors observed in earlier life, usually years before death, which increase the vulnerability to health decline and mortality. Some of these factors cannot be modified, such as chronological age and sex, whereas others are potentially modifiable, such as **functional capacity** and lifestyle.

From an epidemiological perspective, mortality may be studied from several angles. Through such research, we may obtain information about the various biological, psychological, social, economic, and cultural factors that affect the health or aging process of individuals and, consequently, the mortality rate in society. Aging epidemiology usually focuses on indicators of the aging process as predictors of mortality, whereas noncommunicable disease epidemiology focuses on disease risk factors. Whether an indicator describes a disease process or an aging process is typically difficult to separate. Nevertheless, mortality analyses provide knowledge about risk factors and conditions that increase the vulnerability of individuals and predispose them to health declines. Of course, these risk estimates are averages for groups of people, so they may not be meaningful in the context of an individual person.

▶ Definitions and Measurements

Mortality describes how many deaths happen in a population during a given time. Mortality is an important factor underlying population change, along with fertility and migration. *Population* refers to all residents of a given area, such as village, municipality, state, or the planet. Population may sometimes refer to other well-defined groups of people who share something in common, such as age, ethnicity, or language. Historically, mortality has played a dominant role in determining the growth of the world's population, because the size of the population fluctuated largely in response to disease epidemics, famines, or other catastrophes that increased mortality. In more recent times, the single most important contributor to the growth of the global population has been the sharp decline in mortality rates, rather than increases in the fertility rates.

Survival refers to the proportion of people who are still alive a set amount of time after an event. That event may be, for example, the

PEARL 4-1 Death Versus Mortality

The medical definition of *death* is the irreversible cessation of all vital functions, especially as indicated by permanent stoppage of the heart, respiration, and brain activity. *Mortality* describes how many deaths happen in a population during a given time; consequently, it is an important factor underlying population change.

Contributed by Taina Rantanen.

Contributed by Taina Rantanen.

PEARL 4-2 Survival Versus Mortality

Survival refers to the proportion of people who are still alive a set amount of time after an event. This term is commonly used in the context of disease diagnostics and therapies to compare the effectiveness of different therapies. In that case, survival is not simply the opposite of mortality, even though these concepts are related. Reduction in mortality increases survival, but that increase might not necessarily coincide with a decrease in mortality. Survival rates can be increased by making diagnoses earlier in addition to curing diseases and preventing death. Consequently, improved survival among people may not always indicate improved therapy, but rather may result from earlier diagnosis.

90th birthday, in which case survival is the flipside of mortality.

In 1967, the Twentieth World Health Assembly specified that the *cause of death* should be entered in each person's death certificate (World Health Organization [WHO], 1967). Causes of death were defined as "all those diseases, morbid conditions, or injuries which either resulted in or contributed to death and the circumstances of the accident or violence which produced any such injuries."

▸ Epidemiology of Mortality

Methodological Issues

Statistics on births and deaths have been collected over centuries. In 1532, the town council of London, England, started to keep a count of the number of persons dying from the plague. In the 1600s, the clerks of London released a weekly Bill of Mortality. Comprehensive analysis and interpretation of death data was introduced by John Graunt (1620–1674), who quantified the patterns of disease to study the causes of disease (Choi, 2012). Initially, mortality analyses largely concentrated on deaths from infectious diseases with relatively short incubation periods. After World War II, however, modern epidemiological methods advanced rapidly, including the development of basic methods for relative risk estimation and the launch of the first major epidemiological studies of chronic diseases (Choi, 2012).

Mortality analyses are relatively unambiguous, as birth and death dates are registered with practically complete coverage. Underlying causes of death and cause-specific mortality statistics derived from civil registrations systems are instrumental in guiding national and global policies and priorities for health development. Governments and other organizations may use this knowledge to implement and evaluate the need for and effectiveness of various public health policies and programs, such as vaccinations, lifestyle initiatives, nutritional recommendations, or sufficiency of hospital beds.

According to the United Nations, "the population register is a mechanism for the continuous recording of selected information pertaining to each member of the resident population of a country or area." Population registers include data on date of birth, sex, marital status, place of birth, place of residence, citizenship, and language, and potentially other data such as occupation. The population register is updated based on migration. The method and sources of updating should cover all changes so that the characteristics of individuals in the register remain current.

Population registers are useful sources of data for scientists. In human populations, experimental studies on mortality or longevity are almost never feasible due to ethical and practical problems. Instead, it is necessary to rely on "natural experiments"—that is, studies that address the consequences of natural and social disasters (e.g., famine, economic recessions) that people have experienced in a given age or a critical period of development. Natural experiments are most useful when there has been a clearly defined exposure to a risk factor involving a well-defined subpopulation. In such cases, outcomes may be plausibly attributed to the exposure.

Scientists may use population registers for drawing representative study samples in terms of place of residence, age, occupation, sex, ethnicity, and other recorded characteristics. Notably, using the population register as a sampling frame alleviates the problems stemming from reliance on voluntary samples. A voluntary sample is one of the main types of nonprobability sampling methods. It consists of people who self-select into the survey, typically because they have a strong interest in the main topic of the survey—an interest that may, in turn, bias the results.

Knowledge of family relations obtained from the population register provides an opportunity to collect informative samples for studies on genetic or environmental influences on individual differences in health and lifespan. For example, the *Finnish Twin Cohort Study* was launched in the 1970s by researchers who searched the population register for siblings born to the same mother within a short time frame. Another benefit of a population register is that an identification number assigned to each individual in a country makes it possible to link the data in the population register with the study data, thereby enabling complete coverage of vital status in a study cohort.

Crude and Age-Adjusted Mortality Rates, Person-Time, Censoring, and Hazard Ratio

The crude death rate is the number of deaths occurring among the population of a given geographical area during a given year, per 1000 mid-year total population of the given geographical area during the same year (*Handbook of Vital Statistics Systems and Methods*, 1991).

Age adjustment of such data is often necessary, because mortality occurs at different rates in different age groups. An age-adjusted death rate controls for the effects of differences in population age distributions. When comparing populations across geographic areas, some method of age adjustment is typically used to control for the influence that different population age distributions might have on health event rates.

In epidemiology, researchers are often interested in factors that increase or decrease the mortality risk. The length of individuals' follow-ups varies when people enter or exit the study at different times. The problem created by these fluctuations may be solved by expressing the mortality rate relative to the person-time at risk of the outcome. *Person-time* is a measurement combining the number of persons and their time contributions in a study. It is the sum of individual units of time that the persons in the study population are at risk for the conditions of interest. This measure is the most often used denominator in mortality rates.

Some currently available data sets have followed up a cohort until it became completely extinct and the time of death was determined for all members of the cohort. Such comprehensive data are rare, however. More typically, the time to death is not available for all study participants, a situation referred to as *censoring*. A participant is censored when information on the time to the event is not available due to loss of follow-up or non-occurrence of the outcome event before the study ended.

The *hazard ratio* is a measure of how often a particular event (death) happens in one group compared to how often it happens in another group, over time. Hazard ratios measure survival at any point in time in a group of people with an exposure (e.g., smoking, exposed) compared to a reference group without the exposure (nonsmoking, reference). A hazard ratio of 1 means that there was no difference in survival between the groups; a hazard ratio different from 1 indicates that survival differed between the groups. A value greater than 1 means that the risk of the outcome was increased, while a value smaller than 1 indicates that the effect was protective of the outcome. It is important to remember that a hazard ratio is a relation; that is, it is not an absolute value, but rather expresses the risk of one group relative to the risk of another group.

Premature Mortality and Infant Mortality

The goal when measuring *premature mortality* is to draw attention to deaths that could have been prevented. One potential measure of premature mortality is years of potential life lost (YPLL). YPLL, which uses the number of years of life (life-years) lost due to premature death, is calculated against a standard cut-off age of, for example 65, 75, or 85. The idea is to obtain a total sum of the life-years lost before the specified age criterion. Currently, there is no consensus about the age criterion for "premature" death.

Infant mortality is the death of a child younger than one year of age. It is measured as the infant mortality rate (IMR), which is the number of deaths of children before one year of age per 1000 live births. IMR is a widely used indicator of population health and well-being. In 2015, 4.5 million deaths occurred within the first year of life on a worldwide basis. The risk of a child dying before completing the first year of age was highest in Africa (55 deaths per 1000 live births), where the IMR was more than 5 times higher than that in Europe (10 deaths per 1000 live births). Globally, the infant mortality rate has decreased from an estimated 63 deaths per 1000 live births in 1990 to 32 deaths per 1000 live births in 2015. Annual infant deaths have declined from 8.9 million in 1990 to 4.5 million in 2015 (http://www.who.int/gho/child _health/mortality/neonatal_infant_text/en/). For example, in Afghanistan, the infant mortality rate in the 1980s was 160 deaths per 1000 live births, but fell to 66 deaths per 1000 live births in 2011-2015. In the United States,

the corresponding figures were 12 deaths per 1000 live births in the 1980s and 6 deaths per 1000 live births in 2011-2015, and in Finland, they were 7 deaths per 1000 live births in the 1980s and 2 deaths per 1000 live births in 2011-2015 (http://data.worldbank.org). Declining infant mortality rates have had a dramatic effect on the average life expectancy, especially in the developing world, where infant mortality has been and still is quite common.

Selective Mortality and Mortality Risk Factors

Selective mortality is a process whereby disadvantaged individuals die at younger ages than their more advantaged peers. This process gradually changes the composition of cohorts in a systematic way, such that the cohorts appear healthier, wealthier, more educated, and generally better off than they would in the absence of the selection process. Changes in cohort composition over time resulting from selective mortality are relevant to studies of older adults, as selective mortality results in underestimation of the predictive effects. That is, the more strongly a characteristic is related to the risk of dying, the more its prevalence may change over time because those with highest risk experience the highest attrition. The oldest members of the cohort are more likely to die, which makes the characteristics of the group gradually resemble those of the younger individuals. For example, in a study using information provided by respondents at the baseline and including only those respondents who remained in the cohort at later waves, it was shown that over the time of 16 years the prevalence of poor health and the proportions of men, blacks, unmarried people, and smokers declined within a general-population cohort (Zajacova & Burgard 2013). The cohort started with approximately $90,000 in household wealth, but by the last interview the median of the baseline wealth was more than $130,000—an increase that occurred simply because those persons with more wealth were more likely to remain in the study (i.e., remain living).

Because of the effect of selective mortality, it is recommended that gerontological studies focusing on outcomes other than mortality should consider the competing risk of mortality. This step allows the researchers to factor in the consequences of selective mortality.

Changing Causes of Death

High-income countries have systems in place for collecting information on causes of death in the population. In contrast, many low- and middle-income countries do not have such systems, so the numbers of deaths from specific causes in those countries must be estimated from incomplete data. Improvements in producing high-quality cause-of-death data are crucial for improving health and reducing preventable deaths in these countries.

The Global Burden of Disease (GBD) consortium measures disability and death from a multitude of causes worldwide. This organization has grown over the past two decades into an international consortium including more than 1000 researchers in more than 100 countries, and its estimates are updated annually. The GBD was launched in the early 1990s, when the World Bank commissioned the original GBD study. This study had a profound impact on health policy, as it brought global attention to otherwise hidden or neglected health challenges, such as mental illness and the burden of road injuries. The GBD work was institutionalized at the World Health Organization, which has continued updating the GBD findings. GBD 2013 produced estimates for 323 diseases and injuries, 67 risk factors, and 1500 sequelae for 188 countries (http://www.healthdata.org/gbd).

In the GBD 2013, the decomposition of global and regional life expectancy showed reductions in age-standardized death rates

for cardiovascular diseases and cancers in high-income regions, and reductions in child deaths from diarrhea, lower respiratory infections, and neonatal causes in low-income regions. For most communicable causes of death, both numbers of deaths and age-standardized death rates fell. By comparison, for most noncommunicable causes, demographic shifts have increased the numbers of deaths but decreased age-standardized death rates. According to the GBD 2013 data, global deaths from injury increased by 10.7%, from 4.3 million deaths in 1990 to 4.8 million in 2013, but age-standardized rates declined over the same period by 21% (GBD 2013 Mortality and Causes of Death Collaborators, 2015) (**FIGURE 4-1**).

Socioeconomic Disparities in Mortality

The term *disparity* refers to inequality, difference, or dissimilarity. Not all health differences are disparities. Rather, those differences that systematically and negatively impact less socioeconomically advantaged groups are classified as disparities. The term *health disparity* is most often used to refer to health differences stemming from societal inequality, which potentially may be ameliorated with societal measures.

Socioeconomic status (SES) represents a combination of many factors, including (own and spouse's) income, education, childhood

---

PEARL 4-3 Gini Coefficient

The Gini coefficient is the most commonly used measure of inequality. The coefficient's value ranges from 0 to 1, where 0 reflects complete equality and 1 indicates complete inequality (one person has all the income or consumption, all others have none).

Contributed by Taina Rantanen.

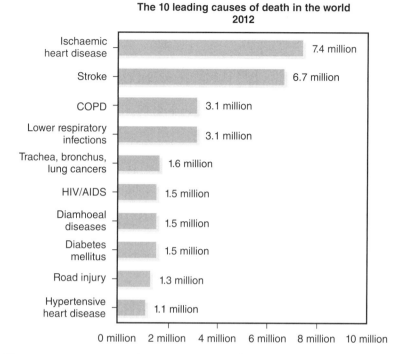

**The 10 leading causes of death in the world
2012**

Ischaemic heart disease	7.4 million
Stroke	6.7 million
COPD	3.1 million
Lower respiratory infections	3.1 million
Trachea, bronchus, lung cancers	1.6 million
HIV/AIDS	1.5 million
Diamhoeal diseases	1.5 million
Diabetes mellitus	1.5 million
Road injury	1.3 million
Hypertensive heart disease	1.1 million

0 million   2 million   4 million   6 million   8 million   10 million

FIGURE 4-1 The most common causes of death in the world in 2012 according to the World Health Organization.

Reproduced from: WHO. 2014. The 10 leading causes of death in the world, 2000 and 2012. Fact sheet 310. Available at http://www.who.int/mediacentre/factsheets/fs310/en/.

income, parental education, wealth, and neighborhood SES. It is not always possible to take into account all of these factors in a single research project, but at least one or two factors are used in most epidemiological studies. It is also possible that SES indicators influence men and women differently, or else that an individual's own SES position may be accentuated or overwhelmed by influences arising from childhood and parental SES. An additional consideration is race and ethnicity, which may modify the SES disparities.

Recently, there has been a preference for using educational attainment as a measure of SES. Information on educational attainment is relatively easy to obtain; thus, it is typically available for everyone in a study. Individuals most often complete their education in young adulthood, and education level remains stable after that point in the life course. Educational attainment is not influenced by subsequent health impairments that can lead to changes in one's occupation, income, and wealth. Thus, education reflects the stock of human capital established relatively early in life that is available to individuals throughout their life course.

Mortality and health outcomes are known to vary by most measures of SES, but the factors that underlie these differences are less clearly understood. The persistence of SES disparities in various surroundings suggests that social position shapes exposures to multiple biomedical, environmental, and psychosocial risk factors for health. Evidence suggests that SES disparities in adulthood may be propelled by disparities in childhood and that the socioeconomic characteristics of residential neighborhoods may influence the health gradients in complex ways. Whether selection versus causation underlies the mortality disparities remains a topic of debate.

The literature on social class differences in mortality is vast and spans a long historical period in developed countries, with a more recent emphasis on this topic emerging in less developed regions. A global example of how **socioeconomic disparities** affect mortality concerns the differences in life expectancy between countries. As indicated in **TABLE 4-1**, the life expectancy at birth is lower in poorer countries with lower per-capita cross-domestic product, and this disparity persists to age 80 and beyond.

Disparities in All-Cause Mortality

In Europe, an extensive study in 22 European countries during the 1990s and early 2000s found that health disparities are present everywhere, but their magnitude is highly variable, particularly in terms of mortality (Mackenbach et al., 2008). Some variations may be attributable to socioeconomic differences in smoking, excessive alcohol consumption, and access to health care. The role of consumption of large amounts of alcohol among men in Eastern Europe has been well documented to underlie SES disparities in mortality in that region. Hazardous drinking is more common in the lower-SES groups than in their higher-SES counterparts. Low levels of social

TABLE 4-1 Cross-Domestic Product per Capita in 2012 and Life Expectancy at Birth in Different Countries in 1990, 2000, and 2012, and Life Expectancy at Ages of 60 and 80 Years

Country	Cross-Domestic Product per Capita (U.S. Dollars)	Life Expectancy at Birth (Both Sexes)			Life Expectancy at Age 60		Life Expectancy at Age 80	
	2012	1990	2000	2012	Men	Women	Men	Women
Afghanistan	690	49	55	60	13	15	5	5
China	6,265	69	71	75	18	20	7	7
Cuba	6,448	74	77	79	20	23	8	9
Ethiopia	470	45	51	64	15	16	5	6
Finland	47,416	75	78	81	19	24	7	9
Japan	46,679	79	81	84	22	27	8	11
United States	51,457	75	77	79	20	24	8	10

Reproduced from: World bank data http://data.worldbank.org and WHO data http://data.un.org. Accessed December 9, 2015.

support, lack of control over one's life, and material hardship, combined with a culture that approves of excessive alcohol consumption, are the factors likely to be involved in creating this disparity.

In Northern European countries, SES disparities in mortality are still evident, but they are systematically smaller than those found in other parts of Europe (Mackenbach et al., 2008). These countries have long histories of egalitarian policies, which provide a high level of social security protection to all residents of the country, resulting in smaller income inequalities and lower poverty rates. A reasonable level of social security and public services may alleviate inequalities in mortality, but lifestyle-related risk factors still contribute to the persistence of inequalities in mortality in the northern region.

Disparities in Age-Specific Mortality

Studies of underlying SES disparities in infant mortality rates have concentrated on either individual or family indicators or ecological (area) disparities. In many countries, data are publicly available on socioeconomic characteristics of different areas; such data may, in turn, be linked with health data from different sources. For example, in Australia, infant mortality rates are elevated in those areas with disproportionately higher concentrations of low-income and single-parent families, unemployed persons, crowded dwellings, public housing, persons with limited educational attainment, and persons in unskilled occupations (Turrella & Mengersen, 2000). Among household factors contributing to infant mortality are birth out of wedlock, maternal age younger than 20 years, alcohol use during pregnancy, and not having access to prenatal care (Khanani, Hearn, & Maseru, 2010). The mother's level of education, environmental conditions, and political and medical infrastructure also contribute to risk of infant mortality.

Socioeconomic mortality disparities among older adults have been less discussed than disparities among younger age groups, but this topic is drawing increasing interest from researchers. Most deaths occur during old age, and any amount of inequality in mortality should be analyzed to indicate how to improve health in the population. In Europe (populations pooled), relative inequalities in mortality have been shown to decrease with increasing age, but still persist. Absolute educational mortality differences increase until persons reach age 90 or older. In some European populations, relative inequalities among older women have been found to be as large as those among middle-aged women. The decline of relative educational inequalities has been largest in Norway (men and women) and in Austria (men). Relative educational inequalities have not decreased, or have hardly decreased, with age in England and Wales (men) and in Belgium, Switzerland, Austria, and Turin (women) (Huisman et al., 2004).

During midlife, relative disparities in mortality are largest due to the higher risk of premature death among those more disadvantaged groups. However, in a recent review of SES disparities in old age, Huisman et al. (2013) concluded that the absolute differences in mortality rates are usually largest in the "oldest old," because the mortality rate is so high in this group. For the same reason, the relative inequalities expressed in rate ratio measures are small in the "oldest old." Nevertheless, studies that have estimated the magnitude of relative inequalities in all-cause mortality rate in the oldest populations (80 years or older) have shown that inequalities generally persist into very old age.

Aging Molecular Biomarkers and Mortality

Aging changes the structure and functioning of most physiological systems, thereby increasing the individual's susceptibility to diseases and death. An important line of research in aging biology is the work seeking to identify biomarkers of aging. The definition of an aging biomarker is related to our understanding of the mechanisms of aging. A biomarker of aging should meet the following criteria:

- Reflect the underlying aging process rather than disease
- Be based on mechanisms described by major theories of aging
- Be reproducible in cross-species comparison
- Be available by noninvasive means and be objectively measured by well-established laboratory assays on easily obtainable body specimens (often saliva, blood, or urine)
- Predict remaining length of life more accurately than chronological age

Of course, some people may have less favorable "starting values" for a biomarker and, consequently, may reach a critical threshold earlier than others, even though their rate of change is not unusually fast. Life course studies that include data from early life to midlife and end of life may address these issues.

A topic of ongoing discussion is whether it is possible to distinguish indicators of aging from indicators of disease process. The line between "normal" and pathological changes is still the subject of debate and may never be pinpointed. Many age-related changes are considered pathological when they become more pronounced. Several biochemical measures have been established as predictors of mortality, but metabolic indicators such as serum levels of glycosylated hemoglobin and lipids such as triglycerides and high- and low-density lipoprotein may actually be more representative of disease processes than aging per se. Currently, a number of molecular aging biomarkers are under intensive investigation, with a body of evidence on their utility being accumulated. Low-grade inflammation and telomere shortening, for example, are under investigation for their potential as aging biomarkers.

Low-grade inflammation is characteristic of human aging (Franceschi et al., 2000). This phenomenon differs from acute-phase inflammation, which is part of the healing process of injuries and diseases. Low-grade subclinical inflammation is a risk factor for both morbidity and mortality in elderly people, but may not be linked with specific diseases. Common inflammatory markers include interleukin-6 (IL-6), C-reactive protein (CRP), and tumor necrosis factor alpha (TNF-α). IL-6 is a proinflammatory cytokine that is produced by the liver. The level of CRP rises when inflammation is present throughout the body. Tumor necrosis factor is involved in systemic inflammation and is a component of the acute-phase reaction; this cytokine is produced chiefly by activated macrophages.

Most of the recent large epidemiological studies of older adults have included collection of serum IL-6, CRP, and TNF-α samples. For example, Harris et al. (1999) published a study based on a sample of 1293 healthy, nondisabled participants aged 65 years or older. Plasma IL-6 and CRP were measured in specimens obtained from 1987 to 1989, and the mortality was followed up prospectively for a mean of 4.6 years. A twofold greater risk of death for the study participants in the highest quartile for IL-6 (3.19 pg/mL or greater) compared with the participants in the lowest quartile was observed. Higher CRP levels (2.78 mg/L or greater) were also associated with 60% higher risk of death. People with elevations in both their IL-6 and CRP levels were 2.6 times more likely to die during follow-up than those with low levels of both **biomarkers**. Similar results were found for cardiovascular and noncardiovascular causes of death, as well as when participants were stratified by sex, smoking status, and prior cardiovascular disease, and for both early (less than 2.3 years) and later follow-up. Elevated levels of circulating IL-6 were reported to be consistently associated with death across multiple causes in the Cardiovascular Health Study and to strongly predict future mortality (Newman et al., 2009; Walston et al., 2009).

The precise etiology of low-grade inflammation and its potential causal role in health declines remain largely unknown (Franceschi & Campisi, 2014). Epidemiological studies illustrate that inflammatory markers in older populations correlate with a number of age-related chronic diseases. Because these markers show unspecific associations with health decline, however, they are not useful as disease diagnostics. Instead, they are useful for identifying individuals at high risk for disability and mortality.

Telomeres are the nucleoprotein caps found flanking DNA at the ends of chromosomes. In somatic cells, telomeres become shortened owing to cell division and oxidative stress. Short telomeres induce cellular senescence. After the telomeres reach a critically short length, functional DNA will be damaged and the cell will lose its ability to further divide. As it is an indicator of a fundamental process of aging, telomere length is hypothesized to be a biomarker of aging. This hypothesis has been tested for more than a decade with epidemiological study methods. Recently, a review was published examining leukocyte telomere length (LTL) as a predictor of mortality (Sanders & Newman, 2013). In that review, the authors included articles reporting on community-dwelling adults or older adults, with LTL being measured in at least 100 participants. The authors concluded that LTL is weakly associated with overall risk of death and possibly more strongly associated with cardiovascular disease- or infectious disease–specific death.

In 2014, further evidence was published based on the Leiden Longevity Study (Deelen et al., 2014). In that study, LTL was measured in 870 nonagenarian siblings (mean age, 93 years), 1580 of their offspring, and 725 of their spouses (mean age, 59 years). This study found that shorter LTL increased mortality in middle to early old age (30 to 80 years) and at very old age (90 years or older). No differences were noted in LTL levels between the middle-aged children of the Leiden Longevity Study participants and their spouses. The scientists then analyzed several other cohorts ($n = 8165$) to explore the relationship of LTL-associated genetic variants with mortality in a prospective meta-analysis. Based in these analyses, the authors concluded that LTL is a marker of prospective mortality from midlife to very old age.

Currently, the general consensus is that more studies are needed on LTL as a potential biomarker for aging. Such investigations will ideally use classic epidemiological techniques, such as studying the extremes of the population and doing so over extended time frames.

Measures of Functional Capacity as Predictors of Mortality

In the context of epidemiology, functional capacity has been studied since the 1950s and the 1960s, when the protocols of large cardiovascular epidemiology studies often included at least some assessments of functional capacity—most often grip strength or questions on activities of daily living. When the members of these pioneer cohorts grew older, many studies shifted their focus from disease risks to aging, while it also became possible to study measures of functional capacity as predictors of mortality. For example, the Honolulu Heart Program was launched in 1965 as a cardiovascular risk factor study, with more than 8000 men participating in this research. In 1991, the cohort was reassembled in the Honolulu-Asia Aging Study, which focused on aging epidemiology.

Another landmark study in the area of functional capacity and mortality was the Established Populations for Epidemiologic Studies of the Elderly (EPESE) project, which was launched in the early 1980s and aimed to identify predictors of mortality, hospitalization, and placement in long-term care facilities and to investigate risk factors for chronic diseases and loss of functioning. The survey elicited information from more 14,000 persons who were 65 years of age and older in four geographic locations: East Boston, Massachusetts;

New Haven, Connecticut; Iowa and Washington Counties, Iowa; and five counties in North Carolina.

Functional capacity is most often evaluated using sets of tests, observations, or self-reports that describe the participant's ability to function in a variety of circumstances. Rehabilitation and sport science studies established functional assessments as their key content more than a century ago, but they used these measures predominantly as outcomes for the treatment or training programs. The first disability-focused model outlining the different levels of functioning was introduced in 1965 by Dr. Saad Nagi. Based on Nagi's outline, tests of functional capacity may be categorized as follows:

- Tests measuring the functioning of an organ system (e.g., muscle strength, postural control, sensory functions, joint range of motion)
- Tests measuring the functioning of the entire body (e.g., walking speed and endurance, ability to lift objects, ability to change and maintain body positions)
- Tests describing the ability of the person to function relative to the requirements of different tasks and environments (e.g., community mobility, activities of daily living [ADLs], instrumental activities of daily living [IADLs])

Tests may aim to assess the highest possible level of performance the person is capable of exhibiting, as in the test of maximal muscle strength. In some cases, the typical performance of the person is of interest, as in the test of customary walking speed or self-reported mobility. Among the objective measures of physical function, the Short Physical Performance Battery (SPPB), the walking speed test, and the hand grip strength are the most commonly used in clinical settings as well as in research.

Measures of functional capacity reflect the combined influences of genetic predisposition, acquired modifications of physical constitution related to lifestyle or work, aging processes, and chronic diseases. Consequently, they capture many of the influences relevant in aging and, therefore, are almost uniformly found to predict mortality. In epidemiological aging studies, it is currently the norm to include at least some measures of functional capacity.

Why muscle strength and other functional measures predict mortality is not totally clear. It may be hypothesized that these measures actually indicate disease severity, which would then explain the association. This potential relationship was studied in the Women's Health and Aging Study (Rantanen et al., 2003). In these researchers' data, the presence of chronic diseases commonly underlying death or the mechanisms behind decline in muscle strength in chronic disease, such as inflammation, poor nutritional status, disuse, and depression, all of which are independent predictors of mortality, did not explain the association between grip strength and mortality. Thus, muscle strength may predict mortality through mechanisms other than those leading directly from disease to muscle impairment. Hand grip strength declines at an annual rate of approximately 1% after midlife, so it may be a good biomarker of aging (Rantanen et al., 1998). High grip strength in midlife may indicate resilience to aging and higher

PEARL 4-4 Measures of Functional Capacity

Measures of functional capacity predict mortality—a relationship that holds across studies and across measures of functioning. Measures of functional capacity reflect the combined influences of genetic predisposition, acquired modifications of the person's physical constitution related to lifestyle or work, aging processes, and chronic diseases.

Contributed by Taina Rantanen.

physiological reserves, increasing the probability of longevity.

Hand grip strength is an example of a variable describing the functioning of the musculoskeletal system. A widely used measure, it indicates total body strength and is a marker of physiological reserves during aging, with good strength protecting the individual from disability and mortality (Rantanen et al., 1999, 2000). Higher midlife grip strength also predicts longevity up to centenarian years (Rantanen et al., 2012). More broadly, measuring the strength of any one muscle group (upper extremity, lower extremity, or trunk) can provide a practically similar predictive value for mortality risk (Portegijs, Rantanen, Sipilä, Laukkanen, & Heikkinen, 2007). Grip strength is an easily performed test and, consequently, is included in most studies. As a biomarker, it predicts all-cause and cause-specific mortality in the general population and in many clinical populations. The muscle strength decline noted in old age may be attributed to disease burden and comorbidity, but is not a distinctive symptom of any one disease. Muscle strength tests, including grip strength tests, may help identify people at increased risk of deterioration of health and mortality.

Life Course Epidemiology of Mortality

A life course approach considers health in adulthood and old age to be—at least partly—a consequence of development and growth taking place during sensitive periods in early life. The approach looks across a cohort's life experiences or across generations for clues to current patterns of health and disease. In epidemiology, a life course approach is being used to study the physical and social hazards during gestation, childhood, adolescence, young adulthood, and midlife that may potentially affect health outcomes in later life (Ben-Shlomo & Kuh, 2002).

An example of a life course approach is the fetal origins hypothesis, which links the intrauterine environment to the later development of adult chronic disease (Barker, 1998). A growing body of evidence suggests that there are critical periods of growth and development during which environmental exposures can damage health on a long-term basis. Additionally, a life course approach considers the long-term health consequences of biological and social experiences in adulthood, which may act interactively with early-life biological and social factors to attenuate or exacerbate long-term risks to health.

The developmental origins of health and disease (DOHaD) paradigm is a multidisciplinary area of study that examines how "environmental factors acting during the phase of developmental plasticity interact with genotypic variation to change the capacity of the organism to cope with its environment in later life" (Gluckman and Hanson, 2006). Thus far, nutritional deficiency has been the main focus of research. The DOHaD paradigm has been debated since the 1960s. Currently, it is recognized that the environment interacts with genes in a way that has implications for adult health. In the 1980s, David Barker identified a link between low birth weight (LBW) and ischemic heart disease in adult life (Barker & Osmond, 1986), with this link between LBW and adult disease risk later being called the Barker hypothesis and being recognized as an important development in the DOHaD field. Further development in the field extended this idea into what became known as fetal origins of adult disease (FOAD). FOAD posits that an organism must make certain developmental tradeoffs to survive under suboptimal conditions. These tradeoffs may be immediately adaptive, in allowing the short-term survival and reproduction of the organism, but at a cost to the organism's long-term health.

The challenge in life course studies on aging lies in the fact that there are only a few data sets in the world that contain data from infancy to old age. The *Helsinki Birth Cohort*

Study (HBCS) includes 13,345 individuals born in Helsinki between 1934 and 1944, who visited child welfare clinics in the city and who were living in Finland in 1971 when a unique personal identification number was assigned to all Finnish residents (Eriksson, Osmond, Kajantie, Forsén, & Barker, 2006; Osmond, Kajantie, Forsén, Eriksson, & Barker, 2007). Data on neonatal characteristics, including weight and length, were extracted from hospital birth records, and infancy and childhood weight and height from child welfare clinics and school health records. In 2000, a random sample of 2003 people aged, on average, 61 years participated in a clinical examination (Barker, Osmond, Forsén, Kajantie, & Eriksson, 2005). From the original clinical study cohort (*n* = 2003), 1404 people who were alive and living within 100-km distance from the study clinic in Helsinki were invited to participate in a new clinical follow-up in 2011. A total of 1094 participants attended the clinical examination between 2011 and 2013. The study data are linked with vital statistics from the population register and other pertinent administrative data, including the hospital discharge database.

An example illustrating how such data can be used in life course research is a study of how naturally occurring body weight changes influence mortality based on the HBCS data (von Bonsdorff et al., 2015). The association between body size in early life and mortality in later life has been little studied, and it is unclear whether the association is driven by adult body size. In the HBCS data, trajectories of body mass index (BMI) development in early life were identified and their mortality risk investigated. Data included serial measures of weight and height from birth to 11 years extracted from healthcare records, weight and height data in adulthood, and register-based mortality data for 2000–2010. The majority of the participants had a similar BMI development pattern in infancy and childhood, which was named "average BMI" by the researchers, but two atypical patterns were also identified:

■ For both men and women, an early BMI trajectory that increased
■ For men, a pattern in which BMI was similar during infancy but later dropped below the average BMI trajectory and, for women, a pattern in which BMI was lower in infancy and childhood but later exceeded the average trajectory

The observed early BMI development patterns were associated with all-cause mortality approximately 70 years later among women, but not among men. Women with an increasing or low-to-high BMI (BMI lower in early childhood, later exceeded average) trajectory had an increased risk of all-cause mortality compared to those with an average BMI trajectory (hazard ratio [HR], 1.55; 95% confidence interval [CI], 1.07–2.23; and HR. 1.57; 95% CI, 1.04–2.37, respectively). Similar associations were observed for cancer mortality. Among men, BMI trajectories were not associated with all-cause mortality, but those with average-to-low BMI (BMI first similar, then dropped below average) had an increased risk of cancer mortality. Adjustment for adult BMI did not affect the results. Based on these data, it appears that an increasing BMI in early life may shorten the lifespan of maturing cohorts as they age, particularly for women (von Bonsdorff et al., 2015).

An example of intergenerational effects discovered through life course research is the findings of the Norwegian Nord-Trøndelag Health Study (HUNT Study), which is one of the largest health studies ever performed. This study utilizes is a unique database of personal and family medical histories. The HUNT1 Survey was carried out in 1984–1986 to establish the health history of 75,000 people. Using family-linkage data, the scientists prospectively examined offspring mortality in relation to parental levels of BMI, height, blood pressure, resting heart rate (RHR), blood glucose and blood lipids, as well as parental smoking, diabetes and cardiovascular disease, and mortality. A detailed description of the procedures and methods can be found at http://www.ntnu.edu/hunt.

The HUNT Study has shown that intergenerational associations of several cardiovascular factors persist into the offspring's adult life, and that parent–offspring associations are largely similar for fathers and mothers. Maternal obesity has been related to increased mortality in adult offspring. Notably, parental cardiovascular risk factors predicted offspring mortality in this study.

The parent–offspring associations might potentially be explained by genetic factors and shared environment. It is possible that different risk factors interact, and it has been reported that obesity may lead to clustering of other cardiovascular risk factors. The intergenerational relationship for cardiovascular risk factors could have its origin in early-life exposures, possibly mediated by low birth weight. However, the similarity between father-offspring and mother-offspring associations in this and other studies argues against a strong effect of the intrauterine environment (Vik, Romundstad, Carslake, Davey Smith, & Nilsen, 2014).

Male–Female Survival Paradox

Since 2006, even in the poorest countries, women have been expected to outlive men. Research literature generally suggests that men are physically stronger, report fewer diseases, and have fewer limitations in their activities of daily living at older ages. Nonetheless, female death rates are substantially lower than those for males at all ages. It is difficult to interpret this contradiction that women live longer than men yet experience worse health during their lifetime. The most widely cited explanations for the male-female health-survival paradox include biological endowments, risks acquired through social roles and behaviors (including illness- and health-reporting behaviors), physicians' diagnostic patterns, and differential healthcare access, treatment, and use (Oksyzyan, Juel, Vaupel, & Christensen, 2008).

The most prominent biological explanations for the health-survival paradox have hormonal, autoimmune, and genetic roots. In terms of a hormonal origin, it been hypothesized that estrogen is a central factor in the paradox. Endogenous estrogen decreases serum low-density lipoprotein cholesterol and increases high-density lipoprotein cholesterol levels, lowering the coronary heart disease (CHD) risk in women of reproductive age. Nevertheless, this estrogen hypothesis does not explain the sex differences at older ages. More research is needed to reveal stronger evidence that estrogen partially explains sex differences in health and mortality.

The "immunocompetence" hypothesis suggests that increased male mortality throughout life may partly be due to the greater susceptibility of men to infections. According to the X-chromosome hypothesis, the lack of a second X chromosome in men is associated with increased mortality. It has also been suggested that X-linked genetic factors might influence human hematopoietic stem-cell kinetics and, potentially, organism survival. The fact that women have two cell lines with different potentials may be one reason why they live longer than men (Christensen et al., 2000).

The rate of change in different health indicators has been suggested as one explanation for the male-female survival paradox. In old age, it would be useful to separate the rate of change in health indicators from the initial level of these indicators. For example, grip strength at age 75 years is the function of the lifetime highest value (which occurs at approximately age 30 years) and the changes that have taken place since then. The changes do not occur at a constant rate and may happen into both directions, though decline is the most common pattern. Little is known about sex differences in these changes. If the absolute rate of change in health indicators is the most predictive factor, this may explain part of the health-survival paradox, as men experience a larger absolute rate of decline in physical function compared to women because men's "starting values" are higher (Oksyzyan et al., 2008).

Although unhealthy behaviors contribute to the increased risk of cardiovascular and other chronic diseases and mortality in men, they cannot fully explain the sex differences in health and mortality. Evidence for this includes the presence of sex difference in mortality in the studies restricted to populations with a particular lifestyle profile, such as old Amish and Mormons (Oksyzyan et al., 2008). It has also been suggested that women report more diseases than men—a pattern that might underlie the paradox, although studies do not really support this hypothesis. Some evidence shows that men postpone seeking medical attention and consequently look for medical consultation at the later stages of their illness compared to women.

Although the male–female health-survival paradox has been studied for decades, we still do not fully understand either the reasons for it or its mechanisms. (Oksyzyan et al., 2008).

Lifestyle Versus Genetic Risk Factors for Mortality

Is the length of human lifespan heritable? Or is it determined by acquired influences? The nature-versus-nurture debate has been going on for decades. In this case, "nature" refers to the coding of genes determining individuals' different traits, such as height, weight, muscle strength, and intelligence. The "nurture" theory holds that genetic influence over traits may exist, but environmental factors are the real origins of our behavior. Given the complexity of the human lifespan phenotype, research on genetic versus environmental influences is currently problematic. Surviving to a given age is probably a multifactorial phenotype involving multiple biological processes, environmental influences, and randomness.

Information about aggregation of longevity into families and across generations

supports the idea that shared familial factors may underlie the longevity. For example, Gudmundsson et al. (2000), using population-based genealogy in Iceland, found that the first-degree relatives of those people who lived to an extreme old age (95 percentile) were twice as likely as the controls to survive to the same age. Familial aggregation of longevity was especially addressed in the Long Life Family Study (LLFS), which is an international collaborative study of the genetics and familial components of exceptional survival, longevity, and healthy aging. Respondents in their 90s self-reported on the survival history of their parents and siblings; on the basis of this information, families that showed clustering of exceptional survival were then recruited. Respondents resided in the United States and Denmark. Altogether, 4953 individuals in 539 families took part in the study. The LLFS pedigrees were selected on the basis of longevity per se in the upper generation and the generation above that. The researchers found that the children's generation had significantly lower rates of many major diseases and better healthy aging profiles for many disease phenotypes (Newman et al., 2011).

These studies show that familial aggregation of longevity exists, but are not able to

PEARL 4-5 Randomness

Randomness is an important factor that represents the part of variation in lifespan that cannot be accounted for. In free-living animal populations, variation in lifespan is usually attributed to the combined effects of individual genetic and environmental factors and to causes such as infection, accident, starvation, predation, and cold. Nevertheless, even when a population comprises genetically uniform individuals that are reared in a constant environment and protected from extrinsic mortality, the individuals exhibit very different lifespans (Kirkwood et al., 2005).

Contributed by Taina Rantanen.

determine whether the familial influences begin from shared genes or shared environmental influences originating from childhood families. It is possible that members of a family might also resemble one another in terms of their socioeconomic attainment, eating habits, or exercise habits, all of which correlate with lifespan.

Twin studies provide a feasible way to assess the heritability of human lifespan. During the last few decades, a series of twin studies have shown that approximately 25% of the variation in lifespan is caused by genetic differences. In terms of the exact genetic variants underlying the lifespan, knowledge is still scarce. To date, the only widely reproduced example of a lifespan-modifying gene is *APOE*. It has been argued that the lack of findings in this area might be due to the complexity of the phenotype, which reflects an extreme polygenic architecture, or due to the low statistical power of the studies carried out (Newman et al., 2011).

Among the lifestyle behaviors, the protective effect of physical activity against both all-cause and cause-specific mortality has been reported repeatedly in observational cohort studies. In humans, randomized controlled studies proving causality in the relationship between physical activity behavior and length of life are not feasible: Such studies would take a very long time and it would be impossible to control attrition of participants over the years. Consequently, uncertainty persists about whether genetic selection might, in fact, underlie the association between different lifestyle influences and longevity.

Recently, Hupin et al. (2015) reviewed 835 study reports addressing people aged 60 years and older; the data included a total of 122,417 participants, a mean follow-up of 9.8 ± 2.7 years, and 18,122 reported deaths. In these studies, a low dose of moderate to vigorous physical activity resulted in a 22% reduction in mortality risk. Increased physical activity beyond this threshold brought further benefits, reaching heights of a 28% reduction

PEARL 4-6 Twin Studies

The classic twin study design compares the similarity of monozygotic and dizygotic twins. A monozygotic twin pair has 100% similar genes, whereas dizygotic twins share on average 50% of their genes. Members of a monozygotic twin pair are made different only by environmental factors, while differences between members of a dizygotic twin pair may arise from genetic or environmental factors. If monozygotic twins are considerably more similar than dizygotic twins, it is concluded that genes play an important role in these traits. By comparing many hundreds of families of twins, the roles of genetic effects, shared environment, and unique environment in shaping traits may be understood.

Contributed by Taina Rantanen.

in all-cause mortality in older adults who followed the current recommendations and a 35% reduction among those with the highest physical activity participation beyond the recommended amount. However, the approach used in this investigation was not able to address the possibility of genetic selection into physical activity.

The question of whether genetic selection underlies healthy behaviors, which in turn correlate with longer lifespan, may be addressed by twin studies. For example, genetic and environmental influences may be disentangled by examining monozygotic twins who are discordant for a specific environmental influence, such as smoking, alcohol use, or physical activity. A challenge remains, however: There are only a very few twin studies that are large enough to allow for identifying a sufficient number of twin pairs who are discordant for a key behavior. Discordance means that one member of the pair has the behavior and other does not. As monozygotic twins have similar genes, only differences in environmental factors, such as lifestyle, can underlie their differences in mortality.

Kujala et al. (2002) studied familial aggregation of mortality risk factors and their association with future deaths in the Finnish Twin Cohort. Cohort members (n = 15,904) were aged 24 to 60 years and healthy at the end of 1981 and had responded to questionnaires in 1975 and 1981; they were followed up for death for 20 years. In individual-based analyses, the age- and sex-adjusted risk of death was higher among those persons who were not participating in vigorous leisure physical activity, among those who smoked, and among those who were heavy users of alcohol. Among monozygotic twin pairs discordant for the health behavior, a difference in mortality risk was seen only for smoking. The authors concluded that genetic selection may account for some of the association between mortality and physical activity and heavy use of alcohol. Thus, the same genes that make it easy and fun to exercise may also underlie the decreased mortality risk among persons who engage in physical activity, pointing toward a genetic selection bias as underlying at least part of the association between physical activity and mortality. Note that these data do not indicate that physical activity would not be beneficial for everyone's health, but simply suggest that physical activity may not lengthen life. This is an important point when it comes to compression of morbidity.

Compression of Morbidity

During the 1970s, data from the National Health Interview Survey showed a trend toward worsening self-reported health among older U.S. men and women. This evidence, combined with the significant declines in age-specific mortality observed since the 1960s, led some researchers to suggest that the health of the older population was declining. This scenario was termed "failure of success." The "compression of mortality" hypothesis contrasted with this view. The idea of compression of morbidity in public health was put forth by Professor James Fries, who suggested

that the burden of lifetime illness may be compressed into a shorter period before the time of death if the age at the onset of the first chronic infirmity can be postponed more rapidly than the age of death. If this happens, the lifetime illness burden may be compressed into a shorter period of time nearer to the age of death.

It is currently debatable whether the compression of mortality is really taking place. In Finland, cohort comparisons among 65-year-old people suggested that socioeconomic situation has improved, physical activity is more common, and self-ratings of health and functioning among this age group have improved, even though prevalence of chronic conditions has not changed (Heikkinen et al., 2011). Another study in Finland among 90-year-olds suggests the opposite, showing that disability prevalence is increasing in older cohorts (Sarkeala, Nummi, Vuorisalmi, Hervonen, & Jylhä, 2011). In Denmark, however, cognitive functioning and activities of daily living functioning were found to have improved among nonagenarians, but grip strength and lower extremity performance had not changed (Christensen et al., 2013). All in all, data from the 1990s and 2000s show a reduction in the share of elderly people who report ADL or IADL limitations (Freedman et al., 2013).

Compression of morbidity is an appealing scenario for most individuals—and for policy makers, too. The differing definitions of morbidity and disability, however, make it challenging to draw conclusions about whether compression of morbidity is truly taking place. Studies suggest that reduction in disability is most marked among those persons with many years until death. Health status in the year or two just prior to death has been found to remain relatively constant over time, but health measured three or more years before death has improved in recent decades. This fact, together with the increase in total life-years, suggests that even though disabled life-years may not have decreased, a larger proportion of life is being lived disability-free.

Last Year of Life

Research on predictors of care needs in the last years of life among those persons who die in old age provides us with an idea about which factors might promote compression of morbidity. Utilization of health services increases before death. To compress the period of dependency prior to death, it is important to gain understanding about predictors of care needs in the last period of life. To study this issue, administrative databases with complete coverage of vital status and hospital care use need to be linked with research data for a decedent cohort for whom information is available about their earlier lifestyle.

Is physical activity earlier in life associated with more or less inpatient care preceding death? The longer expected lifespan of physically active people may predispose them to more—rather than less—need for care at the end of life. In contrast, persons who exercise regularly may suffer less from chronic diseases and disability in old age and, therefore, need less health and social care services at the end of life than more sedentary people.

In line with the idea of the compression of morbidity, the association between physical activity earlier in life and the need for inpatient care prior to death was studied among people who died in old age in Finland (von Bonsdorff et al., 2009). The decedent population comprised 846 persons aged 66 to 98 years at death, who, on average 5.8 years prior to death, had participated in an interview about their current and earlier physical activity. The data on their use of care in the last year of life were taken from a register and complete. Men needed, on average, 96 days (standard deviation [SD], 7.0) and women 138 days (SD, 6.2) of inpatient care in the last year of life. Among men, the risk for all-cause hospital care in the last year of life was higher for those who had been sedentary since midlife compared with those who had been consistently physically active, whereas use of long-term care did not correlate with physical activity history. Among

women, the risk for long-term care was higher for those who had been sedentary or only occasionally physically active than for those who had been consistently active from midlife onward, whereas use of hospital care did not correlate with physical activity history. End-of-life inpatient care patterns differed between men and women.

This study and others lend support to the idea that a healthy lifestyle may promote compression of morbidity, at least when inpatient care is used as an indicator of morbidity. Even though physical activity may not be causally linked to length of life, we may say that physically active people are more likely to experience less severely disabled years in old age compared to sedentary people.

▶ Conclusion and Future Directions

Even though practically all indicators of health, functioning, biological aging, and socioeconomic strata can most likely predict mortality, there are still many unknowns.

First, risk factors tend to change over time. In a recent article, Finch et al. (2014) pointed out that the past 200 years have enabled remarkable increases in human lifespans because infections as a cause of death have been nearly eliminated through improved hygiene (public health), medicine, and nutrition. As a result, noncommunicable diseases have become the most common causes of death. These kinds of changes will happen in the future as well. Cures may become available for some of the noncommunicable diseases that now commonly underlie death, such as cancer or Alzheimer's disease. This kind of development will result in new changes in the most widespread causes of death and predictors of mortality may change in tandem.

We have also been witnessing an ongoing increase in human lifespan. Finch et al. (2014) argue, however, that the limit to lifespan may be approaching. Since 1997, no one has exceeded Jean Calment's record of 122.5 years lived, despite an exponential increase in the number of centenarians. Numerous factors may act to limit greater longevity—for example, global warming will have negative influences in that older people are highly vulnerable to heatwaves (Finch et al., 2014).

The life histories of future cohorts of older people will be different from those of the current cohorts. New knowledge will lead to the implementation of new preventive strategies and policies, which may serve to marginalize some mortality risk factors. At the same time, sustainability of service systems may become a challenge whenever an increasing proportion of the population lives to very old age.

To date, we have witnessed the publication of only the first wave of mortality studies made possible by the aging of major cohorts identified in the 1960s and onwards. These studies have produced knowledge on predictors that could be measured when the studies were initiated; that is, we have been able to study only the data that have been available. The "maturing" of new cohorts assessed with more up-to-date methodologies and new conceptual approaches will produce new knowledge on the mechanisms leading from health risks to health decline. For these groups, high-throughput biochemical and molecular analysis will provide novel data.

Finally, knowledge about biomarkers, effect modifications, interactions, additive effects, and selection biases, among others, is still lacking. These issues need to be addressed in the general older population. In the same time, people with specific conditions and disabilities are growing old, and they should not be forgotten in studies either.

References

Barker, D. J. (1998). In utero programming of chronic disease. *Clinical Science (London), 95*, 115-128.

Barker, D. J. P., & Osmond, C. (1986). Infant mortality, childhood nutrition, and ischaemic heart disease in England and Wales. *Lancet, 1*, 1077-1081.

Barker, D. J., Osmond, C., Forsén, T. J., Kajantie, E., & Eriksson, J. G. (2005). Trajectories of growth among children who have coronary events as adults. *New England Journal of Medicine, 353*, 1802-1809.

Ben-Shlomo, Y., & Kuh, D. (2002). A life course approach to chronic disease epidemiology: Conceptual models, empirical challenges, and interdisciplinary perspectives. *International Journal of Epidemiology, 31*, 285-293.

Choi, B. C. K. (2012). The past, present, and future of public health surveillance. *Scientifica, 2012*, 875253.

Christensen, K., Kristiansen, M., Hagen-Larsen, H., Skytthe, A., Bathum, L., Jeune, B.,... Orstavik, K. H. (2000). X-linked genetic factors regulate hematopoietic stem-cell kinetics in females. *Blood, 95*, 2449-2451.

Christensen, K., Thinggaard, M., Oksuzyan, A., Steenstrup, T., Andersen-Ranberg, K., Jeune, B., ... Vaupel, J. W. (2013). Physical and cognitive functioning of people older than 90 years: A comparison of two Danish cohorts born 10 years apart. *Lancet, 382*, 1507-1513.

Deelen, J., Beekman, M., Codd, V., Trompet, S., Broer, L., Hägg, S.,... Slagboom, P. E. (2014). Leukocyte telomere length associates with prospective mortality independent of immune-related parameters and known genetic markers. *International Journal of Epidemiology, 43*, 878-486.

Eriksson, J. G., Osmond, C., Kajantie, E., Forsén, T. J., & Barker, D. J. (2006). Patterns of growth among children who later develop type 2 diabetes or its risk factors. *Diabetologia, 49*, 2853-2858.

Finch, C. E., Beltrán-Sánchez, H., & Crimmins, E. M. (2014). Uneven futures of human lifespans: Reckonings from Gompertz mortality rates, climate change, and air pollution. *Gerontology, 60*, 183-188.

Franceschi, C., Bonafe, M., Valensin, S., Olivieri, F., De, L. M., Ottaviani, E., & De Benedictis, G. (2000). Inflamm-aging: An evolutionary perspective on immunosenescence. *Annals of the New York Academy of Sciences, 908*, 244-254.

Franceschi, C., & Campisi, J. (2014). Chronic inflammation (inflammaging) and its potential contribution to age-associated diseases. *Journals of Gerontology, Series A: Biological Sciences and Medical Sciences, 69*, S4-S9.

Freedman, V. A., Spillman, B. C., Andreski, P. M., Cornman, J. C., Crimmins, E. M., Kramarow, E., ... Waidmann, T. A. (2013). Trends in late-life activity limitations in the United States: An update from five national surveys. *Demography, 50*, 661-671.

GBD 2013 Mortality and Causes of Death Collaborators. (2015). Global, regional, and national age–sex specific all-cause and cause-specific mortality for 240 causes of death, 1990–2013: A systematic analysis for the Global Burden of Disease Study 2013. *Lancet, 385*, 117-171.

Gluckman, P., & Hanson, M. (2006). The developmental origins of health and disease: An Overview, in Developmental Origins of Health and Disease. Peter Gluckman and Mark Hanson, eds. 1–5. Cambridge, UK: Cambridge University Press.

Gudmundsson, H., Gudbjartsson, D. F., Frigge, M., Gulcher, J. R., & Stefánsson, K. (2000). Inheritance of human longevity in Iceland. *European Journal of Human Genetics, 8,* 743-749.

Handbook of vital statistics systems and methods, volume 1: Legal, organisational and technical aspects. (1991). United Nations Studies in Methods, Glossary, Series F, No. 35. New York, NY: United Nations.

Harris, T. B., Ferrucci, L., Tracy, R. P., Corti, M. C., Wacholder, S., Ettinger, W. H. Jr., … Wallace, R. (1999). Associations of elevated interleukin-6 and C-reactive protein levels with mortality in the elderly. *American Journal of Medicine, 106,* 506-512.

Heikkinen, E., Kauppinen, M., Rantanen, T., Leinonen, R., Lyyra, T. M., Suutama, T., & Heikkinen, R. L. (2011). Cohort differences in health, functioning, and physical activity in the young-old Finnish population. *Aging Clinical and Experimental Research, 23,* 126-134.

Huisman, M., Kunst, A. E., Andersen, O., Bopp, M., Borgan, J. K., Borrell, C., … Mackenbach, J. P. (2004). Socioeconomic inequalities in mortality among elderly people in 11 European populations. *Journal of Epidemiology and Community Health, 58,* 468-475.

Huisman, M., Read, S., Towriss, C. A., Deeg, S. J. H., & Grundy, E. (2013). Socioeconomic inequalities in mortality rates in old age in the World Health Organization Europe Region. *Epidemiologic Reviews, 35,* 84-97.

Hupin, D., Roche, F., Gremeaux, V., Chatard, J. C., Oriol, M., Gaspoz, J. M., … Edouard, P. (2015). Even a low-dose of moderate-to-vigorous physical activity reduces mortality by 22% in adults aged ≥60 years: A systematic review and meta-analysis. *British Journal of Sports Medicine, 49,* 1262-1267.

Khanani, J. E., Hearn, J. C., & Maseru, N. (2010). The impact of prenatal WIC participation on infant mortality and racial disparities. *American Journal of Public Health, 100,* S204–S220.

Kirkwood, T. B., Feder, M., Finch, C. E., Franceschi, C., Globerson, A., Klingenberg, C. P., … Westendorp, R. G. (2005). What accounts for the wide variation in life span of genetically identical organisms reared in a constant environment? *Mechanisms of Ageing and Development, 126,* 439-443.

Kujala, U. M., Kaprio, J., & Koskenvuo, M. (2002). Modifiable risk factors as predictors of all-cause mortality: The roles of genetics and childhood environment. *American Journal of Epidemiology, 156,* 985-993.

Mackenbach, J. P., Stirbu, I., Roskam, A. J. K., Schaap, M. M., Menvielle, G., Leinsalu, M., & Kunst, A.E., for the European Union Working Group on Socioeconomic Inequalities in Health. (2008). Socioeconomic inequalities in health in 22 European countries. *New England Journal of Medicine, 358,* 2468-2481.

Newman, A. B., Glynn, N. W., Taylor, C. A., Sebastiani, P., Perls, T. T., Mayeux, R., … Hadley, E. (2011). Health and function of participants in the Long Life Family Study: A comparison with other cohorts. *Aging (Albany, NY), 3,* 63-76.

Newman, A. B., Sachs, M. C., Arnold, A. M., Fried, L. P., Kronmal, R., Cushman, M., … Lumley, T. (2009). Total and cause-specific mortality in the cardiovascular health study. *Journals of Gerontology, Series A: Biological Sciences and Medical Sciences, 64,* 1251-1261.

Oksuzyan, A., Juel, K., Vaupel, J. W., & Christensen, K. (2008). Men: Good health and high mortality. Sex differences in health and aging. *Aging Clinical and Experimental Research, 20,* 91-102.

Osmond, C., Kajantie, E., Forsén, T. J., Eriksson, J. G., & Barker, D. J. (2007). Infant growth and stroke in adult life: The Helsinki Birth Cohort Study. *Stroke, 38,* 264-270.

Portegijs, E., Rantanen, T., Sipilä, S., Laukkanen, P., & Heikkinen, E. (2007). Physical activity compensates for increased mortality risk among older people with poor muscle strength. *Scandinavian Journal of Medicine & Science in Sports, 17,* 473-479.

Rantanen, T., Guralnik, J. M., Foley, D., Masaki, K., Leveille, S., Curb, D. J., & White, L. (1999). Mid-life hand grip strength as a predictor of old age disability. *Journal of the American Medical Association, 286,* 558-560.

Rantanen, T., Harris, T., Leveille, S., Visser, M., Foley, D., Masaki, K., … Guralnik, J. (2000). Muscle strength and body-mass index as long-term predictors of mortality in Japanese-American men. *Journal of Gerontology: Medical Sciences, 55,* M168-M173.

Rantanen, T., Masaki, K., Foley, D., Izmirlian, G., White, L., & Guralnik, J. M. (1998). Grip strength changes over 27 years in Japanese-American men. *Journal of Applied Physiology, 85,* 2047-2051.

Rantanen, T., Masaki, K., He, Q., Ross, G. W., Willcox, B. J., & White, L. (2012). Midlife muscle strength and human longevity up to age 100 years: A 44-year prospective study among a decedent cohort. *Age, 34,* 563-570.

Rantanen, T., Volpato, S., Ferrucci, L., Heikkinen, E., Fried, L. P., & Guralnik, J. M. (2003). Hand grip strength, cause-specific, and total mortality in older disabled women: Exploring the mechanism. *Journal of the American Geriatrics Society, 51,* 636-641.

Sanders, J. L., & Newman, A. B. (2013). Telomere length in epidemiology: A biomarker of aging, age-related disease, both, or neither? *Epidemiologic Reviews, 35,* 112-131.

Sarkeala, T., Nummi, T., Vuorisalmi, M., Hervonen, A., & Jylhä, M. (2011). Disability trends among nonagenarians in 2001–2007: Vitality 90+ Study. *European Journal of Ageing, 8,* 87-94.

Turrella, G., & Mengersen, K. (2000). Socioeconomic status and infant mortality in Australia: A national study of small urban areas, 1985–89. *Social Science & Medicine, 50,* 1209–1225.

Vik, K. L., Romundstad, P., Carslake, D., Davey Smith, G., & Nilsen, T. I. (2014). Transgenerational effects of parental cardiovascular disease and risk factors on offspring mortality: Family-linkage data from the HUNT Study, Norway. *European Journal of Preventive Cardiology.* pii: 2047487314562118. [Epub ahead of print].

von Bonsdorff, M. B., Rantanen, T., Leinonen, R., Kujala, U. M., Törmäkangas, T., Mänty, M., & Heikkinen, E. (2009). Physical activity history and end-of-life hospital and long-term care. *Journals of Gerontology, Series A: Biological Sciences and Medical Sciences, 64,* 778–784.

von Bonsdorff, M. B., Törmäkangas, T., Rantanen, T., Salonen, M. K., Osmond, C., Kajantie, E., & Eriksson, J. G. (2015). Early life body mass trajectories and mortality in older age: Findings from the Helsinki Birth Cohort Study. *Annals of Medicine, 47,* 34-39.

Walston, J. D., Matteini, A. M., Nievergelt, C., Lange, L. A., Fallin, D. M., Barzilai, N., ... Reiner, A. P. (2009). Inflammation and stress-related candidate genes, plasma interleukin-6 levels, and longevity in older adults. *Experimental Gerontology, 44,* 350-355.

World Health Organization (WHO). (1967). *Twentieth World Health Assembly, Geneva, 8-26 May 1967.* Official records of the World Health Organization No. 160. Part I. Resolutions and decisions. Annexes. Geneva, Switzerland: Author.

Zajacova, A., & Burgard, S. A. (2013). Heathier, wealthier, and wiser: A demonstration of compositional changes in aging cohorts due to selective mortality. *Population Research and Policy Review, 32,* 311-324.

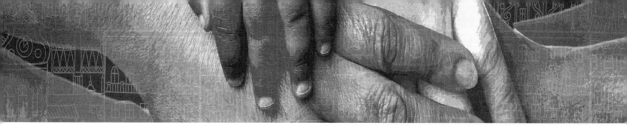

CHAPTER 5

Aging and Late-Life Mobility

Christine M. McDonough, Lori A. Goehring, Molly E. Marino, and **Alan M. Jette**

ABSTRACT

Mobility has been defined as "being able to safely and reliably go where you want, when you want to go, and how you want to get there." Approximately 50% of community-dwelling adults older than age 65 report some limitation in mobility. Mobility limitations predict future problems with walking, activities of daily living, hospitalization, and death. Demographic trends shifting toward increased age of the population, along with the prevalence of obesity and chronic diseases, suggest that the number of people with mobility limitations will increase in the future. The Centers for Disease Control and Prevention has underlined the impact of mobility on older adults: "Lack of mobility in the community or at home significantly narrows an older person's world and ability to do things that bring enjoyment and meaning to life."

This chapter uses the World Health Organization's (WHO) International Classification of Functioning, Disability, and Health (ICF) to explore the role of mobility in aging from the perspective of measurement of mobility limitations for community-dwelling older adults. The ICF is a biopsychosocial model that characterizes disability as resulting from the complex relationships between individual health characteristics, environmental factors, and personal factors, and reflecting the extent to which their interactions affect a person's ability to perform activities and participate in social roles. Using the same core conceptual definition of mobility facilitates international comparisons, dialogue, and collaboration, such as can be found in WHO's 2011 *World Report on Disability*.

This chapter explores the area of aging and mobility with a particular focus on measurements for this population, including self-report, performance-based, and instrumented measurements. Although there is evidence for reliability and validity for all three approaches, these measurement strategies have unique advantages and disadvantages. Self-report measures provide information about respondents' mobility in the context of their activity in the community, and cover a wide range of mobility content. Performance-based measures, such as timed walking distance, focus on more limited aspects of mobility but offer the advantage of standardization—a key advantage for epidemiological research in aging. Instrumented measures, such as accelerometers, have great potential for providing ecologically valid data on the mobility of older adults in their community context, but require further refinement and methodological development.

KEYWORDS

disability	aging	performance-based measures
measurement	physical function	instrumented measures
mobility limitation	self-report measures	

▶ Introduction

Full mobility has been defined as "being able to safely and reliably go where you want, when you want to go, and how you want to get there" (Satariano et al., 2012). In this chapter, we begin with this definition and draw on work from many disciplines to discuss the importance of mobility, and its role in the epidemiology of **aging** from the perspective of **measurement**. Although mobility patterns for institutionalized adults are very important, the scope of this chapter is limited to community-dwelling older adults. In addition to addressing the epidemiology of aging and mobility, one of the main objectives of this chapter is describe the state of the field of mobility measurement as it relates to the study of aging and to provide a comparative review of the most widely used approaches to its measurement. We hope to provide a useful framework for considering how to measure mobility in the epidemiology of aging, and specific guidance to support decision making related to measurement approaches.

▶ Mobility and Aging

Between 1900 and 2000, life expectancy rose from 47 to 77 years in the United States, a relative growth of more than 62%, and there is evidence that this trend is continuing (Molla & Madans, 2010). Today, chronic conditions, which are associated with aging, are the leading cause of death and **disability** in the United States (Institute of Medicine [IOM], 2007; Kung et al., 2008). In contrast, the leading causes of death at the beginning of the 20th century were communicable diseases; thus, the shift to chronic diseases as a key concern is a relatively recent development. Indeed, remarkable shifts in the proportion of older adults in the population are under way. A 2008 Institute of Medicine report predicted that between 2005 and 2030, the number of older adults in the United States would rise from 37 million (12%) to 70 million (20%). The sheer number of older adults at risk for chronic conditions—and consequently at risk for disability—is driving the critical need to address this problem (Brault et al., 2009; Gooloo & Wunderlich, 2009; IOM, 2007; Manton, Corder, & Stallard, 1997; Manton & Gu, 2001; Molla & Madans, 2010; Seeman et al., 2010).

In the 1996 Medical Expenditure Panel Survey, almost 50% of older adults living in the community self-identified as having **mobility limitation** (Rasch et al., 2008). More recently, the 2007 IOM report titled *The Future of Disability in America* reported that 13.5 million people age 65 years and older had a disability, with physical limitations being primarily accountable for that status. Recent trends in diseases and disorders and results from national studies such as the National Health Interview Survey suggest that mobility and other limitations will increase substantially in the coming years (IOM, 2007).

Consequences of mobility limitations are far-reaching, and include limited access to nutritional options and preventive health services, limitations in physical activity, social activity, and worse health outcomes (Satariano et al., 2012). Lower-extremity mobility predicts future problems with walking and performing activities of daily living, and hospitalizations and death (Guralnik et al., 1995, 2000; Hirvensalo, Rantanen, & Heikkinen,

2000; Penninx et al., 2000; von Bonsdorff et al., 2006). The National Report Card on Healthy Aging, which is produced by the Centers for Disease Control and Prevention (CDC), has also highlighted the key role played by mobility for older adults: "Lack of mobility in the community or at home significantly narrows an older person's world and ability to do things that bring enjoyment and meaning to life."

The most common modes of mobility are walking and driving—both activities that are affected by individual-, community- and societal-level factors. Studies of mobility and aging include large population surveys, longitudinal studies of groups affected by specific diseases, and longitudinal studies of aging adults. Important risk factors that have been identified for mobility loss include age, female sex, socioeconomic status, injuries, diseases and chronic conditions, sedentary behavior, and environmental barriers (Satariano et al., 2012). In spite of these serious problems, evidence also indicates that interventions can prevent or decrease mobility limitations in later life (de Vries et al., 2012). There is much work to be done to understand the most effective approaches to maximizing mobility throughout the lifespan. Satariano et al. (2012) highlighted the role of mobility in aging and called for a multidisciplinary approach and "new directions for public health action." They further urged the use of a social-ecological framework that will allow consideration of the full range of important factors determining the trajectory of mobility as people age. This chapter focuses on measurement of mobility to support this call.

▶ Background

Mobility Measures Focused on Older Adults

This chapter draws on recent work funded by the CDC to develop a compendium of measures to support research and practice addressing the mobility of older adults

as they age (McDonough et al., 2014). The compendium provides a description and the properties of each measure based on a comprehensive synthesis of evidence of use focusing on community-dwelling older adults. Like the compendium, this chapter begins with the identification of a conceptual framework developed by the World Health Organization (WHO)—namely, the International Classification of Functioning, Disability, and Health (ICF), which includes individual, social, and environmental factors. Using the ICF as a starting point, evidence is synthesized to report the measurement properties of the selected instruments in community-dwelling older adults, with particular attention being paid to their use in older adults with physical and cognitive impairments as well as the use of assistive devices. The following section provides more detail about the concepts and definitions that underlie the ICF.

This chapter focuses on the three most widely used approaches to measurement: **self-report, performance-based**, and **instrumented measures.** Self-report measures utilize survey methods to elicit a respondent or proxy's assessment of his or her mobility (McDonough et al., 2014). Performance-based measures require an examiner to directly observe performance of a standardized mobility task. Instrumented

PEARL 5-1 Measures of Mobility

Measuring the important dimensions of mobility in gerontological research may require the use of multiple types of measures. Consider the purpose or research question carefully when choosing a measure. For any program, intervention, or study, consider using a combination of self-report, performance-based, and instrumented measures. Each has unique advantages and limitations, and measure triangulation may allow for realizing a combination of their advantages and compensating for the shortcomings of an individual measure.

measures apply electromechanical devices to translate movement into estimated performance (e.g., wearable sensors).

A Biopsychosocial Framework

Mobility limitations are often discussed within the context of concerns about *disability*—a widely used term that includes a broad range of problems with movement, usually caused by a developmental condition, major injury, or disease. Important work of relevance to this chapter comes from the Institute of Medicine's initiative to highlight the extent of disability in the United States and to make recommendations to address it. The 2007 IOM report *The Future of Disability in America* noted the existence of significant confusion about disability and related concepts, and pointed out that conceptual uncertainty was a critical obstacle to progress in research and intervention on disability. The IOM report further identified the need to include socioeconomic and psychosocial factors into a framework for disability, and recommended the adoption and enhancement of the ICF (WHO, 2001).

The ICF is a biopsychosocial model that characterizes the relationships among individual characteristics, health conditions, social and environmental factors in determining a person's ability to perform activities and participate in social roles (WHO, 2001). It was used as the basis for this chapter because it encompasses all of the most relevant perspectives on mobility and aging, including the social and ecological perspectives so critical to the study of aging. The ICF is considered an ecological model because it explicitly addresses social and environmental influence on limitations in functioning and social participation. This perspective is critically important, because to fully include people with physical and other limitations in society, social and environmental contributions must be understood and addressed.

The ICF has been used as the conceptual basis for global studies and evidenced-based policies related to aging and mobility, such as WHO's 2011 *World Report on Disability*. This groundbreaking report found that people with disabilities had worse health and higher poverty rates than those without disabilities, due to barriers to participation and lack of available services. Another notable example of international application of the ICF is the Multi-Country Survey Study and the World Health Survey Program, which has collected data in 71 countries. The multi-county Study on Global AGEing and Adult Health (SAGE) used the ICF framework to studying aging cohorts in methodologically consistent ways to facilitate cross-county comparisons in self-reported health status, including mobility (Naidoo et al., 2010).

In the ICF, *Health conditions* and *contextual factors* are the two broad classes of factors that contribute to health and disability. Diseases, disorders, and injuries are examples of health conditions. Contextual factors may be *personal or environmental*. Examples of personal factors include, age, sex, social, and cultural variables. Environmental factors include physical features of the natural and built environments; legal, organizational, and social policies and structures; and social attitudes.

The ICF describes human functioning at three levels: *body functions and structures, activity,* and *participation*. Body functions include physiological and psychological functioning; body structures consist of organs and systems, and their component parts; activities are specific tasks or actions performed—for example, rising from a chair or walking upstairs; and participation represents "involvement in a life situation" (WHO, 2001, p. 10), such as performing the requirements of social roles. The ICF also highlights the difference between or what one can do, which is called *capacity*, and what one does, which is called *performance*. There is a wide range of complexity of activities and overlap between activities and participation.

The ICF also provides a classification system that breaks down the components of each of the main ICF components (e.g., body structures and functions, activities and participation). Activities and participation are merged within this system and include learning and applying knowledge; general tasks and demands; communication; mobility; self-care; domestic life; interpersonal interactions and relationships; major life areas; and community, social, and civic life.

An important characteristic of the ICF is that the taxonomic system includes both negative and positive terms for each concept. For instance, terms referring to problems with functioning include impairment of body structures and functions, limitations of activity, and restrictions in participation. The coding scheme includes the letters "b", "s", "d", and "e", which denote the components. These letters are followed by a numeric code designating the chapter number (one digit), followed by the second level (two digits), and the third and fourth levels (one digit each). For example, the mobility chapter includes the following code groups: changing and maintaining body position (d410–d429), carrying moving and handling objects (d430–d449), walking and moving (d450–d469), and using transportation (d470–d489). There are 80 available mobility-related activities within the ICF framework.

FIGURE 5-1 illustrates the main concepts included in the ICF, with explication of the mobility components—the focus of this chapter.

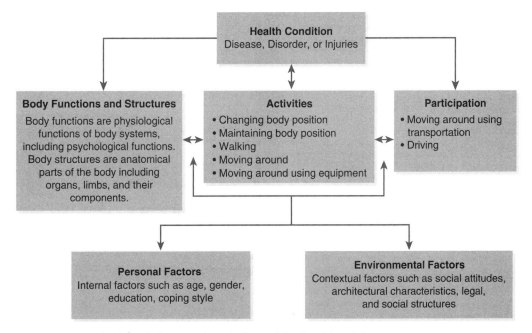

FIGURE 5-1 Example of the ICF framework applied to mobility for older adults.

▶ # Definition and Measurement of Mobility

In this chapter, we define *mobility* as moving by changing body position or location or by transferring from one place or another; by carrying, moving, or manipulating objects; by walking, running, or climbing; and by using various forms of transportation (**FIGURE 5-2**). This definition aligns with the ICF framework, with one exception: It excludes activities of daily living such as dressing, bathing, and grooming that closely relate to upper-extremity fine motor control or dexterity. Excluding some upper-extremity tasks and activities from our definition of mobility is consistent with the evidence that lower-extremity functioning is more strongly related to mobility status (Onder et al., 2005). More expansive constructs such as **physical functioning**, physical health, health-related quality of life, and well-being are not included in our definition of mobility. This omission reflects the objective of this chapter to identify those measures relevant to transportation use, driving, wheeled mobility, and assistive device use, and to report coverage of these dimensions. A second aim is to incorporate evidence from samples of individuals with physical and cognitive impairment.

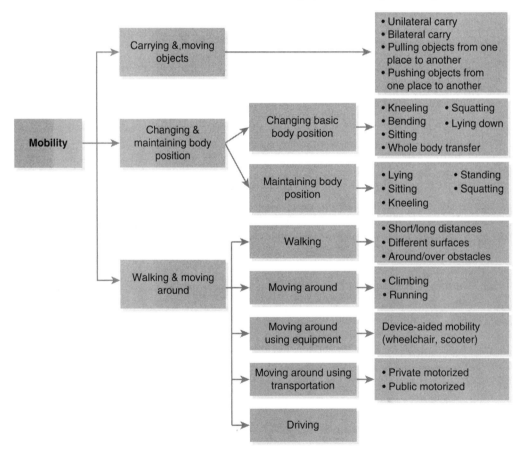

FIGURE 5-2 Components of mobility as defined in McDonough et al.'s (2014) compendium.

Reproduced from: McDonough, C., et al. A Compendium of Mobility Measures Focused on Community-Dwelling Older Adults. 2014 [1/27/2016]. Available from: http://www.bu.edu/bostonroc/instruments /mobilitycompendium/

▸ Approaches to Measurement of Mobility in Aging

Self-Report Measures of Mobility

The self-report measures of mobility consist of two main approaches: (1) traditional fixed-form methods, in which the scores are calculated based on the sum of responses to the total items, and (2) instruments developed using item response theory (IRT). In measures that employ IRT, each item is ordered in a hierarchy along a unidimensional construct, and scores are based on probability models that represent the likelihood that a respondent selects an answer choice, given his or her ability on that construct.

Computerized adaptive testing is a method of administering IRT-based instruments. With such testing, the computer algorithm selects each subsequent question based on the respondent's answer to previous questions. This adaptive approach allows for skipping of items that are irrelevant to a person's functional status, which minimizes the burden of administration without sacrificing measurement precision.

TABLE 5-1 summarizes the self-report measures that have been identified as promising options for use in measuring mobility of community-dwelling older adults. A range of administration methods are possible, including interviewer-, self-, and proxy-based administration, as well as modes such as pencil-and-paper and electronic delivery. Various dimensions of mobility are covered by these measures, including ability, difficulty, activity avoidance, frequency, and intensity. The time required for the respondent to complete the measures ranges from 2 to 15 minutes.

Broadly, the advantages of self-report measures include low respondent and administrative burden (cost, staffing, training, and data management). In addition, self-report measures have high ecological validity, incorporating the lived experience and perspective of the older adult respondent, and in some cases providing explicit measurement of mobility using walking aids or a wheelchair (e.g., Activity Measure for Post Acute Care [AM-PAC] and Late-Life Function and Disability Instrument [LLFDI]). In some cases, there is a licensing cost for use of the measure (e.g., AM-PAC and Short Form-36). Item banks for item-response theory-based self-report measures provide comprehensive coverage of mobility (e.g., changing and maintaining body positions, walking, stair climbing, carrying and moving objects, moving around in different locations, using transportation) compared with traditional self-report measures.

Because they are relatively new and demonstrate promising measurement properties, more evidence is needed on IRT measures of mobility among community-dwelling older adults with physical and cognitive limitations. Computer-adaptive versions of these measures require point-of-contact computers for their administration, which may be difficult to achieve in some settings. However, for all computer-adaptive measures, fixed short forms can be used. Some measures (e.g., AM-PAC) provide for proxy responses to the instrument that could be used for persons with significant cognitive impairment.

Performance-Based Measures of Mobility

Performance-based measures of mobility focus on walking activities, and require some training of the tester to achieve an acceptable level of standardization. These tests can be performed in less than 15 minutes with minimal equipment. In many cases a walking pathway is needed. **TABLE 5-2** summarizes the properties of performance-based measures of mobility.

TABLE 5-1 Properties of Self-Report Mobility Scales

| Mobility Scale | Content Coverage | Mobility Dimensions Measured | Administration | | | | Assistive Device or Wheelchair Items? | Number of Items |
			Versions	Method	Mode	Time		
Activity Measure for Post Acute Care (AM-PAC) (Haley et al., 2008)	✓✓✓	Difficulty doing task, assistance needed	CATs and linked short forms	Electronic, paper and pencil	Interview Self-administered Proxy	Basic mobility CAT: 2–3 minutes	Yes, wheelchair and assistive devices	User defined; available items: 131
Craig Handicap Assessment and Reporting Technique (CHART) (Whiteneck et al., 1992)	✓	Duration, frequency of tasks and activities, adequacy of transportation	Fixed form	Paper and pencil	Interview Self-administered	15 minutes	Not specified	19
Driving Habits Questionnaire (DHQ) (Owsley & McGwin, 1999)	✓	Driving space, avoidance, difficulty, exposure, crashes	Fixed form	Paper and pencil	Interview Self-administered	Not reported	Addresses use of eyeglasses and contact lenses	30
Functional Status Questionnaire (FSQ) (Jette et al., 1986)	✓	Difficulty	Fixed form	Electronic	Self-administered	10–15 minutes	Not specified	9
Late-Life Function and Disability Instrument (LLFDI, LLFDI-CAT) (Jette et al., 2002)	✓✓✓ ✓✓	Difficulty	Fixed form, CATs	Paper and pencil, electronic	Interviewer	Varies by version: 3 minutes (CAT) to 15 minutes	Yes, wheelchair and assistive devices	32 (fixed form); available: 141 total

Measure		Construct	Form	Medium	Administration	Time	Wheelchair/assistive devices	Number of items
Life Space Assessment (LSA) (Baker, Bodner, & Allman, 2003)	✓	Extent, frequency, assistance of movement in life spaces	Fixed form	Paper and pencil	Interviewer	10–15 minutes	Yes, wheelchair and assistive devices	24
Pepper Assessment Tool of Disability (PAT-D) (Rejeski et al., 1995)	✓✓	Difficulty	Fixed form	Paper and pencil	Interviewer or self-administered	5–10 minutes	Not specified	8
PROMIS (Cella et al., 2010)	✓✓✓ ✓✓	Difficulty	Fixed form, CATs	Paper and pencil, electronic	Interviewer or self-administered	2–5 minutes	Separate item bank for mobility aid users	Available: 121 total; 4-, 6-, 8-, 10-, and 20-item short forms
Short-Form 36 PF-10 (PF-10) (Ware & Sherbourne, 1992)	✓✓	Difficulty	Fixed form	Paper and pencil, electronic	Interviewer or self-administered	5–10 minutes	Not specified	10
Wheelchair Skills Test Questionnaire (WST-Q) (Mountain, Kirby, & Smith, 2004)	✓	Ability, difficulty, frequency	Fixed forms: wheelchair and scooter users and caregivers	Paper and pencil	Interviewer or self-administered	10 minutes	Yes, wheelchair only	39
WHO-DAS 2.0 (Chisolm et al., 2005)	✓	Difficulty	Fixed form	Paper and pencil, electronic	Interviewer, self, or proxy administered	2–3 minutes	Not specified	5

Contributed by: McDonough, Goehring, Marino, Jette.

TABLE 5-2 Properties of Performance-Based Measures of Mobility

Instrument	Dimensions of Mobility Measured	Equipment Needed	Administration Time	Assistive Device or Wheelchair Items?	Number of Items
De Morton Mobility Index (DEMMI) (de Morton, Davidson, & Keating, 2008)	✓	Chair, bed, or plinth	< 9 minutes	Individual uses assistive device	15
Dynamic Gait Index (DGI) (Shumway-Cook & Woollacott, 1995)	✓	20-foot walkway, shoebox, cones, 2 stairs	Not reported	Individual uses assistive device	8
Functional Gait Assessment (FGA) (Wrisley et al., 2004)	✓	20-foot walkway, shoebox, cones, 2 stairs	Not reported	Individual uses assistive device	10
5 Times Sit to Stand (5TSS) (Guralnik et al., 1994)	✓	Chair, stopwatch	< 5 minutes	Performed without device	1
30-Second Chair Stand (Jones, Rikli, & Beam, 1999)	✓	Chair, stopwatch	< 5 minutes	Performed without device	1
Gait Speed (Reuben et al., 2013)	✓	Stopwatch, walkway	3 minutes	Not reported	1
6-Minute Walk (6MWT) (Butland et al., 1982)	✓	Stopwatch, cones, measuring tape	10–15 minutes	Not reported	1
2-Minute Walk (2MWT) (Butland et al., 1982)	✓	Stopwatch, cones, measuring tape	4 minutes	Individual uses assistive device	1
Short Physical Performance Battery (SPPB) (Guralnik et al., 1994)	✓	Chair, stopwatch, tape measure,	10–15 minutes	Individual uses assistive device	4
Timed Up and Go (TUG) (Podsiadlo & Richardson, 1991)	✓	Chair, stopwatch, tape measure	< 3 minutes	Individual uses assistive device	2
Stair Climb (Oh-Park, Wang, & Verghese, 2011)	✓	Flight of stairs, stopwatch	< 5 minutes	Not reported	1

Contributed by: McDonough, Goehring, Marino, Jette.

Considerable evidence supports the reliability and validity of performance-based measures of mobility that can be administered in the community by nonclinicians. Performance-based measures are associated with important health outcomes, and the relative standardization of their administration allows comparison to reference values across large epidemiological studies. Disadvantages include the administrative burden of in-person testing in the community and the very limited coverage across the range of mobility activities. For example, carrying and moving objects are typically not addressed by such measures, and there are very limited explicit applications for persons who use walking aids or wheelchairs. In addition, movement in different life spaces, use of wheelchairs, and use of other mobility aids—all of which are important concerns in aging—are not well addressed by performance-based measures.

Instrumented Measures of Mobility

Instrumented measures present a wide range of choices in level of cost, complexity, activities that can be measured, and technical considerations such as battery life. **TABLE 5-3** summarizes the properties of these measures of mobility.

Instrumented measures provide direct measurement of behavior in free-living conditions and have a high degree of ecologic validity. The literature on these measures' reliability and validity focuses on the use of pedometers and accelerometers to measure physical activity, leaving significant gaps in the evidence base for their use in measuring older adults' mobility. There is evolving work to classify body positions and specific activities (e.g., sitting, running, climbing stairs), which also warrants testing among older adults with physical and cognitive limitations.

The wide range of methods used to measure mobility, filter and aggregate the data, and estimate activities, as well as the pace of change

for these devices, provides unique challenges when assessing their reliability and validity. Although there is strong evidence for the reliability and validity of pedometers and accelerometers in measurement of key activities such as walking, actual step counts from different instruments are not comparable. This sort of variation has important implications for the use of reference (normative) values, and it argues for research into such values for older adult populations with physical and cognitive limitations. Instrumented systems that classify activities also tend to be expensive, and require dedicate data management software.

Although a small number of systems have been tested among people who use wheelchairs for mobility, few of these tests have focused on older adults. Therefore, research is needed to establish the evidence base for reliable and valid measurement of mobility in older adults who use devices, including wheelchairs.

Instrumented measures are associated with similar challenges in addressing carrying and moving objects and movement throughout the community as are noted with performance-based measures. Development and testing in these areas is rapidly evolving, however. For example, data from accelerometers may be combined with data from global positioning systems in handheld devices to provide information about where people go. Research is needed to focus these efforts on mobility measurement for older adults.

Comparisons Across Types of Measures

To explore the content coverage of various measures, we classified the content of mobility measures relative to the ICF. Using the previously described ICF coding system, definitions, and examples, **TABLE 5-4** classifies the items, tasks, and features of various measures into their appropriate ICF category. The purpose of such a classification system is to indicate the breadth of use (total number of codes) for such measures.

TABLE 5-3 Properties of Instrumented Report Measures of Mobility

Instrument	Dimensions of Mobility Measured	Location Worn	Output	Data Processing Software Needed	Cost	Battery Life
Pedometers						
New Life series/Kenz (The Pedometer Company)	✓	Waist	Step counts, physical activity levels	Yes	++	2–9 months
StepWatch (SWA)	✓	Ankle	Gait cycles/interval Steps/day 32 variables (e.g., active minutes, maximum steps)	Yes	++	Up to 7 years
Yamax Digiwalker	✓	Waist or shoe	Steps, distance, calories	No	+	3 years
Accelerometers						
Actigraph	✓	Waist	Approximately 35 variables (e.g., step count, activity count, position, physical activity levels)	Yes	++	Approximately 25 days; depends on data sampling settings

Device		Placement	Measures		Rating	Battery
Actical	✓	Depends on measurement goals	Step count, activity counts, energy expenditure	Yes	++	Lithium coin cell—user replaceable
ActivPAL	✓	Anterior thigh	Time in sit, stand, and walking; step count, cadence, sit to stand, calories	Yes	++	Up to 10 days
Dynaport	✓	Waist	Steps, energy expenditure, time in activity levels, time in different body positions	Yes	++	7 days measurement; 7 days standby
IDEEA	✓✓	Chest, thighs, soles of feet	Power, steps, energy expenditure, body positions, transitions, and gaits	Yes	+++	AA batteries
RT6	✓	Depends on measurement goals	Steps, activity counts, calorie expenditure	Yes	++	Not reported
SenseWear	✓	Upper arm	Steps, activity counts, large number of activity and position classification variables	Yes	+++	5–7 days

Contributed by: McDonough, Goehring, Marino, Jette.

TABLE 5-4 Mobility Measure Coverage of the International Classification of Functioning's Health and Disability Mobility Chapter, Ranked from Most to Least Coverage

Measures	d410–d429 Changing and Maintaining Body Position	d430–d449 Carrying, Moving, and Handling Objects	d450 Walking and Moving	d455 Moving Around	d460 Moving Around in Different Locations	d470–d474 Moving Around Using Transportation	d475 Driving	Total Number of ICF Codes Covered
				ICF Mobility Activity Codes				
Self-Report								
AM-PAC Mobility	10	8	4	3	4	0	0	**29**
LLFDI-CAT Function	10	8	3	2	4	0	0	**27**
PROMIS Physical CAT	9	7	3	3	0	0	0	**22**
LLFDI Function	5	7	3	2	2	0	0	**19**
PROMIS SF-10	4	4	1	2	0	0	0	**11**
SF-36 PF-10	2	4	2	2	0	0	0	**10**
PAT-D	4	3	1	1	1	0	0	**10**
FSQ	1	1	2	1	2	1	1	**9**

Measure							Total
WHODAS II	3	0	1	0	2	0	0	6
LSA	0	0	0	0	5	0	0	5
WST-Q	0	0	0	0	5	0	0	5
CHART	0	0	0	0	2	1	0	3
LLFDI-CAT Disability	0	0	0	0	0	1	1	2
DHQ	0	0	0	0	0	0	1	1
Performance-Based								
DEMMI	6	0	1	1	0	0	0	8
DGI	1	0	2	1	0	0	0	4
FGA	1	0	1	1	0	0	0	3
SPPB	3	0	1	0	0	0	0	4
TUG	2	0	1	0	0	0	0	3
Sit to Stand	2	0	0	0	0	0	0	2
Walking Tests	0	0	2	0	0	0	0	2
Stair Climb	0	0	0	1	0	0	0	1

(continues)

TABLE 5-4 Mobility Measure Coverage of the International Classification of Functioning's Health and Disability Mobility Chapter, Ranked from Most to Least Coverage *(continued)*

Instrumented

Pedometers							
Yamax Digiwalker	0	0	2	0	0	0	**2**
New Life series/Kenz	0	0	2	0	0	0	**2**
StepWatch/SWA	0	0	2	0	0	0	**2**
Accelerometers							
IDEEA	7	0	2	3	0	0	**12**
Dynaport	5	0	2	0	0	0	**7**
SenseWear	1	2	2	1	0	1	**7**
ActivPAL	3	0	2	0	0	0	**5**
Actigraph	0	0	2	0	0	0	**2**
Actical	0	0	2	0	0	0	**2**
RT6	0	0	2	0	0	0	**2**

Contributed by: McDonough, Goehring, Marino, Jette.

In general, self-report measures provide more comprehensive coverage of the activities that represent mobility, although there is a considerable variation in the range of coverage for each individual measure. For example, the Driving Habits Questionnaire covers only driving, whereas the computer-adaptive version of the Late-Life Function and Disability Instrument CAT function item bank covers 27 ICF mobility activities. Self-report measures cover carrying and moving objects as well as moving around in different locations, such as in the community. They measure performance (what was done) more than capacity (what could be done). Performance-based measures address capacity; their coverage ranges from 1 to 8 mobility activities. Instrumented measures cover performance of 2 to 12 activities, with a strong focus on changing and maintaining body position and walking. There is little, if any, coverage of carrying, moving objects, or moving in different locations. Pedometers and the simplest accelerometers cover only walking. Multiaxial accelerometer systems are strong in estimating physical activity and walking, but they have limitations in measuring slow movement in older adults with physical limitations. Some systems are able to classify activities, such as lying, sitting, standing, and movement transitions, as well as different walking activities such as stair climbing and running. However, the reliability and validity of these systems in older adults is not well established.

Preliminary evidence is available regarding the validity and reliability of self-report, performance-based, and instrumented measures among older adults with mild cognitive impairment. However, we did not find evidence that might inform use of these measures among older adults with significant cognitive impairment.

All of the self-report, performance-based, and instrumented measures reviewed in this chapter have sufficient evidence of reliability, validity, and feasibility for measurement of mobility, yet each also has distinct advantages and disadvantages. For example, self-report measures integrate the perspective of older adults' mobility in their unique social and physical contexts, across the continuum of life activities. Although this is an important advantage of these measures, the variation inherent in individuals' interpretation and context may contribute to measurement error. For instance, "crossing the street at a traffic light" is subject to several important contextual factors, including wayfinding features, curbs, and noise and traffic levels.

The standardization afforded by performance-based measures allows for comparison of results across individuals and groups, but decreases the resemblance to real-life activity. An interesting study of self-report and performance-based measures by Bean et al. (2011) compared the self-report Late-Life Function and Disability Index (LLFDI) with the performance-based Short Physical Performance Battery (SPPB) in older adults. The LLFDI and the SPPB both measure attributes of exercise tolerance and lower-extremity functioning. Considering additional variables, relationships were found between the SPPB, in terms of lower-extremity activities and age, and between the LLFDI, in terms of chronic conditions, female sex, and falls efficacy. This study suggests that these two measures assess different elements related to functioning (Bean et al., 2011). In another comparison of self-report and performance-based measures among older adults who had sustained a hip fracture, both approaches demonstrated acceptable measurement properties (Latham et al., 2008). This study lends additional support to the notion that the research question or practice objective should guide instrument selection.

Instrumented measures such as pedometers, accelerometers, gyroscopes, and global positioning systems (GPS) have the unique advantage of objectively measuring mobility in real time in the natural environment. Research and practice with instrumented measures is rapidly evolving, due in part to the strong interest in the potential of these measures to solve the problem of fully characterizing mobility in the individual's real-life community context. Notably, there has been great interest in using instruments to measure human movement. From the perspective of mobility, the evidence supporting the use of instrumented measures in older adults is somewhat limited by the heavy focus on characterizing physical activity relative to energy expenditure (e.g., calories expended). Although an in-depth examination of physical activity is beyond the scope of this chapter, the relationships among walking, physical activity, and mobility make physical activity relevant to this discussion. Indeed, Prohaska et al. (2011) describe physical activity as one form of mobility. Ultimately, instrumented measures address a range of physical activity outcomes such as activity counts, duration of time in different levels of energy expenditure, and energy expenditure estimates. At the same time, they measure important mobility parameters such as the number of steps taken and the distance walked.

An exciting and rapidly evolving body of literature focuses on classifying movement postures and activity types—an area that shows promise as a means of measuring mobility in older adults (Culhane et al., 2004; Salarian et al., 2007; Taylor et al., 2014; White, Wagenaar, & Ellis, 2006). The data collected include measures of sitting, standing, walking up stairs, running, and transitions. The evidence for these instruments support their reliability and validity for mobility measurement, albeit with some caveats. There are limitations in measurement accuracy for older adults with very slow mobility patterns, and significant challenges in identifying "moving around using equipment." Additional challenges have been identified in assessing the comparability of estimates from different devices, and even from different models of the same brand/device.

The rapid changes in technology within and between mobility measurement devices, and within and between data processing and analytic methods, pose major challenges to

interpretation of results across studies and populations (Cheung, Gray, & Karunanithi, 2011; de Bruin et al., 2008; Lee & Shiroma, 2014; Lindemann et al., 2013; Taraldsen et al., 2012; Welk, McClain, & Ainsworth, 2012). Development, use, and research for each model, device, and outcome are rapidly changing, but the information provided here should serve as a framework for consideration of current devices.

▸ Conclusion and Future Directions

Although there is no one superior approach to the measurement of mobility for older adults, some important considerations can be applied to guide instrument choice. Self-reported measures have the advantages of broad coverage of mobility content, a high degree of ecologic validity, ease of use, and coverage of both activity and participation outcome domains. In particular, the IRT-based instruments have great potential for meeting the need to measure a wide range of mobility content over the span of aging with limited respondent burden. Several self-report measures explicitly incorporate equipment or assistive device use into the measurement.

Performance-based measures should be chosen when standardization is more important than ecologic validity, and when time and resources allow for training and deployment of testers. The standardization inherent in these measures is an important advantage for comparisons across time and groups in epidemiological research. However, lack of information on actual behavior in the community context should be weighed against these advantages, as well as the fact that performance-based measures do not address more complex aspects of mobility such as transportation.

Instrumented measures show great promise for bridging these two approaches by providing both ecological validity and standardization. Although some of the more sophisticated instruments can characterize a wide range of mobility content, they are expensive and require dedicated data management systems. In addition, limitations in these measures' use for people who use equipment or who move very slowly restrict their application. Although this area is rapidly changing, most of the currently available, easy-to-use instrumented measures focus on a limited range of mobility activities, such as walking.

Our recommendation is to select one of each approach if resources allow, and if not, to prioritize the choice based on the primary objective of measurement. First consider the mobility content of interest, followed by an assessment of the importance of community context and standardization, and then account for dimensions such as equipment use, cognitive impairment, and time and resource availability. Ultimately, using a multifactorial approach to the measurement of mobility guided by a clear conceptual framework will allow consideration of the full range of important factors determining the trajectory of mobility as people age.

This chapter has focused on measuring the mobility of older adults. Our conceptual framework, the ICF, highlights the roles of variables such as health conditions, body functions and structures, and environmental factors in the development of mobility limitations. For example, evolving evidence indicates that age-related central nervous system disorders have important impacts on the development of mobility impairment (Sorond et al., 2015). Experts in the field have recommended central nervous system disorders as a research priority for maintaining older adults' ability to live independently in the community. The built environment also plays a role in the pathway toward disability in aging adults, including considerations related to physical geography; the design, construction, and building products and technology of buildings for public use; architecture and construction;

open space; and transportation services, systems. and policies. We would recommend a focus on measuring the characteristics of the built environment, and research focused on understanding each of their impacts on mobility disability, as topics for future studies (Clarke et al., 2008).

▶ Acknowledgments

Funding for this project was provided by the Centers for Disease Control and Prevention (3U48DP001922-04S2) through the Special Interest Project grant (12-059) and the Boston Roybal Center for Active Lifestyle Interventions (1P30AG048785).

References

Baker, P. S., Bodner, E. V., & Allman, R. M. (2003). Measuring life-space mobility in community-dwelling older adults. *Journal of the American Geriatrics Society*, *51*(11), 1610–1604.

Bean, J. F., Ölveczky, D. D., Kiely, D. K., LaRose, S. I., & Jette, A. M. (2011). Performance-based versus patient-reported physical function: What are the underlying predictors? *Physical Therapy*, *91*(12), 1804–1811.

Brault, M., et al. (2009). Prevalence and most common causes of disability among adults—United States, 2005. *Morbidity and Mortality Weekly Report*, *58*(16), 421–426.

Butland, R.J., Pang, J., Gross, E., Woodcock, A., & Geddes, D. (1982). Two-, six-, and 12-minute walking tests in respiratory disease. *British Medical Journal of Clinical Research*, *284*(6329), 1607–1608.

Cella D., Riley W., Stone A., Rothrock N., Reeve B., Yount S., … & Hays R. (2010). The Patient-Reported Outcomes Measurement Information System (PROMIS) developed and tested its first wave of adult self-reported health outcome item banks: 2005–2008. *Journal of Clinical Epidemiology*, *63*(11), 1179–1194.

Cheung, V. H., Gray, L., & Karunanithi, M. (2011). Review of accelerometry for determining daily activity among elderly patients. *Archives of Physical Medicine & Rehabilitation*, *92*(6), 998–1014.

Chisolm, T. H., Abrams, H. B., McArdle, R., Wilson, R. H., & Doyle, P. J. (2005). The WHO-DAS II: Psychometric properties in the measurement of functional health status in adults with acquired hearing loss. *Trends in Amplification*, *9*(3), 111–126.

Clarke, P., Ailshire, J. A., Bader, M., Morenoff, J. D., & House, J. S. (2008). Mobility disability and the urban built environment. *American Journal of Epidemiology, 168*(5), 506–513.

Culhane, K. M., Lyons, G. M., Hilton, D., Grace, P. A., & Lyons D. (2004). Long-term mobility monitoring of older adults using accelerometers in a clinical environment. *Clinical Rehabilitation, 18*(3), 335_343.

de Bruin, E. D., Hartmann, A., Uebelhart, D., Murer, K., & Zijlstra, W. (2008). Wearable systems for monitoring mobility-related activities in older people: A systematic review. *Clinical Rehabilitation, 22*(10–11), 878_895.

de Morton, N. A., Davidson, M., & Keating, J. L. (2008). The de Morton Mobility Index (DEMMI): An essential health index for an ageing world. *Health & Quality of Life Outcomes, 6*, 63.

de Vries, N. M., Van Ravensberg, C., Hobbelen, J., Rikkert, M. O., Staal, J., & Nijhuis-vander Sanden M. (2012). Effects of physical exercise therapy on mobility, physical functioning, physical activity, and quality of life in community-dwelling older adults with impaired mobility, physical disability, and/or multi-morbidity: A meta-analysis. *Ageing Research Reviews, 11*(1), 136–149.

Gooloo, R., & Wunderlich, S. (Eds.). (2009). *Improving the measurement of late-life disability in population surveys: Beyond ADLs and IADLs. Summary of a Workshop, Committee on National Statistics and Committee on Population, Division of Behavioral and Social Sciences and Education.* Washington, DC: National Research Council.

Guralnik, J. M., Simonsick, E. M., Ferrucci, L., Glynn, R. J., Berkman, L. F., Blazer, D. G., … & Wallace, R. B. (1994). A short physical performance battery assessing lower extremity function: Association with self-reported disability and prediction of mortality and nursing home admission. *Journal of Gerontology, 49*(2), M85–M94.

Guralnik, J. M., Ferrucci, L., Simonsick, E. M., Salive, M. E., & Wallace, R. B. Lower-extremity function in persons over the age of 70 years as a predictor of subsequent disability. *New England Journal of Medicine, 332*(9), 556–561.

Guralnik, J. M., Ferrucci, L., Pieper, C. F., Leveille, S. G., Markides, K. S., Ostir, G., … & Wallace, R. B. (2000). Lower extremity function and subsequent disability: Consistency across studies, predictive models, and value of gait speed alone compared with the short physical performance battery. *Journals of Gerontology Series A: Biological Sciences & Medical Sciences, 55*(4), M221–M231.

Haley, S. M., Gandek, B., Siebens, H., Black-Schaffer, R. M., Sinclair, S. J., Tao, W., … & Jette, A. M. (2008). Computerized adaptive testing for follow-up after discharge from inpatient rehabilitation: II. Participation outcomes. *Archives of Physical Medicine & Rehabilitation, 89*(2), 275–283.

Hirvensalo, M., Rantanen, T., & Heikkinen, E. (2000). Mobility difficulties and physical activity as predictors of mortality and loss of independence in the community-living older population. *Journal of the American Geriatrics Society, 48*(5), 493–498.

Institute of Medicine (IOM). (2007). *The future of disability in America.* Washington, DC: National Academies Press.

Institute of Medicine (IOM). (2008). *Retooling for an aging America: Building the health care workforce.* Washington, DC: National Academies Press.

Jette, A. M., Davies, A. R., Cleary, P. D., Calkins, D. R., Rubenstein, L. V., Fink, A., … & Delbanco, T. L. (1986). The Functional Status Questionnaire: Reliability and validity when used in primary care. *Journal of General Internal Medicine, 1*(3), 143–149. Erratum appears in *Journal of General Internal Medicine, 1*(6), 427.

Jette, A. M., Haley, S. M., Coster, W. J., Kooyoomjian, J. T., Levenson, S., Heeren, T., & Ashba, J. (2002). Late life function and disability instrument: I. Development and evaluation of the disability component. *Journals of Gerontology Series A: Biological Sciences & Medical Sciences, 57*(4), M209–M216.

Jones, C. J., Rikli, R. E., & Beam, W. C. (1999). A 30-s chair-stand test as a measure of lower body strength in community-residing older adults. *Research Quarterly for Exercise and Sport, 70*(2), 113–119.

Kung, H.-C., Hoyert, D. L., Xu, J., Murphy, S. L. (2008). Deaths: Final data for 2005. *National Vital Statistics Reports, 56*(10), 1–120.

Latham, N. K., Mehta, V., Nguyen, A. M., Jette, A. M., Olarsch, S., Papanicolaou, D., & Chandler, J. (2008). Performance-based or self-report measures of physical function: Which should be used in clinical trials of hip fracture patients? *Archives of Physical Medicine & Rehabilitation, 89*(11), 2146–2155.

Lee, I. M., & Shiroma, E. J. (2014). Using accelerometers to measure physical activity in large-scale epidemiological studies: Issues and challenges. *British Journal of Sports Medicine, 48*(3), 197–201.

Lindemann, U., Zilstra, W., Aminian, K., Chastin, S. F., de Bruin, E. D., Helbostad, J. L., & Bussmann, J. B. (2013). Recommendations for standardizing validation procedures assessing physical activity of older persons by monitoring body postures and movements. *Sensors, 14*(1), 1267–1277.

Manton, K. G., Corder, L., & Stallard, E. (1997). Chronic disability trends in elderly United States populations: 1982–1994. *Proceedings of the National Academy of Sciences of the United States of America, 94*(6), 2593–2598.

Manton, K. G., & Gu, X. (2001). Changes in the prevalence of chronic disability in the United States black and nonblack population above age 65 from 1982 to 1999. *Proceedings of the National Academy of Sciences of the United States of America*, 98(11), 6354–6359.

McDonough, C. M, Goehring, L. A., Marino, M. E., & Jette, A. M. (2014). A compendium of mobility measures focused on community-dwelling older adults. Available at: http://www.bu.edu/bostonroc/instruments/mobilitycompendium/

Molla, M. T, & Madans, J. H. (2010). Life expectancy free of chronic condition-induced activity limitations among white and black Americans, 2000–2006. National Center for Health Statistics. *Vital Health Statistics*, 3(34), 1–29.

Mountain, A. D., Kirby, R. L., & Smith, C. (2004). The wheelchair skills test, version 2.4: Validity of an algorithm-based questionnaire version. *Archives of Physical Medicine & Rehabilitation*, 85(3), 416–423.

Naidoo, N., et al. (2010). Ageing and adult health status in eight lower-income countries: The INDEPTH WHO-SAGE collaboration. *Global Health Action, 11.*

Oh-Park, M., Wang, C., & Verghese, J. (2011). Stair negotiation time in community-dwelling older adults: Normative values and association with functional decline. *Archives of Physical Medicine & Rehabilitation*, 92(12), 2006–2011.

Onder, G., Penninx, B. W., Ferrucci, L., Fried, L. P., Guralnik, J. M., & Pahor, M. (2005). Measures of physical performance and risk for progressive and catastrophic disability: Results from the Women's Health and Aging Study. *Journal of Gerontology: Medical Sciences*, 60(1), 74–79.

Owsley, C., & McGwin, G. Jr. (1999). Vision impairment and driving. *Survey of Ophthalmology*, 43(6), 535–550.

The Pedometer Company. Accelerometers and pedometers. Available at: http://www.thepedometercompany.com/pedometers.html

Penninx, B. W., Ferrucci, L., Leveille, S. G., Rantanen, T., Pahor, M., & Guralnik, J. M. (2000). Lower extremity performance in nondisabled older persons as a predictor of subsequent hospitalization. *Journals of Gerontology Series A: Biological Sciences & Medical Sciences*, 55(11), M691–M697.

Podsiadlo, D., & Richardson, S. (1991). The timed "Up & Go": A test of basic functional mobility for frail elderly persons. *Journal of the American Geriatrics Society*, 39(2), 142–148.

Prohaska, T. R., Anderson, L. A., Hooker, S. P., Hughes, S. L., & Belza, B. (2011). Mobility and aging: Transference to transportation. *Journal of Aging Research. Volume* 2011, 1–3. doi:10.4061/2011/392751.

Rasch, E. K., Hochberg, M. C., Magder, L., Magaziner, J., & Altman, B. M. (2008). Health of community-dwelling adults with mobility limitations in the United States: Prevalent health conditions. Part I. *Archives of Physical Medicine & Rehabilitation*, 89(2), 210–218.

Rejeski, W. J., Ettinger, W. H. Jr, Schumaker, S., James, P., Burns, R., & Elam, J. T. (1995). Assessing performance-related disability in patients with knee osteoarthritis. *Osteoarthritis & Cartilage*, 3(3), 157–167.

Reuben, D. B., Magasi, S., McCreath, H. E., Bohannon, R. W., Wang, Y. C., Bubela, D. J., … & Gershon, R. C. (2013). Motor assessment using the NIH Toolbox. *Neurology*, 80(11 suppl 3), S65–S75.

Salarian, A., Russmann, H., Vingerhoets, F. J., Burkhard, P. R., & Aminian, K. (2007). Ambulatory monitoring of physical activities in patients with Parkinson's disease. *IEEE Transactions on Biomedical Engineering*, 54(12), 2296–2299.

Satariano, W. A., Guralnik, J. M., Jackson, R. J., Marottoli, R. A., Phelan, E. A., & Prohaska, T. R. (2012). Mobility and aging: New directions for public health action. *American Journal of Public Health*, 102(8), 1508–1515.

Seeman, T. E, Merkin, S. S., Crimmins, E. M., & Karlamangla, A. S. (2010). Disability trends among older Americans: National Health and Nutrition Examination Surveys, 1988–1994 and 1999–2004. *American Journal of Public Health*, 100(1), 100–107.

Shumway-Cook, A., & Woollacott, M. (1995). *Motor control: Theory and practical applications.* Baltimore, MD: Williams & Wilkins.

Sorond, F. A., Cruz-Almeida, Y., Clark, D. J., Viswanathan, A., Scherzer, C. R., De Jager, P., … & Lipsitz, L. A. (2015). Aging, the central nervous system, and mobility in older adults: Neural mechanisms of mobility impairment. *Journals of Gerontology Series A: Biological Sciences & Medical Sciences*, 70(12), 1526–1532.

Taraldsen, K., Chastin, S. F., Riphagen, I. I., Vereijken, B., Helbostad, J. L. (2012). Physical activity monitoring by use of accelerometer-based body-worn sensors in older adults: A systematic literature review of current knowledge and applications. *Maturitas*, 71(1), 13–19.

Taylor, L. M., Klenk, J., Maney, A. J., Kerse, N., Macdonald, B. M., & Maddison, R. (2014). Validation of a body-worn accelerometer to measure activity patterns in octogenarians. *Archives of Physical Medicine & Rehabilitation*, 95(5), 930–934.

von Bonsdorff, M., Rantanen, T., Laukkanen, P., Suutama, T., Heikkinen, E. (2006). Mobility limitations and cognitive deficits as predictors of institutionalization among community-dwelling older people. *Gerontology*, 52(6), 359–365.

Ware, J. E. Jr., & Sherbourne, C. D. (1992). The MOS 36-item short-form health survey (SF-36). I. Conceptual framework and item selection. *Medical Care*, 30(6), 473–483.

Welk, G. J., McClain, J., & Ainsworth, B. E. (2012). Protocols for evaluating equivalency of acclerometry-based activity monitors. *Medicine & Science in Sports & Exercise*, *44*(1 suppl 1), S39–S49.

White, D. K., Wagenaar, R. C., & Ellis, T. (2006). Monitoring activity in individuals with Parkinson disease: A validity study. *Journal of Neurologic Physical Therapy*, *30*(1), 12–21.

Whiteneck, G. G., Brooks, C. A., Charlifue, S., Gerhart, K. A., Mellick, M. A., Overholser, D., … & Richardson, G. N. (1992). *Guide for use of the CHART: Craig Handicap Assessment and Reporting Technique*. Englewood, CO: Craig Hospital.

World Health Organization (WHO). (2001). *International classification of functioning, disability, and health (ICF)*. Geneva, Switzerland: Author.

World Health Organization (WHO). (2011). *World report on disabilities*. Available at: http://www.who.int /disabilities/world_report/2011/en/

Wrisley, D. M, Marchetti, G. F., Kuharsky, D. K., Whitney, S. L. (2004). Reliability, internal consistency, and validity of data obtained with the functional gait assessment. *Physical Therapy*, *84*(10), 906–918.

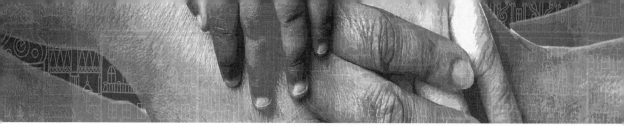

CHAPTER 6

Aging and Cognitive Functioning

Paul Brewster, Julene Johnson, Maria Marquine, Dan Mungas, Bruce Reed, and
Anna Nápoles

ABSTRACT

Cognitive functioning is an important determinant of quality of life and independent functioning in old age. There is significant heterogeneity in late-life cognition such that some individuals remain cognitively stable, some experience mild declines, and others progress to Alzheimer's disease and other forms of dementia. Although genetic and disease factors account for some of the variability in late-life cognition, much remains unknown, especially regarding individual differences in cognitive trajectories over time. A large body of evidence suggests that individual differences in late-life cognition are shaped by experiences across the lifespan, but the pathways linking these exposures to cognitive outcomes several decades later remain unclear. This chapter reviews exposures across the lifespan that have been linked to cognitive ability and dementia risk in old age, and applies a life course perspective to understand their dynamic interplay in relation to late-life cognition. Future directions are proposed for advancing understanding of life course influences on cognitive trajectories in late life, and for applying existing knowledge to interventions against cognitive decline for disadvantaged populations.

KEYWORDS

cognitive aging	dementia	education
cognitive decline	individual differences	ethnicity

▶ Introduction

The term "cognition" refers to a wide range of mental processes (domains) that are critical for independent functioning, including memory, attention, problem solving, and processing speed. Everyday tasks such as meal preparation and management of medication and finances have significant cognitive demands and often become challenging for individuals experiencing cognitive impairment. Cognitive functioning, then, is an important determinant of quality of life and functional independence in older adulthood.

Like other organs, the brain undergoes changes with increasing age. Among these changes are decreases in brain tissue volume due to cell loss in some regions, and widespread reductions in dendritic branching (dynamic cell structures that facilitate communication between neurons). Aging also leads to reduced concentrations of neurotransmitters (chemicals that enable communication between neurons), increases in inflammation (immune response), and changes in blood flow that reduce the brain's energy metabolism. As a result of these changes, most older adults experience changes in some aspects of their cognitive functioning. Nevertheless, the age-related effects on cognition are not uniform within or across cognitive domains. Crystallized intelligence (acquired knowledge), verbal abilities, simple attention, and remote memories tend to remain stable, whereas fluid intelligence (novel problem solving), complex attention, processing speed, executive functions, memory for recent events, and formation of new memories tend to decline. Declines are often noticeable to individuals and their families or caregivers, but normal aging is not associated with cognitive declines significant enough to compromise daily functioning.

Increased public awareness of cognitive impairment and **dementia** has brought about great interest in factors that protect against cognitive decline and reduce dementia risk (see **PEARL 6-1**). Of note, the patterns of age-associated cognitive decline described earlier are based on population-level observations. Significant **individual differences** in cogni-

---

PEARL 6-1 Game-Based Cognitive Training

A multibillion-dollar "brain training" industry, primarily consisting of web-based games designed to target and train players' memory, attention, and multitasking skills, has emerged in response to intense public interest in cognitive health. Developers have marketed these products as effective interventions for delaying or preventing age-associated cognitive declines. The credibility of these claims was brought to public attention in 2015, when a $50 million judgment was imposed on a leading brain training firm by the U.S. Federal Trade Commission, which charged that the company misled the public by marketing its products as capable of reducing or delaying cognitive impairment associated with age and serious health conditions. In the words of the director of the FTC's Bureau of Consumer Protection, the company "preyed on consumers' fears about age-related cognitive decline, suggesting their games could stave off memory loss, dementia, and even Alzheimer's disease… but simply did not have the science to back up its ads." Although experimental research does suggest that intensive game-based cognitive training produces statistically significant improvement in targeted cognitive abilities, there is not yet sufficient evidence to support these games as effective strategies for altering individual cognitive trajectories in a clinically meaningful way. At this juncture, empirical research suggests that consumers of brain training games are likely equally well served—or better off—by prioritizing active, socially, and mentally engaged lifestyles that include work and leisure activities they find challenging and rewarding.

tive ability actually exist throughout the entire lifespan, though these differences become even more marked in old age. Some people remain cognitively stable, some experience gradual declines, and others experience more precipitous declines due to neurodegenerative illness. Although there is great interest in identifying the factors that account for this variability, much remains unknown. A large body of evidence indicates that individual differences in late-life cognition are shaped by experiences across the lifespan. Yet, many aspects of the relationship between various life experiences and late-life cognition are not well understood.

An important advancement in our knowledge of individual differences in late-life cognition was evidence that life experience modifies the impact of age and pathology on cognition. This finding was first observed in patients with Alzheimer's disease, where the brains of highly educated individuals were found to be more resilient to Alzheimer's disease neuropathology compared to those with less **education** (Katzman, 1993). The theory of cognitive reserve was developed around this finding and posits that individual differences in the adaptability of brain networks may allow some people to cope better with brain changes than others (Steffener & Stern, 2012). This concept also applies to healthy aging, such that neuroimaging studies have demonstrated education-associated differences in brain activation during cognitive tasks that underlie the higher cognitive performance of more educated individuals (Steffener & Stern, 2012).

The theory of cognitive reserve has proved useful for understanding why similar structural (e.g., stroke, neuronal loss) and functional (e.g., physiologic or activation) pathologies have variable effects on cognitive outcomes. Currently, little is known about how such a reserve might be acquired or develop over the lifespan. Educational attainment—an exposure that typically occurs many decades before the onset of age-associated cognitive changes—appears to be one of the strongest determinants of cognitive reserve in older adulthood.

Similarly, many socioeconomic and health-related factors from early life and midlife have been shown to directly influence late-life cognitive ability. Nevertheless, the ways in which various risk and protective factors accrue over the lifespan and may interact remain poorly characterized in the **cognitive aging** literature.

A life course epidemiological perspective provides a useful framework for understanding the confluence of life experiences that shape cognitive outcomes in late life. This chapter reviews factors across the lifespan that have been shown to influence late-life cognitive outcomes. We also describe studies that apply a life course framework to understanding the pathways through which these experiences may influence cognitive trajectories in late life. By design, this chapter does not address the rapidly expanding but still indistinctly understood influence of genetic factors on cognitive aging.

▶ Ecological Determinants of Late-Life Cognition: Brain Development in Early Life and Perinatal Factors

Childhood IQ/cognition is an important determinant of adult cognition and brain health and may account for as much as 38% of the variation in cognitive ability in older adulthood (Deary et al., 2012). Although there is a substantial genetic contribution to cognitive ability, environmental exposures also significantly influence developmental trajectories, especially in early life. Neural growth is most rapid during fetal development and remains substantial throughout the first five years of life. Consequently, prenatal and early life exposures can yield significant influences on neurodevelopment and indirectly influence a wide range of adult health outcomes, including lifetime risk of cerebrovascular disease, cardiovascular disease, and type 2 diabetes (Whalley, Dick, & McNeill, 2006). The fetal origins of adult disease hypothesis proposes a causal association exists between negative fetal environmental exposures and the development of heart disease, diabetes, and stroke during adulthood, theorizing that a mismatch between fetal and adult nutritional environments may influence the pathogenesis of cardiovascular disease (Barker, 1990).

With respect to cognitive development, low birth weight is a strong predictor of childhood cognitive ability and is sensitive to environmental factors affecting mothers during pregnancy. For instance, maternal stress, poor nutrition, smoking, and poor prenatal care are all associated with lower birth weight by way of reduced fetal growth and premature birth (Whalley et al., 2006). During childhood, lower birth weight is associated with lower intelligence, poor attention and executive functions, and lower academic achievement (Aarnoudse-Moens, Weisglas-Kuperus, van Goudoever, & Oosterlaan, 2009). These cognitive weaknesses remain measurable in adulthood (Breeman, Jaekel, Baumann, Bartmann, & Wolke, 2015). Although most studies of the association between birth weight and cognitive development have focused on low-birth-weight or very-low-birth-weight infants, normal variations in birth weight have also been shown to predict adult intelligence and brain volume (Shenkin, 2004; Walhovd et al., 2012).

Postnatally, low cognitive stimulation (e.g., being spoken to and read to, having access to educational books and toys), poor nutrition, poor physical health, and limited access to early childhood education all negatively influence cognitive development (Hackman, Farah, & Meaney, 2010).

Childhood Socioeconomic Status

A growing body of literature focuses on childhood socioeconomic status in relation to late-life cognition. Socioeconomic status is strongly associated with birth weight, parental health behaviors, quality of nutrition and physical health, and exposure to cognitive stimulation during early childhood (Parker, Schoendorf, & Kiely, 1994). By age two, the IQs of children born to families of high versus low socioeconomic status differ by six points, and this disparity almost triples by age 16 (Von Stumm, 2015). Socioeconomic status may also moderate genetic contributions to cognitive ability, such that positive genetic influences on cognition are stronger among children from higher-income families relative to lower-income families (Tucker-Drob, Rhemtulla, Harden, Turkheimer, & Fask, 2011). The weaker genetic contribution to cognitive ability in children from low-income families may reflect a suppressive effect driven by negative effects of poverty on neurodevelopment or by associated educational deprivation. Children living in poverty experience lags in brain development such that their brain volume in areas critical for cognition, including the frontal and temporal lobes, is smaller than that of peers of the same age (Hair, Hanson, Wolfe, & Pollak, 2015; Walsh et al., 2014). These poverty-associated brain differences account for as much as 20% of the socioeconomic disparity in academic achievement (Hair et al., 2015), and they remain measurable in adulthood (Walsh et al., 2014).

Several studies have examined the effects of childhood socioeconomic status on cognitive outcomes in late life. A wide range of socioeconomic markers, including county literacy rate (Wilson, 2005), rural upbringing (Zhang, 2008), parental education and occupation (Everson-Rose, 2003), household size, and self-reported childhood socioeconomic status (Wilson, 2005), are associated with cognitive performance and brain volume (Staff et al., 2012) in older adults. Similar findings have been observed across many geographic regions and racial/ethnic groups (Al Hazzouri, Haan, Galea, & Aiello, 2011; Araújo et al., 2014; Kaplan et al., 2001). Moreover, environmental deprivation during childhood may potentially render the brain more vulnerable to Alzheimer's disease-related neuropathologies in later life (Seifan, 2015). Indeed, low socioeconomic status during childhood has been linked to a higher risk of cognitive impairment and dementia in late life (Rogers et al., 2009; Yaffe et al., 2013), and it may partly explain racial/ethnic disparities in dementia risk (Yaffe et al., 2013).

Childhood socioeconomic status seems to primarily influence cross-sectional cognitive ability among older adults (e.g., cognitive performance on a single testing occasion) rather than trajectories of cognitive change. In a striking exception, however, a protective effect has been reported for adverse early-life experiences on cognitive trajectories among blacks/African American adults, such that black older adults who report more extensive early-life adversity experience less cognitive decline than those who report less early-life adversity (Barnes et al., 2012). The same study found no association between early-life experiences and cognitive trajectories among white adults. The authors suggested that among blacks, who as a group report higher levels of adverse early-life experiences, a selective survival effect may contribute to the finding of less cognitive decline among those with the highest levels of early-life adversity (Barnes et al., 2012).

Educational Attainment

Educational attainment is one of the most thoroughly investigated early-life predictors of late-life cognition. Education has a strong positive effect on adult cognition (Clouston et al., 2012) and its influences remain strong in late life (Meng & D'Arcy, 2012). Educational attainment is also associated with reduced risk of developing Alzheimer's disease and other forms of dementia (Meng & D'Arcy, 2012). A meta-analysis examining the effects of education across studies using different cutoffs for low versus high education (e.g., cutoffs ranging from 6 years to 14 years) found that across studies, higher education was associated with a 47% reduction in the risk of dementia

(Valenzuela & Sachdev, 2006). In addition, highly educated individuals who do develop Alzheimer's disease experience a delayed onset of **cognitive decline** relative to those with fewer years of education (Hall, 2007).

Despite the delay in onset of cognitive decline among those with higher education, cohort studies indicate that levels of Alzheimer's disease neuropathology do not seem to differ by education. Rather, the cognitive abilities of individuals with less education seem more vulnerable to Alzheimer's disease neuropathology (Brayne, 2010).

Of note, the majority of studies observing associations between education and late-life cognition have observed this association in relation to cross-sectional cognitive performance. As will be discussed, the association between education and trajectories cognitive change is much less clear.

Although the positive effects of education on adult cognition are clear, the causal pathways are difficult to disentangle (Deary et al., 2012). Education is strongly associated with parental IQ, childhood cognitive ability, and childhood socioeconomic status. Education itself essentially represents a cognitive intervention and, therefore, exerts a direct influence on cognitive ability (Lager, Modin, De Stavola, & Vågerö, 2012). In addition, schooling strongly determines individuals' trajectories in terms of their socioeconomic conditions during adulthood, thereby indirectly influencing adult cognition through positive income-related effects on health and health behaviors. Although likely to influence late-life cognition via multiple pathways, the effects of education on late-life cognition do not seem to be fully explained by life course socioeconomic and lifestyle variables (Brewster et al., 2014). The effects of education on health outcomes appear to be compounded over time, such that health disparities in late life are greater than in midlife or earlier adulthood (Mirowsky & Ross, 2003).

Racial/ethnic, regional, and socioeconomic disparities in access and quality of education have been widely noted (Glymour & Manly, 2008), and income returns on academic qualifications are as much as 30% lower for racial/ethnic minorities relative to non-Latino whites (Williams, Mohammed, Leavell, & Collins, 2010). Thus, systemic factors, such as discrimination, may interrupt many of the pathways linking education with late-life cognition among black and Latino older adults. Indeed, educational attainment is a poorer predictor of cognitive ability and dementia risk among black and Latino older adults relative to non-Latino whites (Fitzpatrick et al., 2004; Harwood et al., 1999)—a finding that may reflect societal discrimination or racial/ethnic differences in access to and quality of education. In a study that matched African American and non-Latino white older adults on level of educational attainment, African American participants performed more poorly on tests of memory, reasoning, executive function, and visuospatial ability (Manly, Jacobs, Touradji, Small, & Stern, 2002). Subsequently, these racial/ethnic differences were greatly reduced after adjusting for group differences in literacy, used here as a measure of quality of education. Thus, the same pathways and mechanisms linking education to cognitive ability are presumed to exist for racial/ethnic minorities, but systematic differences in the links between educational attainment and childhood cognition, cognitive stimulation, and adult socioeconomic status likely attenuate the influence of education on cognitive outcomes in late life among racial/ethnic minorities.

Despite its generally strong effects on baseline cognition, education shares only a tenuous association with cognitive change. In older adults without dementia, most recent studies have not reported an association between educational attainment and rate of cognitive decline. One exception was observed in a multiethnic and socioeconomically diverse cohort of older adults (Zahodne, Nowinski, Gershon, & Manly, 2014). In this sample, associations were observed between educational attainment and rates of global

cognitive decline in individuals with relatively less (0-8) and relatively more (9-20) years of education. Of note, among those study participants with higher education, the influence of education on their cognitive trajectories was fully mediated by adult income. In contrast, the association between education and cognitive trajectory among those study participants with less education was unrelated to socioeconomic factors. The authors interpreted their findings as evidence that elementary education may influence adult cognition by promoting cognitive development during a developmentally sensitive period, whereas high school education may primarily influence adult cognition by way of its effects on socioeconomic status. This study further underscores the complex and multidirectional nature of associations between education and late-life cognition.

Physical Development

Another set of variables related to the early-life environment that have been examined in association with late-life cognition are indicators of physical growth. As much as 20% of variation in adult height is estimated to be due to environmental factors, with childhood disease and malnourishment (especially in regard to vitamin, mineral, and protein intake) representing the probable mechanisms of action due to their effects on childhood growth velocity (Silventoinen, 2003). A relationship between growth indices measured in adulthood (e.g., head circumference, height) and late-life cognition has been demonstrated in a variety of geographic regions and ethnic groups. The majority of these studies have been cross-sectional, and suggest that shorter stature (e.g., Abbot et al., 1998; Maurer, 2010) and smaller head circumference (e.g., de Rooij, Wouters, Yonker, Painter, & Roseboom, 2010; Reynolds, Johnston, Dodge, DeKosky, & Ganguli, 1999) are associated with lower baseline cognition as well as increased risk of developing Alzheimer's disease (Borenstein, Copenhaver, & Mortimer, 2006; Mortimer, Snowdon, &

Markesbery, 2008) in older adulthood. Some, though not all, studies (Brewster et al., 2014; Mak, Kim, & Stuart, 2006) have further demonstrated that morphometric variables predict longitudinal change in memory (Gale, Walton, & Martyn, 2003) and global cognition (Lee, Eom, Cheong, Oh, & Hong, 2010; Melrose et al., 2015). Of note, the association between morphometric variables and cognitive outcomes does not appear to be independent of other proxies for brain development during childhood, such as socioeconomic status (Brewster et al., 2014).

Brain Health in Midlife and Late Life

Physical Exercise

A large body of research demonstrates positive effects of physical exercise across the lifespan on cognitive outcomes in late life. Specifically, cross-sectional studies have identified reduced age effects on cognitive ability among physically active participants (Heisz, Gould, & McIntosh, 2015). On a longitudinal basis, physical activity is consistently associated with reduced cognitive decline among older adults. A meta-analysis of the association between self-reported physical activity and cognitive decline estimated that highly active individuals experience a 38% reduction in the risk of cognitive decline, and those reporting low to moderate activity experience a 35% reduction in risk of decline (Sofi et al., 2011). Studies using objective measures of cardiorespiratory fitness have similarly found less cognitive decline over six years of follow-up among those persons with higher levels of initial fitness (Barnes, Yaffe, Satariano, & Tager, 2003). Intervention studies have provided further support for the positive effects of physical exercise, especially aerobic exercise, on cognition and brain health among older adults (Colcombe & Kramer, 2003).

Several biological mechanisms likely contribute to associations between physical activity and late-life cognition, including improved cerebral blood flow and increased neuronal formation and development. In addition, physical activity may influence cognition through many indirect pathways, including via positive effects on mental health, sleep and diet, and protection against cardiovascular disease (Spirduso, Poon, & Chodzo-Zajko, 2008). Of note, studies examining associations between physical exercise and late-life cognition typically control for potential confounding factors such as education, socioeconomic status, and general health, but it is difficult to rule out possible residual confounding.

Several studies have found that physical activity is associated with reduced risk of cognitive impairment and dementia due to Alzheimer's disease and cerebrovascular disease. Regular engagement in physical activity in midlife has been associated with a 39% reduction in the risk of developing cognitive impairment in later life (Geda et al., 2010). Among those age 65 and older, regular exercise has similarly been associated with a 32% reduction in the risk of cognitive impairment and dementia (Geda et al., 2010; Larson et al., 2006).

Both educational (Clark, 1995) and racial/ethnic (August & Sorkin, 2011) differences in physical activity patterns exist, with racial/ethnic minorities, individuals of low socioeconomic status, and those with low education tending to be less active and to have a higher prevalence of sedentary lifestyles and obesity (Bolen, Rhodes, Powell-Griner, Bland, & Holtzman, 2000). Of note, racial/ethnic and educational differences in the association of physical activity with late-life cognition are eliminated after adjusting for social context and neighborhood effects (Wilson-Frederick et al., 2014). This finding has been attributed to the observation that neighborhoods and communities of lower socioeconomic status tend to possess fewer environmental factors that promote physical activity, such as parks, pedestrian-friendly roads, and proximity to recreation centers (Powell, Slater, & Chaloupka, 2004).

These relationships, however, are complex. For example, in one study, the protective effects of exercise on cognitive decline in African American participants was limited to those with higher baseline cognition and higher educational attainment (Rajan et al., 2015).

Diet

Diet and nutrition, which have direct effects on brain development and physical growth in childhood, remain important determinants during midlife of risk of cognitive decline and Alzheimer's disease (Eskelinen, Ngandu, Tuomilehto, Soininen, & Kivipelto, 2011). Adherence to a Mediterranean diet—that is, high intake of fruits, vegetables, grains, and legumes; low consumption of saturated fats and dairy products; moderate consumption of fish; and low consumption of red meat—may be particularly protective against cognitive decline (Feart et al., 2009; Scarmeas, Stern, Tang, Mayeux, & Luchsinger, 2006). Imaging studies have found reduced brain atrophy (shrinking of the brain due to cell death) in individuals with dietary habits consistent with a Mediterranean diet (Gu et al., 2015), and a recent randomized controlled trial demonstrated improvements in memory and executive control among nondemented older adults who adhered to a Mediterranean diet over four years of follow-up (Valls-Pedret et al., 2015). It is thought that the association between a Mediterranean diet and cognition is due to the protective effects of high fruit and vegetable consumption on cardiovascular health, combined with reductions in intake of high glycemic index foods. Of note, the protective effects of a Mediterranean diet against cognitive decline have been shown to be stronger among African American older adults relative to Caucasians (Koyama, 2015).

Regional, racial/ethnic, educational, and socioeconomic differences in eating patterns have been noted in many studies. For example, a "Southern diet"—that is, a diet high in fried, processed meats and sugared beverages—is more common among African Americans, individuals living in the southeastern United States, and persons with less than a high school education (Judd, 2014). The "Southern diet" has been linked with numerous adverse health outcomes, including heart disease (Shikany, 2015), sepsis (Gutiérrez, 2015), and stroke, and it may partly account for the higher prevalence of these conditions among African Americans (Judd, 2013). As with physical exercise, potential confounding effects of education, socioeconomic status, and health are typically controlled for in studies examining diet and cognition, but residual confounding may still influence the results of this literature.

Locus of Control

Perceptions of the amount of control an individual has over his or her circumstances also contribute to cognitive and other health outcomes in later life. Several studies have demonstrated positive health outcomes associated with internal locus of control—that is, the perception that one's own abilities or resources can be used to control one's circumstances (Lachman, 2006)—such that higher internal locus of control is associated with higher self-rated health and functional ability (Infurna, Gerstorf, Ram, Schupp, & Wagner, 2011 Seeman, Unger, McAvay, & Mendes de Leon, 1999), and reduced cognitive decline (Infurna & Gerstorf, 2013). Internal locus of control is also positively associated with brain size, cortisol regulation, and cognitive function in healthy older adults (Pruessner et al., 2005). In contrast, external locus of control—that is, the attribution of one's fate to external factors—seems to negatively influence health outcomes (Lachman & Weaver, 1998), brain volume, and cognitive performance among older adults (Pruessner et al., 2005). The associations between external locus of control and brain volume have been suggested to stem from the negative effects of chronic cortisol elevations on brain function

(Pruessner et al., 2005). These associations may also reflect control-related differences in engagement in healthy behaviors, social support, and mobilization of existing supports in times of need.

Of note, demographic and socioeconomic differences in control beliefs exist, such that low educational attainment, racial/ethnic minority status, and low socioeconomic status are all associated with higher external locus of control (Lachman, Neupert, & Agrigoraei, 2011). These differences likely reflect individuals' lived experiences of discrimination, employment in occupations with limited independent-judgment and decision-making opportunities (Kohn & Schooler, 1983), and poverty-related restrictions on control. Nevertheless, locus of control appears to modulate some aspects of the negative association between low educational attainment and cognitive performance, such that individuals with low education but high internal locus of control are cognitively similar to individuals with higher levels of education (Zahodne et al., 2014).

Lifetime Cognitive Engagement

Cognitive engagement during adulthood is associated strongly with cognitive outcomes in late life. The concept of "environmental complexity," which suggests that exposure to complex environments at work or during leisure time allows for maintenance and improvement of cognitive skills (Schooler, 1984), has been used as a framework for understanding this relationship. During early and mid-adulthood, occupational complexity and level of attainment are the most commonly examined proxies for cognitive engagement. Both have been associated with higher cognitive ability in late life (Smart, Gow, & Deary, 2014), reduced risk of cognitive impairment and dementia (Karp et al., 2009; Kröger et al., 2008), and attenuated cognitive decline (Marioni et al., 2015).

Using the U.S. Department of Labor's classification system, several studies have examined occupational complexity by quantifying the complexity of work involving people, data (e.g., numbers, words), or things (e.g., tools, machinery). Based on this classification system, work with people and work with data appear to drive the association between occupational complexity and late-life cognition (Andel, 2007). In particular, complexity of work with people has been reported in several studies to share the strongest association with cognitive ability and dementia risk in later life (Finkel, Andel, Gatz, & Pedersen, 2009; Smart et al., 2014; Stern et al., 1995). Although associated strongly with familial socioeconomic status, educational attainment, and cognitive ability, occupational complexity has been shown to influence late-life cognition independent of earlier-life confounds (Smart et al., 2014), and it may, in fact, mitigate the effects of a low educational level as a risk factor for dementia (Karp et al., 2009).

Cognitively demanding leisure activities in midlife and late life are also positively associated with late-life cognition. Leisure activity is typically assessed based on self-reported engagement in cognitively demanding leisure activities, such as reading, writing, and playing games. Higher level of engagement in these activities during midlife and late life has been linked to reduced risk of cognitive impairment and dementia as well as less cognitive decline (Wilson, 2003). In a recent study that examined cognitive activity relative to educational attainment and occupational complexity, associations between cognitive activity and baseline cognitive performance were substantially weaker than those observed for education and occupational complexity, particularly for those persons with high educational and occupational attainment (Vemuri et al., 2014). However, of the examined variables, only cognitive activity was associated with the subsequent trajectory of cognitive change (Vemuri et al., 2014). Similar findings have been reported by other investigators (e.g., Brewster et al., 2014). Although the main effects of cognitive activity were small in this study, particularly among those participants with high educational and occupational attainment, individuals with more limited occupational complexity may experience greater benefits from engaging in demanding cognitive activity in midlife and late life in terms of their late-life cognition (Andel, Finkel, & Pedersen, 2015; Andel, Silverstein, & Kåreholt, 2015). The protective effects of such cognitive activity have been observed across racial/ethnic groups (Rajan et al., 2015; Wilson, 2003) and appear to be independent of socioeconomic status (Singh-Manoux, Richards, & Marmot, 2003).

Some investigators have noted that the relationship between late-life cognition and self-reported cognitive engagement may be somewhat confounded by self-selected reductions in cognitive activity among older adults who are experiencing cognitive decline (Hultsch, Hertzog, Small, & Dixon, 1999). Our group has found that reductions in cognitive activity from midlife to late life are, indeed, associated with increased cognitive decline, but this effect is independent of the protective effects of cognitive activity on cognitive trajectory (Brewster et al., 2014).

Disease-Related Factors

Cerebrovascular Disease

Cerebrovascular disease encompasses a wide range of cerebral blood vessel abnormalities that cause an area of the brain to be damaged by bleeding or lack of oxygen. Cerebrovascular disease represents a leading cause of cognitive impairment in older adults and is thought to be the second most common cause of dementia, after Alzheimer's disease (Fitzpatrick et al., 2004).

Small-vessel disease—the most common form of cerebrovascular disease in older adults—results from weakening of microscopic blood vessels, which in turn causes microscopic bleeds and slows blood flow to affected brain regions (Selnes & Vinters,

2006). Over time, these microscopic changes lead to cell death and decreases in the volume of affected brain tissue. Studies have observed small-vessel disease in 11% to 21% of healthy adults in their 60s, and in 94% of nondemented individuals in their 80s (Ylikosi et al., 1995). Even so, the effects of such disease on cognition are controversial and depend on the areas of the brain that are most severely affected. For example, the area surrounding the lateral ventricles is particularly vulnerable to small-vessel disease, but the effects on cognition from such damage are minimal. Conversely, small-vessel disease affecting the subcortical white matter is associated with progressive cognitive decline, particularly in the domains of memory and executive functioning (Selnes & Vinters, 2006).

In contrast to the gradual course of progression associated with small-vessel disease, stroke is an abrupt blockage or rupture of blood vessels in the brain that results in immediate impairments in speech, vision, motor control, and cognitive function. Stroke is a leading cause of disability and mortality among older adults worldwide (Rosamond et al., 2008). Its cognitive effects depend on the affected brain region, and can range from subtle attentional impairments to dementia. Recovery of at least some cognitive function in the months following stroke is common, but this return to normalcy is slower and more limited among older adults (Selnes & Vinters, 2006).

The onset and course of cerebrovascular disease in older adulthood are strongly influenced by chronic disease factors, including hypertension, diabetes, and hyperlipidemia, and behavioral factors, including smoking and sedentary lifestyle (Sacco, Broderick, Feinberg, & Whisnant, 1997). In keeping with the higher prevalence of chronic disease among racial/ethnic minorities (Bravata et al., 2008) and individuals of lower socioeconomic status (Kapral, Mamdani, & Tu, 2002), significant disparities are noted in the prevalence of cerebrovascular disease as a function of childhood and adult socioeconomic status and educational attainment (Qureshi, Suri, Saad, & Hopkins, 2003). In addition, significant racial/ethnic differences in the prevalence of cerebrovascular disease exist, such that racial/ethnic minorities have higher small-vessel disease burden (Brickman et al., 2008) and experience higher stroke risk (Mozaffarian et al., 2015). Relative to non-Latino whites, African Americans have 2.4-fold higher stroke incidence rates and Latinos have 2-fold higher rates (Sacco et al., 1998), but these racial/ethnic differences have been shown to reflect primarily racial/ethnic differences in lifetime socioeconomic status (Glymour, Avendano, Haas, & Berkman, 2008).

Poor Mental Health

Stress Psychological stress is associated with a wide array of negative health outcomes and has direct effects on cognition. Short-term cognitive effects of stress include reduced attentional resources for information processing (Sliwinski, 2006). Over the longer term, chronically elevated stress hormones lead to dysregulation of endocrine function and increases in inflammatory processes, which in turn cause cell death in the hippocampus (a temporal lobe structure critically involved in the formation of new memories) and the prefrontal cortex. As a result, chronic stress is linked to poorer cognitive function, accelerated cognitive decline (Wilson, 2005), and increased incidence of mild cognitive impairment (Wilson, 2007). The effects of stress on cognitive performance are observed across all domains of cognitive ability, but are most evident on measures of memory and executive functioning (Lagarde, Doyon, & Brunet, 2010). Greater lifelong exposure to chronic stress has been suggested as one potential mechanism linking lower socioeconomic status to adverse health outcomes (Baum, Garofalo, & Yali, 1999); this relationship is supported by evidence of higher levels of stress hormones among individuals of low socioeconomic status (Cohen, Doyle, & Baum, 2006).

Depression Depression is a relatively common condition, estimated to affect 1 in 5 individuals during their lifetime (Kessler, 2005). Depression is associated with many negative health outcomes, including obesity (Ahlberg, 2002), low bone mass (Gebara, 2014), type 2 diabetes (Mezuk, 2008), and coronary heart disease (Lichtman, 2014). Depression is also consistently associated with risk of dementia in case-control and prospective cohort studies (Diniz, Butters, Albert, Dew, & Reynolds, 2013). Onset of depression prior to age 60, as well as duration and frequency of depression in midlife, is associated with a 2- to 4-fold increased risk of developing dementia due to Alzheimer's disease or cerebrovascular disease (Byers & Yaffe, 2011). Evidence for the direct effects of midlife depression on cognitive decline is more limited in nondemented older adults, but depressive symptoms in later life are associated with declines in global cognition (Wilson, 2004), memory (Zahodne et al., 2014), processing speed, and executive function (Royall, 2012).

Several mechanisms have been proposed to explain the association between midlife depression and late-life cognitive outcomes, including chronic inflammation, decreased neurotrophic factors (proteins that support neuron growth and survival), increased cortisol production, and cerebrovascular factors (Byers & Yaffe, 2011). Notably, estimates of the prevalence of depression are higher for some racial/ethnic groups (Dunlop, 2003), individuals of low socioeconomic status (Lorant, 2007), and persons with limited educational attainment (Mezuk, 2008) relative to the general population. The effects of depression on cognition have also been found to differ as a function of race/**ethnicity,** such that depressive symptoms are more strongly associated with performance on tests of memory and executive functions among African Americans relative to non-Latino whites (Zahodne et al., 2014).

▶ Application of Life Course Models to Cognitive Heterogeneity in Late Life

As noted throughout this chapter, a wide range of life experiences appear to make important contributions to cognitive outcomes in late life. Unfortunately, the relationships among the various life experiences and their relative influences on late-life cognition are not well understood because of their confounding nature. For example, educational attainment is strongly associated with cognitive ability and dementia risk in late life, but this variable is intricately interwoven with childhood socioeconomic status, adult occupational attainment, and lifetime cognitive engagement, such that teasing out its specific effects is difficult. A life course perspective is needed to achieve a comprehensive understanding of the pathways linking experiences at various stages of life to cognitive outcomes in late life, and to identify the most fruitful targets for interventions that protect against cognitive decline.

Several studies have employed life course models to examine the ways in which some of the variables described in this chapter may exert their effects on late-life cognition. For instance, Richards and Sacker (2003) applied a life course approach to understanding factors that contribute to cognitive ability at midlife. These authors analyzed data from the 1946 British National Birth Cohort, which is unique in its comprehensive information regarding early-life experiences and objective assessments of childhood cognition. They examined prospectively the relative influences of paternal occupation, cognitive ability assessed at age 8, educational attainment by age 26, and occupational attainment at age 43, on word reading, memory, and visual attention at age 53. The results of this study

provided insight into the mechanisms linking early-life experiences with midlife cognition by demonstrating that paternal occupation—a proxy variable for socioeconomic status—influences midlife cognition indirectly through childhood cognition and educational and occupational attainment. Childhood cognition, education, and occupational attainment, in turn, directly influence memory and intelligence at midlife. Underscoring the ways in which systemic factors can shape social trajectories, occupational attainment was more weakly associated with midlife cognition in women, and education effects were stronger. The authors interpreted this finding as reflective of occupational underachievement, with respect to cognitive ability, of women in this cohort (Richards & Sacker, 2003).

The results obtained from the 1946 British National Birth Cohort provide important insights into the contributions of early-life experiences to adult cognition, particularly by outlining the pathways through which family socioeconomic status influences cognitive ability in midlife. However, Richards and Sacker's (2003) study does not shed any light on the pathways through which peak cognitive ability during adulthood are maintained into later life. Jefferson and colleagues (2011) addressed this question by applying a life course model incorporating information from early life (educational attainment), midlife (adult socioeconomic status), and later life (leisure cognitive activity) to a cohort of older adults for whom more comprehensive neuropsychological test data were available. Even in a model including direct effects of midlife socioeconomic status and late-life cognitive activity on late-life cognitive ability, educational attainment and literacy were the strongest determinants of cognitive ability in their sample. The only exception to this finding was the observation that processing speed was most strongly associated with cognitive activity in late life. This study provides further support for the strong, unique effects of educational attainment and literacy on late-life cognition independent of other markers of socioeconomic status. Notably, educational attainment was the main marker for early-life experience in this study; unmeasured early-life factors, such as childhood socioeconomic status and cognitive ability, may have also potentially contributed to the magnitude of the effect of education on cognition identified by the researchers. In addition, significant direct effects of adult socioeconomic status and late-life cognitive activity were observed on late-life cognition, but their magnitude was weaker than education or word reading. These findings support the strong and robust influence of education on cognitive ability in late life, and suggest that the effects of education on late-life cognition cannot be solely attributed to the influence of education on adult socioeconomic status and late-life cognitive activity.

The studies described in the preceding paragraphs examined cross-sectional cognitive function in late life, so they did not provide information on predictors of cognitive decline over time. This omission is important, because ample evidence supports the contention that predictors of initial cognitive ability are not necessarily the best predictors of subsequent cognitive change (Early et al., 2013). Our group examined the relative influences of a wide range of life course predictors on baseline cognition and within-person changes in a multiethnic sample of older adults (Brewster et al., 2014). Consistent with prior research, we found significant effects of educational attainment and race/ethnicity on baseline cognition, but these effects were greatly attenuated after adjusting for single-word reading. Childhood socioeconomic status and midlife physical activity also positively influenced baseline cognition independent of education and word reading in this sample. With regard to predictors of subsequent cognitive trajectory, a contrasting picture emerged: Age, single-word reading, late-life cognitive activity, and genetic risk of Alzheimer's disease were found to be the primary determinants of longitudinal change. In addition to the positive main effect of late-life cognitive

activity on cognitive trajectory, increased cognitive decline was noted among those study participants who reported a decline in self-reported cognitive activity between midlife and late life. The results of this study suggest that experiences at every stage of life contribute to one's level of cognitive ability in late life, but lifestyle and disease factors in later life are the main determinants of cognitive change.

▶ Interventions to Promote Cognitive Health

Despite a flurry in consumer marketing of a variety of products purported to protect against cognitive decline, including cognitive training programs, supplements, and nutraceuticals, strong evidence to support the beneficial and sustained effects of these interventions on cognition is lacking. Research investigating the effects of interventions to improve cognitive function or slow its decline has largely focused on six areas: cognitive skills training, participation in the arts, technology-assisted cognitive stimulation, electrical simulation, medications, and nootropic drugs/supplements (Institute of Medicine [IOM], 2015).

Regarding cognitive training, two outstanding questions remain to be answered definitively: (1) Does training result in enhanced and maintained cognition as people age? and (2) Do observed benefits transfer to real-world tasks and settings? (IOM, 2015) In the largest randomized controlled trial (RCT) of cognitive training conducted to date (Ball et al., 2002), older adults exhibited gains in memory, reasoning, and speed of processing, but transfer across these processes was limited. Interestingly, the benefits of training for memory and speed of processing were maintained as long as ten years later (Rebok et al., 2014).

Technology-assisted cognitive training RCTs are also being performed. One of the most promising studies, conducted by Anguera and colleagues (2013), tested an adaptive multitasking training video game. The researchers found that among older adults (60 to 85 years), multitasking costs were reduced compared to both an active control group and a no-contact control group; the participants who received the intervention attained proficiency levels beyond those achieved by untrained 20-year-old participants, with their gains persisting for 6 months. The training benefits transferred to untrained cognitive control abilities (enhanced sustained attention and working memory). A larger trial by this group is in process and will extend the study to Spanish-speaking older adults. These results suggest that cognitive training interventions may offer promise as means for cognitive enhancement throughout the life span, but more studies are needed to clarify these effects.

Despite some methodological limitations, studies of active participation in the arts have shown that this activity holds some promise for improving specific aspects of cognition (Noice, Noice, & Kramer, 2014). Nevertheless, these studies have been inconsistent in their design, and no studies have compared one form of artistic participation on a head-to-head basis with another such form (IOM, 2015). The arts-related trials that yielded positive results have focused on theatrical acting, dance, music performance, and choir participation.

The largest trial testing a novel community choir intervention with great translation potential is being conducted in San Francisco (see **PEARL 6-2**) and is enrolling approximately 400 ethnically diverse older adults; Johnson et al. (2015) describe the study design. The cluster-randomized controlled trial is assessing the effects of implementing community choirs in senior centers on social, cognitive, physical, and emotional health and well-being.

Interventions focused on medications, nootropics, and supplements have generally

---

PEARL 6-2   A Community Choir Intervention to Promote Healthy Aging

In contrast to brain-training games that try to isolate and train specific cognitive abilities for the purposes of preventing cognitive decline, arts-based interventions seek to promote physical, mental, and cognitive health by involving seniors in enjoyable, socially engaging, and culturally relevant activities. An indirect benefit of such activities is that they provide opportunities for cognitive engagement. Preliminary evidence suggests that such programs can improve the physical and mental health of participants.

In the most rigorous investigation to date, a National Institutes of Health–funded trial currently under way in San Francisco is directly testing the physical, cognitive, and psychosocial effects of participation in a community choir. Participants in the Community of Voices choir receive vocal training, learn new songs, participate in weekly rehearsals, and perform at community events. The six-month trial includes three waves of assessment that will test the physical mobility, cognitive functioning, and emotional well-being of participants relative to waitlist controls. Unique for cognitive intervention research, a sizable proportion of the Community of Voices sample are racial/ethnic minorities, and both English and Spanish choirs are included in the trial. This diversity was achieved through close partnerships between researchers at the University of California, San Francisco and established community organizations that deliver services to socioeconomically and racial/ethnically diverse older adults in the San Francisco Bay Area. Another likely contributor to the success of this trial in engaging racial/ethnically diverse participants is the centrality of song to cultures all around the world. In this respect, the Community of Voices study stands in stark contrast to typical intervention studies, where examinees are recruited directly by academic institutions and trained to perform highly controlled and unfamiliar tasks. While the outcomes of this trial are forthcoming, the Community of Voices study provides a strong exemplar for engaging diverse elders in cognitive intervention research.

failed to demonstrate important clinical changes as far as enhancing cognition or delaying cognitive declines in nondemented individuals (IOM, 2015). An IOM (2015) report also concluded that transcranial direct current stimulation (applying a weak electrical current to promote cortical brain networks) shows promise in healthy adults for enhancing learning and specific cognitive functions, but that further evidence of its efficacy and safety is needed.

Although much remains to be learned about the maintenance of cognitive health throughout the lifespan, a number of actions to maintain cognitive health have been recommended by experts (IOM, 2015). These measures include engaging in regular physical activity, reducing and managing cardiovascular risk factors, reviewing conditions and medications that may affect cognition with healthcare professionals, remaining socially and intellectually engaged throughout the life course, and ensuring high-quality sleep. Multimodal interventions that have combined physical activity with other promising interventions, such as cognitive training, are emerging as a new approach in the recent literature (IOM, 2015). Unfortunately, almost no attention in testing of interventions has been directed toward vulnerable U.S. subpopulations, such as African Americans and Latinos.

▶ Conclusion and Future Directions

While the precise life experience factors that affect late-life cognition, their interplay, and their time course are not yet well understood, abundant evidence shows that life experiences beginning in utero and extending over the lifespan have a substantial impact on the cognition trajectory in old age. It has been argued that a population's cognitive and emotional health constitutes "mental wealth" that must be optimized to ensure national prosperity and economic competitiveness (Beddington

et al., 2008). This argument, and the life course perspective, is especially relevant given demographic shifts that are projected to result in more than 20% of the American population (almost 84 million people) being older than age 65 by 2050 (Ortman, Velkoff, & Hogan, 2014).

The older population is becoming increasingly racially and ethnically diverse, with projections that it will consist of 39% minorities by 2050, up from 20.7% in 2012. These demographic shifts are relevant due to substantial evidence of disparities among African Americans and Latinos in the United States compared to non-Latino whites with respect to incidence and prevalence of Alzheimer's disease and other dementias (**PEARL 6-3**). As has been illustrated in this chapter, these disparities represent a compounded effect of exposures from every stage of life. Disparities are also evident in the costs, accessibility, and quality of services for diverse elders due to cultural factors, poverty, and limited health insurance. Achieving progress in preserving the cognitive health of the U.S. population and meeting the healthcare needs of those affected by cognitive impairment and dementia will require the active engagement of these subpopulations in research.

Much more is known about the determinants of one's initial level of cognitive ability in late life than is known about those factors that contribute to the trajectory of within-person change. Most of the recent studies suggest that late-life exposures are most reliably associated with cognitive trajectory, with early-life and midlife exposures having less influence over this pathway. Several studies have found attenuated cognitive change among individuals who report high levels of cognitive engagement in later life, and randomized controlled trials support the effectiveness of cognitive engagement for attenuating cognitive and functional declines in late life (Rebok et al., 2014). In addition, our group has observed that reductions in cognitive activity between midlife and late life are associated with late-life cognitive decline. Cognitive activity throughout

PEARL 6-3 Dementia Defined

The term *dementia* is used to describe cognitive changes caused by damage to brain cells that is severe enough to impact a person's ability to perform everyday activities. Alzheimer's disease—the most common cause of dementia—is characterized by progressive declines in memory and other cognitive abilities due to extensive cell death starting in the temporal lobes of the brain, and eventually progressing to affect the entire brain. Vascular dementia, which is often considered the second leading cause of dementia, is characterized by cognitive changes caused by damage to blood vessels that supply the brain. Frontotemporal dementia is characterized by changes in behavior, personality, language, and executive function, due to cell death in the frontal and temporal lobes of the brain. Lewy body dementia and Parkinson's disease dementia are both associated with parkinsonism and changes in memory, attention, and executive functioning due to abnormal protein deposits that develop in the brain.

No cure is currently available for these leading causes of dementia, but the brains of healthier, active, and socially engaged people are typically able to withstand the effects of neuropathology longer, thereby extending these individuals' independence and improving their quality of life. Vascular dementia may be prevented through a healthy lifestyle and aggressive treatment of common causes of cerebrovascular disease, such as high blood pressure, high cholesterol levels, and heart disease.

adulthood, therefore, appears to represent a potentially important and modifiable determinant of cognitive decline among older adults.

A wide range of life experiences make important contributions to cognitive outcomes in late life. Nevertheless, relatively few attempts have been made to comprehensively model the dynamic interplay among the various exposures that occur across the entire human lifespan and influence late-life cognition. We argue that life course approaches can provide a helpful framework for understanding how very distal life experiences such as birth weight and educational attainment can reliably predict risk of cognitive impairment and dementia many decades later. Elucidating this framework can help us identify the most fruitful targets, at every stage of life, for positively influencing cognitive trajectory and resilience and for maintaining optimal cognitive ability.

Many fundamental questions remain regarding the precise causal mechanisms that contribute to the development of cognitive impairment and dementia. To understand the determinants of cognitive heterogeneity in late life, the basic mechanisms that contribute

to normal and pathological cognitive change need to be better understood.

Understanding the multifactorial etiology and heterogeneity of cognitive functioning requires well-powered, multiethnic-cohort studies to identify risk and protective factors, as these factors may potentially vary across subpopulations. Standard recruitment practices are insufficient to recruit samples characterized by cognitive heterogeneity and socioeconomic and racial/ethnic diversity. Several studies have successfully engaged diverse communities by forging close partnerships with community and cultural organizations, engaging in community outreach, and hiring research staff who are members of those communities that the investigators sought to recruit (e.g., Mungas et al., 2010). Unless deliberate efforts such as these are made to recruit populations with a wide range of life experiences, life course models are unlikely to gain meaningful insight into the effects of adversity during childhood and adulthood on cognitive outcomes in late life.

Studies relying upon retrospective reporting in midlife and late life have been criticized due to apparent inconsistencies in retrospective self-reporting of experiences of negative events (Ayalon, 2015). To avoid this problem, future life course aging research should seek to incorporate objective measures from across the lifespan. There are obvious challenges to obtaining such measurements in aging research cohorts, but several groups have successfully incorporated such information into their longitudinal cohorts. These investigations are typically follow-up studies of individuals who underwent cognitive evaluations during childhood or early adulthood, as with military intelligence testing data collected during World War II and the British National Birth Cohort in 1946.

A large body of research has documented the socioeconomic determinants of childhood cognitive ability. It has been argued that these influences likely persist across the adult lifespan, ultimately influencing late-life cognition. Although empirical evidence supporting these claims is sparse, the existing research strongly supports an ongoing influence of childhood cognition on brain size and cognitive ability later in life. As appropriate research cohorts become available, the indirect effects of social and educational interventions for children and families on socioeconomic trajectory and cognitive health in old age should be examined. Current projections estimate that the trend of aging of the overall population will continue through 2050, so characterizing the lifelong cognitive gains associated with optimal cognitive development during childhood and adolescence may be particularly important from a public policy perspective.

Neighborhood effects and the geographic patterning of cognitive health disparities remain poorly understood. The accessibility of social services, health care, and quality education differ greatly across neighborhoods, cities, and geographic regions, and the effects of these factors in mitigating the adverse effects of poverty and social disadvantage on cognitive outcomes should be addressed in future life course aging research. In addition, further research regarding intergenerational transmission of risk by way of regional differences in diet and health behaviors needs to be undertaken, especially in relation to racial/ethnic minority populations.

The effects of education on adult cognition are well documented. To date, however, progress toward understanding the precise mechanisms through which education influences cognition has been limited by the crude measures of educational attainment that are collected in most epidemiological studies (e.g., high school graduation rates). Such measures tell us little about the educational processes and specific skills or acquired knowledge that promote cognitive health. Future research examining associations between education and cognition should seek to directly test the multiple avenues reviewed in this chapter through which education is thought to influence cognition.

References

Aarnoudse-Moens, C. S., Weisglas-Kuperus, N., van Goudoever, J. B., & Oosterlaan, J. (2009). Meta-analysis of neurobehavioral outcomes in very preterm and/or very low birth weight children. *Pediatrics*, *124*(2), 717-228.

Abbott, R. D., White, L. R., Ross, G. W., Petrovitch, H., Masaki, K. H., Snowdon, D. A., & Curb, J. D. (1998). Height as a marker of childhood development and late-life cognitive function: The Honolulu-Asia Aging Study. *Pediatrics*, *102*(3 Pt 1), 602-609.

Al Hazzouri, A. Z., Haan, M. N., Galea, S., & Aiello, A. E. (2011). Life-course exposure to early socioeconomic environment, education in relation to late-life cognitive function among older Mexicans and Mexican Americans. *Journal of Aging and Health*, *23*(7), 1027-1049.

Ahlberg, A. C., Ljung, T., Rosmond, R., McEwen, B., Holm, G., Akesson, H. O., & Björntorp, P. (2002). Depression and anxiety symptoms in relation to anthropometry and metabolism in men. *Psychiatry Research*, *112*(2), 101-110.

Andel, R., Finkel, D., & Pedersen, N. (2015). Effects of preretirement work complexity and postretirement leisure activity on cognitive aging. *Journals of Gerontology, Series B: Psychological Sciences & Social Sciences*. pii: gbv026

Andel, R., Kåreholt, I., Parker, M. G., Thorslund, M., & Gatz, M. (2007). Complexity of primary lifetime occupation and cognition in advanced old age. *Journal of Aging and Health*, *19*(3), 397-415.

Andel, R., Silverstein, M., & Kåreholt, I. (2015). The role of midlife occupational complexity and leisure activity in late-life cognition. *Journals of Gerontology, Series B: Psychological Sciences & Social Sciences*, *70*(2), 314-321.

Anguera, J. A., Boccanfuso, J., Rintoul, J. L., Al-Hashimi, O., Faraji, F., Janowich, J.,... Gazzaley, A. (2013). Video game training enhances cognitive control in older adults. *Nature*, *501*(7465), 97-101.

Araújo, L. F., Giatti, L., Chor, D., Passos, V. M., & Barreto, S. M. (2014). Maternal education, anthropometric markers of malnutrition and cognitive function (ELSA-Brasil). *BMC Public Health*, *14*, 673.

August, K. J., & Sorkin, D. H. (2011). Racial/ethnic disparities in exercise and dietary behaviors of middle-aged and older adults. *Journal of General Internal Medicine*, *26*(3), 245–250.

Ayalon, L. (2015). Retrospective reports of negative early life events over a 4-year period: A test of measurement invariance and response consistency. *Journals of Gerontology, Series B: Psychological Sciences and Social Sciences*. pii: gbv087. [Epub ahead of print].

Ball, K., Berch, D. B., Helmers, K. F., Jobe, J. B., Leveck, M. D., Marsiske, M.,...Willis, S. L. (2002). Effects of cognitive training interventions with older adults: A randomized controlled trial. *Journal of the American Medical Association*, *288*(18), 2271-2281.

Barnes, D. E., Yaffe, K., Satariano, W. A., & Tager, I. B. (2003). A longitudinal study of cardiorespiratory fitness and cognitive function in healthy older adults. *Journal of the American Geriatrics Society*, *51*(4), 459-465.

Barnes, L. L., Wilson, R. S., Everson-Rose, S. A., Hayward, M. D., Evans, D. A., & Mendes de Leon, C. F. (2012). Effects of early-life adversity on cognitive decline in older African Americans and whites. *Neurology*, *79*(24), 2321-2327.

Barker, D. J. (1990). The fetal and infant origins of adult disease. *BMJ*, *301*(6761), 1111.

Baum, A., Garofalo, J. P., & Yali, A. M. (1999). Socioeconomic status and chronic stress: Does stress account for SES effects on health? *Annals of the New York Academy of Sciences*, *896*, 131-144.

Beddington, J., Cooper, C. L., Field, J., Goswami, U., Huppert, F. A., Jenkins, R.,... Thomas, S. M. (2008). The mental wealth of nations. *Nature*, *455*(7216), 1057-1060.

Bolen, J. C., Rhodes, L., Powell-Griner, E. E., Bland, S. D., & Holtzman, D. (2000). State-specific prevalence of selected health behaviors, by race and ethnicity— Behavioral Risk Factor Surveillance System, 1997. *MMWR CDC Surveillance Summaries*, *49*(2), 1-60.

Borenstein, A. R., Copenhaver, C. I., & Mortimer J. A. (2006). Early-life risk factors for Alzheimer disease. *Alzheimer Disease and Associated Disorders*, *20*, 63–72.

Bravata, D. M., Wells, C. K., Gulanski, B., Kernan, W. N., Brass, L. M., Long, J., & Concato, J. (2005). Racial disparities in stroke risk factors: The impact of socioeconomic status. *Stroke, 36*(7), 1507-1511.

Bravata, D. M., Wells, C. K., Gulanski, B., Kernan, W. N., Brass, L. M., Long, J., & Concato, J. (2008). Racial disparities in stroke risk factors: The impact of socioeconomic status. *Stroke, 36*, 1507–1511.

Brayne, C., Ince, P. G., Keage, H. A., McKeith, I. G., Matthews, F. E., Polvikoski, T., & Sulkava, R. (2010). Education, the brain and dementia: Neuroprotection or compensation? *Brain, 133*, 2210-2216.

Breeman, L. D., Jaekel, J., Baumann, N., Bartmann, P., & Wolke, D. (2015). Preterm cognitive function into adulthood. *Pediatrics*, *136*(3), 415-423.

Brewster, P. W., Melrose, R. J., Marquine, M. J., Johnson, J. K., Napoles, A., MacKay-Brandt, A.,... Mungas, D. (2014). Life experience and demographic influences on cognitive function in older adults. *Neuropsychology*, *28*(6), 846-858.

Brickman, A. M., Schupf, N., Manly, J. J., Luchsinger, J. A., Andrews, H., Tang, M. X.,... Brown, T. R. (2008). Brain morphology in older African Americans, Caribbean Hispanics, and whites from northern Manhattan. *Archives of Neurology*, *65*(8), 1053–1061.

Byers, A. L., & Yaffe, K. (2011). Depression and risk of developing dementia. *Nature Reviews: Neurology*, *7*(6), 323–331.

Clark, D. O. (1995). Racial and educational differences in physical activity among older adults. *Gerontologist*, *35*(4), 472–480.

Clouston, S. A., Kuh, D., Herd, P., Elliott, J., Richards, M., & Hofer, S. M. (2012). Benefits of educational attainment on adult fluid cognition: International evidence from three birth cohorts. *International Journal of Epidemiology*, *41*(6), 1729-1736.

Cohen, S., Doyle, W. J., & Baum, A. (2006). Socioeconomic status is associated with stress hormones. *Psychosomatic Medicine*, *68*(3), 414-420.

Colcombe, S., & Kramer, A. F. (2003). Fitness effects on the cognitive function of older adults: A meta-analytic study. *Psychological Science*, *14*(2), 125-130.

Deary, I. J., Yang, J., Davies, G., Harris, S. E., Tenesa, A., Liewald, D.,... Visscher, P. M. (2012). Genetic contributions to stability and change in intelligence from childhood to old age. *Nature*, *482*(7384), 212-215.

de Rooij, S. R., Wouters, H., Yonker, J. E., Painter, R. C., & Roseboom, T. J. (2010). Prenatal undernutrition and cognitive function in late adulthood. *Proceedings of the National Academy of Sciences USA*, *107*(39), 16881–16886.

Diniz, B. S., Butters, M. A., Albert, S. M., Dew, M. A., & Reynolds, C. F. (2013). Late-life depression and risk of vascular dementia and Alzheimer's disease: Systematic review and meta-analysis of community-based cohort studies. *British Journal of Psychiatry*, *202*(5), 329-335.

Dunlop, D. D., Song, J., Lyons, J. S., Manheim, L. M., & Chang, R. W. (2003). Racial/ethnic differences in rates of depression among preretirement adults. *American Journal of Public Health*, *93*(11), 1945–1952.

Early, D. R., Widaman, K. F., Harvey, D., Beckett, L., Park, L. Q., Farias, S. T.,... Mungas, D. (2013). Demographic predictors of cognitive change in ethnically diverse older persons. *Psychology and Aging, 28*(3), 633-645.

Eskelinen, M. H., Ngandu, T., Tuomilehto, J., Soininen, H., & Kivipelto, M. (2011).Midlife healthy-diet index and late-life dementia and Alzheimer's disease. *Dementia and Geriatric Cognitive Disorders, 1*(1), 103-112.

Everson-Rose, S. A., Mendes de Leon, C. F., Bienias, J. L., Wilson, R. S., & Evans, D. A. (2003). Early life conditions and cognitive functioning in later life. *American Journal of Epidemiology, 158*(11), 1083–1089.

Feart, C., Samieri, C., Rondeau, V., Amieva, H., Portet, F., Dartigues, J.-F.,… Barberger-Gateau, P. (2009). Adherence to a Mediterranean diet, cognitive decline, and risk of dementia. *Journal of the American Medical Association, 302*(6), 638–648.

Finkel, D., Andel, R., Gatz, M., & Pedersen, N. (2009). The role of occupational complexity in trajectories of cognitive aging before and after retirement. *Psychology and Aging, 24*(3), 563-573.

Fitzpatrick, A. L., Kuller, L. H., Ives, D. G., Lopez, O. L., Jagust, W., Breitner, J. C.,… Dulberg, C. (2004). Incidence and prevalence of dementia in the Cardiovascular Health Study. *Journal of the American Geriatric Society, 52*, 195–204.

Gale, C. R., Walton, S., & Martyn, C. N. (2003). Foetal and postnatal head growth and risk of cognitive decline in old age. *Brain, 126*(Pt 10), 2273–2278.

Gebara, M. A., Shea, M. L., Lipsey, K. L., Teitelbaum, S. L., Civitelli, R., Müller, D. J.,… Lenze, E. J. (2014). Depression, antidepressants, and bone health in older adults: A systematic review. *Journal of the American Geriatrics Society, 62*(8), 1434-1441.

Geda, Y. E., Roberts, R. O., Knopman, D. S., Christianson, T. J. H., Pankratz, V. S., Ivnik, R. J.,… Rocca, W. A. (2010). Physical exercise and mild cognitive impairment: A population-based study. *Archives of Neurology, 67*(1), 80–86.

Glymour, M., Avendano, M., Haas, S., & Berkman, L. (2008). Lifecourse social conditions and racial disparities in incidence of first stroke. *Annals of Epidemiology, 18*(12), 904–912.

Glymour, M. M., & Manly, J. J. (2008). Lifecourse social conditions and racial and ethnic patterns of cognitive aging. *Neuropsychology Review, 18*(3), 223-254.

Gu, Y., Brickman, A. M., Stern, Y., Habeck, C. G., Razlighi, Q. R., Luchsinger, J. A.,… Scarmeas, N. (2015). Mediterranean diet and brain structure in a multiethnic elderly cohort. *Neurology, 85*(20), 1744-1751.

Gutiérrez, O. M., Judd, S. E., Voeks, J. H., Carson, A. P., Safford, M. M., Shikany, J. M., & Wang, H. E. (2015). Diet patterns and risk of sepsis in community-dwelling adults: A cohort study. *BMC Infectious Diseases, 15*, 231.

Hackman, D. A., Farah, M. J., & Meaney, M. J. (2010). Socioeconomic status and the brain: Mechanistic insights from human and animal research. *Nature Reviews Neuroscience, 11*, 651–659.

Hall, C. B., Derby, C., LeValley, A., Katz, M. J., Verghese, J., & Lipton, R. B. (2007). Education delays accelerated decline on a memory test in persons who develop dementia. *Neurology, 69*(17), 1657-1664.

Hair, N. L., Hanson, J. L., Wolfe, B. L., & Pollak, S. D. (2015). Association of child poverty, brain development, and academic achievement. *JAMA Pediatrics, 169*(9), 822-829.

Harwood, D. G., Barker, W. W., Loewenstein, D. A., Ownby, R. L., St George-Hyslop, P., Mullan, M., & Duara, R. (1999). A cross-ethnic analysis of risk factors for AD in white Hispanics and white non-Hispanics. *Neurology, 52*(3), 551-556.

Heisz, J. J., Gould, M., & McIntosh, A. R. (2015). Age-related shift in neural complexity related to task performance and physical activity. *Journal of Cognitive Neuroscience, 27*(3), 605-613.

Hultsch, D. F., Hertzog, C., Small, B. J., & Dixon, R. A. (1999). Use it or lose it: Engaged lifestyle as a buffer of cognitive decline in aging? *Psychology and Aging, 14*(2), 245-263.

Infurna, F. J., & Gerstorf, D. (2013). Linking perceived control, physical activity, and biological health to memory change. *Psychology and Aging, 28*(4), 1147-1163.

Infurna, F. J., Gerstorf, D., Ram, N., Schupp, J., & Wagner, G. G. (2011). Long-term antecedents and outcomes of perceived control. *Psychology & Aging, 26*, 559–575.

Institute of Medicine (IOM). (2015). Committee on the Public Health Dimensions of Cognitive Aging. *Cognitive aging: Progress in understanding and opportunities for action.* D. G. Blazer, K. Yaffe, & C. T. Liverman (Eds.). Washington, DC: Committee on the Public Health Dimensions of Cognitive Aging, Board on Health Sciences Policy, Institute of Medicine of the National Academies.

Jefferson, A. L., Gibbons, L. E., Rentz, D. M., Carvalho, J. O., Manly, J., Bennett, D. A., & Jones, R. N. (2011). A life course model of cognitive activities, socioeconomic status, education, reading ability, and cognition. *Journal of the American Geriatrics Society, 59*(8), 1403–1411.

Johnson, J. K., Nápoles, A. M., Stewart, A. L., Max, W. B., Santoyo-Olsson, J., Freyre, R.,… Gregorich, S. E. (2015). Study protocol for a cluster randomized trial of the Community of Voices choir intervention to promote the health and well-being of diverse older adults. *BMC Public Health, 15*, 1049.

Judd, S. E., Letter, A. J., Shikany, J. M., Roth, D. L., & Newby, P. K. (2014). Dietary patterns derived using exploratory and confirmatory factor analysis are stable and generalizable across race, region, and gender subgroups in the REGARDS study. *Frontiers in Nutrition, 1*, 29.

Kaplan, G. A., Turrell, G., Lynch, J. W., Everson, S. A., Helkala, E. L., & Salonen, J. T. (2001). Childhood socioeconomic position and cognitive function in adulthood. *International Journal of Epidemiology, 30*(2), 256-263.

Kapral, M. K., Mamdani, M., & Tu, J. V. (2002). Effect of socioeconomic status on treatment and mortality after stroke. *Stroke, 33*, 268-273.

Karp, A., Andel, R., Parker, M. G., Wang, H. X., Winblad, B., & Fratiglioni, L. (2009). Mentally stimulating activities at work during midlife and dementia risk after age 75: follow-up study from the Kungsholmen Project. *American Journal of Geriatric Psychiatry, 17*(3), 227-236.

Katzman, R. (1993). Education and the prevalence of dementia and Alzheimer's disease. *Neurology, 44*(1), 13-20.

Kessler, R. C., Berglund, P., Demler, O., Jin, R., Merikangas, K. R., & Walters, E. E. (2005). Lifetime prevalence and age-of-onset distributions of *DSM-IV* disorders in the National Comorbidity Survey replication. *Archives of General Psychiatry, 62*(6), 593-602.

Kohn, M. L., & Schooler, C. (1983). *Work and personality: An inquiry into the impact of social stratification.* Norwood, NJ: Ablex.

Koyama, A., Houston, D. K., Simonsick, E. M., Lee, J. S., Ayonayon, H. N., Shahar, D. R.,… Yaffe, K. (2015). Association between the Mediterranean diet and cognitive decline in a biracial population. *Journals of Gerontology, Series A: Biological Sciences and Medical Sciences, 70*(3), 354-359.

Kröger, E., Andel, R., Lindsay, J., Benounissa, Z., Verreault, R., & Laurin, D. (2008). Is complexity of work associated with risk of dementia? The Canadian Study of Health And Aging. *American Journal of Epidemiology, 167*(7), 820-830.

Lachman, M. E. (2006). Perceived control over aging-related declines. *Current Directions in Psychological Science, 15,* 282-286.

Lachman, M. E., Neupert, S. D., & Agrigoroaei, S. (2011). The relevance of control beliefs for health and aging. In K. W. Schaie & S. L. Willis SL (Eds.), Handbook of the psychology of aging (7th ed., pp. 175-190). San Diego, CA: Academic Press.

Lachman, M. E., & Weaver, S. L. (1998). The sense of control as a moderator of social class differences in health and well-being. *Journal of Personality and Social Psychology, 74,* 763-773.

Lagarde, G., Doyon, J., & Brunet, A. (2010). Memory and executive dysfunctions associated with acute posttraumatic stress disorder. *Psychiatry Research, 177*(1-2), 144-149.

Lager, A. C., Modin, B. E., De Stavola, B. L., & Vågerö, D. H. (2012). Social origin, schooling and individual change in intelligence during childhood influence long-term mortality: A 68-year follow-up study. *International Journal of Epidemiology, 41*(2), 398-404.

Larson, E. B., Wang, L., Bowen, J. D., McCormick, W. C., Teri, L., Crane, P., & Kukull, W. (2006). Exercise is associated with reduced risk for incident dementia among persons 65 years of age and older. *Annals of Internal Medicine, 144*(2), 73-81.

Lee, K. S., Eom, J. S., Cheong, H. K., Oh, B. H., & Hong, C. H. (2010). Effects of head circumference and metabolic syndrome on cognitive decline. *Gerontology, 56*(1), 32-38.

Lichtman, J. H., Froelicher, E. S., Blumenthal, J. A., Carney, R. M., Doering, L. V., Frasure-Smith, N.,… Wulsin, L.; American Heart Association Statistics Committee of the Council on Epidemiology and Prevention and the Council on Cardiovascular and Stroke Nursing. (2014). Depression as a risk factor for poor prognosis among patients with acute coronary syndrome: Systematic review and recommendations: A scientific statement from the American Heart Association. *Circulation, 129*(12), 1350-1369.

Lorant, V., Croux, C., Weich, S., Deliège, D., Mackenbach, J., & Ansseau, M. (2007). Depression and socio-economic risk factors: 7-year longitudinal population study. *British Journal of Psychiatry, 190*(4), 293-298.

Mak, Z., Kim, J. M., & Stewart, R. (2006). Leg length, cognitive impairment and cognitive decline in an African-Caribbean population. *International Journal of Geriatric Psychiatry, 21*(3), 266-272.

Manly, J. J., Jacobs, D. M., Touradji, P., Small, S. A., & Stern, Y. (2002). Reading level attenuates differences in neuropsychological test performance between African American and white elders. *Journal of the International Neuropsychology Society, 8*(3), 341-348.

Marioni, R. E., Proust-Lima, C., Amieva, H., Brayne, C., Matthews, F. E., Dartigues, J. F., & Jacqmin-Gadda, H. (2015). Social activity, cognitive decline and dementia risk: A 20-year prospective cohort study. *BMC Public Health, 24*(15), 1089.

Maurer, J. (2010). Height, education and later-life cognition in Latin America and the Caribbean. *Economics & Human Biology, 8*(2), 168-176.

Melrose, R. J., Brewster, P., Marquine, M. J., MacKay-Brandt, A., Reed, B., Farias, S. T., & Mungas, D. (2015). Early life development in a multiethnic sample and the relation to late life cognition. *Journals of Gerontology, Series B: Psychological Sciences and Social Sciences, 70*(4), 519-531.

Meng, X., & D'Arcy, C. (2012). Education and dementia in the context of the cognitive reserve hypothesis: A systematic review with meta-analyses and qualitative analyses. *PLoS One, 6,* e38268. doi: 10.1371/journal.pone.0038268

Mezuk, B., Eaton, W. W., Albrecht, S., & Golden, S. H. (2008). Depression and type 2 diabetes over the lifespan: A meta-analysis. *Diabetes Care, 31*(12), 2383-2390.

Mezuk, B., Eaton, W. W., Golden, S. H., & Ding, Y. (2008). The influence of educational attainment on depression and risk of type 2 diabetes. *American Journal of Public Health, 98*(8), 1480-1485.

Mirowsky, J., & Ross, C. (2003). *Education, social status, and health.* New York, NY: Aldine de Gruyter.

Mortimer, J. A., Snowdon, D. A., & Markesbery, W. R. (2008). Small head circumference is associated with less education in persons at risk for Alzheimer disease in later life. *Alzheimer Disease and Associated Disorders, 22,* 249-254.

Mozaffarian, D., Benjamin, E. J., Go, E. S., Arnett, D. K., Blaha, M. J., Cushman, M.,… Turner, M. B.; American Heart Association Statistics Committee and Stroke Statistics Subcommittee. (2015). Heart disease and stroke statistics—2015 update: A report from the American Heart Association. *Circulation, 131* (4), e329-e322.

Mungas, D., Beckett, D., Harvey, D., Farias, S., Reed, B., Carmichael, O.,… DeCarli, C. (2010). Heterogeneity of cognitive decline trajectories in diverse older persons. *Psychology and Aging, 25*(3), 606-619.

Noice, T., Noice, H., & Kramer, A. F. (2014). Participatory arts for older adults: A review of benefits and challenges. *Gerontologist, 54*(5), 741-753.

Ortman, J., Velkoff, V. A., & Hogan, H. (2014). *An aging nation: The older population in the United States.* Current Population Reports, P25-1140. Washington, DC: U.S. Census Bureau. Available at: http://www.census.gov/library/publications/2014/demo/p25-1140.html

Parker, J. D., Schoendorf, K. C., & Kiely, J. L. (1994). Associations between measures of socioeconomic status and low birth weight, small for gestational age, and premature delivery in the United States. *Annals of Epidemiology, 4*(4), 271-278.

Powell, L. M., Slater, S., & Chaloupka, F. J. (2004). The relationship between community physical activity settings and race, ethnicity and socioeconomic status. *Evidence Based Preventive Medicine, 1,* 135–144.

Pruessner, J. C., Baldwin, M. W., Dedovic, K., Renwick, R., Mahani, N. K., Lord, C.,… Lupien, S. (2005). Self-esteem, locus of control, hippocampal volume, and cortisol regulation in young and old adulthood. *Neuroimage, 28*(4), 815-826.

Qureshi, A. I., Suri, M. F., Saad, M., & Hopkins, L. N. (2003). Educational attainment and risk of stroke and myocardial infarction. *Medical Science Monitor, 9,* CR466–CR473.

Rajan, K. B., Barnes, L. L., Skarupski, K. A., Mendes de Leon, C. F., Wilson, R. S., & Evans, D. A. (2015). Physical and cognitive activities as deterrents of cognitive decline in a biracial population sample. *American Journal of Geriatric Psychiatry, 23*(12), 1225-1233.

Rebok, G. W., Ball, K., Guey, L. T., Jones, R. N., Kim, H.-Y., King, J. W.,… Willis, S. L. (2014). Ten-year effects of the ACTIVE cognitive training trial on cognition and everyday functioning in older adults. *Journal of the American Geriatrics Society, 62*(1), 16–24.

Reynolds, M. D., Johnston, J. M., Dodge, H. H., DeKosky, S. T., & Ganguli, M. (1999). Small head size is related to low Mini-Mental State Examination scores in a community sample of nondemented older adults. *Neurology, 53*(1), 228–229.

Richards, M., & Sacker, A. (2003). Lifetime antecedents of cognitive reserve. *Journal of Clinical and Experimental Neuropsychology, 25,* 614–624. doi: 10.1076/jcen.25.5.614.14581

Rogers, M. A., Plassman, B. L., Kabeto, M., Fisher, G. G., McArdle, J. J., Llewellyn, D. J.,… Langa, K. M. (2009).Parental education and late-life dementia in the United States. *Journal of Geriatric Psychiatry and Neurology, 22*(1), 71-80.

Rosamond, W., Flegal, K., Furie, K., Go, A., Greenlund, K., Haase, N.,… Hong, Y.; American Heart Association Statistics Committee and Stroke Statistics Subcommittee. (2008). Heart disease and stroke statistics—2008 update: A report from the American Heart Association Statistics Committee and Stroke Statistics Subcommittee. *Circulation, 117*(4), e25-146.

Royall, D. R., Palmer, R., Chiodo, L. K., & Polk, M. J. (2012). Depressive symptoms predict longitudinal change in executive control but not memory. *International Journal of Geriatric Psychiatry, 27,* 89–96.

Sacco, R. L., Boden-Albala, B., Gan, R., Chen, X., Kargman, D. E., Shea, S.,… Hauser, W. A. (1998). Stroke incidence among white, black, and Hispanic residents of an urban community: The Northern Manhattan Stroke Study. *American Journal of Epidemiology, 147*(3), 259-268.

Sacco, R. L., Broderick, J., Feinberg, W., & Whisnant, J. (1997). American Heart Association Prevention Conference, IV: Prevention and rehabilitation of stroke: Risk factors. *Stroke, 28,* 1507–1517.

Scarmeas, N., Stern, Y., Tang, M.-X., Mayeux, R., & Luchsinger, J. A. (2006). Mediterranean diet and risk for Alzheimer's disease. *Annals of Neurology, 59*(6), 912–921.

Schooler, C. (1984). Psychological effects of complex environments during the life span: A review and theory. *Intelligence, 8,* 259-281.

Seeman, T. E., Unger, J. B., McAvay, G., & Mendes de Leon, C. F. (1999). Self-efficacy beliefs and perceived declines in functional ability: MacArthur Studies of Successful Aging. *Journals of Gerontology: Psychological Sciences, 54B,* P214–P222.

Seifan, A., Schelke, M., Obeng-Aduasare, Y., & Isaacson, R. (2015). Early life epidemiology of Alzheimer's disease: A critical review. *Neuroepidemiology, 45*(4), 237-254.

Selnes, O. A., & Vinters, H. V. (2006). Vascular cognitive impairment. *Nature Clinical Practice Neurology, 2,* 538-547.

Shenkin, S. D., Starr, J. M., & Deary, I. J. (2004). **Birth weight** and cognitive ability in childhood: A systematic review. *Psychological Bulletin, 130*(6), 989–1013.

Shikany, J. M., Safford, M. M., Newby, P. K., Durant, R. W., Brown, T. M., & Judd, S. E. (2015). Southern dietary pattern is associated with hazard of acute coronary heart disease in the Reasons for Geographic and Racial Differences in Stroke (REGARDS) study. *Circulation, 132*(9), 804-814.

Silventoinen, K. (2003). Determinants of variation in adult body height. *Journal of Biosocial Science, 35*(2), 263–285.

Singh-Manoux, A., Richards, M., & Marmot, M. (2003). Leisure activities and cognitive function in middle age: Evidence from the Whitehall II study. *Journal of Epidemiology and Community Health, 57*(11), 907-913.

Sliwinski, M. J., Smyth, J. M., Hofer, S. M., & Stawski, R. S. (2006). Intraindividual coupling of daily stress and cognition. *Psychology and Aging, 21*(3), 545-557.

Smart, E. L., Gow, A., & Deary, I. J. (2014). Occupational complexity and lifetime cognitive abilities. *Neurology, 83*(24), 2285-2291.

Sofi, F., Valecchi, D., Bacci, D., Abbate, R., Gensini, G. F., Casini, A., & Macchi, C. (2011). Physical activity and risk of cognitive decline: A meta-analysis of prospective studies. *Journal of Internal Medicine, 269*(1), 107-117.

Spirduso, W., Poon, L., & Chodzo-Zajko, W. (2008). Using resources and reserves in an exercise-cognition model. In W. Spirduso, L. Poon, & W. Chodzo-Zajko (Eds.), *Exercise and its mediating effects on cognition* (pp. 3-11). Champaign, IL: Human Kinetics.

Staff, R. T., Murray, A. D., Ahearn, T. S., Mustafa, N., Fox, H. C., & Whalley, L. J. (2012). Childhood socioeconomic status and adult brain size: Childhood socioeconomic status influences adult hippocampal size. *Annals of Neurology, 71*(5), 653-660.

Stern, Y., Alexander, G. E., Prohovnik, I., Stricks, L., Link, B., Lennon, M. C., & Mayeux, R. (1995). Relationship between lifetime occupation and parietal flow: Implications for a reserve against Alzheimer's disease pathology. *Neurology, 45*(1), 55-60.

Steffener, J., & Stern, Y. (2012). Exploring the neural basis of cognitive reserve in aging. *Biochimica et Biophysica Acta, 1822*(3), 467-473.

Tucker-Drob, E. M., Rhemtulla, M., Harden, K. P., Turkheimer, E., & Fask, D. (2011). Emergence of a gene × socioeconomic status interaction on infant mental ability between 10 months and 2 years. *Psychological Science, 22*(1), 125-133. doi: 10.1177/0956797610392926

Valenzuela, M. J., & Sachdev, P. (2006). Brain reserve and dementia: A systematic review. *Psychological Medicine, 36*(4), 441-454.

Valls-Pedret, C., Sala-Vila, A., Serra-Mir, M., Corella, D., de la Torre, R., Martínez-González, M. Á.,… Ros, E. (2015). Mediterranean diet and age-related cognitive decline: A randomized clinical trial. *JAMA Internal Medicine, 175*(7), 1094-1103.

Vemuri, P., Lesnick, T. G., Przybelski, S. A., Machulda, M., Knopman, D. S., Mielke, M. M.,… Jack, C. R. Jr. (2014). Association of lifetime intellectual enrichment with cognitive decline in the older population. *JAMA Neurology, 71*(8), 1017-1024.

Von Stumm, S., & Plomin, R. (2015). Socioeconomic status and the growth of intelligence from infancy through adolescence. *Intelligence, 48*, 30-36.

Walhovd, K. B., Fjell, A. M., Brown, T. T., Kuperman, J. M., Chung, Y., Hagler, D. J. Jr.,… Dale, A. M.; Pediatric Imaging, Neurocognition, and Genetics Study. (2012). Long-term influence of normal variation in neonatal characteristics on human brain development. *Proceedings of the National Academy of Sciences, 109*(49), 20089-20094.

Walsh, N. D., Dalgleish, T., Lombardo, M. V., Dunn, V. J., Van Harmelen, A. L., Ban, M., & Goodyer, I. M. (2014). General and specific effects of early-life psychosocial adversities on adolescent grey matter volume. *NeuroImage: Clinical, 11*(4), 308-318.

Whalley, L. J., Dick, F. D., & McNeill, G. (2006). A life-course approach to the aetiology of late-onset dementias. *Lancet Neurology, 5*(1), 87-96.

Williams, D. R., Mohammed, S. A., Leavell, J., & Collins, C. (2010). Race, socioeconomic status and health: Complexities, ongoing challenges and research opportunities. *Annals of the New York Academy of Sciences, 1186*, 69-101.

Wilson, R. S., Bennett, D. A., Bienias, J. L., Mendes de Leon, C. F., Morris, M. C., & Evans, D. A. (2003). Cognitive activity and cognitive decline in a biracial community population. *Neurology, 61*(6), 812-816.

Wilson, R., Mendes de Leon, C. F., Bennett, D., Bienias, J., & Evans, D. (2004). Depressive symptoms and cognitive decline in a community population of older persons. *Journal of Neurology, Neurosurgery, and Psychiatry, 75*(1), 126-129.

Wilson, R. S., Schneider, J. A., Boyle, P. A., Arnold, S. E., Tang, Y., & Bennett, D. A. (2007). Chronic distress and incidence of mild cognitive impairment. *Neurology, 68*(24), 2085-2092.

Wilson, R. S., Boyle, P. A., Yu, L., Barnes, L. L., Schneider, J. A., & Bennett, D. A. (2013). Life-span cognitive activity, neuropathologic burden, and cognitive aging. *Neurology, 81*(4), 314-321.

Wilson, R. S., Scherr, P. A., Hoganson, G., Bienias, J. L., Evans, D. A., & Bennett, D. A. Early life socioeconomic status and late life risk of Alzheimer's disease. *Neuroepidemiology.* 2005;25(1):8-14. Epub 2005 Apr 25.

Wilson-Frederick, S. M., Thorpe, R. J. Jr., Bell, C. N., Bleich, S. N., Ford, J. G., & LaVeist, T. A. (2014). Examination of race disparities in physical inactivity among adults of similar social context. *Ethnicity & Disease, 24*(3), 363-369.

Yaffe, K., Falvey, C., Harris, T. B., Newman, A., Satterfield, S., Koster, A.,… Simonsick, E.; Health ABC Study. (2013). Effect of socioeconomic disparities on incidence of dementia among biracial older adults: Prospective study. *British Medical Journal, 34*, 7051.

Ylikoski, A., Erkinjuntti, T., Raininko, R., Sarna, S., Sulkava, R., & Tilvis, R. (1995). White matter hyperintensities on MRI in the neurologically nondiseased elderly: Analysis of cohorts of consecutive subjects aged 55 to 85 years living at home. *Stroke, 26*, 1171-1177.

Zahodne, L. B., Nowinski, C. J., Gershon, R. C., & Manly, J. J. (2014). Depressive symptoms are more strongly related to executive functioning and episodic memory among African American compared with non-Hispanic white older adults. *Archives of Clinical Neuropsychology, 29*(7), 663-669. doi: 10.1093/arclin/acu045

Zhang, Z., Gu, D., & Hayward, M. D. (2008). Early life influences on cognitive impairment among oldest old Chinese. *The Journals of Gerontology Series B: Psychological Sciences and Social Sciences, 63*(1),S25-33.

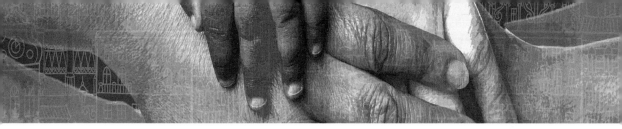

CHAPTER 7

Aging and the Epidemiology of Depression

Mark Snowden and **Lesley Steinman**

ABSTRACT

Late-life depression is a key public health issue, representing a leading cause of death and disability across the globe. A multitude of biological, social, and psychological factors across the lifespan have been identified as risks for late-life depression. Depression is more likely to occur after the onset of common conditions of old age and often negatively impacts the outcome of those conditions. Increasingly, studies are also identifying depression as a risk factor for conditions ranging from dementia to cardiovascular disease. Effective tools are available for screening and identification of depression as well as for monitoring the outcomes of treatment. Although public health agencies have begun to endorse depression screening, providing easy access to evidence-based programs remains the challenge. Effective treatments for depression exist and are being integrated into primary care, behavioral health settings, and aging provider networks. Given that more than two in three older adults now live with multiple chronic conditions, it is important to combine treatment approaches for depression with those for patients' other conditions. More research is also needed to identify the most efficient means of dissemination and implementation of effective treatment models. Finally, research is needed to improve the depression outcomes of people living with dementia, to improve outcomes for their care partners and caregivers, and to address disparities in depression risk and access to treatment.

KEYWORDS

depression	depressive symptoms	older adults
major depressive disorder	screening	life course
minor depression	interventions	multiple chronic conditions

Image: Hands © Shutterstock, Inc./Dewald Kirsten; Buildings © Shutterstock, Inc./Bariskina.

▶ Introduction

Late-life **depression** is a key public health issue across the globe, associated with both increased morbidity and mortality in **older adults** worldwide (McCall & Kintziger, 2013). Depressive disorders in older adults are associated with increased burden of physical illness, impaired functioning, and risk of suicide, all of which are linked to increased mortality (Blazer, 2003), increased use of health services and higher costs to society (Alexopoulos, 2005), and greater family caregiving burden (Charney et al., 2003). Depression is also a leading cause of disease burden and disability both in the United States and globally, second only to heart disease in contributing to disability-adjusted life-years (DALYs) (Chapman, 2008; McKenna et al., 2005). In fact, the global burden of depressive disorders increased by 37.5% between 1990 and 2010 because of population growth and aging (Ferrari et al., 2013).

This chapter covers current definitions of depressive disorders and validated measurement tools. The fifth edition of the *Diagnostic and Statistical Manual of Mental Disorders* (*DSM-5*) (American Psychiatric Association, 2013) includes the following diagnoses as types of depressive disorders: disruptive mood dysregulation disorder; **major depressive disorder,** single and recurrent episodes; persistent depressive disorder (dysthymia); premenstrual dysphoric disorder; substance/medication-induced depressive disorder; depressive disorder due to another medical condition; other specified depressive disorder; and unspecified depressive disorder. In addition, late-life depression can include minor or subsyndromal depression and clinically significant **depressive symptoms.** While these are less severe manifestations of depressive disorders, similar risk and protective factors have been associated with both (Fiske, 2009).

Depression in late life is complex. It is the "quintessential biopsychosocial disorder," with often multiple biological, psychological, and social factors contributing to its development (Aziz & Steffens, 2013). As such, this chapter describes demographic, social, psychological, and other risk and protective factors for late-life depression, as well as some of the comorbidities that depression affects and is affected by. Depression in older adults differs in important ways from depression in younger adults. It is important to understand how age may affect factors that are associated with both the onset and the maintenance of depression so as to effectively treat depression in older adults (Fiske, Loebach, & Gatz, 2009).

Lastly, this chapter reviews effective treatments and programs for depression, and describes future directions for better understanding, preventing, and treating late-life depression worldwide. Public health approaches are essential for helping to destigmatize the diagnosis and treatment of depression and to better enable older adults and their healthcare providers to recognize late-life depression (Chapman, 2008).

▶ Definition and Measurement

Definitions

In defining epidemiologically relevant forms of depression, it is important to recognize that depression exists across a continuum that starts with normal sadness and extends to severe major depression, which may involve suicidality and significant functional impairment. Quantitative instruments for measuring depression have been developed for both epidemiological and clinical purposes. Typically, the cutoff scores used to define relevant depression are based on depression severity as noted in the *DSM* diagnosis of major depression (American Psychiatric Association, 2013). *DSM-5* defines major depression as a syndrome, involving multiple symptoms, not just emotional sadness. The cardinal or required symptoms include (1) depressed mood or

(2) loss of interest or pleasure that is present most of the day, nearly every day, over a sustained two-week period and that results in significant distress or functional decline. Additional symptoms include (3) appetite changes that may result in weight change, (4) sleep changes, (5) motor agitation or retardation that is noticeable by others, (6) fatigue, (7) feelings of worthlessness or inappropriate guilt, (8) decreased concentration or indecisiveness, and (9) recurrent thoughts of death (American Psychiatric Association, 2013). Five or more of these symptoms are required for a diagnosis of a major depression syndrome, and at least one of the symptoms must be depressed mood or loss of interest. The severity of the syndrome can vary from mild to severe, and is typically determined in the *DSM* approach by looking at the number of symptoms and the severity of distress and functional impairment caused.

Most relevant to older adults, the *DSM* approach specifically instructs the clinician not to include symptoms that are clearly caused by another medical condition. Given that older adults often have **multiple chronic conditions,** and many of these conditions produce symptoms that overlap with the depression syndrome symptoms (e.g., heart failure–related fatigue, Parkinson's disease–related motor retardation, cancer-related appetite and weight changes), making a diagnosis of major depression more complicated in some older adults.

Older adults may also be more likely to experience grief and bereavement, which are generally considered normal expressions of sadness. Previous editions of the *DSM* ruled out making a diagnosis of major depression in the immediate bereavement period, out of recognition that wide variations in the character of bereavement exist across different cultures and depend on the nature of the relationship to the deceased. *DSM-5*, however, no longer prohibits making a diagnosis of major depression during this period, but instead suggests some qualities that may distinguish sadness experienced in grief (e.g., episodic "pangs"

of emptiness and loss) from sadness of major depression (e.g., persistent depressed mood) and suggests that a major depression may develop or coexist with grief. Many clinicians continue to recommend caution in diagnosing major depression in the immediate 2 to 4 weeks after a significant loss. These clinicians also support the *DSM-5* suggestion that when full major depression syndrome symptoms appear and persist for months during bereavement, it is important to consider the additional diagnosis of major depression.

There is an acknowledged component of arbitrariness in defining major depression as requiring five or more symptoms, as some people who have fewer than five symptoms may experience significant distress and functional impairment. The terms **minor depression** and subsyndromal depression have been used to label these conditions. In *DSM* terminology, it has always been recognized that other depressive conditions of clinical significance may develop, with these conditions being labeled "depression not otherwise specified" (depression NOS). Epidemiological data have often shown that while older adults often have lower rates of major depression compared to younger adults, their rates of subsyndromal depression are often higher than those seen in younger adults (Judd, Schettler, & Akiskal, 2002). Additionally, the degree of functional impairment related to subsyndromal depression may be quite important from a population and public health standpoint (Lyness et al., 2006).

Measures

Instruments for measuring depression were initially developed for quantifying treatment outcomes. The initial outcome studies most commonly performed and published were antidepressant treatment trials that were greatly concerned with efficacy evaluations and internal validity considerations. These considerations favored instruments that allowed a trained clinician to interview a subject and quantify the subject's responses around specific depression symptoms (e.g., Hamilton Rating Scale for Depression). As treatment trials moved from trials of individual drugs or psychotherapies in relatively small samples to effectiveness or pragmatic trials concerned with a broader range of outcomes across significantly larger samples, shorter, self-report instruments were developed (e.g., Beck Depression Inventory, Patient Health Questionnaire-9 [PHQ-9]). Similarly, in epidemiological studies focused primarily on case identification, the use of self-report instruments that could be administered easily by a person without extensive clinical experience gained favor. Although self-reported data might potentially be biased by factors leading patients or subjects to over-report or under-report symptoms, there are no laboratory-based approaches for identification of depression—thus, a self-report aspect is common across all depression measures. Studies aimed at both screening and outcome determinations prioritized selection of an instrument that could be used for both aspects. As sample sizes increased, investigators sought the development of shortened versions of these instruments that could be used for screening and used the longer, full versions for treatment outcome determination (e.g., the PHQ-2 and PHQ-9). When depression assessment was included in Global Burden of Disease estimates, in contrast, the methodology used combined various surveys and administrative data such that no single set of screening instruments was readily identified (Global Burden of Disease Study Collaborators 2013, 2015).

Investigators in both clinical trials and epidemiological studies recognized the difficulty of identifying depression in older adults, primarily because of the significant overlap of depression symptoms with other chronic conditions. This understanding led to the development of more geriatric-specific instruments (e.g., Geriatric Depression Scale). Difficulties inherent in getting valid self-reports from older adults with significant cognitive impairment, like that seen in major neurocognitive disorders such as Alzheimer's dementia, prompted the development of another, more specialized instrument (i.e., the Cornell Scale for Depression in Dementia) for use with this population, in which a caregiver or other informant with knowledge of the subject's daily function is also queried about specific depression syndrome items.

Evidence for Utility of Screening

In January 2016, the U.S. Preventive Services Task Force (USPSTF) recommended **screening** for depression of adults in the general population, including older adults (Siu & USPSTF, 2016; USPSTF, 2016). It found grade "B" evidence for screening, concluding that "the net benefit of screening for depression in the general adult population is moderate." Unlike in its 2009 recommendation, the USPSTF did not limit the 2016 recommendation for screening to settings with adequate systems in place to assure that effective diagnosis and treatment could be provided to those with screens indicating depression. Although the new recommendation continued to emphasize the importance of linking screening to effective systems of care, it concluded that such systems are much more common in mental health and primary care treatment settings since the 2009 recommendation was made.

Other organizations have also supported the screening of adults, including older adults. Based on expert panel consensus systematic review and recommendations, the Community Preventive Services Task Force has recommended collaborative care treatment approaches for older adults and recognized that such approaches should employ active screening for depression using validated screening instruments (Frederick, 2007; Snowden, Steinman, Frederick, & Wilson, 2009; Thota et al., 2012). The utility of screening instruments for older adults is determined based on common screening statistics including sensitivity, specificity, likelihood ratio statistics, and area under the curve (AUC) found in receiver operating characteristic (ROC) curves. Studies specific to analyses of older adults are more limited in numbers of participants compared to the analyses carried out in younger adults, yet many studies have found acceptable screening characteristics for the accuracy of instruments in older adults (Dennis et al., 2012; Phelan et al., 2010; Snowden et al., 2009; USPSTF, 2016).

Center of Epidemiological Studies Depression Scale

The Center of Epidemiological Studies Depression Scale (CES-D) was one of the first depression scales developed for epidemiological studies (Radloff, 1977). Though not specifically deployed with older adults, it has been found to be appropriate for older adults, and several systematic reviews have recommended it for this population. A shortened, 10-item version has also been validated and used in multiple studies (Boey, 1999; Kohout, Berkman, Evans, & Cornoni-Huntley, 1993; Robison, Gruman, Gaztambide, & Blank, 2002). The 20-item version uses a 4-choice response format, whereas the 10-item version uses yes/no responses.

Both of these instruments have been translated into several languages and are commonly used in epidemiological studies and in some treatment trials. Neither version explicitly covers the nine *DSM* major depression criteria, so additional questions as well as diagnostic evaluation would need to be performed to establish a diagnosis of major depression. The full version is clearly responsive to change over time, but the shortened version obtains fewer data on responsiveness to change over time. For the 20-item version, a commonly accepted cutoff score for depression is 16 or higher; for the 10-item version, a cutoff score of 4 or higher is often recommended. Because the CES-D has often been used by investigators performing epidemiological studies, scholars wishing to repeat or advance prior epidemiological studies would find that using this same instrument is most amenable for comparing changes in the epidemiology of depression over time.

Geriatric Depression Scale

The Geriatric Depression Scale (GDS) was the first depression scale specifically designed for use in older adult populations (Yesavage, 1983). The authors of the GDS consciously attempted to remove items found in the *DSM* diagnostic criteria and other instruments that were more somatically based and, therefore, more likely to overlap with symptoms of the physical illnesses commonly seen in geriatric populations. Although some somatic items remain (e.g., energy level), the GDS items are felt by many to capture the more psychological aspects of depression as perceived by older adults.

The original 30-item instrument has been shortened to a commonly used 15-item version (Sheik & Yesavage, 1986) and an even briefer, though less commonly seen, 5-item version (Hoyl et al., 1999). Commonly used cut-points for the 30-item and 15-item versions are scores of 10 or higher and 6 or higher, respectively.

The items for all versions use a yes/no response format and ask the subject to respond based on recollections of the past week. As in the CES-D, the instruments do not directly address all nine items of the *DSM*, so additional questions and approaches are needed to establish a clinical diagnosis of major depression. For some subjects the yes/no format is easier, in that the individual does not need to recall numbers of days over a longer 2-week period (as in the PHQ-9). Other subjects find it difficult to categorically answer questions about their feelings in a dichotomous yes/no format. The yes/no format does lend itself to verbal administration of the instrument, as when investigators conduct epidemiological surveys via telephone interviews, especially if the investigator can accommodate for the hearing impairments commonly seen in older adult populations.

Patient Health Questionnaire Nine-Item Depression Scale

The PHQ-9 was developed as part of a larger instrument, the Prime-MD, designed to screen adults for the most common psychiatric disorders in a primary care setting (Spitzer et al., 1994). The nine questions specific to depression were subsequently removed from the full Prime-MD and validated as an independent depression measure in a study that included significant numbers of elderly patients (Kroenke, Spitzer, & Williams, 2001). These nine items correspond directly to the nine symptoms identified in the *DSM* major depression syndrome diagnostic criteria.

The response format of the PHQ-9 is ordinal, with subjects being asked to rate how often they have been bothered by symptoms over the last 2 weeks, ranging from not at all to nearly every day. Although commonly used in younger adult populations, the instrument compares favorably to the Geriatric Depression Scale, suggesting that there is no clear advantage of the instrument designed specifically for older adults (Phelan et al., 2010).

The first two items of the PHQ-9, which ask about loss of interests and sad mood, have been separated into an even briefer instrument, the PHQ-2. Though its brevity lends itself to screening, the limited range of the PHQ-2 presents significant limitations on use for tracking change over time. More often, the PHQ-2 is used as the first step in a two-part screening protocol, such that subjects with positive PHQ-2 scores are then given the remaining items of the PHQ-9.

Two approaches are used for interpreting the scores. In the simplest approach, a total score cut-point of 10 or greater is used to identify people with clinically relevant depression. In the second, more diagnostic approach, subjects are required to have one of the first two items (anhedonia, sadness) for more than half of the 2-week period, and then required to have a total of five or more items scored as more than half the days or nearly every day.

▶ Depression in Different Settings

The prevalence of late-life depression varies considerably depending on where an older

adult lives. For example, in community-dwelling samples of older adults (age 65 or older) who are living independently at home and have a wider range of overall health status, including many people with good health, the prevalence of major depressive disorder ranges from 1% to 5% in large epidemiological studies that have been conducted in the United States and internationally (Fiske et al., 2009). Meanwhile, clinically significant depressive symptoms that might not meet the full criteria for major depression are evident in approximately 15% of community-based older adults (Blazer, 2003). Rates of major depression in late life are much higher in other settings, including among medical outpatients (5% to 10% overall, though a wider range of estimates exist), medical inpatients (10% to 15%), hospice and palliative care patients (10% to 25%, based on limited research), and residents of long-term care facilities (14% to 49%); all of these settings include higher proportions of significantly ill persons than home-based epidemiological studies (Blazer, 2003; Djernes, 2006; Institute of Medicine [IOM], 2012; King, Heisel, & Lyness, 2005). It is believed that it is not the institutionalized or congregate living situation that causes depression (e.g., older kibbutz residents have lower rates of depression than community samples [Blumstein et al., 2004]); rather, the move to these types of settings is often prompted by health issues and/or the loss of a spousal care partner. Indeed, older adults who have voluntarily moved to an institution have lower rates of depression than those who have been involuntarily institutionalized (Fiske et al., 2009).

A recent meta-analysis estimated the prevalence of lifetime major depressive disorder at 16.52%, with specific rates ranging from 9.8% to 26.5% (Volkert, 2013). Far fewer studies have examined the incidence of late-life depression. The first systematic review on this topic was recently released and included 20 studies with adults aged 70 and older. The incidence rate of major depressive disorder ranged from 0.2 to 12.1 per 100 person-years, and the incidence rate of clinically relevant depressive symptoms was 6.8 per 100 person-years (Büchtemann, 2012).

▶ **Demographic Patterns**

A Life Course Perspective

A **life course** perspective is increasingly being applied to late-life depression, aiming to recognize the points at which key risk and protective factors develop over the lifespan (**FIGURE 7-1**). It makes sense to examine late-life depression using a life course approach, as multiple factors lead to depression in older adults, many of which interact over time (Colman & Ataullahjan, 2010). Risk factors for the development of late-life depression likely involve complex interactions among genetic vulnerabilities, cognitive diathesis, age-associated neurobiological changes, and stressful events (Fiske et al., 2009). Risks change as people age, with some risk factors declining and others increasing. Protective factors may emerge as well, such as age-related increases in psychological resilience, engagement in meaningful activities, and religious or spiritual involvement (Fiske et al., 2009). These protective factors may help explain why rates of depression tend to decrease in old age. A developmental perspective on depression across the lifespan can also help identify opportunities for prevention of this mental health disorder (Reynolds, 2009).

Age

Contrary to common perceptions, the severity and prevalence of depression are lower in older adults when compared to younger populations. That said, less-severe depressive symptoms in older adults can have real consequences (e.g., impacting how they manage other chronic conditions or whether they are physically active) and can be treated (Judd & Akiskal, 2002). In addition, late-life depressive disorders may be undercounted in epidemiological studies and surveys, as older adults tend to underreport depressed mood (Gallo & Rabins, 1999) or attribute their depressive symptoms to other medical conditions or life crises (Eaton, Neufield, Chen, & Cai, 2000).

The prevalence of late-life depression increases as older adults age (Aziz & Steffens, 2013). In a recent meta-analysis and systematic review of elders aged 75 or older, the pooled point prevalence of major depression was 7.2% and the pooled point prevalence of clinically significant depressive symptoms was 17.1%. While the prevalence of clinically significant depressive symptoms increased by 20% to 26% in people aged 85 years and older and by 30% to 50% in persons aged 90 and older, this trend was not seen for people with major or minor depression (Leach, 2012; Luppa et al., 2012). In some cases, older adults may score higher on depressive symptom checklists due to symptoms from bereavement or physical illnesses rather than as the result of actual depression (Newmann, 1989). Studies suggest that the increase in late-life depression as older adults age may be explained by characteristics that are associated with aging, such as a greater proportion of women, more physical disability, loss of function, higher cognitive impairment, more chronic conditions, and lower socioeconomic status (Blazer, 2003; Roberts, Kaplan, Shema, & Strawbridge, 1997). Healthy, normally functioning older adults are at no greater risk for depression than younger adults (Satariano, 2006). In addition, people who experience depression as adolescents are at elevated risk to develop depression later in life, including as older adults.

Late-Life Depression Often Includes Both Late and Early Onset

More than half of late-life depression cases involve "late-onset depression," meaning that their first onset occurs after age 60 (Fiske

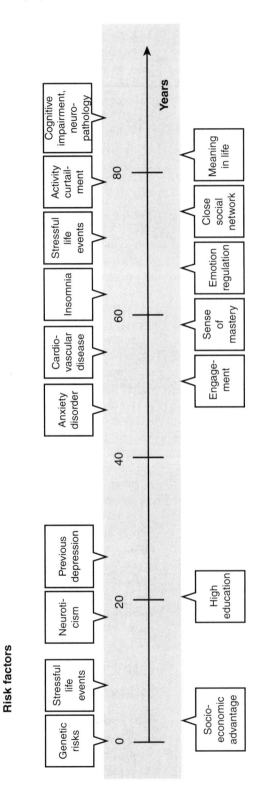

FIGURE 7-1 Lifespan perspective on risk and protective factors for late-life major depression. The schematic illustrates risk and protective factors corresponding to when they emerge over the lifespan.

Reproduced with permission of Annual Review of Clinical Psychology, Vol. 5, pp. 363–89, © 2009 by Annual Reviews, http://www.annualreviews.org.

PEARL 7-1 Life-Course Perspective

It is important to apply a life course perspective when examining the epidemiology of late-life depression to better understand the multiple risk and protective factors that exist over people's lives. Late-life depression is the "quintessential biopsychosocial disorder," with multiple biological, psychological, and social factors contributing to its development (Aziz & Steffens, 2013). It is particularly important to target the modifiable risk factors, including social determinants of health that impact both risk for depression and access to and effectiveness of treatment. In addition, some risk factors for depression can be consequences of late-life depression.

et al., 2009). Many studies do not distinguish between early-onset and late-onset depression, and the age at which an older adult is diagnosed with "late-onset" depression can vary (Fiske et al., 2009)—though typically it is characterized as occurring after age 60 or 65 (Aziz & Steffens, 2013). Older adults with late-onset depression have discrete risk factors and presentation of symptoms. For instance, those with late-onset depression may be less likely to have a family history of depression (e.g., Heun, Papassotiropoulos, Jessen, Maier, & Breitner, 2001) and a lower prevalence of personality

PEARL 7-2 Depression Is a Leading Cause of Disability

Depression is a leading cause of disability both locally and globally, increasing the risk for other chronic conditions and mortality. Even minor depression and clinically significant depressive symptoms are serious for older adults— though less severe symptomatically, they are as impactful as major depression in terms of their effects on health and quality of life.

disorder (e.g., Brodaty et al., 2001) when compared to those with early-onset depression. In addition, older adults with late-onset depression may be more likely to have vascular risk factors (Hickie et al., 2001), and to have concomitant cognitive deficits and later develop dementia (Schweitzer, Tuckwell, O'Brien, & Ames, 2002). While some consensus has emerged around this literature that links structural brain changes to late-life depression, even a recent meta-analysis described the heterogeneity of findings and need for further research (Sexton, Mackay, & Ebmeier, 2013). Furthermore, some attributes of late-onset depression may be evident in older patients with a previous episode of depression as well (Alexopoulos, 2005). In this chapter, we use the term "late-life depression" to capture both early- and late-onset cases unless studies make a distinction between the two.

Gender

Older women are at greater risk for late-life depression than older men (Cole & Dendukuri, 2003; Djernes, 2006; Riedel-Heller, Busse, & Angermeyer, 2006). The Cache County Study, one of the often cited epidemiological studies of community-dwelling elderly persons, reports that the prevalence of major depressive disorder is greater among older women (4.4%) than among older men (2.7%) (Steffens et al., 2000). For older elders (age 75 and older), a recent systematic review and meta-analysis found that the prevalence of major depression was between 4.0% and 10.3% for women and between 2.8% and 6.9% for men (Luppa et al., 2012). Recurrence of depressive syndromes has also been found to be higher for older women (73.1 per 1000 patient-years) than for men (51.6 per 1000 patient-years) (Luijendijk et al., 2008). The gender gap is narrower in older adults (particularly among the oldest old) than the twofold difference seen across the adult life span (Djernes, 2006). Findings from a recent systematic literature review reported female incidence rates of late-life depression that were generally higher than male incidence, though these findings were not statistically significant (Buchtemann, 2012).

The differences between older men and women may partly result from different social factors (e.g., roles, support, chronic life stressors) and psychological factors (e.g., coping style, low sense of mastery control) for these groups (Bebbington, 1996; Nolen-Hoeksema, Larson, & Grayson, 1999). Some life stressors are more prevalent for older women (e.g., widowhood and caretaking), whereas other life stressors decrease as women age (e.g., childbearing, social isolation, balancing multiple roles of worker and homemaker [Blazer, 2003]). It has also been suggested that the gender differences are somewhat artificial, whether due to bias in case identification (Blazer, 2003) or because women are more likely to share their dysphoric feelings than men, whereas men are more likely to deny and act out these feelings through alcoholism and suicide (Koenig & Blazer, 2007; Sonnenberg, Beekman, Deeg, & van Tilburg, 2000).

Race and Ethnicity

There are less consistent data on racial/ethnic differences in late-life depression. In a recently conducted literature review (Pickett, 2013), some studies reported lower prevalence of major depression in older African Americans than in older Caucasians and Latinos (Aranda et al., 2011; Steffens, Fisher, Langa, Potter, & Plassman, 2009; Woodward et al., 2012), while other studies found no significant racial differences (e.g., Byers, Yaffe, Covinsky, Friedman, & Bruce, 2010; Fyffe, Sirey, Heo, & Bruce, 2004; Somervell, Leaf, Weissman, Blazer, & Bruce, 1989). However, older African Americans (Williams et al., 2007) and older Hispanics (Swenson, Baxter, Shetterly, Scarbro, & Hamman, 2000) have reported greater depressive symptoms when compared to older Caucasians (Busse & Blazer, 1989; Spence, Adkins, & Dupre, 2011), with Hispanics reporting the highest levels (Blazer, 2003; Liang, Xu, Quiñones, Bennett, & Ye, 2011). Other data show that older African Americans have lower rates of recognition of and treatment for depression (particularly with antidepressants) as compared to white populations (Pickett, 2013).

Other factors have been shown to mediate or moderate the effects of race on late-life depression. A recent analysis of data from the National Longitudinal Survey of Mature Women (NLSMW; mean age 67, $N = 3182$) demonstrated that physical health and socioeconomic status accounted for much of the racial gap in depressive symptoms and that marital status moderated racial differences between Caucasian and African American women (Spence et al., 2011). While most longitudinal studies have shown that racial/ethnic differences in the level of depressive symptoms between whites and blacks or nonwhites were considerably weaker when socioeconomic status and health were used to adjust the data (Blazer, Landerman, Hays, Simonsick, & Saunders, 1998; Cole, Kawachi, Maller, & Berkman, 2000; Klein, Shankman, & Rose, 2008; Lynch & George, 2002; Yang, 2007), some studies have found persistent racial/ethnic differences even after adjusting for these factors (Kim & Durden, 2007; Liang et al., 2011; Skarupski et al., 2005).

The weathering hypothesis (Geronimus, 2001) posits that differences in both exposure to and response to stress may further differentiate older black and white adults in terms of their depressive symptomology, and the persistent inequality hypothesis suggests that racial disadvantages may be so deeply entrenched by later in life that they are immutable to changes in other factors (Ferraro & Farmer, 1996). In contrast, the age-as-leveler hypothesis (Xu, Liang, Bennett, Quinones, & Ye, 2010) may explain the smaller racial/ethnic differences in late-life depressive disorders, suggesting that the relative social advantage of being white may become less influential given that all women face worsening health as they age.

Other factors at play include acculturation (one study showed that older Hispanic women with lower acculturation had greater depressive symptoms [Swenson et al., 2000]), immigration status (which may increase depression risk, particularly for female immigrants [Black, Markides, & Miller, 1998]), and neighborhood density (e.g., the Hispanic EPESE found that Mexican Americans living in higher-density neighborhoods had lower levels of depression [Ostir, 2003]). Further research is needed to better understand late-life depression in racial/ethnic minority groups—particularly in Native Americans, Asian Americans, and Pacific Islanders—and to examine the variations within these large racial/ethnic constructs. It is particularly important to better understand racial/ethnic differences in late-life depression as the U.S. population becomes increasingly diverse (Coffee & Cummings, 2000) and these communities remain underserved.

Socioeconomic Status

Socioeconomic stressors such as lower income and less education have a strong influence on the development of late-life depression. Declining financial status is one of the most common stressors experienced by older adults (Fiske, 2003). The chronic nature of stressors related to having a low income, such as financial strain and exposure to unsafe and unstable environments, means that older adults who are economically disadvantaged are more likely to experience persistent depressive symptoms (Mojtabai & Olfson, 2004). Financial strain (irrespective of income bracket) in adulthood has also been linked to depression in late life (Wang, Schmitz, & Dewa, 2010; Zimmerman & Katon, 2005).

As compared with older adults with more education, those with lower education have a higher risk of depression (relative risk [RR] = 1.49) (Chang-Quan et al., 2010). Findings from the Work, Family, and Well-Being Study suggest that the relationship between depression and education becomes stronger with increasing age, and physical health problems among adults with lower education account for most (80%) of the diverging gap in depression (Miech & Shanahan, 2000). Meanwhile, widowhood, retirement, and declines in internal sense of control and social support have been found to explain little of the divergence (Miech & Shanahan, 2000). Low levels of education were also significantly associated with higher rates of depressive symptoms in a multiethnic sample of older women (Myers, 2002). In addition, the gap between different education groups and their risk for depression has been shown to widen as age increases (Miech & Shanahan, 2000).

There are two possible pathways through which low socioeconomic status (SES) during the lifespan can increase risk for late-life depression. First, socioeconomic disadvantage earlier in life can increase exposure to social, behavioral, and environmental stressors over the lifetime, such as poor nutrition, reduced opportunities for education, less access to health care, and other mechanisms (Fiske et al., 2009) (**FIGURE 7-2**). Second, older low-SES adults have fewer resources with which to address the stressors in their life or reduce their effects. Lower income has been associated with poorer access to health and mental health services, making it hard for older adults with depression to adhere to treatment or attend appointments (Areán & Reynolds, 2005). Not surprisingly, higher education and SES are protective factors for late-life depression (Fiske et al., 2009), suggesting that larger public health **interventions** to impact social determinants of health are needed to reduce the risk for late-life depression. Neighborhood SES may also be a factor for late-life depression: A recent systematic literature review (Kim, 2008) found some relationship between neighborhood SES (e.g., percentage of neighbors with incomes below the poverty level) and depression in older adults, while other studies produced insignificant findings relative to this link.

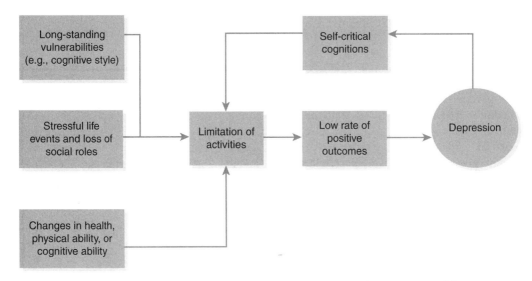

FIGURE 7-2 Behavioral model of late-life depression, depicting the onset and maintenance of depression in older age.

Reproduced with permission of Annual Review of Clinical Psychology, Vol. 5, pp. 363–89, © 2009 by Annual Reviews, http://www.annualreviews.org.

▶ Social Factors

Stressful Events

In addition to SES, acute stressful events can increase the risk of late-life depression. Common stressors in late life include death of a spouse or loved one (bereavement), a new physical illness or disability in self or a family member, change in the individual's living situation, financial difficulties, and interpersonal conflict (Areán & Reynolds, 2005; Fiske et al., 2009; Wright, 2006). The number of stressful life events a person experiences is associated with late-life depression (as is depression at other ages) (Nolen-Hoeksema & Ahrens, 2002). Several life stressors have been identified in longitudinal cohort studies as risk factors for late-life depressive disorders, including adverse life events and ongoing difficulties; bereavement; medical illness, especially diseases of the cardiovascular system, and injuries; and disability and functional decline (Areán & Reynolds, 2005; Wright, 2006). Functional decline is particularly an issue: For community-dwelling older adults, the

presence of disabilities (defined as an activities of daily living score of 1 to 4) increased the risk of depression more than threefold (3.7) over a 1-year period, after adjusting for age, gender, marital status, loneliness, contact with friends, and index depression score (Prince et al., 1998). In most older adults, retirement is not associated with late-life depression, with one exception: Men who retire early have elevated risk for depression (Butterworth et al., 2006).

Studies demonstrate that the greatest impact from a recent life stressor occurs within six months of the event, suggesting that most people are fairly resilient. Past events, however, can still contribute to depression risk. For example, late-life depression has been associated with emotional abuse and neglect in childhood (Blazer, 2003; Pesonen et al., 2007), early loss of a parent (Kivela, 1998), and being raised in foster care (Pesonen et al., 2007)—providing evidence that traumatic experiences in childhood increase the risk of depressive symptoms in older adulthood.

Life stressors can lead to late-life depression in multiple ways. They can necessitate hospitalization or stint in a nursing home or other residential facility, reduce participation in social activities, increase disability, shift the nature of social relationships, or even result in residential relocation (Wright, 2006). Poor social support can decrease resilience and promote a depressive response to life stressors. Maladaptive coping strategies for stressful events, such as unhelpful patterns of thinking and behaving, can lead to dysphoric mood states as well (Aziz & Steffens, 2013). Cognitive style also influences a person's response to stressful events, which fluctuates based on the interaction between cognitive style and type of event. For instance, among older adults with a need for close relationships, interpersonal dependency, and a concern about approval (a constellation of styles called sociotropy), stressful events that are interpersonal in nature have been most closely associated with depression. For older adults with high autonomy (e.g., which highlights personal control and success), negative events that are associated with achievement (e.g., loss of long-term residence) were more strongly associated with depression (Mazure, Maciejewski, Jacobs, & Bruce, 2002).

Bereavement

Bereavement is one of the most significant risk factors for late-life depression (Areán & Reynolds, 2005), and a stressful life event that occurs more frequently as people age. How one copes with the loss, how traumatic or unexpected the death is, and the degree to which the death results in social isolation may be among the factors that link loss and late-life depression (Aziz & Steffens, 2013). Depressive symptoms are a normal reaction to the loss of a loved one, but persistent symptoms that last more than two months may indicate a depressive disorder. A meta-analysis of prospective studies of depressive symptoms and disorders in adults age 50 or older found that bereavement more than tripled the risk of depression and had the largest effect size of any risk factors examined (Cole & Dendukuri, 2003); one study reported that the loss of a spouse or partner increased the adjusted odds of late-life depression by 12.1

(Bruce et al., 1990). The prevalence of major depression after the second year of bereavement is 14%, compared to 2% to 5% in the older adult population overall (Blazer, 2003).

Compared to women, men are more likely to become depressed following the loss of a spouse, and to remain depressed longer (Fiske et al., 2009). This difference may occur because losing a spouse involves different stressors for men and women due to their different roles in the marriage: For widowed women, financial strain is the main mediator of depressive symptoms; for men, the chief mediator is household management (Umberson et al., 1992).

Interestingly, bereavement confers less risk of depression on older adults than it does on middle-aged adults. This discrepancy may reflect the fact that older adults are more likely than younger adults to resolve regrets associated with loss, and this resolution has been associated with better adaptation after a loss (Torges, Stewart, & Nolen-Hoeksema, 2008). In addition, one study of 1810 community-based older adults found that depression onset was best predicted by the death of a partner or other relatives, whereas the onset of anxiety was best predicted by having a partner who developed a major illness (De Beurs et al., 2001).

Caregiving

Caring for a relative with an illness or disability is another life stressor that is more common later in life and may increase the risk of depression for the care partner (formerly referred to as a caregiver). Care partners for older adults with disabilities are twice as likely as non-care partners to develop symptoms of depression (Alexopoulos, 2004). The real proportion may be even greater, as male care partners and African American care partners tend to under-report depressive symptoms (Farran, Miller, Kaufman, & Davis, 1997). Estimates of depression among care partners vary widely, and high rates are based mainly on help-seeking samples (Fiske et al., 2009). Notably, increased risk for late-life depression is found among care partners for older adults with dementia (compared to care partners for older adults with a physical disability) and/or greater severity of behavioral problems and distress (Schulz, 2008), as well as those providing care over the long term (Collins, Stommel, Wang, & Given, 1994) and those who have limited help from others (Clyburn, Stones, Hajistravropoulos, & Tuokko, 2000). Having to limit their typical activities may help explain why care partners are at increased risk for late-life depression (Williamson & Shaffer, 2000).

Social Support

Social support is another significant risk factor for late-life depression. Social support involves perceptions (e.g., satisfaction with social support), structures (e.g., social networks), and behaviors (e.g., helping others). Research suggests that the quality—not the quantity—of social support plays a greater role in developing depression: Perceived social support, also called emotional support, is one of the stronger social predictors for late-life depression (Bruce, 2002). Other social support–related factors that may contribute to late-life depression include social network size, network composition, social contact frequency, satisfaction of social support, instrumental/emotional support, having a confidante, and helping others (Aziz & Steffens, 2013; Chi & Chou, 2001), as well as troubled relationships (e.g., marital conflict), perceived family criticism, and depression in the spouse (Nolen-Hoeksema & Ahrens, 2002). Loneliness is another important social factor: The increased risk of depression caused by lack of contact with friends has been estimated at 2.5, and the increased risk caused by loneliness at 3.6 (Prince et al., 1998). The effects of social support factors may also be affected by both the person and the context; for instance, one study showed that receiving social support was associated with increased depressive symptoms in older men with physical limitations and a greater desire for independence (Nagurney, Reich, & Newsom, 2004). It can be difficult to tease out when social support is the cause of or the effect of late-life depression (Fiske et al., 2009).

Psychological Factors

As with social factors, psychological factors (e.g., self-efficacy and sense of control) are important contributors to depression in older adults. Aziz and Steffens' (2013) recent review paper on key causes of late-life depression found that psychological factors are just as important (or perhaps even more important) to understand what we traditionally think of as risk factors, such as medical illness or disability. For example, one cross-sectional review found that environmental mastery (a sense of self-efficacy and competence in managing one's environment), purpose in life, and autonomy could be used to distinguish between patients with and without major depressive disorder 80% of the time (Davison et al., 2012). Psychological factors often intersect with social factors as risk factors for late-life depression, as they play a role in how well (or badly) older adults cope with stressful life events, including caregiving. These psychological factors include behaviors (e.g., learned helplessness) and cognition (e.g., negative thinking, cognitive distortions) that influence how stressful life events are experienced. Findings from another literature review (Fiske et al., 2009) suggest that a common pathway to depression in older adults may be limiting daily activities, regardless of which predisposing risks are most prominent. When self-critical thinking is present, a depressed state may be further aggravated and sustained (Fiske et al., 2009).

▶ Disease and Comorbidities

Dementia

Depression is a common condition in older adults and frequently comorbid with other chronic conditions. Although individual studies are not universally consistent on this front, recent reviews demonstrate that depression is a risk factor for dementia of both the vascular and Alzheimer's types (Jorm, 2001; Ownby, Crocco, Acevedo, John, & Loewenstein, 2006; Sullivan et al., 2013). Increasingly, public health efforts to encourage behaviors that might prevent dementia are identifying depression as one of the most modifiable risk factors for dementia (Deckers et al., 2015).

The pathophysiology of the association of depression and dementia is not fully understood, however, and it is not clear whether depression plays a causal role or represents a risk vulnerability. Leading theories to explain the association include the stress model, in which significant stress experienced by individuals with impaired hypothalamic–pituitary-adrenal axis systems leads to increased levels of corticotropin-releasing factor and subsequently increased levels of glucocorticoids. Increased glucocorticoids have been associated with smaller hippocampal volumes, depressive features, and dementia (Palazidou, 2012; Raadsheer, Hoogendijk, Stam, Tilders, & Swaab, 1994). In contrast, proponents of the inflammation theory suggest that based on the increased levels of inflammatory markers (e.g., C-reactive protein and interleukins) found in individuals with depression and dementia, inflammation might be the common pathway leading to both depression and later dementia. The lack of consistency in study results may reflect differences in how studies define the specific dementia types and variations in how depression is defined and operationalized (Craft, Cholerton, & Baker, 2013; Hermida, McDonald, Steenland, & Levey, 2012).

Other studies point to the increased risk for depression seen in those who develop dementia. Whether this relationship is pathophysiologically based or represents an emotional reaction to development of dementia is not known. Rates of depression as determined by GDS scores have been found to be significantly higher in patients with cognitive impairment—defined as either mild cognitive impairment or dementia at time of enrollment in dementia centers. When patients without a history of depression were followed over time, incidence rates of depression were significantly higher for patients with mild cognitive impairment or dementia compared to normal controls followed in these Alzheimer's disease research centers (Snowden et al., 2015). These findings suggest that efforts to engage and treat older adults with dementia will also need to address treatment of depression.

Cardiovascular Disease

Since the seminal studies published by Frasure-Smith, Lesperance, and Talajic in 1993, it has been known that depression after myocardial infarction has a significant negative impact on mortality following a heart attack. In these authors' study of a group with a mean age of 60 years, the 6-month hazard ratio for death was 5.74 (95% confidence interval, 4.61 to 6.87) and all deaths were cardiac related. The findings persisted in studies that included control of heart function and other clinical variables. More recent studies have confirmed this association and suggested that the association is more linear and related to severity of depression, rather than a categorical diagnosis (Kozela et al., 2016).

Subsequent treatment interventions have failed to show that treatment for depression significantly lowers subsequent mortality endpoints. For example, in the Enhancing Recovery in Coronary Heart Disease randomized controlled trial of cognitive-behavioral therapy (CBT), participants showed improvements in depression but not decreased rates of all-cause or cardiac mortality or lower rates of subsequent heart attacks. A secondary analysis suggested that antidepressants, particularly selective serotonin reuptake inhibitors, were associated with lower mortality. Nevertheless, as the authors noted, this trial was not designed to test the effectiveness of antidepressants based on the randomization protocols used.

Similarly, a later study of 331 subjects found no difference in cardiac and all-cause mortality for patients randomized to antidepressant treatment after a myocardial infarction compared to those randomized to usual care. Interestingly, the researchers noted that the subjects who received usual care were able to get depression treatment (16%) and might be more motivated to seek out treatment than people who have not had a heart attack, making it difficult to have a true control group without antidepressants in these types of trials. Again, for those patients taking antidepressants (independent of randomization group), all-cause mortality rates were lower than the rates for patients receiving usual care (Zuidersma, Conradi, van Melle, Ormel, & de Jonge, 2013).

As is true for the relationship between dementia and depression, the relationship between cardiovascular disease and depression is bidirectional. Meta-analysis shows a significant increased risk of development of heart disease in patients with depression (Katon et al., 2004). This again leads to considerations of causal mechanisms beyond psychological stress, which is inherent to many serious chronic conditions, whereby increased stress produces depression. In the case of cardiovascular disease, biological mechanisms implicated in the relationship with depression include sympathetic nervous system overactivity and hypothalamic–pituitary–adrenal axis pathology that produces cardiac-specific pathology such as arrhythmias and ventricular hypertrophy, as well as triggers the release of pro-inflammatory cytokines. Of more importance from a behavioral health perspective, persons suffering from depression are less able to adequately address the lifestyle factors that might prevent and alleviate cardiac disease, such as increasing exercise, stopping smoking or excessive alcohol consumption, losing weight, or adhering to medications for heart disease (Dhar & Barton, 2016).

▶ Interventions

Effective treatment of late-life depression has been associated with improved emotional, social, and physical functioning; increased quality of life; better self-care for chronic medical conditions; and reduced mortality (Bruce et al., 2004; Gallo et al., 2007; Unützer et al., 2002; Unützer et al., 2006). The good news is that effective treatments for late-life depression exist, including for older adults with dementia and for older adults who are care partners/caregivers. Research studies show that effective psychological treatments include behavioral therapy, cognitive-behavioral therapy, cognitive bibliotherapy, problem-solving therapy, brief psychodynamic therapy, and life review/reminiscence therapy. **TABLE 7-1** summarizes both evidence-based and promising psychological interventions for late-life depression.

Approximately two-thirds of older adults who present with depressive disorders respond to antidepressant treatment (Andreescu & Reynolds, 2011). Recent reviews, meta-analyses, and consensus statements have found strong evidence for tricyclic antidepressants (TCAs), selective serotonin reuptake inhibitors (SSRIs), monoamine oxidase (MAO) inhibitors, and non-TCAs to treat late-life depression (Nelson, Delucchi, & Schneider, 2008; Wilson et al., 2001), with SSRIs rated as the most tolerable and efficacious (Alexopoulos et al., 2001; Bartels et al., 2002). Older, frail elders are vulnerable to the side effects from pharmacotherapy (particularly cardiovascular and anticholinergic side effects), which can negatively impact both adherence to and the effectiveness of treatment (Mottram, Wilson, & Strobl, 2006).

Late-life depression is often resistant to antidepressant treatment and may have a slower resolution of symptoms compared to mid-life depression (Whyte et al., 2004). Several studies have examined the biological, clinical, and psychosocial predictors of antidepressant treatment response in late-life

TABLE 7-1 Psychological Interventions for Depression in Late Life

Evidence-Based Interventions

Behavioral therapy
Cognitive-behavioral therapy
Cognitive bibliotherapy
Problem-solving therapy
Brief psychodynamic therapy
Life review therapy

Promising Interventions

Interpersonal therapy[a]
Clinical case management[b]
Personal construct therapy[b]
Coping Together group therapy[b]
Interpersonal counseling[b]
Behavioral bibliotherapy[b]
Goal-focused therapy[b]

Evidence-Based Interventions for Caregivers

Cognitive-behavioral therapy
Multicomponent interventions

Evidence-Based Interventions for Persons with Dementia

Behavioral therapy
Social engagement approaches
Sensory/environmental approaches

[a] Efficacy has been demonstrated for continuation treatment of older adult patients who responded to acute treatment with pharmacotherapy or pharmacotherapy + interpersonal therapy.
[b] Efficacy has been demonstrated by only one study or only one set of investigators.

Reproduced with permission of Annual Review of Clinical Psychology, Vol. 5, pp. 363–89, © 2009 by Annual Reviews, http://www.annualreviews.org.

depression (Andreescu, 2011), with higher social support (Dew et al., 1997; Martire et al., 2008), income (Cohen et al., 2006), and self-esteem (Gildengers et al., 2005) each being correlated with better treatment response. Identifying these predictors of treatment response may help clinicians to select the best treatment options earlier during the course of treatment.

Most guidelines recommend supporting antidepressant medication treatment with psychosocial interventions, given the higher likelihood of pharmacotherapy-related side effects in older adults (Wilson, Mottram, & Vassilas, 2008). Effect sizes were comparable in the few studies that have compared pharmacologic and psychological interventions, and may favor psychotherapy as an intervention (Pinquart,

Duberstein, & Lyness, 2006). In practice, however, evidence-based psychological treatments are often combined with pharmacologic interventions, even though the research on combined treatment lags behind practice (Fiske et al., 2009; Wilson et al., 2008).

Electroconvulsive therapy (ECT) is used more frequently in older adults than in any other age group, as it is appropriate when depression is not responsive to medications, when antidepressants are not tolerated due to side effects, or when depression is accompanied by life-threatening complications such as severe weight loss or catatonia such that a rapid definitive response is required (Kelly & Zisselman, 2000). ECT is also considered a low-risk procedure that can be successfully undertaken in medically ill older adults. Its efficacy rates range from 60% to 80%, as demonstrated in several randomized controlled trials (Dombrovski & Mulsant, 2007; Flint & Rifat, 1998; Kujala, Rosenvinge, & Bekkeland, 2002; Sackeim, 2004; van der Wurff, Stek, Hoogendijk, & Beekman, 2003). ECT is often recommended for older adults with depression that is resistant to other treatments and for those at risk for serious harm because of psychotic depression, suicidal ideation, or severe malnutrition (Unützer, 2007). Although still viewed as controversial, ECT has also been shown to be effective in older adults with comorbid cardiovascular disease, dementia, or Parkinson's disease (Rice et al., 1994). Common side effects of this therapy include headaches and temporary confusion or memory impairment, with memory loss and falls occurring less frequently (Fiske et al., 2009; Unützer, 2007).

The greatest challenge to effectively treating late-life depression are issues with treatment access and delivery (Blazer, 2005), which especially impacts men and people of color (Unützer et al., 2003). Reasons for undertreatment or lack of treatment include the challenges in detecting and adequately treating depression in older adults (Alexopoulos & Kelly, 2009; Fiske et al., 2009), stigma associated

with depression (Sirey et al., 2001), the belief that depression is a normal part of aging (Sarkisian, Lee-Henderson, & Mangione, 2003), and access to treatment issues, as many older adults seek care for depression in primary care rather than specialty mental health settings (Bartels et al., 2004). Collaborative care models, in which a trained depression care manager delivers evidence-based psychological and pharmacologic treatments in the primary care setting (Bruce et al., 2004; Unützer et al., 2002) or in the elder's home (Ciechanowski, 2004), have demonstrated greater improvement in depression outcomes (including reduced suicidal ideation) when compared to the primary care physician managing the depression treatment on his or her own (usual care). Recommended by the Guide to Community Preventive Services ("The Community Guide"), collaborative care (or depression care management) models may also increase access and adherence to effective depression treatment services by meeting older adults where they are. Notably, collaborative or integrative care models have been shown to be effective in reducing depression among older Latinos and African Americans, although further research is needed with heterogeneous racial/ethnic minority groups, including those who are English language learners (Fuentes, 2012).

Some research also suggests that exercise can be a complementary or alternative medicine (CAM) treatment for late-life depression (Barbour & Blumenthal, 2005; Sjösten & Kivelä, 2006). A recent systematic review and meta-analysis of randomized controlled trials (RCTs) found a moderate effect size for exercise on depressive symptoms in older adults, suggesting that physical exercise may be a feasible additional intervention for late-life depression (Heinzel, 2015). This finding is important because many older adults with depression are not receiving adequate treatment and, as such, may benefit from additional, low-threshold treatments.

Limitations of studies of exercise interventions for late-life depression include limited follow-up periods and small sample sizes. Moreover, many have not included clinically depressed subjects, making it is unclear whether clinically significant changes can be expected in this population (Frederick, 2007). In addition, while exercise programs can be a first-line strategy for older adults with mild to moderate depression who prefer this approach, it may be difficult for patients with depression to engage in exercise programs, suggesting that additional treatment with antidepressants or psychotherapy may be warranted in this population (Fiske et al., 2009; Unützer 2007). Recent data suggest that exercise may be used to augment other effective depression treatments: In a recent RCT, a greater proportion of older adults with major depression who received both a nonprogressive group exercise intervention and antidepressant treatment (sertraline) achieved remission (81% versus 45%) and experienced a shorter time to remission than the medication-only group (Belvederi Murri et al., 2015).

Evidence is limited but growing for other physical treatments for late-life depression, such as yoga and tai-chi (Nyer et al., 2013). Preliminary evidence from a recent systematic literature review and meta-analysis of exercise interventions indicated that these types of exercises produced the highest effect sizes (although the sample sizes for many of the included RCTs were small), suggesting that including the "mental" treatment aspects may go beyond the physical components of the treatment effect (Heinzel, 2015). Group interventions such as these may also provide the added benefit of social interaction, which many elders often lack (Nicholson, 2012). Limited evidence exists for some other CAM interventions, such as massage therapy, natural remedies, music therapy, and religious and spiritual interventions; studies of these interventions are often hampered by similar limitations as those described for exercise (Nyer et al., 2013).

Prevention strategies may also be appropriate both to reduce the risk for late-life depressive disorders (e.g., among persons with subsyndromal depressive symptoms [Schoevers et al., 2006]) and to lower the risk of adverse outcomes from late-life depression (e.g., by reducing suicidal thoughts [Bruce et al., 2004]). Preventive interventions are also recommended given the challenges in achieving remission of late-life depressive disorders (Andreescu & Reynolds, 2011). A recent literature review found evidence for selective primary prevention (i.e., targeting individuals at risk for, but not presenting with, depression) for older adults with stroke and macular degeneration (but not for older adults with hip fracture) and for caregiving in dementia, using antidepressant medication treatment in standard doses and problem-solving treatment (Baldwin, 2010). Preventive interventions that include education for individuals with chronic illness, behavioral activation, cognitive restructuring, skills training, group support, and life review have also received support (Fiske et al., 2009).

▶ Conclusion and Future Directions

Depression remains a significant condition for older adults, consistently ranking in the top five causes of all age disability worldwide in Global Burden of Disease Studies over the last several years. Of significant importance to older adults, this mental health disorder is more likely to occur after onset of common conditions of old age and often negatively impacts the outcome of those conditions. Increasingly, studies are also identifying depression as a risk factor for conditions ranging from dementia to cardiovascular disease. Effective tools exist for screening and identification of depression as well as for monitoring the outcomes of treatment. Public health organizations have begun to endorse depression screening, but providing easy access to evidence-based treatments remains a challenge. Nevertheless, effective treatments for depression exist and are being integrated into primary care, behavioral health settings, and aging provider networks. As comorbidity is quite common among older adults, combining treatment approaches for multiple conditions, as opposed to providing sequential treatment of one condition at a time, is needed. More research is also needed to identify the most efficient means of dissemination and implementation of effective treatment models.

Unfortunately, many models of care focus on cognitively normal or minimally impaired subjects. Given the growing epidemic of dementia and the interplay between depression and dementia, different treatment approaches will be necessary for improving outcomes of depression in patients with significant cognitive impairment. Elderly care partners are also a growing population at increased risk for depression. The stakes are significantly higher for this group: If a care partner becomes disabled by depression or develops a chronic condition as a result of depression, that person will no longer be able to provide care for the partner. Thus, more research is needed to explore practical means of providing care to prevent development of depression and accessible treatments for care partners suffering from depression. Access to care remains a product of social determinants of health for many people. Thus, as preventive

and treatment services are developed, policy makers will need to assure that persons whose sociodemographic factors increase their risk for development of depression are not also less able to access care because of those same social determinants of care.

References

Alexopoulos, G. S. (2004). Late-life mood disorders. In J. Sadavoy, L. F. Jarvik, G. T. Grossberg, & B. S. Meyers (Eds.), *Comprehensive textbook of geriatric psychiatry* (3rd ed., pp. 609-653). New York, NY: W. W. Norton and Company.

Alexopoulos, G. S. (2005). Depression in the elderly. *Lancet, 365,* 1961–1970.

Alexopoulos, G. S., Katz, I. R., Reynolds, C. F. 3rd, Carpenter, D., Docherty, J. P., & Ross, R. W. (2001). Pharmacotherapy of depression in older patients: A summary of the expert consensus guidelines. *Journal of Psychiatric Practice, 7,* 361–376.

Alexopoulos, G. S., & Kelly, R. E. (2009). Research advances in geriatric depression. *World Psychiatry, 8,* 140-149.

American Psychiatric Association. (2013). *Diagnostic and statistical manual of mental disorders* (5th ed.). Washington, DC: Author.

Andreescu, C., & Reynolds, C. F. 3rd. (2011). Late-life depression: Evidence-based treatment and promising new directions for research and clinical practice. *Psychiatric Clinics of North America, 34*(2), 335-355, vii-viii.

Aranda, M. P., Chae, D. H., Lincoln, K. D., Taylor, R. J., Woodward, A. T., & Chatters, L. M. (2011). Demographic correlates of *DSM-IV* major depressive disorder among older African Americans, black Caribbeans, and non-Hispanic whites: Results from the National Survey of American Life. *International Journal of Geriatric Psychiatry, 27*(9), 940-947.

Areán, P. A., & Reynolds, C. F. 3rd. (2005).The impact of psychosocial factors on late-life depression. *Biology and Psychiatry, 58*(4), 277–282.

Aziz, R., & Steffens, D. C. (2013). What are the causes of late-life depression? *Psychiatric Clinics of North America, 36*(4), 497-516.

Baldwin, R. C. (2010). Preventing late-life depression: A clinical update. *International Psychogeriatrics, 22*(8), 1216-1224.

Barbour, K. A., & Blumenthal, J. A. (2005). Exercise training and depression in older adults. *Neurobiology and Aging, 26*(suppl 1), 119–123.

Bartels, S. J., Coakley, E. H., Zubritzky, C., Ware, J. H., Miles, K. M., Areán, P. A.,... PRISM-E Investigators. (2004). Improving access to geriatric mental health

PEARL 7-3 Depression Is Treatable

The good news is that effective screening instruments and interventions for late-life depression exist. Particularly promising are those collaborative care programs that integrate both screening and treatment. We need public health, healthcare reform, integrated primary care and behavioral health, community-based social and aging service providers, and other innovation models to prioritize and pay for these essential services, thereby helping older adults maintain their independence and quality of life.

services: A randomized trial comparing treatment engagement with integrated versus enhanced referral care for depression, anxiety, and at-risk alcohol use. *American Journal of Psychiatry, 161*, 1455–1462.

Bartels, S. J., Dums, A. R., Oxman, T. E., Scheider, T. E., Areán, P. A., Alexopolous, G. S., & Jeste, D. V. (2002). Evidence-based practices in geriatric mental health care. *Psychiatric Services, 53*, 1419–1431.

Bebbington, P. (1996). The origins of sex differences in depressive disorder: Bridging the gap. *International Reviews of Psychiatry, 8*, 295–332.

Belvederi Murri, M., Amore, M., Menchetti, M., Toni, G., Neviani, F., Cerri, M.,… Zanetidou, S. (2015). Safety and Efficacy of Exercise for Depression in Seniors (SEEDS) Study Group. Physical exercise for late-life major depression. *British Journal of Psychiatry, 207*(3), 235–242.

Black, S. A., Markides, K. S., & Miller, T. Q. (1998). Correlates of depressive symptomatology among older community-dwelling Mexican Americans: The Hispanic EPESE. *Journals of Gerontology, Series B: Psychological Sciences and Social Sciences, 53B*(4), S198–S208.

Blazer, D. G. (2003). Depression in late life: Review and commentary. *Journals of Gerontology: Medical Sciences, 56A*, 249–265.

Blazer, D. G., Hybels, C. F., Fillenbaum, G. G., & Pieper, C.F. (2005). Predictors of antidepressant use among older adults: Have they changed over time? *American Journal of Psychiatry, 162*, 705–10.

Blazer, D. G., Landerman, L. R., Hays, J. C., Simonsick, E. M., & Saunders, W. B. (1998). Symptoms of depression among community-dwelling elderly African-American and white older adults. *Psychological Medicine, 28*(6), 1311–1320.

Blumstein, T., Benyamini, Y., Fuchs, Z., Shapira, Z., Novikov, I., Walter-Ginzburg, A., & Modan, B. (2004). The effect of a communal lifestyle on depressive symptoms in late life. *Journal of Aging and Health, 16*, 151–174.

Boey, K. (1999). Cross-validation of a short form of the CES-D in Chinese elderly. *Journal of Geriatric Psychiatry, 14*(8), 608–617.

Brodaty, H., Luscombe, G., Parker, G., Wilhelm, K., Hickie, I., Austin, M. P., & Mitchell, P. (2001). Early and late onset depression in old age: Different aetiologies, same phenomenology. *Journal of Affective Disorders, 66*, 225–236.

Bruce, M. L. (2002). Psychosocial risk factors for depressive disorders in late life. *Biological Psychiatry, 52*(3), 175–184.

Bruce, M. L., Kim, K., Leaf, P. J., & Jacobs, P. (1990). Depressive episodes and dysphoria resulting from conjugal bereavement in a prospective community sample. *American Journal of Psychiatry, 147*(5), 608–611.

Bruce, M. L., Ten Have, T. R., Reynolds, C. F. 3rd, Katz I. I., Schulberg, H. C., Mulsant, B. H., … Alexopolous, G.S. (2004). Reducing suicidal ideation and depressive

symptoms in depressed older primary care patients: A randomized controlled trial. *Journal of the American Medical Association, 291*, 1081-1091.

Büchtemann, D., Luppa, M., Bramesfeld, A., & Riedel-Heller, S. (2012). Incidence of late-life depression: A systematic review. *Journal of Affective Disorders, 142*(1–3), 172–9.

Busse, E. W., & Blazer, D. G. (1989). *Geriatric psychiatry.* Washington, DC: American Psychiatric Press.

Butterworth, P., Gill, S. C., Rodgers, B., Anstey, K. J., Villamil, E., & Melzer, D. (2006). Retirement and mental health: Analysis of the Australian national survey of mental health and well-being. *Social Science and Medicine, 62*, 1179–1191.

Byers, A. L., Yaffe, K., Covinsky, K. E., Friedman, M. B., & Bruce, M. L. (2010). High occurrence of mood and anxiety disorders among older adults: The National Comorbidity Survey Replication. *Archives of General Psychiatry, 67*, 489–496.

Chang-Quan, H., Zheng-Rong, W., Yong-Hong, L., Yi-Zhou, X., & Qing-Xiu, L. (2010). Education and risk for late life depression: A meta-analysis of published literature. *International Journal of Psychiatry in Medicine, 40*(1), 109–124.

Chapman, D. P., & Perry, G. S. (2008). Depression as a major component of public health for older adults. *Preventing Chronic Disease, 5*(1).

Charney, D. S., Reynolds, C. F. 3rd, Lewis, L., Lebowitz, B. D., Sunderland, T., Alexopoloulos, G. S.,… Young, R. C. (2003). Depression and bipolar support alliance consensus statement on the unmet needs in diagnosis and treatment of mood disorders in late life. *Archives of General Psychiatry, 60*, 664-672.

Chi, I., & Chou, K. L. (2001). Social support and depression among elderly Chinese people in Hong Kong. *International Journal of Aging and Human Development, 52*(3), 231–252.

Ciechanowski, P., Wagner, E., Schmaling, K., Schwartz, S., Williams, B., & Diehr P. (2004). Community-integrated home-based depression treatment in older adults: A randomized controlled trial. *Journal of the American Medical Association, 291*, 1569–1577.

Clyburn, L. D., Stones, M. J., Hajistravropoulos, T., & Tuokko, H. (2000). Predicting caregiver burden and depression in Alzheimer's disease. *Journals of Gerontology, Series B: Psychologic Sciences and Social Sciences, 55*, S2–S13.

Coffee, C. E., & Cummings, J. L. (2000). *Textbook of geriatric psychiatry* (2nd ed.). Washington, DC American Psychiatric Press.

Cohen, A., Houck, P. R., Szanto, K., Dew, M. A., Gilman, S. E., & Reynolds, C. F. 3rd. (2006). Social inequalities in response to antidepressant treatment in older adults. *Archives of General Psychiatry, 63*, 50–56.

Cole, M. G., & Dendukuri, N. (2003). Risk factors for depression among elderly community subjects: A systematic review and meta-analysis. *American Journal of Psychiatry, 160*, 1147–1156.

Cole, S. R., Kawachi, I., Maller, S. J., & Berkman, L. F. (2000). Test of item-response bias in the CES-D scale: Experience from the New Haven EPESE study. *Journal of Clinical Epidemiology, 53*(3), 285–289.

Collins, C. E., Stommel, M., Wang, S., & Given, C. W. (1994). Caregiving transitions: Changes in depression among family caregivers of relatives with dementia. *Nursing Research, 43*, 220–225.

Colman, I., & Ataullahjan, A. (2010). Life course perspectives on the epidemiology of depression. *Canadian Journal of Psychiatry, 55*(10), 622–632.

Craft, S., Cholerton, B., & Baker, L. D. (2013). Insulin and Alzheimer's disease: Untangling the web. *Journal of Alzheimer's Disease, 33*(suppl 1), S263–S275.

Davison, T. E., McCabe, M. P., Knight, T., & Mellor, D. (2012). Biopsychosocial factors related to depression in aged care residents. *Journal of Affective Disorders, 142*(1–3), 290–296.

De Beurs, E., Beekman, A., Geerlings, S., Deeg, D., Van Dyck, R., & Van Tilburg, W. (2001). On becoming depressed or anxious in late life: Similar vulnerability factors but different effects of stressful life events. *British Journal of Psychiatry, 179*(5), 426–431.

Deckers, K. van Boxtel, M. P. J., Schiepers, O. J. G., de Vugt, M., Muños Sànchez, J. L., Anstey, K. J.,... Köhler, S. (2015). *International Journal of Geriatric Psychiatry, 30*(3), 234–246.

Dennis, M., Kadri, A., & Coffey, J. (2012). *Age and Ageing, 41*(2), 148–154.

Dew, M. A., Reynolds, C. F. 3rd, Houck, P. R., Hall, M., Buysse, D. J., Frank, E., & Kupfer, D. J. (1997). Temporal profiles of the course of depression during treatment: Predictors of pathways toward recovery in the elderly. *Archives of General Psychiatry, 54*, 1016–1024.

Dhar, A. K., & Barton, D. A. (2016). Depression and the link with cardiovascular disease. *Frontiers in Psychiatry, 7*, 33.

Djernes, J. K. (2006). Prevalence and predictors of depression in populations of elderly: A review. *Acta Psychiatrica Scandinavica, 113*, 372–387.

Dombrovski, A. Y., & Mulsant, B. H. (2007). The evidence for electroconvulsive therapy (ECT) in the treatment of severe late-life depression: ECT: The preferred treatment for severe depression in late life. *International Psychogeriatrics, 19*, 10–14, 24.

Eaton, W. W., Neufeld, K., Chen, L., & Cai, G. (2000). A comparison of self-report and clinical diagnostic interviews for depression: Diagnostic interview schedule and schedules for clinical assessment in neuropsychiatry in the Baltimore Epidemiologic Catchment Area Follow-up. *Archives of General Psychiatry, 57*(3), 217–222.

Farran, C. J., Miller, B. H., Kaufman, J. E., & Davis, L. (1997). Race, finding meaning, and caregiver distress. *Journal of Aging and Health, 9*, 316–333.

Ferrari, A. J., Charlson, F. J., Norman, R. E., Patten, S. B., Freedman, G. D., Murray, C. J. L.,... Whiteford, H. A. (2013). Burden of depressive disorders by country, sex, age, and year: Findings from the Global Burden of Disease Study 2010. *PLoS Medicine, 10*(11), e1001547.

Ferraro, K. F., & Farmer, M.M. (1996). Double jeopardy, aging as leveler, or persistent health inequality? A longitudinal analysis of white and black Americans. *The Journal of Gerontology Series B Psychological Sciences and Social Sciences, 51*(6), S319-28.

Fiske, A., Gatz, M., & Pedersen, N.L. (2003). Depressive symptoms and aging: The effects of illness and non-health-related events. *Journals of Gerontology, Series B: Psychological Sciences and Social Sciences, 58*, P320–8.

Fiske, A., Loebach, W., & Gatz, M. (2009). Depression in older adults. *Annual Review of Clinical Psychology*, 363–389.

Flint, A. J., & Rifat, S. L. (1998). The treatment of psychotic depression in later life: A comparison of pharmacotherapy and ECT. *International Journal of Geriatric Psychiatry, 13*, 23–28.

Frasure-Smith, N., Lespérance, F., & Talajic, M. (1993). *Journal of the American Medical Association, 270*(15), 1819–1825.

Frederick, J. F. (2007). Community-based treatment of late-life depression: An expert panel-informed literature review. *American Journal of Preventive Medicine, 33*(3), 222–249.

Fuentes, D., & Aranda, M. P. (2012). Depression interventions among racial and ethnic minority older adults: A systematic review across 20 years. *The American Journal of Geriatric Psychiatry, 20*(11), 915–931.

Fyffe, D. C., Sirey, J. A., Heo, M., & Bruce, M. L. (2004). Late-life depression among black and white elderly homecare patients. *American Journal of Geriatric Psychiatry, 12*, 531–535.

Gallo, J. J., Bogner, H. R., Morales, K. H., Post, E. P., Lin, J. Y., & Bruce, M. L. (2007). The effect of a primary care practice-based depression intervention on mortality in older adults: A randomized trial. *Annals of Internal Medicine, 146*, 689–698.

Gallo, J. J., & Rabins, P. V. (1999). Depression without sadness: Alternative presentations of depression in late life. *American Family Physician, 60*(3), 820–826.

Geronimus, A. T. (2001). Understanding and eliminating racial inequalities in women's health in the United States: The role of the weathering conceptual framework. *Journal of the American Medical Women's Association, 56*(4), 133–136, 149–150.

Gildengers, A. G., Houck, P. R., Mulsant, B. H., Dew, M. A., Alzenstein, H. J., Jones, B. L., ... Reynolds, C. F. 3rd. (2005). Trajectories of treatment response in late-life depression: psychosocial and clinical correlates. *Journal of Clinical Psychopharmacology, 25*, S8–S13.

Global Burden of Disease Study Collaborators 2013. (2015). Global, regional, and national prevalence and years lived with disability for 301 acute and chronic conditions and injuries in 108 countries, 1990-2013: A systematic analysis for the Global Burden of Disease 2013. *Lancet, 386*(9995), 743-800.

Heinzel, S., Lawrence, J.B., Kallies, G., Rapp, M.A., & Heissel A. (2015). Using exercise to fight depression in older adults: A systematic review and meta-analysis. *The Journal of Gerontopsychology and Geriatric Psychiatry, 28*(4), 149-162.

Hermida, A. P., McDonald, W. M., Steenland, K., & Levey, A. (2012). The association between late-life depression, mild cognitive impairment and dementia: Is inflammation the missing link? *Expert Reviews of Neurotherapy, 12*(11), 1339-1350.

Heun, R., Papassotiropoulos, A., Jessen, F., Maier, W., & Breitner, J. C. (2001). A family study of Alzheimer's disease and early- and late-onset depression in elderly patients. *Archives of General Psychiatry, 58*, 190–196.

Hickie, I., Scott, E., Naismith, S., Ward, P., Turner, K., Parker, J., Mitchell, P., & Wilhelm, K. (2001). Late-onset depression: Genetic, vascular and clinical contributions. *Psychological Medicine, 31*, 1403–1412.

Hoyl, M. T., Alessi, C. A., Harker, J. O., Josephson, K. R., Pietruszka, F. M., Koelfgen, M.,... Rubenstein, L. Z. (1999). Development and testing of a five-item version of the Geriatric Depression Scale. *Journal of the American Geriatric Society, 47*(7), 873-878.

Institute of Medicine (IOM). (2012). *The mental health and substance use workforce for older adults: In whose hands?* Washington, DC: National Academies Press.

Jorm, A. F. (2001). History of depression as a risk factor for dementia: An updated review. *Australian & New Zealand Journal of Psychiatry, 35*(6), 776-781.

Judd, L. L., & Akiskal, H. S. (2002). The clinical and public health relevance of current research on subthreshold depressive symptoms in elderly patients. *American Journal of Geriatric Psychiatry, 10*(3), 233-238.

Judd, L. L., Schettler, P. J., & Akiskal, H. S. (2002). The prevalence, clinical relevance, and public health significance of subthreshold depressions. *Psychiatric Clinics of North America, 25*, 685–698.

Katon, W. J., Lin, E. H. B., Russo, J., Von Koff, M., Ciechanowski, P., Simon, G.,... Young, B. (2004). Cardiac risk factors in patients with diabetes mellitus and major depression. *Journal of General Internal Medicine, 19*(12), 1192-1199.

Kelly, K. G., & Zisselman, M. (2000). Update on electroconvulsive therapy (ECT) in older adults. *Journal of the American Geriatric Society, 48*, 560–566.

Kim, D. (2008). Blues from the neighborhood? Neighborhood characteristics and depression. *Epidemiologic Reviews, 30*, 101-117.

Kim, J., & Durden, E. (2007). Socioeconomic status and age trajectories of health. *Social Science & Medicine, 65*(12), 2489–2502.

King, D. A., Heisel, M. J., & Lyness, J. F. (2005). Assessment and psychological treatment of depression in older adults with terminal or life-threatening illness. *Clinical Psychology Science and Practice, 12*, 339–353.

Kivelä, S. L., Luukinen, H., Koski, K., Viramo, P., & Pahkala, K. (1998). Early loss of mother or father predicts depression in old age. *International Journal of Geriatric Psychiatry, 13*(8), 527-30.

Klein, D. N., Shankman, S. A., & Rose, S. (2008). Dysthymic disorder and double depression: Prediction of 10-year course trajectories and outcomes. *Journal of Psychiatric Research, 42*(5), 408–415.

Koenig, H.G., Blazer, D.G. (2007). Mood Disorders. In: Blazer, D.G., Steffens, D.C., Busse, E.W. (Eds.), *Essential of geriatric psychiatry*. American Psychiatric Pub, Washington, DC, pp. 145–176.

Kohout, F. J., Berkman, L. F., Evans, D. A., & Cornoni-Huntley, J. (1993). Two shorter forms of the CES-D (Center for Epidemiological Studies Depression) depression symptoms index. *Journal of Aging and Health, 5*(2), 179-193.

Kozela, M., Bobak, M., Besala, A., Kubinova, R., Malyutina, S., Denisova, D.,... Pajak, A. (2016). The association of depressive symptoms with cardiovascular and all-cause mortality in Central and Eastern Europe: Prospective results of the HAPIEE study. *European Journal of Preventive Cardiology, 23*(17), 1839-1847.

Kroenke, K., Spitzer, R. L., & Williams, J. B. (2001). The PHQ-9: Validity of a brief depression severity measure. *Journal of General Internal Medicine, 16*(9), 606-613.

Kujala, I., Rosenvinge, B., & Bekkelund, S. I. (2002). Clinical outcome and adverse effects of electroconvulsive therapy in elderly psychiatric patients. *Journal of Geriatric Psychiatry and Neurology, 15*, 73-76.

Leach, L. S. (2012). Review: major depression affects about 7% of adults aged 75 and above. *Evidence-Based Mental Health, 15*(3), 64.

Liang, J., Xu, X., Quiñones, A. R., Bennett, J. M., & Ye, W. (2011). Multiple trajectories of depressive symptoms in middle and late life: Racial/ethnic variations. *Psychology and Aging, 26*(4), 761-777.

Luijendijk, H. J., van den Berg, J. F., Dekker, M. J., van Tuijl, H. R., Otte, W., Smit, F.,... Tiemeier, H. (2008). Incidence and recurrence of late-life depression. *Archives of General Psychiatry, 65*(12), 1394–1401.

Luppa, M., Sikorski, C., Luck, T., Ehreke, L., Konnopka, A., Wiese, B.,... Riedel-Heller, S. G. (2012). Age- and gender-specific prevalence of depression in latest life: Systematic review and meta-analysis. *Journal of Affective Disorders, 136*(3), 212–221.

Lynch, S. M., & George, L. K. (2002). Interlocking trajectories of loss-related events and depressive symptoms among elders. *Journal of Gerontology: Social Sciences, 57B*(2), S117–S125.

Lyness, J. M., Heo, M., Datto, C. J., Ten Have, T. R., Katz, I. R., Drayer, R.,… Bruce, M. L. (2006). Outcomes of minor and subsyndromal depression among elderly patients in primary care settings. *Annals of Internal Medicine, 144*(7), 496–504.

Martire, L. M., Schulz, R., Reynolds, C. F. 3rd., Morse, J. Q., Butters, M. A., Hinrichsen, G. A. (2008). Impact of close family members on older adults' early response to depression treatment. *Psychology and Aging, 23*, 447–452.

Mazure, C. M., Maciejewski, P. K., Jacobs, S. C., & Bruce, M. L. (2002). Stressful life events interacting with cognitive/personality styles to predict late-onset major depression. *American Journal of Geriatric Psychiatry, 10*, 297–304.

McCall, W. V., & Kintziger, K. W. (2013). Late life depression: A global problem with few resources. *Psychiatric Clinics of North America, 36*(4), 475–481.

McKenna, M. T., Michaud, C. M., Murray, C. J. L., & Marks, J. S. (2005). Assessing the burden of disease in the United States using disability-adjusted life years. *American Journal of Preventive Medicine, 28*, 415–423.

Miech, R. A., & Shanahan, M. J. (2000). Socioeconomic status and depression over the life course. *Journal of Health and Social Behavior, 41*(2), 162–176.

Mojtabai, R., & Olfson, M. (2004). Major depression in community-dwelling middle-aged and older adults: Prevalence and 2-year and 4-year follow-up symptoms. *Psychological Medicine, 34*, 623–34.

Mottram, P., Wilson, K., & Strobl, J. (2006). Antidepressants for depressed elderly. *Cochrane Database of Systematic Reviews, 1*, CD003491.

Myers, H. F., Lesser, I., Rodriguez, N., Mira, C. B., Hwang, W-C., Anderson, C. C., D.,… Wohl, M. Ethnic differences in clinical presentations of depression in adult women. *Cultural Diversity and Ethnic Minority Diversity, 8*(2), 138–156.

Nagurney, A. J., Reich, J. W., & Newsom, J. T. (2004). Gender moderates the effects of independence and dependence desires during the social support process. *Psychology and Aging, 19*, 215–218.

Nelson, J. C., Delucchi, K., & Schneider, L. S. (2008). Efficacy of second generation antidepressants in late-life depression: A meta-analysis of the evidence. *American Journal of Geriatric Psychiatry, 16*, 558–567.

Newmann, J. P. (1989). Aging and depression. *Psychology and Aging, 4*, 150–165.

Nicholson, N. R. (2012). A review of social isolation: An important but under-assessed condition in older adults. *Journal of Primary Prevention, 33*, 137–152.

Nolen-Hoeksema, S., & Ahrens, C. (2002). Age differences and similarities in the correlates of depressive symptoms. *Psychology and Aging, 17*, 116–124.

Nolen-Hoeksema, S., Larson, J., & Grayson, C. (1999). Explaining the gender difference in depressive symptoms. *Journal of Personality and Social Psychology, 77*(5), 1061–1072.

Nyer, M., Doorley, J., Durham, K., Yeung, A. S., Freeman, M. P., & Mischoulon, D. (2013). What is the role of alternative treatments in late-life depression? *Psychiatric Clinics of North America, 36*(4), 577–596.

Ostir, G. V., Eschbach, K., Markides, K.S., & Goodwin, J. S. (2003). Neighbourhood composition and depressive symptoms among older Mexican Americans. *Journal of Epidemiology and Community Health, 57*(12), 987–92.

Ownby, R. L., Crocco, E., Acevedo, A., John, V., & Loewenstein, D. (2006). Depression and risk for Alzheimer disease: systematic review, meta-analysis, and metaregression analysis. *Archives of General Psychiatry, 63*(5), 530–538.

Palazidou, E. (2012). The neurobiology of depression. *British Medical Bulletin, 101*, 127–145.

Pesonen, A. K., Räikkönen, K., Heinonen, K., Kajantie, E., Forsén, T., & Eriksson, J. G. (2007). Depressive symptoms in adults separated from their parents as children: A natural experiment during World War II. *American Journal of Epidemiology, 166*, 1126–1133.

Phelan, E., Williams, B., Meeker, K., Bonn, K., Frederick, J., Logerfo, J., & Snowden, M. (2010). A study of the diagnostic accuracy of the PHQ-9 in primary care elderly. *BMC Family Practice, 11*, 63.

Pickett, Y. R., Bazelais, K. N., & Bruce, M. L. (2013). Late-life depression in older African Americans: A comprehensive review of epidemiological and clinical data. *International Journal of Geriatric Psychiatry, 28*(9), 903–913.

Pinquart, M., Duberstein, P. R., & Lyness, J. M. (2006). Treatments for later-life depressive conditions: A meta-analytic comparison of pharmacotherapy and psychotherapy. *American Journal of Psychiatry, 163*, 1493–1501.

Prince, M. J., Harwood, R. H., Thomas, A., & Mann, A. H. (1998). A prospective population-based cohort study of the effects of disablement and social milieu on the onset and maintenance of late-life depression. The Gospel Oak Project VII. *Psychological Medicine, 28*(2), 337–350.

Raadsheer, F. C., Hoogendijk, W. J., Stam, F. C., Tilders, F. J., & Swaab, D. F. (1994). Increased number of corticotropin-releasing hormone expressing neurons in the hypothalamic paraventricular nucleus of depressed patients. *Neuroendocrinology, 60*(4), 436–444.

Radloff, L. S. The CES-D scale: A self-report depression scale for research in the general population. (1997). *Applied Psychological Measurement, 1*(3), 385–401.

Reynolds, C. F. 3rd (2009). The cutting edge: Prevention of depressive disorders. *Depression and Anxiety, 26*, 1062–1065.

Rice, E. H., Sombrotto, L. B., Markowitz, J. C., & Leon, A. C. (1994). Cardiovascular morbidity in high-risk patients during ECT. *American Journal of Psychiatry*, *151*, 1637-1641.

Riedel-Heller, S. G., Busse, A., & Angermeyer, M. C. (2006). The state of mental health in old-age across the "old" European Union: A systematic review. *Acta Psychiatrica Scandinavica*, *113*, 388-401.

Roberts, R. E., Kaplan, G. A., Shema, S. J., & Strawbridge, W. J. (1997). Does growing old increase the risk for depression? *American Journal of Psychiatry*, *154*(10), 1384-1390.

Robison, J., Gruman, C., Gaztambide, S., & Blank, K. (2002). Screening for depression in middle-aged and older Puerto Rican primary care patients. *Journals of Gerontology, Series A: Biological Sciences & Medical Sciences*, *57*(5), M308-M314.

Sackeim, H. A. (2004). Electroconvulsive therapy in late-life depression. In C. Salzman (Ed.), *Clinical geriatric psychopharmacology* (4th ed.). Baltimore, MD: Lippincott Williams & Wilkins, pp. 385–422.

Sarkisian, C. A., Lee-Henderson, M. H., & Mangione, C. M. (2003). Do depressed older adults who attribute depression to "old age" believe it is important to seek care? *Journal of General Internal Medicine*, *18*, 1001-1005.

Satariano, W. (2006). *Epidemiology of Aging: An Ecological Approach*. Jones and Bartlett Publishers. 424 pages. Sudbury, MA.

Schoevers, R. A., Smit, F., Deeg, D. J. H., Cuijpers, P., Dekker, J., van Tilburg, W., & Beekman, A. T. (2006). Prevention of late-life depression in primary care: Do we know where to begin? *American Journal of Psychiatry*, *163*, 1611–1621.

Schulz, R., & Sherwood, P. R. (2008). Physical and Mental Health Effects of Family Caregiving. *American Journal of Nursing*, *108*(9 Suppl), 23–27.

Schweitzer, I., Tuckwell, V., O'Brien, J., & Ames, D. (2002). Is late onset depression a prodrome to dementia? *International Journal of Geriatric Psychiatry*, *17*, 997–1005.

Sexton, C. E., Mackay, C.E., & Ebmeier, K. P. (2013). A systematic review and meta-analysis of magnetic resonance imaging studies in late-life depression. American Journal of Geriatric Psychiatry, 21(2),184–195.

Sheikh, J. I., & Yesavage, J. A. (1986). Geriatric Depression Scale (GDS): Recent evidence and development of a shorter version. *Clinical Gerontologist*, *5*, 165-173.

Sirey, J. A., Bruce, M. L., Alexopoulos, G. S., Perlick, D. A., Friedman, S. J., & Meyers, B. S. (2001). Stigma as a barrier to recovery: Perceived stigma and patient-rated severity of illness as predictors of antidepressant drug adherence. *Psychiatric Services*, *52*, 1615-1620.

Siu, A. L. & U.S. Preventive Services Task Force (USPSTF). (2016). Screening for depression in adults: U.S. Preventive Services Task Force recommendation statement. *Journal of the American Medical Association*, *315*(4), 380-387.

Sjösten, N., & Kivelä, S. L. (2006). The effects of physical exercise on depressive symptoms among the aged: A systematic review. *International Journal of Geriatric Psychiatry*, *21*, 410–418.

Skarupski, K. A., Mendes de Leon, C. F., Bienias, J. L., Barnes, L. L., Everson-Rose, S. A., Wilson, R. S., & Evans, D. A. (2005). Black-white differences in depressive symptoms among older adults over time. *Journal of Gerontology: Psychological Sciences*, *60B*(3), P136–P142.

Snowden, M. B., Atkins, D. C., Steinman, L. E., Bell, J. F., Bryant, L. L., Copeland, C., & Fitzpatrick, A. L. (2015). Longitudinal association of dementia and depression. *American Journal of Geriatric Psychiatry*, *23*(9), 897-905.

Snowden, M., Steinman, L., Frederick, J., & Wilson, N. (2009). Screening for depression in older adults: Recommended instruments and considerations for community-based practice. *Clinical Geriatrics*, 1-7.

Somervell, P. D., Leaf, P. J., Weissman, M. M., Blazer, D. G., & Bruce, M. L. (1989). The prevalence of major depression in black and white adults in five United States communities. *American Journal of Epidemiology*, *130*, 725–735.

Sonnenberg, C. M., Beekman, A. T., Deeg, D. J., & van Tilburg, W. (2000). Sex differences in late-life depression. *Acta Psychiatrica Scandinavica*, *101*, 286–292.

Spence, N. J., Adkins, D. E., & Dupre, M. E. (2011). Racial differences in depression trajectories among older women: Socioeconomic, family, and health influences. *Journal of Health and Social Behavior*, *52*(4), 444-459.

Spitzer, R. L., Williams, J. B., Kroenke, K., Linzer, M., deGruy III, F. V., Hahn, S. R.,… Johnson, J. G. (1994). Utility of a new procedure for diagnosing mental disorders in primary care: The PRIME-MD 1000 study. *Journal of the American Medical Association*, *272*(22), 1749–1756.

Steffens, D. C., Fisher, G. G., Langa, K. M., Potter, G. G., & Plassman, B. L. (2009). Prevalence of depression among older Americans: The Aging, Demographics and Memory Study. *International Psychogeriatrics*, *21*, 879–888.

Steffens, D. C., Skoog, I., Norton, M. C., Hart, A. D., Tschanz, J. T., Plassman, B. L.,… Breitner, J. C. (2000). Prevalence of depression and its treatment in an elderly population: The Cache County Study. *Archives of General Psychiatry*, *57*(6), 601–607.

Sullivan, M. D., Katon, W. J., Lovato, L. C., Miller, M. E., Murray, A. M., Horowitz, K. R.,… Launer, L. J. (2013). Association of depression with accelerated cognitive decline among patients with type 2 diabetes in the ACCORD-MIND trial. *JAMA Psychiatry*, *70*(10), 1041-1047.

Swenson, C. J., Baxter, J., Shetterly, S. M., Scarbro, S. L., & Hamman, R. F. (2000). Depressive symptoms in

Hispanic and non-Hispanic white rural elderly: The San Luis Valley Health and Aging Study. *American Journal of Epidemiology, 152,* 1048–1055.

Thota, A. B., Sipe, T. A., Byard, G. J., Zometa, C. S., Hahn, R. A., McKnight-Eily, L. R.,... Williams, S. P.; Community Preventive Services Task Force. (2012). Collaborative care to improve the management of depressive disorders: A Community Guide systematic review and meta-analysis. *American Journal of Preventive Medicine, 42*(5), 525–538.

Torges, C. M., Stewart, A. J., & Nolen-Hoeksema, S. (2008). Regret resolution, aging, and adapting to loss. *Psychology and Aging, 23,* 169–180.

Umberson, D., Wortman, C. B., & Kessler, R. C. (1992). Widowhood and depression: explaining long-term gender differences in vulnerability. *Journal of Health and Social Behavior, 33*(1), 10-24.

United States Preventive Services Task Force (USPSTF). (2016). Final recommendation statement: Depression in adults: Screening. *Journal of the American Medical Association, 315*(4), 380-387.

Unützer, J. (2007). Late-life depression. *New England Journal of Medicine, 357,* 2269-2276.

Unützer, J., Katon, W., Callahan, C. M., Williams, J. W., Jr., Hunkeler, E., Harpole, L.,... IMPACT Investigators. (2002). Collaborative care management of late-life depression in the primary care setting: A randomized controlled trial. *Journal of the American Medical Association, 288,* 2836-2845.

Unützer, J., Katon, W., Callahan, C. M., Williams, J. W., Jr., Hunkeler, E., Harpole, L.,... Oishi, S. (2003). Depression treatment in a sample of 1,801 depressed older adults in primary care. *Journal of the American Geriatric Society, 51,* 505-514.

Unützer, J., Tang, L., Oishi, S., Katon, W., Williams, J. W., Jr., Hunkeler, E.,... IMPACT Investigators. (2006). Reducing suicidal ideation in depressed older primary care patients. *Journal of the American Geriatric Society, 54,* 1550-1556.

van der Wurff, F. B., Stek, M. L., Hoogendijk, W. J., & Beekman, A. T. (2003). The efficacy and safety of ECT in depressed older adults: A literature review. *International Journal of Geriatric Psychiatry, 18,* 894-904.

Volkert, J., Schulz, H., Härter, M., Wlodarczyk, O., & Andreas, S. (2013). The prevalence of mental disorders in older people in Western countries—a meta-analysis. *Ageing Research Reviews, 12*(1), 339-353.

Wang, J. L., Schmitz, N., & Dewa, C. S. (2010). Socioeconomic status and the risk of major depression: The Canadian National Population Health Survey. *Journal of Epidemiology and Community Health, 64*(5), 447-452.

Whyte, E. M., Dew, M. A., Gildengers, A., Lenze, E., J., Bharucha, A., Mulsant, B. H., & Reynolds, C. F., 3rd. (2004). Time course of response to antidepressants in late-life major depression: Therapeutic implications. *Drugs and Aging, 21,* 531-554.

Williams, D. R., Gonzalez, H. M., Neighbors, H., Nesse, R., Abelson, J. M., Sweetman, J., & Jackson, J. S. (2007). Prevalence and distribution of major depressive disorder in African Americans, Caribbean blacks, and non-Hispanic whites: Results from the National Survey of American Life. *Archives of General Psychiatry, 64,* 305-315.

Williamson, G. M., & Shaffer, D. R. (2000). The activity restriction model of depressed affect: Antecedents and consequences of restricted normal activities. In G. M. Williamson, D. R, Shaffer, & P. A. Parmelee (Eds.), *Physical illness and depression in older adults: A handbook of theory, research, and practice* (pp. 173–200). New York, NY: Kluwer Academic/Plenum.

Wilson, K., Mottram, P., Sivanranthan, A., & Nightingale, A. (2001). Antidepressant versus placebo for depressed elderly. *Cochrane Database of Systematic Reviews,* 1, CD000561.

Wilson, K. C., Mottram, P. G., & Vassilas, C.A. (2008). Psychotherapeutic treatments for older depressed people. *Cochrane Database of Systematic Reviews, 1,* CD004853.

Woodward, A. T., Taylor, R. J., Bullard, K. M., Aranda, M. P., Lincoln, K. D., & Chatters, L. M. (2012). Prevalence of lifetime DSM-IV affective disorders among older African Americans, black Caribbeans, Latinos, Asians and non-Hispanic white people. *International Journal Of Geriatric Psychiatry, 27,* 816-827.

Wright, J. H. (2006). Cognitive behavior therapy: Basic principles and recent advances. *Focus, 4*(2), 173.

Xu, X., Liang, J., Bennett, J. M., Quinones, A. R., & Ye, W. (2010). Ethnic differences in the dynamics of depressive symptoms in middle aged and older Americans. *Journal of Aging and Health, 22*(5), 631–652.

Yang, Y. (2007). Is old age depressing? Growth trajectories and cohort variations in late-life depression. *Journal of Health and Social Behavior, 48*(1), 16–32.

Yesavage, J. A., Brink T. L., Rose, T. L., Lum, O., Huang, V., Adey, M. B. & Leirer, V. O. (1983). Development and validation of a geriatric depression screening scale: A preliminary report. *Journal of Psychiatric Research, 39,* 37–49.

Zimmerman, F. J., & Katon, W. (2005). Socioeconomic status, depression disparities, and financial strain: What lies behind the income-depression relationship? *Health Economics, 14*(12), 1197-1215.

Zuidersma, M., Conradi, H. J., van Melle, J. P., Ormel, J., & de Jonge, P. (2013). Depression treatment after myocardial infarction and long-term risk of subsequent cardiovascular events and mortality: A randomized controlled trial. *Journal of Psychosomatic Research, 74*(1), 25-30.

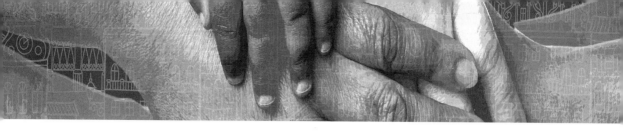

CHAPTER 8

Disease, Comorbidity, and Multimorbidity

Martin Fortin, Aline Ramond, Cynthia Boyd, and **Jose Almirall**

ABSTRACT

This chapter focuses on multimorbidity (MM), which refers to several coexisting health conditions in a single individual. MM negatively affects individuals' health-related outcomes (functional status, social participation, quality of life, life expectancy) and is also responsible for numerous impacts on society (healthcare utilization, direct and indirect costs). MM is now acknowledged as a research priority in health care, and in-depth understanding of its main determinants is required as a first step in this direction. After identifying MM-related essential definitions and concepts, this chapter successively addresses the role of sociodemographics, socioeconomic factors, social networks, social capital, genetics, lifestyle, psychological and psychosocial factors, and polypharmacy as potential risk factors for MM, following an ecological model of health. Finally, this chapter highlights current gaps in the literature as well as specific challenges, and suggests future directions for MM epidemiology research.

KEYWORDS

multimorbidity	measurement	polypharmacy
comorbidity	socioeconomic status	biopsychosocial
aging	lifestyle	treatment burden

▶ Introduction

This chapter focuses on **multimorbidity** (MM), which refers to several coexisting health conditions in a single individual. MM has generated growing interest in the last decades (Fortin, Soubhi, Hudo C, Bayliss, & van den Akker, 2007; Starfield, 2007) and is now acknowledged as a research priority in health care (Hummers-Pradier et al., 2010; Valderas, Starfield, & Roland, 2007). MM is very prevalent in the general population (Partnership

for Solutions, 2004; Rapoport, Jacobs, Bell, & Klarenbach, 2004); in fact, it now occurs so frequently that it is more the rule than the exception in both primary care (Fortin, Bravo, Hudon, Vanasse, & Lapointe, 2005) and hospital care (Steiner & Friedman, 2013).

MM is responsible for multiple individual consequences (Marengoni et al., 2011) (**FIGURE 8-1**). Patients living with MM experience a higher level of disability and functional decline (Garin et al., 2014; Jones, Amtmann, & Gell, 2015; McDaid et al., 2013; Ryan, Wallace,

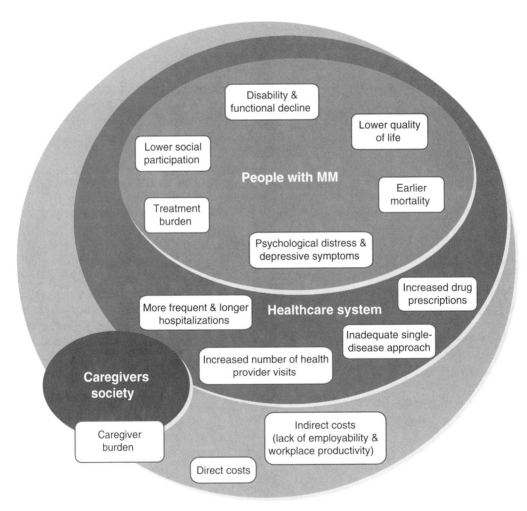

FIGURE 8-1 The impact of multimorbidity on people, the healthcare system, and society.
Contributed by: Martin Fortin, Aline Ramond, Cynthia Boyd, and Jose Almirall.

chronicity itself is still debated. Duration (with thresholds most often varying from 3 to 12 months) as well as other characteristics such as etiology, onset, need for medical attention, recurrence/pattern, prognosis, sequelae, severity, nonamenability to cure, and prevalence have all been suggested as means by which to determine whether a condition is chronic (Goodman, Posner, Huang, Parekh, & Koh, 2013; O'Halloran, Miller, & Britt, 2004).

Finally, another source of variability in the definition of MM is the number of conditions considered as "multiple." Consensual agreement on a given number is not essential for clinical purpose, of course, because the situations with multiple long-term conditions that patients and clinicians may face are arrayed on a continuum rather than appearing on an "on-off" scale. In contrast, the operational definition of MM, including a minimal number of conditions, is crucial for research purposes (Fortin, Mercer, & Salisbury, 2014). Most authors have used either a minimum of two or three conditions to define MM (Goodman et al., 2013; Harrison, Britt, Miller, & Henderson, 2014), but others have proposed four or even five conditions as valuable cutoffs (Almirall & Fortin, 2013; Fortin et al., 2014). Researchers must acknowledge that the meaning of a specific number of conditions depends both on the number of possible conditions considered and on the specific conditions that are present.

Finally, MM should be distinguished from several related concepts. *Disability* can be defined as any restriction, difficulty, or dependency in carrying out activities "in the manner or within the range considered normal for a human being" (WONCA Classification Committee, 1995). *Frailty* has been suggested to be "a dynamic state affecting an individual who experiences losses in one or more domains of human functioning (physical, psychological, social), which is caused by the influence of a range of variables and which increases the risk of adverse outcomes" (Gobbens, Luijkx, Wijnen-Sponselee, & Schols, 2010). *MM burden* refers to "the overall impact of the different diseases in an individual taking into account their severity" (Valderas, Starfield, Sibbald, Salisbury, & Roland, 2009). *Patient complexity* encompasses MM burden as well as non-health-related factors, such as socioeconomic, cultural, environmental, and patient behavior characteristics that interact "to make clinical management more or less challenging, time-consuming, and resource intensive" (Valderas et al., 2009). Finally, *serious illness* has been recently defined as "a condition that carries a high risk of mortality, negatively impacts quality of life and daily function, and/or is burdensome in symptoms, treatments, or caregiver stress" (Kelley, 2014).

All of these concepts are strongly interrelated but should be cautiously distinguished to better understand health and improve care services (Fried, Ferrucci, Darer, Williamson, & Anderson, 2004; Valderas et al., 2009). A significant portion of people whose situation matches one or more of these definitions have MM. On the other side, people with MM do not always experience disability, frailty, complexity, or serious illness. Operational definitions of MM based on the number of conditions present encompass people with highly varying levels of health status, including some with extremely severe medical conditions and others who experience far less disease burden. This continuum of severity implies that everyone with MM does not need the same type of care. Nevertheless, some general principles (such as continuity, coordination, and patient-centeredness) may apply to the organization and the delivery of health care for the benefit of everyone with MM.

Measurement

Many MM measurement tools have been proposed and used in the literature, in different populations, with more or less evaluation of their validity and reliability (de Groot, Beckerman, Lankhorst, & Bouter, 2003; Diederichs, Berger, & Bartels, 2011; Huntley, Johnson, Purdy, Valderas, & Salisbury, 2012). Some examples are presented in **TABLE 8-1**.

TABLE 8-1 Examples of Tools or Lists Used to Measure Multimorbidity and Their Main Characteristics

	Modified CIRS	DBMA	Barnett's List	Tonelli's List	Charlson
Nature of items	Body systems	Chronic conditions	Chronic conditions	Chronic conditions	Diseases or group of diseases
Number of items	14	25	40	30	30
Type of tool	Index	Index	Count	Count	Index
Weighting of items	Provider's assessment of severity	Interference with daily activities	None	None	Empirically derived relative risk for 1-year mortality
Source of data	Medical records	Patient's self-report	Medical records	Administrative data	Medical records
Main publication	Salvi et al., 2008	Bayliss, Ellis, & Steiner, 2005	Barnett et al., 2012	Tonelli et al., 2015	Charlson, Pompei, Ales, & MacKenzie, 1987

Abbreviations: CIRS=Cumulative Illness Rating Scale; DBMA=Disease Burden Morbidity Assessment.

Contributed by: Martin Fortin, Aline Ramond, Cynthia Boyd, and Jose Almirall.

A wide heterogeneity exists in the preestablished lists of conditions considered to measure MM. As few as 4 conditions to as many as 102 conditions have been included in such lists (Diederichs et al., 2011), and some authors have even suggested the use of open lists of conditions for a more comprehensive evaluation (Fortin et al., 2005). Most tools consider individual conditions, groups of conditions, or body systems (e.g., diseases of the respiratory system), whereas others consider proxies for the existence of chronic conditions, especially classes of medications (Fishman et al., 2003). All of these measures can be classified into two main categories: those that are based on a simple count of conditions, often called "diseases counts," and those that apply weighting to each condition, often called "indexes" (Diederichs et al., 2011). For indexes, three main methods of weighting have been applied to the conditions identified: based on the patient's self-reported impact of each condition (Bayliss, Ellis, & Steiner, 2005); on the severity of each condition, as assessed by a care provider (Linn, Linn, & Gurel, 1968); or on empirically derived weights according to the individual impact of each disease on specific outcomes (e.g., mortality) (Byles, D'Este, Parkinson,

O'Connell, & Treloar, 2005; Charlson, Pompei, Ales, & MacKenzie, 1987).

Sources of data used to measure MM also vary among the studies. Some use patients' self-reports, whereas others rely on patient interviews conducted by providers, medical chart reviews, or medico-administrative data (Diederichs et al., 2011).

Finally, the results from these instruments can be used in different ways—that is, as binary, ordinal, or continuous variables. In the case of binary variables derived from counts of conditions, different cutoffs have been proposed for the number of conditions required to meet the MM designation (most often two or three, rarely four, but sometimes even five).

Use of different measurement tools has resulted in large variation in MM prevalence estimates (Fortin, Stewart, Poitras, Almirall, & Maddocks, 2012; Harrison et al., 2014)

(**FIGURE 8-3**), in quality of life estimates (Fortin et al., 2005; Ramond-Roquin, Haggerty, Lambert, Almirall, & Fortin, 2016), and in validity of MM to predict functioning, healthcare utilization, or mortality (Boeckxstaens et al., 2015; Brilleman SL, Salisbury, 2013). The large number of available measurement tools has, therefore, made it very difficult to compare results from different studies and especially to determine to what extent the differences observed are attributable to real population differences versus methodological differences in relation to MM measures (Fortin et al., 2012; Stewart, Fortin, Britt, Harrison, & Maddocks, 2013). This ambiguity calls for some standardization in MM measurement, along with careful consideration of these methodological aspects of the research when studying MM. At the same time, it is important to acknowledge that different definitions of MM may be relevant, depending on the

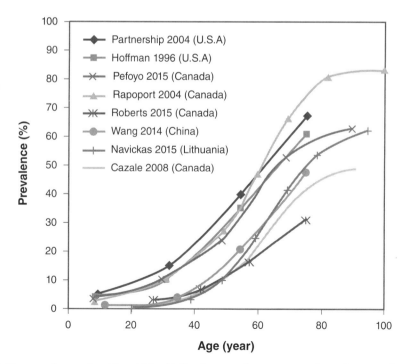

FIGURE 8-3 The prevalence of multimorbidity (defined as two diseases or more) as a function of age, in the general population.

Contributed by Martin Fortin, Aline Ramond, Cynthia Boyd, and Jose Almirall based on previously published data (5, 6, 85, 89, 96, 100, 208, 209), and using the methodology described in a previous literature review (78). Prevalence data have been estimated in the primary studies either using lists from 7 to 40 conditions, or taking into account all chronic conditions classified in ICD-9 codes.

PEARL 8-1 Randomized Controlled Trials for the Study of MM

In the Cochrane systematic review of interventions to improve outcomes for people with MM in primary care and community settings, Smith et al. (2016) identified 18 generally well-designed randomized controlled trials meeting the eligibility criteria. The majority of studies examined interventions that involved changes to the organization of care delivery, although some studies had more patient-focused interventions. Overall, the results regarding the effectiveness of interventions were mixed, but suggested that interventions designed to target specific risk factors and those that focus on difficulties that people experience with daily functioning may be more effective.

According to Susan Smith, "This review identifies the emerging evidence to support policy for the management of people with multimorbidity in primary care and community settings. There are remaining uncertainties about the effectiveness of interventions for people with multimorbidity given the relatively small number of randomized controlled trials conducted in this area to date, with mixed findings overall. However, several large ongoing studies were identified that will add to the slowly emerging evidence base."

objective of the research. Having two or more of a long list of conditions may be a relevant definition for epidemiological purposes in active adults from the general population, whereas using indexes that evaluate both number and impact of conditions may be more appropriate for some clinical purposes, such as identifying people with serious illness who need a high-intensity intervention (Harrison et al., 2014; Marengoni et al., 2011; Valderas et al., 2009).

Epidemiology of MM

Prevalence of MM is known to be high in the general population, especially in aging people, but estimates vary significantly depending on both the samples and the methods used to measure it (Marengoni et al., 2011; Fortin et al., 2012). Prevalence of MM, defined as two or more chronic conditions, has been estimated in people older than 65 years in many different countries. It was found to vary between 3% and 45% when considering only a limited number of conditions (five to nine) (Afshar, Roderick, Kowal, Dimitrov, & Hill, 2015; Alaba & Chola, 2013; Cazale & Dumitru, 2008; Menotti et al., 2001; Taylor et al., 2010), and between 33% and 72% when using longer lists (14 or more conditions) (Barnett et al., 2012; Diaz, Poblador-Pou, et al., 2015; Partnership for Solutions,

2004; Schram et al., 2008; Uijen & van de Lisdonk, 2008; van den Akker, Buntinx, Metsemakers, & Knottnerus, 1998; van den Bussche et al., 2011; Wang et al., 2014).

Prevalence of MM, defined as having two or more chronic conditions among a list of 10 conditions, increased from 21.8% to 26.0% between 2001 and 2010 in the noninstitutionalized U.S. adult population (Ward & Schiller, 2013). Such a significant increase in prevalence has also been reported in other countries over the last two decades, both in the general population and in populations receiving primary care (Fu, Huang, & Chou, 2014; Pefoyo et al., 2014; Uijen & van de Lisdonk, 2008; Vos et al., 2015). Studies suggest that the proportion of people with three or more conditions has increased the most, while the proportion of people with one or two conditions has remained quite stable. Interestingly, the highest increases in MM were reported in young people (in persons younger than 18 years, followed by persons age 18 to 45 years).

Prevalence of MM may be higher in Western (developed) countries (Barnett et al., 2012; Britt, Harrison, Miller, & Knox, 2008; Fuchs, Busch, Lange, & Scheidt-Nave, 2012; Roberts, Rao, Bennett, Loukine, & Jayaraman, 2015; Ward, Schiller, & Goodman, 2014) than in non-Western (emerging) countries (Afshar et al., 2015; Pati et al., 2014), but this suspicion is mainly supported by indirect comparisons between methodologically heterogeneous studies. Some international studies, based on a single protocol, also suggest that prevalence of MM varies significantly depending on region of the world (Afshar et al., 2015; Arokiasamy et al., 2015; Garin et al., 2015). However, these studies have limitations in relation to either the number of countries studied or the MM measure, which prevents researchers from drawing firm conclusions in this regard. Beyond the figures, the nature of the chronic conditions contributing to MM also differs according to the region of the world (Garin et al., 2015). For example, even if prevalence of MM in adults older than 50 years was only slightly higher in South Africa (63.4%) than in India (57.9%), the prevalence of hypertension (78.3% versus 37.5%) and obesity (46.9% versus 2.5%) were much higher, whereas the prevalence of cataracts (6.4% versus 47.4%) was dramatically lower. These findings illustrate the need for considering a large range of conditions, some of which may be more or less prevalent or impactful depending on the country, when measuring MM prevalence on an international scale.

Incidence of MM has been studied less often than prevalence (Marengoni et al., 2011). In 1998, van den Akker estimated the 1-year incidence of MM to be 1.3% in a study sample comparable to the Dutch population, but the incidence was defined as the number of people with two or more new diagnoses during a given year divided by the total number of people, including a significant part already having MM (van den Akker, Buntinx, Metsemakers, Roos, & Knottnerus, 1998). More recently, St Sauver et al. (2015) estimated the incidence of MM, defined as the proportion of people with newly diagnosed MM (i.e., diagnosed with two or more conditions) among U.S. people with no or only one condition at baseline. Based on a cohort with a mean follow-up of 10.8 years, they found the MM incidence to be 3.7 cases per 100 person-years. Aging people

were at higher risk for incident MM in both of these studies. In comparison to the figures for the general population presented earlier, the 1-year "incidence" was 3.5% for those persons between 60 and 79 years old and 5.9% in those older than 80 years (van den Akker et al., 1998), while incident rates were 19.7 cases per 100 person-years in people older than 65 years (St Sauver et al., 2015). Unsurprisingly, incidence of MM is higher in people who already have a chronic condition than in those without any condition (Melis, Marengoni, Angleman, & Fratiglioni, 2014; Wikstrom, Lindstrom, Harald, Peltonen, & Laatikainen, 2015).

Patterns and Classifications of MM

The nature of the chronic conditions combined in individuals define different patterns of MM. Better description of the frequent patterns of MM might be expected to improve diagnosis and management of patients with MM as well as to ensure better alignment of the care organization and services with population needs (Schäfer et al., 2010; Violan, Foguet-Boreu, Flores-Mateo, et al., 2014). Unsurprisingly, combinations of the most frequently occurring individual conditions (such as hypertension, dyslipidemia, diabetes, and osteoarthritis) account for a significant part of total MM (Steinman et al., 2012; van den Bussche et al., 2011; Violan, Foguet-Boreu, Flores-Mateo, et al., 2014). Three categories of patterns have been consistently suggested to be very prevalent in the elderly (cumulative prevalence from 33% to 50%), involving (1) cardiometabolic diseases, (2) psychogeriatric problems, and (3) mechanical and somatoform disorders (Abad-Diez et al., 2014; Cornell et al., 2007; Poblador-Plou et al., 2014; Prados-Torres et al., 2012; Schäfer et al., 2010; van den Bussche et al., 2011; Violan, Foguet-Boreu, Roso-Llorach, et al., 2014) (**FIGURE 8-4**). The most frequent patterns of MM probably slightly differ between countries (Garin et al., 2015).

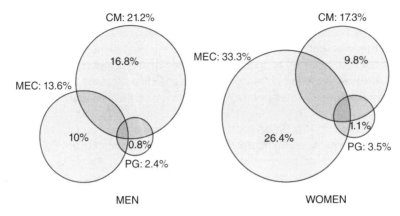

FIGURE 8-4 Overlapping of the main multimorbidity patterns, in older men and women.

To further characterize the diversity of MM patterns, several classifications have been proposed, based on the type of link between the co-occurring conditions. Unfortunately, the inconsistency in the terms used in the literature regarding these classifications has led to some confusion. A first group of classifications has distinguished between any situation where several conditions coexist (called "concurrent" or "simple" MM), situations where conditions coexist more frequently than what would be expected from a random distribution of each condition (called "cluster" or "associative" MM), and situations where conditions share risk factors or a physiopathological pathway, or where one condition is a prerequisite for the occurrence of the other (called "causal" MM) (Schellevis, 1993; van den Akker et al., 1996). Exploration of cluster and causal MM is especially important from an etiological perceptive, as it may be possible to prevent MM development in some cases (Violan, Foguet-Boreu, Flores-Mateo, et al., 2014). Comparisons between the distribution of patterns observed in large populations and the distribution expected by random chance have allowed exploration of cluster of MM. Patterns that include gout or osteoarthritis, for example, have been shown to be among the combinations with the highest ratios observed/

expected (van den Bussche et al., 2011). Moreover, certain conditions (such as hypertension and dyslipidemia) have been found more frequently than expected in patterns including a limited number of conditions, while other conditions (such as chronic low back pain and peripheral arterial occlusive disease) have been suggested to be more frequent than expected in patterns including a large number of conditions (Schafer, 2012).

Other classifications have been designed from a clinical management perspective. Concordant MM refers to combinations of conditions that can be managed synergistically (e.g., diabetes, hypertension, and coronary atherosclerosis), whereas discordant MM comprises conditions that do not share the same clinical management (Magnan et al., 2015; Piette & Kerr, 2006; Valderas et al., 2014). Quality of care may be better in the case of concordant MM and worse in the case of discordant MM, due to the increased complexity faced by the patient's providers (Lagu et al., 2008; Magnan et al., 2015; Zulman et al., 2014). This distinction may inform the definition of priorities when efforts are made to improve care for people with MM.

Different patterns of MM result in different impacts. This reality has been especially demonstrated with quality of life (Fortin, Dubois,

Hudon, Soubhi, & Almirall, 2007; Mujica-Mota et al., 2015; Rijken, van Kerkhof, Dekker, & Schellevis, 2005; Vos, Bor, Rangelrooij-Minkels, Schellevis, & Lagro-Janssen, 2013) and with healthcare-associated costs (Schoenberg, Kim, Edwards, & Fleming, 2007). The variable effects argue for in-depth characterization of MM in the population of interest when studying MM and its related outcomes.

Only recently has research on MM patterns been undertaken in earnest, and its implications for improving health practices and policies have yet to be demonstrated. Moreover, this approach faces an important methodological challenge in relation to the data needed to study MM patterns. Characterizing patterns based on a limited number of conditions will lead to the same flaws as when studying MM and related outcomes—namely, missing potentially important health problems and producing biased estimates. On the other side, using long lists of conditions can become counterproductive. Indeed, the number of different patterns grows exponentially with the number of candidate conditions considered. Analyzing such detailed data often requires drastic simplification methods to reduce it to an understandable level. As an example, van den Bussche et al. (2011) studied MM patterns based on a list of 46 candidate conditions and identified 15,024 (from the theoretically possible 15,180) different triads of conditions and 832,589 (from the theoretically possible 1,370,754) different combinations of five conditions! These researchers finally focused their analyses first on the 10 most prevalent triads, and then on the 100 most prevalent triads. The optimal degree of granularity for analysis related to patterns is not known, however, and some standardization on other methodological aspects is required to make the results comparable between different studies (Boyd et al., 2010; Sorace et al., 2011; Weiss, Boyd, Yu, Wolff, & Leff, 2007).

The next section presents in detail the current knowledge about the diverse determinants of MM. Sociodemographics and socio-economic factors have been extensively studied as potential risk factors for MM. In contrast, research focusing on social networks, social capital, genetics, lifestyle, psychological and psychosocial factors, and **polypharmacy** has been undertaken only more recently and remains fragmented. Finally, some other factors, such as the physical environment or biological factors, may be worthy of consideration as potential determinants of MM, as either etiologic or modulating factors (Marengoni et al., 2011).

▶ Sociodemographics

Age and MM

Age is certainly the most frequently studied risk factor of MM (Violan, Foguet-Boreu, Flores-Mateo, et al., 2014). All research results converge to show that prevalence and incidence of MM steeply increase with age (Fortin et al., 2012; Marengoni et al., 2011; St Sauver et al., 2015; Violan, Foguet-Boreu, Flores-Mateo, et al., 2014) (Figure 8-3). Although prevalence highly varies across studies, it is estimated to be approximately 20% to 30% for the adult population as whole, and between 55% and 98% among the elderly (Marengoni et al., 2011). Compared to incidence rates for 40- to 49-year-old people, incidence rates have been estimated to be about 3 to 5 times higher in the 60- to 69-year-old group, and about 5 to 8 times in those older than 80 years (St Sauver et al., 2015).

When using "having two or more conditions" to define MM, prevalence particularly increases between 25 and 75 years of age, but then reaches a plateau; in contrast, when using "having three or more conditions" as the definition of MM, prevalence is lower but still increases with age after 75 years (Brett et al., 2013; Fortin et al., 2012; Harrison et al., 2014). Certain regions of the world, however, present quite different patterns in this regard, due to specific morbidity. For example, MM prevalence gradually decreases after 60 years in South Africa—a phenomenon that has been attributed to the prevalence of HIV, whose rates are extremely high in young people but much lower in the elderly (Garin et al., 2015).

Interestingly, the absolute number of people with prevalent MM, and especially those with incident MM, is much larger among young people (younger than age 65 years) than among older ones, making the situation of MM not specific to elderly people (Barnett et al., 2012; St Sauver et al., 2015).

MM leads to very heterogeneous clinical situations. Beyond prevalence or incidence, aging is associated with both a larger number of chronic conditions (Pefoyo et al., 2015; van den Bussche et al., 2011; Vos, van den Akker, Boesten, Robertson, & Metsemakers, 2015) and a larger number of morbidity domains (Britt et al., 2008). Patterns of MM also differ with age (St Sauver et al., 2015; Steinman et al., 2012; Violan, Foguet-Boreu, Roso-Llorach, et al., 2014). In particular, among people older than 65 years, prevalence of conditions from the cardiometabolic and psychogeriatric patterns still increases with age, while prevalence of those associated with musculoskeletal and pain-related patterns is not correlated with age (Abad-Diez et al., 2014; Prados-Torres et al., 2012; Schafer et al., 2012). Moreover, conditions within patterns also evolve with age: Within the cardiometabolic pattern, for example, young adults mainly present with cardiometabolic risk factors, while combinations including cardiovascular complications are more frequently encountered in older people (Prados-Torres et al., 2012).

Finally, aging progressively results in increased burden of MM. Compared to middle-aged people with a similar number of conditions, those older than 75 years experience greater limitation in their daily activities and lower self-rated health status (McDaid et al., 2013). Perhaps differences in the nature of conditions themselves (e.g., risk factors in middle age versus symptomatic complications in older people) or the higher frequency of frailty in older people is the factor that increases their risk of adverse outcomes for a given situation. Interestingly, although experiencing greater limitation and lower health status (McDaid et al., 2013), older people in this study report a similar level of quality of life when they co-occur in the presence of other conditions (McDaid et al., 2013). This suggests older people with MM possess some sort of resilience—namely, an ability to face and positively adapt to their impaired health status, which may include an increasing level of disability (Coatta, 2008). The literature has also suggested that increasing age is associated with increasing healthcare utilization, in terms of number of visits, medications received, and hospitalizations.

Gender and MM

MM may be slightly more frequent in women than in men (Uijen & van de Lisdonk, 2008; Violan, Foguet-Boreu, Roso-Llorach, et al., 2014; Walker, 2007) but this association has been found inconsistently in the literature (Britt et al., 2008; Prados-Torres et al., 2012; Schafer et al., 2012; van den Bussche et al., 2011). Moreover, incidence of MM seems to be quite similar in men and women (St Sauver et al., 2015; van den Akker et al., 1998).

More interestingly, men and women present some significant differences in terms of patterns of MM (Figure 8-4). Although these patterns are frequent and largely overlap in both genders, mechanical patterns are the most prevalent in old women, while cardiometabolic patterns dominate in old men, (Abad-Diez et al., 2014, Schafer et al., 2012; Schafer et al., 2014). Some (less prevalent) patterns seem to be quite specific to persons of one gender, such as psychiatric–substance abuse in (young) men and depressive patterns in women (Prados-Torres et al., 2012).

Ethnicity and MM

Research results have been consistent in suggesting that ethnicity is a determinant of MM.

Indeed, prevalence of MM differs between populations of different ethnicities living in the same geographic area, and this difference persists even after taking into account the main sociodemographic determinants of MM. This issue has been especially studied in the United States, where African Americans present with higher rates of MM while Hispanics, Asians, and Pacific Islanders present with lower rates of MM in comparison to non-Hispanic Caucasians (Cabassa et al., 2013; Lochner & Cox, 2013; Ward & Schiller, 2013). Within the Canadian general population, Aboriginal status is associated with higher prevalence of MM, especially in the oldest groups of individuals (50 to 64 years, and to an even greater extent in the 65-plus population) (Roberts et al., 2015). Higher risk of MM in Aboriginal people was also found in a sample of marginalized people in Australia (Brett et al., 2014). In a rare study that explored the link between ethnicity and incidence, the results were aligned with those related to prevalence: Incidence was found to be higher in blacks and lower in Asians, compared to whites, in the United States (St Sauver et al., 2015).

Differences in the prevalence and incidence of MM according to ethnicity are not unexpected, given that several frequently observed chronic conditions show comparable patterns in relation to ethnic groups. For example, African Americans have especially elevated prevalence of hypertension, kidney disease, diabetes, and asthma (Blackwell & Lucas, 2014; Centers for Disease Control and Prevention [CDC], 2011; Gold & Wright, 2005). Genetic determinants, as well as cultural elements, may partly explain the differences observed. In addition, socioeconomic factors probably play a significant role in these ethnic minorities, either directly or indirectly. Indeed, deprived people often have more difficulties engaging in healthy lifestyles. Moreover, they often experience poorer access to health care and receive poorer quality of medical care, as described in the inverse care law (Mercer, Guthrie, Furler, Watt, & Hart, 2012; Mercer & Watt, 2007).

▶ Socioeconomic Factors

Socioeconomic Status and MM

Socioeconomic status (SES) constitutes a major risk factor for MM. People with lower education and those with lower income present with significantly higher prevalence of MM (Marengoni et al., 2011; Violan, Foguet-Boreu, Flores-Mateo, et al., 2014). This association has been shown to exist based on many different individual indicators, such as low number of years of education, low income, childhood financial hardship, social assistance, consulting in a mobile street health clinic (rather than in a mainstream primary healthcare setting), or illiteracy (Alaba & Chola, 2013; Brett et al., 2014; Ha, Le, Khanal, & Moorin, 2015; Marengoni, Winblad, Karp, & Fratiglioni, 2008; Schafer et al., 2012; Sinnott, McHugh, Fitzgerald, Bradley, & Kearney, 2015; Taylor et al., 2010; Tucker-Seeley, Li, Sorensen, & Subramanian, 2011; Uijen & van de Lisdonk, 2008; van den Akker et al., 1998; van den Bussche et al., 2011). Similarly, at an ecological level, prevalence of MM is higher in highly deprived areas, characterized by lack of car ownership, overcrowded households, households that are not owner-occupied, and unemployment (Barnett et al., 2012; Salisbury, Johnson, Purdy, Valderas, & Montgomery, 2011). Finally, at a country level, an international study has observed that there is a positive relationship between national gross domestic product per capita and MM prevalence, at least among low- and middle-income countries (Afshar et al., 2015).

This socioeconomic gradient (i.e., the progressive increase in prevalence of MM with lower SES) exists across all age groups but seems to be more important in middle-aged individuals (Barnett et al., 2012; Brett et al., 2014; Britt et al., 2008) (**FIGURE 8-5**). Moreover, the gradient is quite consistent within different populations over the world (Afshar et al., 2015; Arokiasamy et al., 2015), including within marginalized and impoverished populations (Habib, Hojeij, Elzein, Chaaban, &

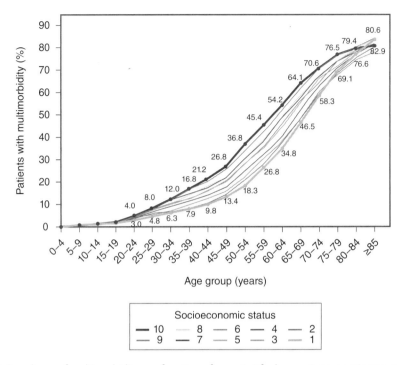

FIGURE 8-5 Prevalence of multimorbidity as a function of age, stratified on socioeconomic status.

Reproduced from: Barnett K, Mercer SW, Norbury M, Watt G, Wyke S, Guthrie B. Epidemiology of multimorbidity and implications for health care, research, and medical education: a cross-sectional study. Lancet. 2012;380(9836):37-43.

Seyfert, 2014), despite large differences in MM prevalence.

Low SES is also associated with earlier onset (Barnett et al., 2012; Brett et al., 2014), with MM occurring 10 to 15 years earlier in the most deprived people in comparison to the most affluent, and with a larger number of chronic conditions (Brett et al., 2014; Jackson, Dobson, Tooth, & Mishra, 2015). Different patterns of MM can be observed depending on SES. Cardiometabolic patterns and patterns including mental health problems or musculoskeletal disorders, for example, seem to be more frequent in more deprived and less educated people (Barnett et al., 2012; Brett et al., 2014; Schafer et al., 2012).

This association between SES and MM may be explained by several complementary hypotheses. Individuals with lower SES often present higher levels of exposure to other risk factors for MM. In particular, obesity may be a significant mediator between SES and MM (Nagel et al., 2008). Individuals with lower SES also more often experience the "inverse care law," which states that "the availability of good medical care tends to vary inversely with the need for it in the population served" (Hart, 1971). As a consequence, these patients present to their providers with situations of higher complexity (mixing MM burden and non-health-related factors), on the one hand, and they have poorer access to the healthcare system, the lengths of their patient–provider consultations are shorter, they have more difficulty discussing their health issues with their physicians, and they feel less enabled, on the other hand (Mercer et al., 2012; Mercer & Watt, 2007). Collectively, these elements may contribute to individuals with low SES receiving poorer preventive and curative care, which in turn may increase their risk of MM and related outcomes.

▸ Immigration and MM

Two recent studies have suggested that being an immigrant is associated with lower risk of MM. In comparison to a Canadian-born population, immigrants to Canada presented with lower risk of MM, especially when their immigration was recent (i.e., living in Canada for less than 5 years) (Britt et al., 2008). In Norway, compared to Norwegian-born individuals, first-generation migrants also presented with lower risk, depending on the area of origin. Indeed, the risk difference was small for people from Western Europe and North America, and more importantly for those from Eastern Europe, Asia, Africa, and Latin America (Diaz, Poblador-Pou, et al., 2015).

These observations may seem surprising given that immigrants more often face socioeconomic challenges, such as financial difficulties, unemployment, or lack of health insurance (Singh & Hiatt, 2006). Nevertheless, several phenomena may contribute to these results. First, immigrants generally represent a healthy subgroup of the population of their original country and are healthier than the population of their new country, as suggested by the "healthy immigrant theory" (Razum, Zeeb, & Rohrmann, 2000). Aligned with that theory, they have healthier lifestyles than the host population (Singh & Hiatt, 2006). Moreover, according to the "salmon bias" theory, some older and sicker migrants come back to their country of birth, leading to a decrease in the morbidity patterns observed within the (remaining) migrant population (Razum et al., 2000). Finally, some important differences probably exist between immigrants whose resettlement is motivated by labor and education concerns, on the one hand, and refugees, on the other hand, with the latter group being exposed to many more health problems in general and higher risk of MM in particular (Diaz, Kumar, et al., 2015; Pfortmueller et al., 2013).

▸ Living Arrangements, Social Networks, Social Support, and MM

Living alone or being separated, divorced, or widowed has been associated with higher prevalence of MM (Arokiasamy et al., 2015; Taylor et al., 2010; van den Akker, Buntinx, Metsemakers, van der Aa, & Knottnerus, 2001; van den Bussche et al., 2011). This association remains after adjusting on the main other predictors of MM and seems to exist within different age groups (Taylor et al., 2010). Moreover, being involved in multiple social networks (such as those related to work and study activities, or to sports and leisure activities) may protect individuals from having or from developing MM (van den Akker, Buntinx, Metsemakers, & Knottnerus, 2000; van den Akker et al., 2001). To our knowledge, no study has explored the link between social support and MM prevalence or incidence. Rather, several different studies have shown that social support may contribute to better outcomes in individuals with MM (Sells et al., 2009; Warner et al., 2011).

▸ Social Capital and MM

Social capital refers to "those features of social structures—such as levels of interpersonal trust and norms of reciprocity and mutual aid—which act as resources for individuals and facilitate collective action" (Berkman & Kawachi, 2000). Thus, it is a characteristic of populations and communities, rather than a characteristic of individuals.

Some works suggest that social capital may be associated with higher self-rated health or with better health outcomes in individuals with chronic conditions, including MM (Hu et al., 2014; Waverijn et al., 2014). To date, few studies have investigated social capital as a risk factor for MM.

PEARL 8-2 Caring for People with MM: Complexity for People with Multiple Chronic Conditions, Their Family and Friends, and Their Providers

Providing person-centered, evidence-based care for older adults with MM is challenging. Although evidence-based clinical practice guidelines exist for many conditions, most focus on the management of the disease as a stand-alone entity and do not address the question of how to integrate care for people with MM. The cumulative effects of following single-disease clinical practice guidelines in older adults with MM may result in care that is impractical, irrelevant, or even harmful.

More than 40% of community-dwelling older adults may experience treatment burden, and 30% of older adults share or delegate what is commonly thought of as "self-management" to family members or friends (Wolff & Boyd, 2015). Strategies to address this population include that proposed by the American Geriatrics Society's Guiding Principles for the Care of Older Adults with Multimorbidity (http://www.americangeriatrics.org/files/documents/MCC.principles.pdf).

Five guiding principles apply when caring for people with MM:

- Elicit and incorporate patient preferences into medical decision-making for older adults with MM.
- While recognizing the limitations of the evidence base, interpret and apply the medical literature specifically to older adults with MM.
- Frame clinical management decisions within the context of risks, burdens, benefits, and prognosis (e.g., remaining life expectancy, functional status, quality of life) for older adults with MM.
- Consider treatment complexity and feasibility when making clinical management decisions for older adults with MM.
- Use strategies for choosing therapies that optimize benefit, minimize harm, and enhance quality of life for older adults with MM.

Civic participation, as measured by individual associational involvement, was found not to be associated with MM prevalence in two different studies in South Africa (Alaba & Chola, 2013) and in Canada (Veenstra et al., 2005).

▶ Genetics and MM

As mentioned earlier, some chronic conditions coexist more frequently than would be expected from a random distribution of each condition. In line with this observation, certain genetic variants have been identified as risk factors for co-occurrence of specific conditions, or specific patterns of MM, in the case of both mental and somatic MM.

In the case of mental MM, nicotine dependence and alcohol dependence have been associated with a candidate single-nucleotide polymorphism (Wen, Schaid, & Lu, 2013). Also, evidence strongly suggests that the coexistence of autism spectrum disorders with coordination disorders, tic disorders, and learning problems is due to a common genetic liability in the majority of children with this MM (Lichtenstein, Carlstrom, Rastam, Gillberg, & Anckarsater, 2010).

Among the somatic clusters of MM, metabolic syndrome—in which central obesity coexists with two or more factors that include dyslipidemia, hypertension, and diabetes (International Diabetes Federation, 2006)—has been associated with genetic polymorphisms predisposing individuals to this syndrome (Chang et al., 2016; Herrera et al., 2016). Also, some findings suggest that the concomitant presence of allergic diseases (asthma, rhinitis, and atopic dermatitis), which is often observed in children and known as allergic MM, may be the result of common causal mechanisms and risk factors that are only partly mediated by immunoglobulin E (IgE) (Bousquet et al., 2015). In this sense, it has been hypothesized that common causal mechanisms of allergic MM may be associated with fetal genes from the mesoderm (Th2 signaling) (Bousquet et al., 2015).

▶ Lifestyle

The association between lifestyle risk factors and MM has been explored for obesity (as a proxy of dietetic lifestyle) (Agborsangaya, Ngwakongnwi, Lahtinen, Cooke, & Johnson, 2013; Alaba & Chola, 2013; Booth, Prevost, & Gulliford, 2014; Britt et al., 2008; de Souza Santos Machado et al., 2013; de Souza Santos Machado, Valadares, da Costa-Paiva, Moraes, & Pinto-Neto, 2012; Fortin et al., 2014; Jackson et al., 2015; Nagel et al., 2008; Sinnott et al., 2015; Taylor et al., 2010; van den Akker et al., 2000; Wikstrom et al., 2015), lack of physical activity (Autenrieth et al., 2013; Britt et al., 2008; Fortin et al., 2014; Jackson et al., 2015; Sinnott et al., 2015; van den Akker et al., 2000; Wikstrom et al., 2015), nutrition (Britt et al., 2008; Fortin et al., 2014; Nagel et al., 2008; Ruel et al., 2014; Sinnott et al., 2015; Wikstrom et al., 2015), smoking (Alaba & Chola, 2013; Britt et al., 2008; Fortin et al., 2014; Jackson et al., 2015; Nagel et al., 2008; Sinnott et al., 2015; Taylor et al., 2010; van den Akker et al., 2000; Wikstrom et al., 2015), and at-risk alcohol consumption (Fortin et al., 2014; Jackson et al., 2015; Nagel et al., 2008; Sinnott et al., 2015; van den Akker et al., 2000).

Obesity has consistently been found to be a major predictor of MM, mainly in studies using body mass index (BMI) as a criterion for obesity, but also using other indicators such as waist circumference or waist/hip ratio (Arokiasamy et al., 2015; Taylor et al., 2010). This relationship has been demonstrated both in cross-sectional studies (Agborsangaya et al.,

2013; de Souza Santos Machado et al., 2013; Fortin et al., 2014) and in longitudinal studies (Jackson et al., 2015; Wikstrom et al., 2015). Obesity has been associated with clinical trajectories in which chronic diseases accumulate with time, especially in middle-aged women (Jackson et al., 2015). The prevalence of MM has been shown to progressively increase with higher degree of obesity (Booth et al., 2014; Jackson et al., 2015). Moreover, obesity is more strongly associated with severe MM, in terms of the number of chronic conditions experienced (Booth et al., 2014). This association between obesity and MM has been reported for both sexes (Fortin et al., 2014; Wikstrom et al., 2015), across all age groups (Agborsangaya et al., 2013; Britt et al., 2008), and within different income categories (Agborsangaya et al., 2013). Although it has been most often reported in high-income countries, similar patterns have been found in low- and middle-income countries (Alaba & Chola, 2013; Arokiasamy et al., 2015; de Souza Santos Machado et al., 2012).

As an explanation for these observations, it has been hypothesized that obesity leads to a low-grade chronic inflammatory state that facilitates the genesis and progression of obesity complications (Cancello & Clement, 2006). This low-grade chronic inflammatory state is thought to be the result of the expanding adipose tissue that elicits macrophage accumulation for controlling and eventually limiting the fat mass development; at the same time, however, the proliferation in macrophages leads to increased secretion of chemokines and inflammatory cytokines. This hypothesis is rooted in the moderate increase of circulatory inflammatory factors observed in obese subjects, and in the identification of macrophage cells infiltrating the white adipose tissue (Cancello & Clement, 2006).

Lack of physical activity seems to be moderately associated with MM prevalence, and this association may be more significant in older people (Britt et al., 2008). Greater consumption of fruits and vegetables appeared to lower the risk of MM in several recent studies, including a longitudinal study (Ruel et al., 2014;

Sinnott et al., 2015). This relationship may be supported by current observations and hypotheses related to the potential protective effects of fruits and vegetables consumption against certain chronic diseases. Nevertheless, this association has been inconsistently reported in the literature (Britt et al., 2008; Fortin et al., 2014; Wikstrom et al., 2015).

Smoking has been associated with increased risk for MM (Britt et al., 2008; Fortin et al., 2014). In terms of age groups, the association with smoking (daily or occasional) seems to be more important in young adults (younger than 50 years) than in elderly subjects (Britt et al., 2008). In terms of sex, the association of present or past smoking with increased risk for MM has been observed in men but not in women (Fortin et al., 2014).

Finally, **at-risk alcohol consumption** has been found not to be associated with MM prevalence in most cross-sectional studies (Fortin et al., 2014; Sinnott et al., 2015; Taylor et al., 2010; van den Akker et al., 2000). Nevertheless, it was predictive of delayed but rapidly increasing MM trajectories in a large longitudinal study in middle-aged women (Jackson et al., 2015).

Not only lifestyle risk factors in isolation have been found to be related with MM: The accumulation of unhealthy lifestyle habits has also been associated with a progressively higher likelihood of MM (Fortin et al., 2014). This finding concurs with the observation that the accumulation of healthy lifestyle habits is associated with morbidity and mortality benefits (Breslow & Enstrom, 1980; King, Mainous, Matheson, & Everett, 2013; Matheson, King, & Everett, 2012; Odegaard, Koh, Gross, Yuan, & Pereira, 2011; Sasazuki et al., 2012).

▶ Psychological Factors

As for previously mentioned factors, the analysis of the role of psychological factors in the development of MM should be explored while keeping in mind that most disease processes are likely multifactorial. Thus, a genetic predisposition to the disease, interaction with the environment, developmental processes related to age, hormonal differences, and other factors, including those related to personality, may all be involved in the etiology of disease.

Mental Health and Physical MM

Even if mental conditions are frequently included in definitions of MM, the medical literature has traditionally distinguished between mental and physical conditions. This section focuses on the abundant and interesting literature related to the association between mental conditions and physical MM, which may be also considered as physical "comorbidity" of mental health problems.

There is a strong association between mental health disorders and physical MM (**FIGURE 8-6**). This has been demonstrated in both sexes, in older people as well as in middle-aged adults, in different socioeconomic groups, and in different countries including non-Western countries (Alaba & Chola, 2013; Barnett et al., 2012; Jones et al., 2015). Higher prevalence of physical MM has been found not only in those populations who have specific and severe mental diseases (such as bipolar affective disorder or schizophrenia) (Woodhead, Ashworth, Schofield, & Henderson, 2014), but also in those with more common mental disorders (such as depression or anxiety) (Cabassa et al., 2013; Jones et al., 2015; Sinnige et al., 2015). Interestingly, the risk of MM progressively increases when a stricter MM definition is used. In a large study in Scottish primary care patients, in comparison to those without depression, the odds ratios in those with depression were 1.55 for two physical conditions, 1.84 for three physical conditions, 2.06 for four physical conditions, and 2.65 for five or more physical conditions (Smith et al., 2014).

Most studies related to the association between mental health and physical MM have been cross-sectional, a design that prevents researchers from making any causal

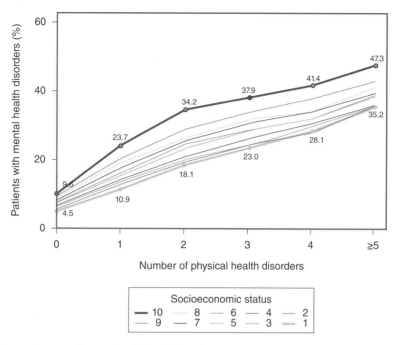

FIGURE 8-6 Co-occurrence of mental and physical conditions.

Reproduced from: Barnett K, Mercer SW, Norbury M, Watt G, Wyke S, Guthrie B. Epidemiology of multimorbidity and implications for health care, research, and medical education: a cross-sectional study. Lancet. 2012;380(9836):37-43.

inferences. Several causal or non-causal pathways probably coexist, explaining the associations observed. On one side, physical MM and related impairment may cause reactive depression (O'Dowd, 2014). On the other side, mental health disorders may increase the risk of MM through various mechanisms, including higher exposition to health risk factors, lower level of motivation and self-management in the case of existing risk factors, cardiometabolic adverse effects of the drugs prescribed for mental health disorders, and poorer access to and lower quality of care (Cabassa et al., 2013; Newcomer & Hennekens, 2007). Finally, physical MM and mental health disorders share some risk factors, especially socioeconomic factors that may bring confusion.

Exploring the link between mental health disorders and physical MM, as well as the potential pathways explaining the associations observed, is very important from a preventive perspective. It is also highly relevant for clinical

purposes, since healthcare systems have long been structured to have distinct organizations and services for physical and mental disorders. Considering that people with mental health disorders frequently have physical MM, and that mental health disorders and physical MM seem to share determinants and to interact with each other, their intertwined nature strongly calls for better integration of physical and mental healthcare delivery (Newcomer & Hennekens, 2007; O'Dowd, 2014; van den Brink, Gerritsen, Oude Voshaar, & Koopmans, 2014).

Health Locus of Control and MM

For some time, researchers have advocated for the idea of a generic disease-prone personality (Friedman & Booth-Kewley, 1987; Friedman & VandenBos, 1992; Thomas, 1988), but this hypothesis has not been sufficiently validated. However, some studies have provided evidence about the relationship between the health locus of control and MM. The health locus of control can be divided in internal locus (when one believes that one has control over one's own health), an external locus (when one's own health is attributed to powerful others, such as doctors), and a chance locus (when health is believed to be a matter of luck) (van der Linden, van der Akker, & Buntinx, 2001). Cross-sectional studies have found that MM is associated with an external locus of control (van den Akker et al., 2000; van den Akker et al., 2001), and an increasing morbidity burden is associated with a progressively more external locus of control (Henninger, Whitson, Cohen, & Ariely, 2012).

In spite of these interesting findings, it is not possible from these studies to determine whether locus of control is a cause or a consequence of MM because of the cross-sectional study design. However, in a cohort of 3460 patients who were followed for a period of 2 years, an internal health locus of control was prospectively associated with a decreased risk for general disease susceptibility, in addition to—and independent of—other factors including coping styles and occurrence of positive life events (van den Akker, Vos, & Knottnerus, 2006). General disease susceptibility was defined in this study as the "co-occurrence of diseases that cannot (yet) be explained with current pathophysiological knowledge." The authors concluded that the distinction between patients with general disease susceptibility and disease-related susceptibility, according to their psychological characteristics, was feasible and may be useful in research and clinical practice.

▸ Psychosocial Factors

Adverse Childhood Experiences and MM

An interesting study, conducted in a large population-based cohort, showed that patients with MM more often had experienced adverse childhood experiences, in comparison to those having a single disease or no disease at all (Sinnott et al., 2015). The adverse childhood experiences considered in this study included a wide range of abuse, neglect, and household dysfunction. This association between adverse childhood experiences and MM was present even after taking into account potential confounding factors, including social, behavioral, and other psychological factors. This finding is consistent with recent literature suggesting an impact of adverse childhood experiences on a wide range of chronic diseases and related outcomes (McCrory, Dooley, Layte, & Kenny, 2015).

Psychosocial Factors in Adults and MM

Negative life events that threaten important personal goals or that negatively influence an individual's self-image, as well as long-term difficulties, such as problems with housing, work, school, finances, and relationship with parents, have been studied as potential determinants of MM (van den Akker et al., 2000). Both types of psychosocial factors have been found to occur significantly more frequent in persons living with MM, in comparison to those with a single condition or no chronic conditions. However, this association seems to be at least partly explained by other sociodemographic factors, such as occupational status, coping style, health locus of control, living arrangement, or social network (van den Akker et al., 2000; van den Akker et al., 2001).

▸ Polypharmacy and MM

Acknowledging the difficulties associated with the definition of polypharmacy (Davies & O'Mahony, 2015; Reeve, Shakib, Hendrix, Roberts, & Wiese, 2014; Tjia, Velten, Parsons, Valluri, & Briesacher, 2013), we will use here *polypharmacy* as a broad term meaning multidrug therapy that includes unnecessary drugs as well. Polypharmacy is well known as one of the most striking and problematic effects resulting from MM. The increase in the number of chronic diseases in older people leads to increased prescribing in these patients, which brings with it many negative consequences, including adverse drug events, increased healthcare utilization and related costs, and geriatric syndromes (Maher, Hanlon, & Hajjar, 2014; Shah & Hajjar, 2012).

Given these potential negative outcomes, then, polypharmacy may be considered a risk factor for MM. In older patients, polypharmacy sometimes generates or worsens geriatric syndromes, which constitute specific patterns of MM. Geriatric syndromes that have been considered to result from polypharmacy include cognitive impairment (which includes delirium and dementia), falls and their consequences, urinary incontinence, and malnourishment (Maher et al., 2014; Shah & Hajjar, 2012). Collectively, these factors may create a vicious cycle in which the presence of multiple conditions leads to multidrug therapy and then to even more conditions. Reduction of medication exposure in older adults, also referred as "deprescribing," is a concern that has been addressed in several studies, but rigorous research on this subject is still needed (Gnjidic, Le Couteur, Kouladjian, & Hilmer, 2012; Reeve et al., 2014; Tjia et al., 2013).

▶ Conclusion and Future Directions

Sociodemographics and socioeconomic factors have been extensively studied as potential risk factors for MM. In contrast, research focusing on social networks, social capital, genetics, lifestyle, psychological and psychosocial factors, and polypharmacy has been undertaken only more recently and publications remain sparse. In addition, some other factors, such as physical environment or biological factors, may be worth being considered as potential determinants of MM (Marengoni et al., 2011).

Along with these gaps in the current literature, the research community faces certain specific challenges in its efforts to better understand the mechanisms underlying the development of MM. The development and use of a common definition of MM and of standardized measurement tools are required for greater comparability of results from different studies (Fortin et al., 2012; Huntley et al., 2012). Moreover, clusters of MM conditions have recently generated growing interest, but the potential implications of focusing research efforts on this issue (in terms of both benefits and potential harms) should be carefully clarified.

In conclusion, MM is a rapidly moving and increasing health problem. Prevalence of MM will continue to increase, due to aging of the population, increases in unhealthy lifestyle habits, the emergence of "new" chronic diseases (e.g., communicable diseases that are no longer life threatening in the short term), and earlier detection of, and progress in treatment of, chronic conditions. Better understanding of the diverse determinants of MM and of their complex interrelations, in line with an ecological model of health, is definitely needed. It certainly constitutes the first step toward the concerted mobilization of all health actors (including health care as well as social care, education, and other types of entities) that is required to adequately address the complex issue of MM.

References

Abad-Diez, J. M., Calderon-Larranaga, A., Poncel-Falco, A., Poblador-Plou, B., Calderon-Meza, J. M., Sicras-Mainar, A.,... Prados-Torres, A. (2014). Age and gender differences in the prevalence and patterns of multimorbidity in the older population. *BMC Geriatrics, 14*, 75.

Afshar, S., Roderick, P. J., Kowal, P., Dimitrov, B. D., & Hill, A. G. (2015). Multimorbidity and the inequalities of global ageing: A cross-sectional study of 28 countries using the World Health Surveys. *BMC Public Health, 15*(1), 776.

Agborsangaya, C. B., Ngwakongnwi, E., Lahtinen, M., Cooke, T., & Johnson, J. A. (2013). Multimorbidity prevalence in the general population: The role of obesity in chronic disease clustering. *BMC Public Health*, *13*, 1161.

Alaba, O., & Chola, L. (2013). The social determinants of multimorbidity in South Africa. *International Journal for Equity in Health*, *12*(1), 63.

Almirall, J., & Fortin, M. (2013). The coexistence of terms to describe the presence of multiple concurrent diseases. *Journal of Comorbidity*, *3*(1), 4–9.

Arokiasamy, P., Uttamacharya, U., Jain, K., Biritwum, R. B., Yawson, A. E., Wu, F.,... Kowal, P. (2015). The impact of multimorbidity on adult physical and mental health in low- and middle-income countries: What does the Study on Global Ageing and Adult Health (SAGE) reveal? *BMC Medicine*, *13*, 178.

Atun, R. (2015). Transitioning health systems for multimorbidity. *Lancet*, *386*(9995), 721–722.

Autenrieth, C. S., Kirchberger, I., Heier, M., Zimmermann, A. K., Peters, A., Doring, A., & Thorand, B. (2013). Physical activity is inversely associated with multimorbidity in elderly men: Results from the KORA-Age Augsburg Study. *Preventive Medicine*, *57*, 17–19.

Bahler, C., Huber, C. A., Brungger, B., & Reich, O. (2015). Multimorbidity, health care utilization and costs in an elderly community-dwelling population: A claims data based observational study. *BMC Health Services Research*, *15*(1), 23.

Barnett, K., Mercer, S. W., Norbury, M., Watt, G., Wyke, S., & Guthrie, B. (2012). Epidemiology of multimorbidity and implications for health care, research, and medical education: A cross-sectional study. *Lancet*, *380*(9836), 37–43.

Bayliss, E. A., Ellis, J. L., & Steiner, J. F. (2005). Subjective assessments of comorbidity correlate with quality of life health outcomes: Initial validation of a comorbidity assessment instrument. *Health and Quality of Life Outcomes*, *3*, 51.

Berkman, L. F., & Kawachi, I. (2000). *Social epidemiology*. New York, NY: Oxford University Press.

Blackwell, D., & Lucas, J. (2014). *Summary health statistics for U.S. adults: National Health Interview Survey, 2012*. Washington, DC: National Center for Health Statistics.

Boeckxstaens, P., Vaes, B., Van Pottelbergh, G., De Sutter, A., Legrand, D., Adriaensen, W.,... Degryse, J. (2015). Multimorbidity measures were poor predictors of adverse events in patients aged >/=80 years: A prospective cohort study. *Journal of Clinical Epidemiology*, *68*(2), 220–227.

Boeing, H., Bechthold, A., Bub, A., Ellinger, S., Haller, D., Kroke, A.,... Watzl, B. (2012). Critical review: Vegetables and fruit in the prevention of chronic diseases. *European Journal of Nutrition*, *51*(6), 637–663.

Bookman, A., & Harrington, M. (2007). Family caregivers: A shadow workforce in the geriatric health care system? *Journal of Health Politics, Policy and Law*, *32*(6), 1005–1041.

Booth, H. P., Prevost, A. T., & Gulliford, M. C. (2014). Impact of body mass index on prevalence of multimorbidity in primary care: Cohort study. *Family Practice*, *31*(1), 38–43.

Bousquet, J., Anto, J. M., Wickman, M., Keil, T., Valenta, R., Haahtela, T.,... von Hertzen, L. (2015). Are allergic multimorbidities and IgE polysensitization associated with the persistence or re-occurrence of foetal type 2 signalling? The MeDALL hypothesis. *Allergy*, *70*(9), 1062–1078.

Boyd, C. M., & Fortin, M. (2010). Future of multimorbidity research: How should understanding of multimorbidity inform health system design? *Public Health Reviews*, *32*(2), 451–474.

Boyd, C., Leff, B., Weiss, C., Wolff, J., Clark, R., & Richards, T. (2010). Clarifying multimorbidity to improve targeting and delivery of clinical services for Medicaid populations 2010. Available at: http://www.chcs.org/media/Clarifying_Multimorbidity_for_Medicaid_report-FINAL.pdf

Boyd, C. M., Wolff, J. L., Giovannetti, E., Reider, L., Weiss, C., Xue, Q. L.,... Rand, C. (2014). Healthcare task difficulty among older adults with multimorbidity. *Medical Care*, *52*(suppl 3), S118–S225.

Breslow, L., & Enstrom, J. E. (1980). Persistence of health habits and their relationship to mortality. *Preventive Medicine*, *9*(4), 469–483.

Brett, T., Arnold-Reed, D. E., Popescu, A., Soliman, B., Bulsara, M. K., Fine, H.,... Moorhead, R. G. (2013). Multimorbidity in patients attending 2 Australian primary care practices. *Annals of Family Medicine*, *11*(6), 535–542.

Brett, T., Arnold-Reed, D. E., Troeung, L., Bulsara, M. K., Williams, A., & Moorhead, R. G. (2014). Multimorbidity in a marginalised, street-health Australian population: A retrospective cohort study. *BMJ Open*, *4*(8), e005461.

Brilleman, S. L., & Salisbury, C. (2013). Comparing measures of multimorbidity to predict outcomes in primary care: A cross sectional study. *Family Practice*, *30*(2), 172–178.

Britt, H. C., Harrison, C. M., Miller, G. C., & Knox, S. A. (2008). Prevalence and patterns of multimorbidity in Australia. *Medical Journal of Australia*, *189*, 72–77.

Byles, J. E., D'Este, C., Parkinson, L., O'Connell, R., & Treloar, C. (2005). Single index of multimorbidity did not predict multiple outcomes. *Journal of Clinical Epidemiology*, *58*, 997–1005.

Cabassa, L. J., Humensky, J., Druss, B., Lewis-Fernández, R., Gomes, A. P., Wang, S., & Blanco, C. (2013). Do race, ethnicity, and psychiatric diagnoses matter in the prevalence of multiple chronic medical conditions? *Medical Care, 51*(6), 540-547.

Cancello, R., & Clement, K. (2006). Is obesity an inflammatory illness? Role of low-grade inflammation and macrophage infiltration in human white adipose tissue. *BJOG, 113*(10), 1141-1147.

Caracciolo, B., Gatz, M., Xu, W., Marengoni, A., Pedersen, N. L., & Fratiglioni, L. (2013). Relationship of subjective cognitive impairment and cognitive impairment on dementia to chronic disease and multi-morbidity in a nation-wide twin study. *Journal of Alzheimer's Disease, 36*(2), 275-284.

Cazale, L., & Dumitru, V. (2008, March). Chronic diseases in Quebec: Some striking facts -[French]. *Zoom Santé*, 1-4.

Centers for Disease Control and Prevention. (2011). *National diabetes fact sheet: National estimates and general information on diabetes and prediabetes in the United States, 2011*. Atlanta, GA: U.S. Department of Health and Human Services.

Chang, H. W., Lin, F. H., Li, P. F., Huang, C. L., Chu, N. F., Su, S. C.,... Hsieh, C. H. (2016). Association between a glucokinase regulator genetic variant and metabolic syndrome in Taiwanese adolescents. *Genetic Testing and Molecular Biomarkers, 20*(3), 137-142.

Charlson, M. E., Pompei, P., Ales, K. L., & MacKenzie, C. R. (1987). A new method of classifying prognostic comorbidity in longitudinal studies: Development and validation. *Journal of Chronic Disease, 40*, 373-383.

Coatta, K. L. (2008). *A conceptual and theoretical analysis of resilience in the context of aging with multiple morbidities*. University of Toronto.

Cornell, J., Pugh, J., Williams, J., Kazis, L., Parchman, M., & Zeber, J. (2007). Multimorbidity clusters: Clustering binary data from a large administrative medical database. *Applied Multivariate Research, 12*(3), 163-182.

Cottrell, E., & Yardley, S. (2015). Lived experiences of multimorbidity: An interpretative meta-synthesis of patients', general practitioners' and trainees' perceptions. *Chronic Illness, 11*(4), 279-303.

Davies, E. A., & O'Mahony, M. S. (2015). Adverse drug reactions in special populations: The elderly. *British Journal of Clinical Pharmacology, 80*(4), 796-807.

de Groot, V., Beckerman, H., Lankhorst, G. J., & Bouter, L. M. (2003). How to measure comorbidity: A critical review of available methods. *Journal of Clinical Epidemiology, 56*, 221-29.

de Souza Santos Machado, V., Valadares, A. L., Costa-Paiva, L. H., Osis, M. J., Sousa, M. H., & Pinto-Neto, A. M. (2013). Aging, obesity, and multimorbidity in women 50 years or older: A population-based study. *Menopause, 20*(8), 818-224.

de Souza Santos Machado, V., Valadares, A. L., da Costa-Paiva, L. S., Moraes, S. S., & Pinto-Neto, A. M. (2012). Multimorbidity and associated factors in Brazilian women aged 40 to 65 years: A population-based study. *Menopause, 19*(5), 569-575.

Diaz, E., Kumar, B. N., Gimeno-Feliu, L. A., Calderon-Larranaga, A., Poblador-Pou, B., & Prados-Torres, A. (2015). Multimorbidity among registered immigrants in Norway: The role of reason for migration and length of stay. *Tropical Medicine and International Health, 20*(12), 1805-1814.

Diaz, E., Poblador-Pou, B., Gimeno-Feliu, L.-A., Calderón-Larrañaga, A., Kumar, B. N., & Prados-Torres, A. (2015). Multimorbidity and its patterns according to immigrant origin: A nationwide register-based study in Norway. *PLoS One, 10*(12), e0145233.

Diederichs, C., Berger, K., & Bartels, D. B. (2011). The measurement of multiple chronic diseases: A systematic review on existing multimorbidity indices. *Journals of Gerontology, Series A: Biological Sciences & Medical Sciences, 66*, 301-311.

Doessing, A., & Burau, V. (2015). Care coordination of multimorbidity: A scoping study. *Journal of Comorbidity, 5*, 15–28.

Duff, K., Mold, J. W., Roberts, M. M., & McKay, S. L. (2007). Medical burden and cognition in older patients in primary care: Selective deficits in attention. *Archives of Clinical Neuropsychology, 22*, 569-575.

Fabbri, E., Zoli, M., Gonzalez-Freire, M., Salive, M. E., Studenski, S. A., & Ferrucci, L. (2015). Aging and multimorbidity: New tasks, priorities, and frontiers for integrated gerontological and clinical research. *Journal of the American Medical Directors Association, 16*(8), 640-647.

Feinstein, A. R. (1970). The pre-therapeutic classification of co-morbidity in chronic diseases. *Journal of Chronic Diseases, 23*, 455-469.

Fishman, P. A., Goodman, M. J., Hornbrook, M. C., Meenan, R. T., Bachman, D. J., & O'Keeffe Rosetti, M. C. (2003). Risk adjustment using automated ambulatory pharmacy data: The RxRisk model. *Medical Care, 41*(1), 84-99.

Fortin, M., Bravo, G., Hudon, C., Lapointe, L., Dubois, M. F., & Almirall, J. (2006). Psychological distress and multimorbidity in primary care. *Annals of Family Medicine, 4*(5), 417-422.

Fortin, M., Bravo, G., Hudon, C., Vanasse, A., & Lapointe, L. (2005). Prevalence of multimorbidity among adults seen in family practice. *Annals of Family Medicine, 3*, 223-228.

Fortin, M., Dubois, M.-F., Hudon, C., Soubhi, H., & Almirall, J. (2007). Multimorbidity and quality of life: A closer look. *Health Quality of Life Outcomes, 5*, 52.

Fortin, M., Haggerty, J., Almirall, J., Bouhali, T., Sasseville, M., & Lemieux, M. (2014). Lifestyle factors and multimorbidity: A cross sectional study. *BMC Public Health, 14*(1), 686.

Fortin, M., Hudon, C., Dubois, M.-F., Almirall, J., Lapointe, L., & Soubhi, H. (2005). Comparative assessment of three different indices of multimorbidity for studies on health-related quality of life. *Health Quality of Life Outcomes, 3*, 74.

Fortin, M., Lapointe, L., Hudon, C., Ntetu, A. L., Maltais, D., & Vanasse, A. (2004). Multimorbidity and quality of life in primary care: A systematic review. *Health Quality of Life Outcomes, 2*, 51.

Fortin, M., Mercer, S. W., & Salisbury, C. (2014). Introducing multimorbidity. In: S. W. Mercer, C. Salisbury, & M. Fortin (Eds.), ABC of multimorbidity (pp. 1–4). Chichester, UK: BMJ Books (Wiley Blackwell).

Fortin, M., Soubhi, H., Hudon, C., Bayliss, E. A., & van den Akker, M. (2007). Multimorbidity's many challenges. *BMJ, 334*, 1016–1017.

Fortin, M., Stewart, M., Poitras, M. E., Almirall, J., & Maddocks, H. (2012). A systematic review of prevalence studies on multimorbidity: Toward a more uniform methodology. *Annals of Family Medicine, 10*(2), 142–151.

Fried, L. P., Ferrucci, L., Darer, J., Williamson, J. D., & Anderson, G. (2004). Untangling the concepts of disability, frailty, and comorbidity: Implications for improved targeting and care. *Journals of Gerontology, Series A: Biological Sciences & Medical Sciences, 59*, 255–263.

Friedman, H. S., & Booth-Kewley, S. (1987). The "disease-prone personality": A meta-analytic view of the construct. *American Psychologist, 42*(6), 539–555.

Friedman, H. S., & VandenBos, G. R. (1992). Disease-prone and self-healing personalities. *Hospital and Community Psychiatry, 43*(12), 1177–1179.

Fu, S., Huang, N., & Chou, Y. J. (2014). Trends in the prevalence of multiple chronic conditions in Taiwan from 2000 to 2010: A population-based study. *Prevention of Chronic Disease, 11*, E187.

Fuchs, J., Busch, M., Lange, C., & Scheidt-Nave, C. (2012). Prevalence and patterns of morbidity among adults in Germany: Results of the German telephone health interview survey German Health Update (GEDA) 2009. *Bundesgesundheitsblatt Gesundheitsforschung Gesundheitsschutz, 55*(4), 576–586.

Gallacher, K., May, C. R., Montori, V. M., & Mair, F. S. (2011). Understanding patients' experiences of treatment burden in chronic heart failure using normalization process theory. *Annals of Family Medicine, 9*(3), 235–243.

Garin, N., Koyanagi, A., Chatterji, S., Tyrovolas, S., Olaya, B., Leonardi, M.,… Haro, J. M. (2015). Global multimorbidity patterns: A cross-sectional, population-based, multi-country study. *Journals of Gerontology, Series A: Biological Sciences & Medical Sciences, 71*(2), 205–214.

Garin, N., Olaya, B., Moneta, M. V., Miret, M., Lobo, A., Ayuso-Mateos, J. L., & Haro, J. M. (2014). Impact of multimorbidity on disability and quality of life in the Spanish older population. *PLoS One, 9*(11), e111498.

Gill, A., Kuluski, K., Jaakkimainen, L., Naganathan, G., Upshur, R., & Wodchis, W. P. (2014). "Where do we go from here?" Health system frustrations expressed by patients with multimorbidity, their caregivers and family physicians. *Healthcare Policy, 9*(4), 73–89.

Giovannetti, E. R., Wolff, J. L., Xue, Q. L., Weiss, C. O., Leff, B., Boult, C.,… Boyd, C. M. (2012). Difficulty assisting with health care tasks among caregivers of multimorbid older adults. *Journal of General Internal Medicine, 27*(1), 37–44.

Gnjidic, D., Le Couteur, D. G., Kouladjian, L., & Hilmer, S. N. (2012). Deprescribing trials: Methods to reduce polypharmacy and the impact on prescribing and clinical outcomes. *Clinics in Geriatric Medicine, 28*(2), 237–253.

Gobbens, R. J., Luijkx, K. G., Wijnen-Sponselee, M. T., & Schols, J. M. (2010). In search of an integral conceptual definition of frailty: Opinions of experts. *Journal of the American Medical Directors Association, 11*(5), 338–343.

Gold, D. R., & Wright, R. (2005). Population disparities in asthma. *Annual Review of Public Health, 26*, 89–113.

Goodman, R. A., Posner, S. F., Huang, E. S., Parekh, A. K., & Koh, H. K. (2013). Defining and measuring chronic conditions: Imperatives for research, policy, program, and practice. *Prevention of Chronic Disease, 10*, E66.

Gunn, J. M., Ayton, D. R., Densley, K., Pallant, J. F., Chondros, P., Herrman, H. E., & Dowrick, C. F. (2012). The association between chronic illness, multimorbidity and depressive symptoms in an Australian primary care cohort. *Social Psychiatry and Psychiatric Epidemiology, 47*(2), 175–184.

Ha, N. T., Le, N. H., Khanal, V., & Moorin, R. (2015). Multimorbidity and its social determinants among older people in southern provinces, Vietnam. *International Journal for Equity in Health, 14*(1), 50.

Habib, R. R., Hojeij, S., Elzein, K., Chaaban, J., & Seyfert, K. (2014). Associations between life conditions and multi-morbidity in marginalized populations: The case of Palestinian refugees. *European Journal of Public Health, 24*(5), 727–733.

Harrison, C., Britt, H., Miller, G., & Henderson, J. (2014). Examining different measures of multimorbidity, using a large prospective cross-sectional study in Australian general practice. *BMJ Open, 4*(7), e004694.

Hart, J. T. (1971). The inverse care law. *Lancet, 1*(7696), 405–412.

Henninger, D. E., Whitson, H. E., Cohen, H. J., & Ariely, D. (2012). Higher medical morbidity burden is associated with external locus of control. *Journal of the American Geriatrics Society, 60*(4), 751–755.

Herrera, C. L., Castillo, W., Estrada, P., Mancilla, B., Reyes, G., Saavedra, N.,… Salazar, L. A. (2016). Association of polymorphisms within the renin–angiotensin system with metabolic syndrome in a cohort of Chilean subjects. *Archives of Endocrinology and Metabolism, 60*(3), 190-198.

Hu, F., Hu, B., Chen, R., Ma, Y., Niu, L., Qin, X., & Hu, Z. (2014). A systematic review of social capital and chronic non-communicable diseases. *BioScience Trends, 8*(6), 290-296.

Hughes, L. D., McMurdo, M. E., & Guthrie, B. (2013). Guidelines for people not for diseases: The challenges of applying UK clinical guidelines to people with multimorbidity. *Age and Ageing, 42*(1), 62-69.

Hummers-Pradier, E., Beyer, M., Chevallier, P., Eilat-Tsanani, S., Lionis, C., Peremans, L.,... van Royen, P. (2010). Series: The research agenda for general practice/family medicine and primary health care in Europe. Part 4. Results: Specific problem solving skills. *European Journal of General Practice, 16*(3), 174-181.

Huntley, A. L., Johnson, R., Purdy, S., Valderas, J. M., & Salisbury, C. (2012). Measures of multimorbidity and morbidity burden for use in primary care and community settings: A systematic review and guide. *Annals of Family Medicine, 10*(2), 134-141.

International Diabetes Federation. (2006). The IDF consensus worldwide definition of the metabolic syndrome. Available at: http://www.idf.org/webdata/docs/MetS_def_update2006.pdf

Jackson, C. A., Dobson, A., Tooth, L., & Mishra, G. D. (2015). Body mass index and socioeconomic position are associated with 9-year trajectories of multimorbidity: A population-based study. *Preventive Medicine, 81*, 92-98.

Jones, S. M., Amtmann, D., & Gell, N. M. (2015). A psychometric examination of multimorbidity and mental health in older adults. *Aging and Mental Health*, 1-9.

Joshi, K., Kumar, R., & Avasthi, A. (2003). Morbidity profile and its relationship with disability and psychological distress among elderly people in Northern India. *International Journal of Epidemiology, 32*, 978-987.

Kelley, A. S. (2014). Defining "serious illness." *Journal of Palliative Medicine, 17*(9), 985.

King, D. E., Mainous, A. G., 3rd, Matheson, E. M., & Everett, C. J. (2013). Impact of healthy lifestyle on mortality in people with normal blood pressure, LDL cholesterol, and C-reactive protein. *European Journal of Preventive Cardiology, 20*(1), 73-79.

Knottnerus, J. A., Metsemakers, J., Hoppener, P., & Limonard, C. (1992). Chronic illness in the community and the concept of "social prevalence." *Family Practice, 9*, 15-21.

Kuo, R. N., & Lai, M. S. (2013). The influence of socioeconomic status and multimorbidity patterns on healthcare costs: A six-year follow-up under a universal healthcare system. *International Journal for Equity in Health, 12*(1), 69.

Lagu, T., Weiner, M. G., Hollenbeak, C. S., Eachus, S., Roberts, C. S., Schwartz, J. S., & Turner, B. J. (2008). The impact of concordant and discordant conditions on the quality of care for hyperlipidemia. *Journal of General Internal Medicine, 23*(8), 1208-1213.

Le Reste, J. Y., Nabbe, P., Manceau, B., Lygidakis, C., Doerr, C., Lingner, H.,... Lietard, C. (2013). The European General Practice Research Network presents a comprehensive definition of multimorbidity in family medicine and long term care, following a systematic review of relevant literature. *Journal of the American Medical Directors Association, 14*(5), 319-325.

Lichtenstein, P., Carlstrom, E., Rastam, M., Gillberg, C., & Anckarsater, H. (2010). The genetics of autism spectrum disorders and related neuropsychiatric disorders in childhood. *American Journal of Psychiatry, 167*(11), 1357-1363.

Linn, B. S., Linn, M. W., & Gurel, L. (1968). Cumulative illness rating scale. *Journal of the American Geriatrics Society, 16*, 622-626.

Lochner, K. A., & Cox, C. S. (2013). Prevalence of multiple chronic conditions among Medicare beneficiaries, United States, 2010. *Prevention of Chronic Disease, 10*, E61.

Luijks, H., Lucassen, P., van Weel, C., Loeffen, M., Lagro-Janssen, A., & Schermer, T. (2015). How GPs value guidelines applied to patients with multimorbidity: A qualitative study. *BMJ Open, 5*(10), e007905.

Machlin, S. R., & Soni, A. (2013). Health care expenditures for adults with multiple treated chronic conditions: Estimates from the medical expenditure panel survey, 2009. *Prevention of Chronic Disease, 10*, E63.

Magnan, E. M., Gittelson, R., Bartels, C. M., Johnson, H. M., Pandhi, N., Jacobs, E. A., & Smith, M. A. (2015). Establishing chronic condition concordance and discordance with diabetes: A Delphi study. *BMC Family Practice, 16*, 42.

Magnan, E. M., Palta, M., Johnson, H. M., Bartels, C. M., Schumacher, J. R., & Smith, M. A. (2015). The impact of a patient's concordant and discordant chronic conditions on diabetes care quality measures. *Journal of Diabetes Complications, 29*(2), 288-294.

Maher, R. L., Hanlon, J., & Hajjar, E. R. (2014). Clinical consequences of polypharmacy in elderly. *Expert Opinion on Drug Safety, 13*(1), 57-65.

Marengoni, A., Angleman, S., Melis, R., Mangialasche, F., Karp, A., Garmen, A.,... Fratiglioni, L. (2011). Aging with multimorbidity: A systematic review of the literature. *Ageing Research Reviews, 10*(4), 430-439.

Marengoni, A., & Onder, G. (2015). Guidelines, polypharmacy, and drug-drug interactions in patients with multimorbidity. *BMJ, 350*, h1059.

Marengoni, A., Winblad, B., Karp, A., & Fratiglioni, L. (2008). Prevalence of chronic diseases and multimorbidity among the elderly population in

Sweden. *American Journal of Public Health*, *98*, 1198–1200.

Matheson, E. M., King, D. E., & Everett, C. J. (2012). Healthy lifestyle habits and mortality in overweight and obese individuals. *Journal of the American Board of Family Medicine*, *25*(1), 9–15.

McCrory, C., Dooley, C., Layte, R., & Kenny, R. A. (2015). The lasting legacy of childhood adversity for disease risk in later life. *Health Psychology*, *34*(7), 687–696.

McDaid, O., Hanly, M. J., Richardson, K., Kee, F., Kenny, R. A., & Savva, G. M. (2013). The effect of multiple chronic conditions on self-rated health, disability and quality of life among the older populations of Northern Ireland and the Republic of Ireland: A comparison of two nationally representative cross-sectional surveys. *BMJ Open*, *3*(6), 1–9.

Melis, R., Marengoni, A., Angleman, S., & Fratiglioni, L. (2014). Incidence and predictors of multimorbidity in the elderly: A population-based longitudinal study. *PLoS One*, *9*(7), e103120.

Menotti, A., Mulder, I., Nissinen, A., Giampaoli, S., Feskens, E. J., & Kromhout, D. (2001). Prevalence of morbidity and multimorbidity in elderly male populations and their impact on 10-year all-cause mortality: The FINE study (Finland, Italy, Netherlands, Elderly). *Journal of Clinical Epidemiology*, *54*(7), 680–686.

Mercer, S. W., Guthrie, B., Furler, J., Watt, G. C. M., & Hart, J, T. (2012). Multimorbidity and the inverse care law in primary care. *BMJ (Clinical Research Ed.)*, *344*, e4152-e.

Mercer, S. W., Smith, S. M., Wyke, S., O'Dowd, T., & Watt, G. C. (2009). Multimorbidity in primary care: Developing the research agenda. *Family Practice*, *2*, 79–80.

Mercer, S. W., & Watt, G. C. (2007). The inverse care law: Clinical primary care encounters in deprived and affluent areas of Scotland. *Annals of Family Medicine*, *5*(6), 503–510.

Mujica-Mota, R. E., Roberts, M., Abel, G., Elliott, M., Lyratzopoulos, G., Roland, M., & Campbell, J. (2015). Common patterns of morbidity and multi-morbidity and their impact on health-related quality of life: Evidence from a national survey. *Quality of Life Research*, *24*(4), 909–918.

Muth, C., van den Akker, M., Blom, J. W., Mallen, C. D., Rochon, J., Schellevis, F. G.,… Glasziou, P. P. (2014). The Ariadne principles: How to handle multimorbidity in primary care consultations. *BMC Medicine*, *12*, 223.

Nagel, G., Peter, R., Braig, S., Hermann, S., Rohrmann, S., & Linseisen, J. (2008). The impact of education on risk factors and the occurrence of multimorbidity in the EPIC-Heidelberg cohort. *BMC Public Health*, *8*, 384.

Newcomer, J. W., & Hennekens, C. H. (2007). Severe mental illness and risk of cardiovascular disease.

Journal of the American Medical Association, *298*(15), 1794–1796.

Noel, P. H., Chris Frueh, B., Larme, A. C., & Pugh, J. A. (2005). Collaborative care needs and preferences of primary care patients with multimorbidity. *Health Expectations*, *8*(1), 54–63.

Odegaard, A. O., Koh, W. P., Gross, M. D., Yuan, J. M., & Pereira, M. A. (2011). Combined lifestyle factors and cardiovascular disease mortality in Chinese men and women: The Singapore Chinese health study. *Circulation*, *124*, 2847–2854.

O'Dowd, T. Depression and multimorbidity in psychiatry and primary care. *The Journal of clinical psychiatry*. 2014;*75*(11):e1319-20.

O'Halloran, J., Miller, G. C., & Britt, H. (2004). Defining chronic conditions for primary care with ICPC-2. *Family Practice*, *21*, 381–386.

Partnership for Solutions. (2004). *Chronic conditions: Making the case for ongoing care*. Baltimore, MD: Johns Hopkins, Bloomberg School of Public Health University. Available at: http://www.partnershipforsolutions.org/

Pati, S., Agrawal, S., Swain, S., Lee, J. T., Vellakkal, S., Hussain, M. A., & Millett, C. (2014). Noncommunicable disease multimorbidity and associated health care utilization and expenditures in India: Cross-sectional study. *BMC Health Services Research*, *14*, 451.

Pefoyo, A. J., Bronskill, S. E., Gruneir, A., Calzavara, A., Thavorn, K., Petrosyan, Y.,… Woodchis, W. P. (2015). The increasing burden and complexity of multimorbidity. *BMC Public Health*, *15*, 415.

Pfortmueller, C. A., Stotz, M., Lindner, G., Muller, T., Rodondi, N., & Exadaktylos, A. K. (2013). Multimorbidity in adult asylum seekers: A first overview. *PLoS One*, *8*(12), e82671.

Piette, J. D., & Kerr, E. A. (2006). The impact of comorbid chronic conditions on diabetes care. *Diabetes Care*, *29*(3), 725–731.

Poblador-Plou, B., van den Akker, M., Vos, R., Calderon-Larranaga, A., Metsemakers, J., & Prados-Torres, A. (2014). Similar multimorbidity patterns in primary care patients from two European regions: Results of a factor analysis. *PLoS One*, *9*(6), e100375.

Prados-Torres, A., Poblador-Plou, B., Calderon-Larranaga, A., Gimeno-Feliu, L. A., Gonzalez-Rubio, F., Poncel Falco, A.,… Alcalá-Nalvaiz, J. T. (2012). Multi-morbidity patterns in primary care: Interactions among chronic diseases using factor analysis. *PLoS One*, *7*(2), e32190.

Ramond-Roquin, A., & Fortin, M. (2016). Towards increased visibility of multimorbidity research. *Journal of Comorbidity*, *6*, 42–45.

Ramond-Roquin, A., Haggerty, J., Lambert, M., Almirall, J., & Fortin, M. (2016). Different multimorbidity measures result in varying estimated levels of physical quality of life in individuals with multimorbidity:

A cross-sectional study in the general population. *Biomedical Research International, 2016,* 7845438.

Rapoport, J., Jacobs, P., Bell, N. R., & Klarenbach, S. (2004). Refining the measurement of the economic burden of chronic diseases in Canada. *Chronic Diseases in Canada, 25,* 13-21.

Razum, O., Zeeb, H., & Rohrmann, S. (2000). The "healthy migrant effect": Not merely a fallacy of inaccurate denominator figures. *International Journal of Epidemiology, 29*(1), 191-192.

Reeve, E., Shakib, S., Hendrix, I., Roberts, M. S., & Wiese, M. D. (2014). Review of deprescribing processes and development of an evidence-based, patient-centred deprescribing process. *British Journal of Clinical Pharmacology, 78*(4), 738-747.

Reeve, J., Blakeman, T., Freeman, G. K., Green, L. A., James, P. A., Lucassen, P.,... van Weel, C. (2013). Generalist solutions to complex problems: Generating practice-based evidence: The example of managing multi-morbidity. *BMC Family Practice, 14,* 112.

Ridgeway, J. L., Egginton, J. S., Tiedje, K., Linzer, M., Boehm, D., Poplau, S.,... Eton, D. T. (2014). Factors that lessen the burden of treatment in complex patients with chronic conditions: A qualitative study. *Patient Preference and Adherence, 8,* 339-351.

Rijken, M., van Kerkhof, M., Dekker, J., & Schellevis, F. G. (2005). Comorbidity of chronic diseases: Effects of disease pairs on physical and mental functioning. *Quality of Life Research, 14,* 45-55.

Roberts, K. C., Rao, D. P., Bennett, T. L., Loukine, L., & Jayaraman, G. C. (2015). Prevalence and patterns of chronic disease multimorbidity and associated determinants in Canada. *Health Promotion and Chronic Disease Prevention in Canada, 35*(6), 87-94.

Roland, M., & Paddison, C. (2013). Better management of patients with multimorbidity. *BMJ, 346,* f2510.

Ruel, G., Shi, Z., Zhen, S., Zuo, H., Kroger, E., Sirois, C.,... Taylor, A. W. (2014). Association between nutrition and the evolution of multimorbidity: The importance of fruits and vegetables and whole grain products. *Clinical Nutrition, 33*(3), 513-520.

Ryan, A., Wallace, E., O'Hara, P., & Smith, S. M. (2015). Multimorbidity and functional decline in community-dwelling adults: A systematic review. *Health Quality of Life Outcomes, 13*(1), 168.

Salisbury, C., Johnson, L., Purdy, S., Valderas, J. M., & Montgomery, A. A. (2011). Epidemiology and impact of multimorbidity in primary care: A retrospective cohort study. *British Journal of General Practice, 61,* e12-e21.

Salvi, F., Miller, M. D,, Grilli, A., Giorgi, R., Towers, A. L., Morichi, V.,... Dessì-Fulgheri, P. (2008). A manual of guidelines to score the modified cumulative illness rating scale and its validation in acute hospitalized elderly patients. *Journal of the American Geriatrics Society, 56,* 1926-1931.

Sasazuki, S., Inoue, M., Iwasaki, M., Sawada, N., Shimazu, T., Yamaji, T., & Tsugane, S.; JPHC Study Group. (2012). Combined impact of five lifestyle factors and subsequent risk of cancer: The Japan Public Health Center Study. *Preventive Medicine, 54,* 112-116.

Satariano, W. (2006). *Epidemiology of aging: An ecological approach.* Sudbury, MA: Jones and Bartlett.

Schafer, I. (2012). Does multimorbidity influence the occurrence rates of chronic conditions? A claims data based comparison of expected and observed prevalence rates. *PLoS One, 7*(9), e45390.

Schafer, I., Hansen, H., Schon, G., Hofels, S., Altiner, A., Dahlhaus, A.,... Wiese, B. (2012). The influence of age, gender and socio-economic status on multimorbidity patterns in primary care: First results from the multicare cohort study. *BMC Health Services Research, 12,* 89.

Schafer, I., Kaduszkiewicz, H., Wagner, H. O., Schon, G., Scherer, M., & van den Bussche, H. (2014). Reducing complexity: A visualisation of multimorbidity by combining disease clusters and triads. *BMC Public Health, 14,* 1285.

Schäfer, I., von Leitner, E. C., Schön, G., Koller, D., Hansen, H., Kolonko, T.,... van den Bussche, H. (2010). Multimorbidity patterns in the elderly: A new approach of disease clustering identifies complex interrelations between chronic conditions. *PLoS One, 5,* e15941.

Schellevis, F. G. (1993). *Chronic disease in general practice: Comorbidity and quality of care.* Utrecht, Netherlands: Drukkerij Pascal.

Schoenberg, N. E., Kim, H., Edwards, W., & Fleming, S. T. (2007). Burden of common multiple-morbidity constellations on out-of-pocket medical expenditures among older adults. *Gerontologist, 47*(4), 423-437.

Schram, M. T., Frijters, D., van de Lisdonk, E. H., Ploemacher, J., de Craen, A. J., de Waal, M. W.,... Schellevis, F. G. (2008). Setting and registry characteristics affect the prevalence and nature of multimorbidity in the elderly. *Journal of Clinical Epidemiology, 61,* 1104-1112.

Sells, D., Sledge, W. H., Wieland, M., Walden, D., Flanagan, E., Miller, R., & Davidson, L. (2009). Cascading crises, resilience and social support within the onset and development of multiple chronic conditions. *Chronic Illness, 5*(2), 92-102.

Shah, B. M., & Hajjar, E. R. (2012). Polypharmacy, adverse drug reactions, and geriatric syndromes. *Clinical Geriatric Medicine, 28*(2), 173-186.

Singh, G. K., & Hiatt, R. A. (2006). Trends and disparities in socioeconomic and behavioural characteristics, life expectancy, and cause-specific mortality of native-born and foreign-born populations in the United States, 1979-2003. *International Journal of Epidemiology, 35*(4), 903-919.

Sinnige, J., Korevaar, J. C., Westert, G. P., Spreeuwenberg, P., Schellevis, F. G., & Braspenning, J. C. (2015). Multimorbidity patterns in a primary care population aged 55 years and over. *Family Practice*, 32(5), 505-513.

Sinnott, C., McHugh, S., Browne, J., & Bradley, C. (2013). GPs' perspectives on the management of patients with multimorbidity: Systematic review and synthesis of qualitative research. *BMJ Open*, 3(9), e003610.

Sinnott, C., McHugh, S., Fitzgerald, A. P., Bradley, C. P., & Kearney, P. M. (2015). Psychosocial complexity in multimorbidity: The legacy of adverse childhood experiences. *Family Practice*, 32(3), 269-275.

Smedley, B. D., & Syme, S. L. (Eds.). (2000). *Promoting health: Intervention strategies from social and behavioral research*. Washington DC: National Academies Press.

Smith, D. J., Court, H., McLean, G., Martin, D., Langan Martin, J., Guthrie, B.,… Mercer, S. W. (2014). Depression and multimorbidity: A cross-sectional study of 1,751,841 patients in primary care. *Journal of Clinical Psychiatry*, 75(11), 1202-1208; quiz 8.

Smith, S. M., Wallace, E., O'Dowd, T., & Fortin, M. (2016). Interventions for improving outcomes in patients with multimorbidity in primary care and community settings. *Cochrane Database of Systematic Reviews*, 3, CD006560.

Sondergaard, E., Willadsen, T. G., Guassora, A. D., Vestergaard, M., Tomasdottir, M. O., Borgquist, L.,… Reventlow, S. (2015). Problems and challenges in relation to the treatment of patients with multimorbidity: General practitioners' views and attitudes. *Scandinavian Journal of Primary Health Care*, 33(2), 121-126.

Sorace, J., Wong, H. H., Worrall, C., Kelman, J., Saneinejad, S., & MaCurdy, T. (2011). The complexity of disease combinations in the Medicare population. *Population Health Management*, 14(4), 161-166.

Starfield, B. (2007). Global health, equity, and primary care. *Journal of the American Board of Family Medicine*, 20(6), 511-513.

Steiner, C. A., & Friedman, B. (2013). Hospital utilization, costs, and mortality for adults with multiple chronic conditions, nationwide inpatient sample, 2009. *Prevention of Chronic Disease*, 10, E62.

Steinman, M, A., Lee, S. J., John Boscardin, W., Miao, Y., Fung, K. Z., Moore, K. L., & Schwartz, J. B. (2012). Patterns of multimorbidity in elderly veterans. *Journal of the American Geriatrics Society*, 60(10), 1872-1880.

Stewart, M., Fortin, M., Britt, H. C., Harrison, C. M., & Maddocks, H. L. (2013). Comparisons of multimorbidity in family practice: Issues and biases. *Family Practice*, 30(4), 473-480.

St Sauver, J. L., Boyd, C. M., Grossardt, B. R., Bobo, W. V., Finney Rutten, L. J., Roger, V. L.,… Rocca, W. A.

(2015). Risk of developing multimorbidity across all ages in an historical cohort study: differences by sex and ethnicity. *BMJ Open*, 5(2), e006413.

Taylor, A. W., Price, K., Gill, T. K., Adams, R., Pilkington, R., Carrangis, N.,… Wilson, D. (2010). Multimorbidity: Not just an older person's issue. Results from an Australian biomedical study. *BMC Public Health*, 10, 718.

Thomas, S. P. (1988). Is there a disease-prone personality? Synthesis and evaluation of the theoretical and empirical literature. *Issues in Mental Health Nursing*, 9(4), 339-352.

Tjia, J., Velten, S. J., Parsons, C., Valluri, S., & Briesacher, B. A. (2013). Studies to reduce unnecessary medication use in frail older adults: A systematic review. *Drugs and Aging*, 30(5), 285-307.

Tonelli, M., Wiebe, N., Fortin, M., Guthrie, B., Hemmelgarn, B. R., James, M. T.,… Quan, H.; Alberta Kidney Disease Network. (2015). Methods for identifying 30 chronic conditions: Application to administrative data. *BMC Medical Informatics and Decision Making*, 15, 31.

Tran, V. T., Montori, V. M., Eton, D. T., Baruch, D., Falissard, B., & Ravaud, P. (2012). Development and description of measurement properties of an instrument to assess treatment burden among patients with multiple chronic conditions. *BMC Medicine*, 10, 68.

Treadwell, J. (2015). Coping with complexity: Working beyond the guidelines for patients with multi-morbidities. *Journal of Comorbidity*, 5, 11-14.

Tucker-Seeley, R. D., Li, Y., Sorensen, G., & Subramanian, S. (2011). Lifecourse socioeconomic circumstances and multimorbidity among older adults. *BMC Public Health*, 11, 313.

Uijen, A. A., & van de Lisdonk, E. H. (2008). Multimorbidity in primary care: Prevalence and trend over the last 20 years. *European Journal of General Practice*, 1(14 suppl), 28-32.

Valderas, J. M., Starfield, B., & Roland, M. (2007). Multimorbidity's many challenges: A research priority in the UK. *BMJ*, 334, 1128.

Valderas, J. M., Starfield, B., Sibbald, B., Salisbury, C., & Roland, M. (2009). Defining comorbidity: Implications for understanding health and health services. *Annals of Family Medicine*, 7, 357-363.

van den Akker, M., Buntinx, F., & Knottnerus, J. A. (1996). Comorbidity or multimorbidity: What's in a name? A review of literature. *European Journal of General Practice*, 2, 65-70.

van den Akker, M., Buntinx, F., Metsemakers, J. F., & Knottnerus, J. A. (1998). Morbidity in responders and non-responders in a register-based population survey. *Family Practice*, 15, 261-263.

van den Akker, M., Buntinx, F., Metsemakers, J. F., & Knottnerus, J. A. (2000). Marginal impact of psychosocial factors on multimorbidity: Results of an explorative nested case-control study. *Social Science & Medicine, 50*(11), 1679-1693.

van den Akker, M., Buntinx, F., Metsemakers, J. F., Roos, S., & Knottnerus, J. A. (1998). Multimorbidity in general practice: Prevalence, incidence, and determinants of co-occurring chronic and recurrent diseases. *Journal of Clinical Epidemiology, 51,* 367-375.

van den Akker, M., Buntinx, F., Metsemakers, J. F., van der Aa, M., & Knottnerus, J. A. (2001). Psychosocial patient characteristics and GP-registered chronic morbidity: A prospective study. *Journal of Psychosomatic Research, 50*(2), 95-102.

van den Akker, M., Vos, R., & Knottnerus, J. A. (2006). In an exploratory prospective study on multimorbidity general and disease-related susceptibility could be distinguished. *Journal of Clinical Epidemiology, 59*(9), 934-939.

van den Brink, A. M., Gerritsen, D. L., Oude Voshaar, R. C., & Koopmans, R. T. (2014) Patients with mental-physical multimorbidity: Do not let them fall by the wayside. *International Psychogeriatrics, 26*(10), 1585-1589.

van den Bussche, H., Koller, D., Kolonko, T., Hansen, H., Wegscheider, K., Glaeske, G.,... Schön, G. (2011). Which chronic diseases and disease combinations are specific to multimorbidity in the elderly? Results of a claims data based cross-sectional study in Germany. *BMC Public Health, 11,* 101.

van den Bussche, H., Schön, G., Kolonko, T., Hansen, H., Wegscheider, K., Glaeske, G.,... Koller, D. (2011). Patterns of ambulatory medical care utilization in elderly patients with special reference to chronic diseases and multimorbidity: Results from a claims data based observational study in Germany. *BMC Geriatrics, 11,* 54.

van der Linden, M., van der Akker, M., & Buntinx, F. (2001). The relation between health locus of control and multimorbidity: A case-control study. *Personality and Individual Differences, 30,* 1189-1197.

van Oostrom, S. H., Picavet, H. S., de Bruin, S. R., Stirbu, I., Korevaar, J. C., Schellevis, F. G., & Baan, C. A. (2014). Multimorbidity of chronic diseases and health care utilization in general practice. *BMC Family Practice, 15*(1), 61.

Veenstra, G., Luginaah, I., Wakefield, S., Birch, S., Eyles, J., & Elliott, S. (2005). Who you know, where you live: Social capital, neighbourhood and health. *Social Science & Medicine,* 0277-9536.

Violan, C., Foguet-Boreu, Q., Flores-Mateo, G., Salisbury, C., Blom, J., Freitag, M.,... Valderas, J. M. (2014). Prevalence, determinants and patterns of multimorbidity in primary care: A systematic review of observational studies. *PLoS One, 9*(7), e102149.

Violan, C., Foguet-Boreu, Q., Roso-Llorach, A., Rodriguez-Blanco, T., Pons-Vigues, M., Pujol-Ribera, E.,... Valderas, J. M. (2014). Burden of multimorbidity, socioeconomic status and use of health services across stages of life in urban areas: A cross-sectional study. *BMC Public Health, 14,* 530.

Vos, H. M., Bor, H. H., Rangelrooij-Minkels, M. J., Schellevis, F. G., & Lagro-Janssen, A. L. (2013). Multimorbidity in older women: The negative impact of specific combinations of chronic conditions on self-rated health. *European Journal of General Practice, 19*(2), 117-122.

Vos, R., van den Akker, M., Boesten, J., Robertson, C., & Metsemakers, J. (2015). Trajectories of multimorbidity: Exploring patterns of multimorbidity in patients with more than ten chronic health problems in life course. *BMC Family Practice, 16*(1), 2.

Vos, T., Barber, R. M., Bell, B., Bertozzi-Villa, A., Biryukov, S., Bolliger, I.,... Murray, C. J. (2015). Global, regional, and national incidence, prevalence, and years lived with disability for 301 acute and chronic diseases and injuries in 188 countries, 1990-2013: A systematic analysis for the Global Burden of Disease Study 2013. *Lancet, 386*(9995), 743-800.

Walker, A. E. (2007). Multiple chronic diseases and quality of life: Patterns emerging from a large national sample, Australia. *Chronic Illness, 3*(3), 202-218.

Wang, H., Wang, J., Wong, S., Wong, M., Li, F., Wang, P.,... Mercer, S. W. (2014). Epidemiology of multimorbidity in China and implications for the healthcare system: Cross-sectional survey among 162,464 community household residents in southern China. *BMC Medicine, 12*(1), 188.

Ward, B. W., & Schiller, J. S. (2013). Prevalence of multiple chronic conditions among US Adults: Estimates from the National Health Interview Survey, 2010. *Prevention of Chronic Disease, 10,* E65.

Ward, B. W., Schiller, J. S., & Goodman, R. A. (2014). Multiple chronic conditions among US adults: A 2012 update. *Prevention of Chronic Disease, 11,* E62.

Warner, L. M., Ziegelmann, J. P., Schüz, B., Wurm, S., Tesch-Römer, C., & Schwarzer, R. (2011). Maintaining autonomy despite multimorbidity: Self-efficacy and the two faces of social support. *European Journal of Ageing, 8*(1), 3-12.

Waverijn, G., Wolfe, M. K., Mohnen, S., Rijken, M., Spreeuwenberg, P., & Groenewegen, P. (2014). A prospective analysis of the effect of neighbourhood and individual social capital on changes in self-rated health of people with chronic illness. *BMC Public Health, 14*(1), 1-11.

Weiss, C. O., Boyd, C. M., Yu, Q., Wolff, J. L., & Leff, B. (2007). Patterns of prevalent major chronic disease among older adults in the United States. *Journal of the American Medical Association, 298*(10), 1160-1162.

Wen, Y., Schaid, D. J., & Lu, Q. (2013). A bivariate Mann-Whitney approach for unraveling genetic variants and interactions contributing to comorbidity. *Genetic Epidemiology, 37*(3), 248-255.

Wikstrom, K., Lindstrom, J., Harald, K., Peltonen, M., & Laatikainen, T. (2015). Clinical and lifestyle-related risk factors for incident multimorbidity: 10-year follow-up of Finnish population-based cohorts 1982-2012. *European Journal of Internal Medicine*, 26(3), 211-216.

Wilkie, R., Peat, G., Thomas, E., & Croft, P. (2007). Factors associated with participation restriction in community-dwelling adults aged 50 years and over. *Quality of Life Research*, 16(7), 1147-1156.

Wolff, J. L., & Boyd, C. M. (2015). A look at person- and family-centered care among older adults: Results from a national survey [corrected]. *Journal of General Internal Medicine*, 30(10), 1497-1504.

WONCA Classification Committee. (1995). An international glossary for general/family practice. *Family Practice*, 12(3), 341-369.

Woodhead, C., Ashworth, M., Schofield, P., & Henderson, M. (2014). Patterns of physical co-/multi-morbidity among patients with serious mental illness: A London borough-based cross-sectional study. *BMC Family Practice*, 15(1), 117.

Zulman, D. M., Asch, S. M.., Martins, S. B., Kerr, E. A., Hoffman, B. B., & Goldstein, M. K. (2014). Quality of care for patients with multiple chronic conditions: The role of comorbidity interrelatedness. *Journal of General Internal Medicine*, 29(3), 529-537.

Zulman, D. M., Pal Chee, C., Wagner, T. H., Yoon, J., Cohen, D. M., Holmes, T. H.,... Asch, S. M. (2015). Multimorbidity and healthcare utilisation among high-cost patients in the US Veterans Affairs Health Care System. *BMJ Open*, 5(4), :e007771.

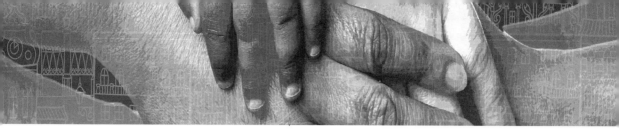

CHAPTER 9

Frailty and Geriatric Syndromes

Qian-Li Xue, Brian Buta, Ravi Varadhan, Sarah L. Szanton, Paulo Chaves, Jeremy D. Walston, and **Karen Bandeen-Roche**

ABSTRACT

One of the biggest challenges in health care worldwide is the medical and economic burden of caring for vulnerable older adults who are ravaged by physical and cognitive impairments. One of the most common geriatric conditions, frailty syndrome, affects 15% of the older non-nursing-home population aged 65 and older in the United States and between 3.5% and 27.3% of the elderly population worldwide. Frailty is known to be a strong predictor of poor health outcomes including disability, hospitalization, institutionalization, and mortality. Although significant progress has been made in frailty research over the last two decades, spanning from theory development to construct development and validation, and from intervention design and testing to clinical translation, there are still great challenges to be met. In this chapter, we provide a brief overview of three common geriatric syndromes—falls, incontinence, and delirium—and their operational definitions, risk factors, and treatments. Next, we offer an introduction to frailty research covering theories, biology, and assessment tools, followed by a discussion of conceptual differences between frailty and geriatric syndromes as well as epidemiological and biological evidence of their linkages. We then provide a summary of recent findings from frailty research including updated prevalence and incidence, natural history of clinical manifestations, results from intervention trials, and current applications in clinical practice. We conclude the chapter with a discussion of current issues and challenges and future directions of frailty research.

KEYWORDS

aging	measurement	resilience
compensation	medical syndrome	vulnerability
frailty		

▶ Introduction

The combination of increased lifespan and reduced fertility rates is leading to the rapid **aging** of populations around the world. For example, according to the World Health Organization's *World Report on Aging and Health* (WHO, 2015), the life expectancy of a child born in Brazil or Myanmar in 2015 is 20 years longer than that of a child born in those countries 50 years ago. Unfortunately, the increases in longevity are not always being accompanied by an extended period of health and vigorous life at older ages—that is, compression of morbidity (Crimmins & Beltran-Sanchez, 2011; Fries, 1980). To the contrary, length of life with disease and mobility functioning loss in older adults increased between 1998 and 2008, with age-specific prevalence of a number of physiologic risk factors, including dysregulated markers of inflammation and glucose processing, largely being unmoved (Crimmins & Beltran-Sanchez, 2011). So far, little evidence supports the claim that "70 is the new 60," which is a central tenet underpinning the compression of morbidity hypothesis. Nevertheless, the trajectory of functional decline is highly heterogeneous and is not fully determined by a person's chronological age. This heterogeneity is believed to arise from a person's innate functioning ability, physical and social environments, as well as interactions between them. The fact that there is no "typical" older person makes it critically important to identify the most vulnerable subset so as to better guide intervention targeting, optimize resource allocation and delivery, and improve person-centered outcomes. The conceptualization of frailty and the proliferation of research on this topic and its application are the focus of a recent effort to tackle the issue of heterogeneity in late-life **vulnerability**.

Frailty is theoretically defined as a clinically recognizable state of increased vulnerability, resulting from an aging-associated decline in reserve and function across multiple physiologic systems, such that the ability to cope with everyday or acute stressors is compromised (Morley et al., 2013). In reality, however, there is still no consensus on the operational definition of frailty for research and clinical uses. In the geriatric literature, frailty is often considered a geriatric syndrome, and its relationships with other geriatric syndromes such as delirium, falls, and incontinence have not been well articulated. The goals of this chapter, then, are fivefold:

■   Summarize commonalities of assessment and shared etiologies among geriatric syndromes
■   Review the evolution of frailty research including theories, operational definitions, assessment tools, and translational efforts
■   Discuss potential biological links between frailty and common geriatric syndromes
■   Explicate cross-cutting issues and challenges of assessing and studying frailty and geriatric syndromes, and propose solutions to these challenges
■   Outline future directions in this field

▶ Geriatric Syndromes

The healthcare needs of geriatric patients can be complex. In addition to disease- and organ-specific problems, older adults commonly experience health conditions that "defy conventional medical wisdom by crossing traditional organ- and discipline-based boundaries" (Kuchel, 2009). Geriatric syndromes, or what Sir Bernard Isaacs originally dubbed the "geriatric giants," are therefore used to refer to the health conditions commonly occurring in older adults that do not fit into discrete disease categories (Morley, 2004). Falls, immobility, incontinence, delirium, dizziness, and syncope are examples of geriatric syndromes. Though diverse, these syndromes share several common features. Geriatric syndromes are highly prevalent among older adults and are associated with poor outcomes in quality of life, disability, and morbidity (Inouye, Studenski, Tinetti, & Kuchel, 2007; Kuchel, 2009). Another feature is the multifactorial origin of these syndromes. Unlike traditional medical syndromes driven by a single underlying factor, geriatric syndromes are conceived as resulting from a number of interacting intrinsic, external, and iatrogenic factors (Bergman et al., 2007; Flacker, 2003). The complex roots of these syndromes can pose significant challenges for clinicians and researchers alike in elucidating their etiology, natural history, presentation, and outcomes. Four shared risk factors have been identified among common geriatric syndromes: (1) increased age, (2) cognitive impairments, (3) functional impairments, and (4) mobility impairment (Inouye et al., 2007).

PEARLS 9-1, **9-2**, and **9-3** provide a brief overview of three common geriatric syndromes—falls, incontinence, and delirium—and their

---

PEARL 9-1 Geriatric Syndrome of Falls

Definition: "An event that results in a person coming to rest inadvertently on the ground or floor or other lower level" (WHO, 2007).

Prevalence

- Approximately one-third of community-dwelling older adults worldwide experience a fall each year (Gillespie et al., 2012; WHO, 2007).
- As many as 50% of older adults (over 80 years old or with institutionalization) worldwide experience a fall each year annually (Martin, 2011; Rubenstein & Josephson, 2002; Soriano, DeCherrie, & Thomas, 2007; WHO, 2007).

Burden

- As many as 20% of falls result in serious health outcomes (Gillespie et al., 2012; Rubenstein, 2006).
- Falls are the leading cause of injury-related deaths among adults ages 65 and older in the United States (Sleet, Moffett, & Stevens, 2008).
- Direct U.S. medical costs for fall injuries are estimated at $34 billion annually (Stevens, Corso, Finkelstein, & Miller, 2006), and they are anticipated to exceed $50 billion per year by 2020 due to aging of the population (Shubert, Smith, Prizer, & Ory, 2014).

Risk Factors (Nonphysiologic)

- Risk factors include declines in muscle strength and physical, neurologic, and sensory function; polypharmacy; environmental hazards; and history of or fear of falling (Campbell, Borrie, & Spears, 1989; Martin, 2011; Panel on Prevention of Falls in Older Persons, 2011; Rubenstein, 2006).
- The majority of falls are due to nonspecific interacting factors listed above (Campbell et al., 1989; Campbell & Robertson, 2006).

Preventions and Treatments

Interventions may include multifactorial interventions to improve muscle function and stability, increase physical activity, reduce psychological concerns, decrease medications, and address environmental hazards (Campbell & Robertson, 2006), although the effectiveness of these interventions in trials has been mixed (Panel on Prevention of Falls in Older Persons, 2011). Other interventions include Tai Chi, certain medications, and anti-slip devices (Gillespie et al., 2012).

PEARL 9-2   Geriatric Syndrome of Incontinence

Definition: The leakage or involuntary loss of control of the bladder (urinary incontinence [UI]) and/or bowel (fecal incontinence [FI]).

Prevalence

- The estimated mean global prevalence of UI is 27.6% (range: 4.8–58.4%) in females and 10.5% (range: 1–34.1%) in males (Minassian, Drutz, & Al-Badr, 2003).
- Non-institutionalized older adults 65 years and older in the United States have a 43% estimated UI prevalence and a 17% FI prevalence (Gorina, Schappert, Bercovitz, Elgaddal, & Kramarow, 2014).
- Among institutionalized older adults, nearly 50% of short-term (length of stay < 100 days) nursing home residents and 75% of long-term care residents surveyed experienced incontinence (Gorina et al., 2014).

Burden

Annual costs of managing UI in the United States are estimated at $26 billion (Levy & Muller, 2006).

Risk Factors (Nonphysiologic)

- Risk factors include bladder/sphincter dysfunction and interacting risk factors such as chronic diseases and conditions (arthritis, diabetes, stroke), impairments in cognition (dementia, delirium) and mood (anxiety, depression), impairments in physical function and mobility limitations, and body weight (Gorina et al., 2014; Markland, Richter, Fwu, Eggers, & Kusek, 2011).
- Certain drugs and medications, as well as polypharmacy, are also associated with incontinence (Gibson et al., 2014; Talley, Wyman, & Shamliyan, 2011).

Preventions and Treatments

Lifestyle and behavioral treatments include multicomponent behavioral interventions. For UI, these include pelvic floor muscle exercise and bladder training (Talley et al., 2011). Pharmacologic and surgical treatments have been considered, but there are concerns about complications, especially among frail older adults (Gibson et al., 2014; Wagg et al., 2015).

---

operational definitions, risk factors, and treatments. The selection of these syndromes for discussion here is meant to be exemplary in terms of their clinical significance, potentially shared risk factors, and methodological challenges.

▶ Frailty: Theories and Definitions

The term "frail elderly" was first introduced by Monsignor Charles F. Fahey and the U.S. Federal Council on Aging (FCA) in 1970s to focus attention on a particular segment of the older population "over the age of 75, who because of an accumulation of various continuing problems often require one or several supportive services in order to cope with daily life." Early definitions for the "frail elderly" bear a close resemblance to the definition of disability; indeed, the two terms were at times used interchangeably (Hogan, MacKnight, & Bergman, 2003). Theories of frailty etiology started to emerge in early 1990s, including Buchner and Wagner's vulnerability theory, Bortz's "use it or loss it" theory, Fried's cycle of frailty, Ferrucci's homeostatic dysregulation theory, Lipsitz's loss of complexity theory,

PEARL 9-3 Geriatric Syndrome of Delirium

Definition: "An acute decline in cognitive functioning," (Inouye, Westendorp, & Saczynski, 2014), including disorientation, inattention, and cognitive disturbances, that commonly occurs among older adults in hospital and long-term care settings and can last for a few hours up to several days or longer (Clegg, Siddiqi, Heaven, Young, & Holt, 2014; Davis et al., 2013; Inouye et al., 2014).

Prevalence

- Delirium is most common in clinical settings: Prevalence is 10–35% among older hospitalized adults (Inouye et al., 2014; Siddiqi, House, & Holmes, 2006) and as high as 50% in patients in intensive care units (Inouye et al., 2014).
- Among community-dwelling older adults, prevalence is approximately 1–2%, though it increases to approximately 10% in persons age 85 and older (de Lange, Verhaak, & van der Meer, 2013).

Burden

The burden on the U.S. healthcare system due to delirium is estimated at $38 billion annually, at a minimum (Leslie & Inouye, 2011).

Risk Factors (Nonphysiologic)

- Risk factors include surgical procedures, infections and sepsis, environmental changes, nutrition and dehydration, and certain medications (Clegg et al., 2014; Collier, 2012; Inouye et al., 2014).
- Presence of dementia, comorbidities, and function limitations are predisposing factors for elevated delirium risk (Collier, 2012; Inouye et al., 2014).

Preventions and Treatments

- Nonpharmacologic approaches are considered to be the best intervention strategies (Inouye et al., 2014).
- Multicomponent interventions were found to reduce delirium incidence by 40% (Flaherty, 2011; Inouye, 2006; Quinlan et al., 2011).
- Pharmacologic approaches, namely antipsychotic medications, have not been found effective and are not generally recommended (Flaherty, 2011; Flaherty, Gonzales, & Dong, 2011; Inouye et al., 2014).

Varadhan's dynamical system theory, and Rockwood's cumulative deficit theory. In this section, we discuss each of these theories in brief.

A universal biological feature of aging is progressive decline in the capacity of an organism to withstand stress. Buchner and Wagner (1992) posited that such age-related declines will be generally larger with so-called stress tests (e.g., glucose and insulin response to glucose load) than with resting or basal measures (e.g., fasting blood glucose and fasting blood insulin levels). This loss of physiologic reserves in older adults can deprive them of a "margin of safety." Buchner and Wagner defined frailty

as the state of reduced physiologic reserve associated with increased susceptibility to disability. For the purposes of prevention, they restricted frailty to include those losses of physiologic reserve that increase the risk of disability. Thus, they viewed frailty as a precursor state representing a loss of physiologic capacity that is either not severe enough to interfere with major activities of daily living or is compensated for by alternative strategies.

Bortz (1993) hypothesized that frailty is the result of uncoupling of an organism from its environment that leads to a break in the forward-feedback cycle of stimulus to growth and increased functional competence. For this cycle to continue, there needs to be correspondence between structure and function. A modulated energy flow of appropriate intensity and duration is anabolic; either too much or too little energy is catabolic. Frailty, then, can be envisioned as the loss of structural integrity that results when an organism is uncoupled from its environment. Bortz proposed that disease, disuse, and aging all contributed in the aggregate to diminished vitality and increased frailty—a phenomenon he termed disuse syndrome (**FIGURE 9-1**). The phrase "use it or lose it" captures the essence of this idea (Bortz, 1993, 2002). Most of the body serves movement purposes, so diminished movement is a principal pathogenic mechanism for human frailty. According to Bortz's theory, lifestyle is the greatest contributor to frailty. Bortz argued that a substantial portion of previously established declines are reversible by reestablishment of an optimal energy flow— that is, by increasing levels of activity.

Fried and Walston conceptualized frailty as a state of increased vulnerability that arises from multisystem dysregulation, leading to decline in physiologic reserves, and therefore to diminished capacity to cope with everyday or acute stressors (Fried et al., 2005; Fried et al., 1998). This decline in multiple systems affects the normal complex adaptive behavior that is essential to health (Fried et al., 2009) and eventually results in a self-perpetuating

"cycle of frailty" that includes skeletal muscle decline (i.e., sarcopenia), lower levels of energy production, and altered nutritional intake and processing (**FIGURE 9-2**). Fried and Walston's theory enabled the development of a specific physical frailty phenotype (PFP) with five binary-coded criteria indicating the presence or absence of weakness, slowness, reduced activity, low energy, and unintended weight loss (Bandeen-Roche et al., 2006). It has been postulated that frailty may be clinically identified as a critical mass of these five phenotypic criteria consistent with a **medical syndrome**. Specifically, the PFP defines frailty as meeting three out of the five criteria. A pre-frail stage, in which one or two criteria are present, identifies a subset of the population at high risk of progressing to frailty. It is becoming widely accepted that physical frailty represents a unique construct that is distinct from disability and multimorbidity (Fried, Ferrucci, Darer, Williamson, & Anderson, 2004; Morley et al., 2013). Chronic diseases likely increase the risk of frailty. Frailty itself increases the risk of disability, such that disability is viewed as a consequence of frailty by some sources (Abellan van Kan, Rolland, Bergman, et al., 2008; Vellas et al., 2013). The PFP has provided a useful working model for frailty and has facilitated the development and testing of a number of more specific biological hypotheses related to dysregulations in the innate immune system, endocrine axes, and neuroendocrine systems.

Ferrucci et al. (2005) define frailty as the core biological dysregulation that is facilitated by aging. Examples of such core biological dysregulation include cellular damage due to oxidative stress and heat, and the inability to shut off the inflammatory response once an inciting event has resolved, which results in a chronic, low-grade, pro-inflammatory state. The biological dysregulation may remain present yet not manifest as clinical disease until the homeostatic mechanisms become overwhelmed. When this occurs, disease and eventually disability become clinically apparent. Ferrucci et al. posit that the same processes responsible for aging-related progressive

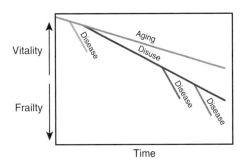

FIGURE 9-1 Aging, disease, and disuse as contributors to frailty.

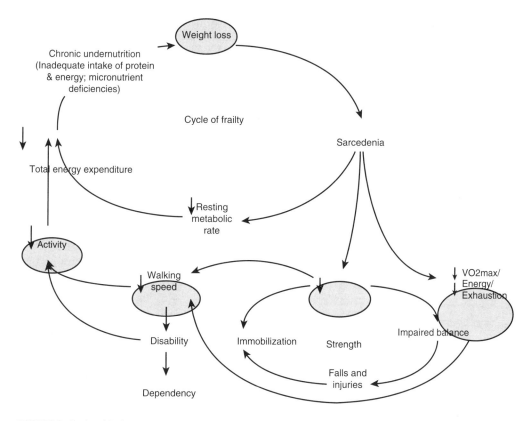

FIGURE 9-2 Cycle of frailty.

Modified from Fried, L. P., Walston, J., Hazzard, W. R., et al. Frailty and failure to thrive. Principles of Geriatric Medicine and Gerontology. Vol 4th, 1998:1392 (Figure 109-5). Reprinted by permission of McGraw-Hill Education.

dysregulation and dysfunction of the biological mechanisms that maintain a stable homeostasis may also be responsible for the progressive decline of physical function with aging. Accordingly, disease and functional declines may be viewed as parallel outcomes of the dysregulation in core homeostatic mechanisms, or frailty. Ferrucci et al. state that intrinsic causes of frailty should be searched for in common pathways for multiple impairments—for example, hormones, inflammation, equilibrium between production and scavenging of free radicals, and balance between sympathetic and parasympathetic systems.

Lipsitz (2002, 2004) theorized that healthy physiologic systems exhibit complex nonlinear dynamics when at rest. When the organism is perturbed, however, the physiologic systems evoke closed-loop responses over relatively short time scales in an effort to reestablish homeostasis. Compared to the resting dynamics, the transient stimulus–response dynamics is less complex, occurring in a dominant response mode called reactive tuning. Lipsitz postulated that frailty is due to the loss of complexity under resting conditions and dysregulated reactive tuning response to perturbations. He suggested that nonlinear mathematical techniques that quantify physiological dynamics may predict onset of frailty (e.g., fractals and power-law scaling in temporal response of physiologic systems). A limitation of Lipsitz's approach is that it can be applied only to the study of physiologic systems whose temporal behavior can be sampled at high frequency (e.g., heart rate, pulse pressure, center-of-pressure of human gait).

Varadhan, Seplaki, and colleagues (2008) proposed that frailty might be identified using a classical, linear dynamical systems approach. According to this approach, frailty is due to the loss of **resilience** in homeostatic regulation. This loss of resilience can be evaluated and quantified using features of a physiologic system's dynamic response when the system is perturbed or stressed by a stimulus. Some of the key features of this approach include time to peak response, time to recovery, and amplitude of response. An important mechanism for loss of resilience is impaired negative feedback mechanisms, which can lead to longer time to recovery from a stressor. An example is the hypothalamus–pituitary–adrenal (HPA) axis.

Varadhan, Seplaki, and colleagues (2008) considered a simplified model of a hypothetical physiologic system that, despite its simplicity, captures the rich stimulus–response patterns postulated in the literature (**FIGURE 9-3**). Assume there are two biomarkers (of any closed-loop physiologic system), "neurotransmitter A" and "hormone B." Y1 is the concentration of the neurotransmitter A produced by the brain in response to a stimulus of strength k1, which then stimulates the production of a hormone B (represented by parameter k3), whose concentration is denoted by Y2. The hormone cannot only inhibit its own production locally, but also inhibit the production of neurotransmitter via a negative feedback mechanism (represented by k2). This system can produce a variety of responses as the parameters k2, k3, and k4 vary. In particular, the negative feedback parameters k2 and k4 can have a large impact on the time to recover the system following a stressor.

Mitnitski, Mogilner, and Rockwood (2001) adopted a very different approach to characterizing frailty. They examined the aging process as comprising the accumulation of deficits that, while age related, are not necessarily known as risks for diminished life expectancy, such as impaired vision/hearing or skin problems. These researchers derived a quantitative measure called the frailty index, which elucidates the accumulation of deficits, and proposed it as a means of assessing individual aging. Although this approach is used in studies of frailty, the frailty index might be viewed more as a measure of biological aging than as a syndrome of physiologic vulnerability to stressors.

Despite the conceptual differences underlying the different theories discussed in this section, it is generally agreed that declines in physiologic reserves and resilience are the essence of being frail (Fried, 1992; Fried et al., 2001; Varadhan, Seplaki, et al., 2008), and that frailty is a fundamental state depicting vulnerability to poor outcomes in the face of a stressor. Similarly, scientists agree that the risk of frailty increases with age and with the incidence of diseases. Beyond that, some evidence now supports the theory that the development of frailty involves declines in the function of many different physiologic systems (Fried et al., 2009).

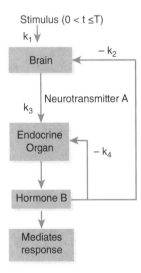

FIGURE 9-3 A schematic showing the components and parameters of a hypothetical dynamic system.

Reprinted from Mechanisms of Ageing and Development, 129(11), Varadhan, R., Seplaki, C. L., Xue, Q. L., Bandeen-Roche, K., & Fried, L. P. Stimulus-response paradigm for characterizing the loss of resilience in homeostatic regulation associated with frailty, pages 666-670. Copyright 2008, with permission from Elsevier.

▶ Biology of Frailty

The early studies addressing the biological underpinnings of frailty were epidemiological in nature. One line of work demonstrated that frailty status is strongly related to elevated levels of inflammatory cytokines, including interleukin 6 (IL-6) and C-reactive protein (CRP), and suggested chronic activation of the innate immune system occurs in frail individuals as compared to nonfrail older adults (Leng, Xue, Tian, Walston, & Fried, 2007; Walston et al., 2002). A large cohort study of frail compared to nonfrail older adults also demonstrated a strong relationship between frailty status and high levels of fibrinogen and d-dimers, suggesting an ongoing low-grade activation of coagulation systems in frail versus nonfrail older adults that is likely driven by inflammatory mediators (Walston et al., 2002). Additional early studies showed a significant association between lower serum levels of insulin-like growth factor 1 (IGF-1) and dehydroepiandrosterone sulfate (DHEA-S), suggesting an important role for endocrine systems in frailty (Leng et al., 2004). These circulating endocrine factors are important in the maintenance of skeletal muscle. Cortisol secretion, which is part of the HPA axis and stress response system, is chronically higher in frail compared to nonfrail older adults (Johar et al., 2014; Varadhan, Walston, et al., 2008). Autonomic nervous system activity appears to be altered as well, as measured by declines in appropriate heart rate variability associated with frailty (Varadhan et al., 2009). These studies have highlighted the reality that frail older adults often have dysregulation in stress response systems, which may put them at higher risk for the development of adverse health outcomes of any type. Further, the chronic exposure to inflammatory mediators, cortisol, and autonomic nervous system tone in and of itself drives pathophysiologic changes in skeletal muscle, cardiac, lung, and likely other tissues over time, setting up the frail individual for the development or worsening of acute and chronic disease states as well as functional decline and the development of disability.

Underlying the multisystem dysregulation that characterizes frailty are likely many aging-related biological changes. Altered telomeres, epigenetic changes, autophagy, mitochondrial decline, cell senescence, nutrient

sensing, protein processing, and DNA alterations have all been hypothesized to drive many age-related changes and perhaps drive frailty and late-life vulnerability (Kaminskyy & Zhivotovsky, 2014; Tchkonia et al., 2010; Walston, 2015). Investigators have utilized mouse models to explore the etiologies of frailty related to these factors. For example, a mouse that is missing the gene that produces the anti-inflammatory cytokine interleukin 10 (IL-10) has been extensively utilized as a model of frailty. This mouse gradually develops inflammatory pathway activation in early life, which leads to chronic muscle weakness, endocrine abnormalities, lower levels of activity, lower mitochondrial energy production, altered mitophagy, and ultimately early mortality. Because the mouse experiences only mild inflammation early in life, it survives well into older age so that the impact of its chronic inflammation on the development of frailty can be studied. This and other mouse models may facilitate the identification of specific etiologies that drive frailty, eventually allowing for the development of a more targeted prevention and treatment approach in older adults (Akki et al., 2014; Ko et al., 2012; Walston et al., 2008).

Finally, chronic disease is likely a very important biological driver of frailty and late-life vulnerability. Indeed, frailty is highly associated with diabetes, congestive heart failure, and hypertension in epidemiological studies of older adults (Newman et al., 2001). These disease states and conditions drive inflammatory pathway activation, mitochondrial abnormalities, and energy production pathways that may worsen the biological processes described earlier. This, in turn, makes the chronically ill older adult more likely to develop frailty and its related vulnerability to adverse health outcomes. Further investigation into the interplay among aging-related biological decline, chronic disease, and frailty would be helpful in the attempt to identify potential points for intervention strategies aimed at preventing frailty and late-life decline.

▶ Frailty Instruments and Measurement

Frailty is widely recognized as measure of vulnerability to adverse outcomes, but lack of consensus persists over which instrument should be used to measure frailty in research and clinical settings. Over the past two decades, efforts to distinguish frail from nonfrail older adults have led to the introduction of dozens of operational definitions (Gobbens, Luijkx, Wijnen-Sponselee, & Schols, 2010b; Hogan et al., 2003), each with variations in its theoretical basis, clinical feasibility, and included domains and assessment items (Bouillon et al., 2013; de Vries et al., 2011; Gobbens et al., 2010b; Sternberg, Wershof Schwartz, Karunananthan, Bergman, & Mark Clarfield, 2011). This variability has resulted in debate over which frailty assessment is appropriate in a given context, which then raises important questions about (1) whether to include certain measures, such as disability and comorbidity, in frailty instruments and (2) how much concordance exists between instruments. Despite challenges, some general agreement has been reached that operational definitions of frailty should aim to be multidimensional, exclusive of disability and possibly comorbidity, dynamic, predictively valid for adverse outcomes, and feasible (Gobbens et al., 2010b; Hogan et al., 2003).

The authors of a recent literature review identified 67 distinct published frailty instruments; of these, nine were highly cited (200 or more citations; Buta et al., 2016):

- Physical Frailty Phenotype (PFP, also called CHS frailty phenotype) (Fried et al., 2001)
- Deficit Accumulation Index (DAI, also called Frailty Index) (Mitnitski et al., 2001; Mitnitski, Song, & Rockwood, 2004; Rockwood, Andrew, & Mitnitski, 2007; Rockwood & Mitnitski, 2007; Rockwood, Mitnitski, Song, Steen, & Skoog, 2006)

- Gill Frailty Measure (Gill et al., 2002)
- Frailty/Vigor Assessment (Speechley & Tinetti, 1991)
- Clinical Frailty Scale (Rockwood et al., 2005)
- Brief Frailty Instrument (Rockwood et al., 1999)
- Vulnerable Elders Survey (VES-13) (Saliba et al., 2001)
- FRAIL Scale (Abellan van Kan, Rolland, Bergman, et al., 2008; Abellan van Kan, Rolland, Morley, & Vellas, 2008)
- Winograd Screening Instrument (Winograd et al., 1991)

The first two were developed based respectively on the "cycle of frailty" theory by Fried et al. and the accumulation of deficits theory by Rockwood and Mitnitski. The PFP was found to be the most used instrument in the research literature, followed by the Deficit Accumulation Index (**FIGURE 9-4**). Therefore, although the notion of frailty as vulnerability to poor outcomes is a commonality, the operationalization of the measures employed is unique for each of the numerous frailty instruments that have been utilized in research studies and clinics.

Among highly cited instruments, the inclusion of some measure of physical function has been common, whereas the inclusion of other domains (e.g., physical activity, cognition) has varied (Buta et al., 2016) (**TABLE 9-1**). Eight major categories of use for frailty instruments have been identified in the literature: risk assessment for adverse health outcomes (31% of all uses); etiologic studies of frailty (22%); methodology studies (14%); biomarker studies (12%); study inclusion/exclusion criteria (10%); estimating prevalence as primary goal (5%); clinical decision making (2%); and interventional targeting (2%) (Buta et al., 2016) (**FIGURE 9-5**). The most common assessment context has been observational studies of older community-dwelling adults.

While the frequency and patterns of use are notable when selecting a frailty assessment instrument, consideration must also be given to the following items: (1) the intended purpose of the assessment, (2) the theoretical

a. Physical Frailty Phenotype
Measures
➤ Weight loss: ≥10 pounds of weight lost unintentionally in prior year at baseline; 5% of body weight lost in prior year at follow-up
➤ Weakness: Measured hand grip strength (kg) in the lowest quintile at baseline, stratified by gender and body mass index
➤ Exhaustion: Self-reported questions on exhaustion from the CES–D depression scale
➤ Slow walking speed: Timed walk over a 15-foot course in the lowest 20%, stratified by gender and height
➤ Low physical activity: Self-reported questionnaire to calculate a weighted score of kilocalories expended per week in the lowest quintile at baseline, stratified by gender
Scoring (categorical) Not Frail: 0 present Pre-frail: 1-2 present Frail: ≥3 present

b. Deficit Accumulation Index
Measures
➤ 20+ health deficits, selected from various categories that include: o chronic conditions o physical disability and dependence o physical impairments o cognitive impairments o psychosocial dysfunction o sensory impairments o other signs, symptoms, measures
➤ Number of deficits may vary
➤ Types of deficits may vary
Scoring (continuous) Calculated as the proportion of the number of deficits present divided by the number of deficits total. Higher proportion = higher level of frailty.

FIGURE 9-4 (a) Biologic syndrome model of frailty. (b) Deficit accumulation model of frailty.

a. Fried, L. P., Tangen, C. M., Walston, J., et al. Frailty in older adults: evidence for a phenotype. b. Mitnitski, Mogilner, and Rockwood, 2001. J. Gerontol. A. Biol. Sci. Med. Sci. 2001;56(3):M146-M156, Table 1, by permission of Oxford University Press.

basis and validation of the constructs included in the assessment, and (3) the feasibility of the assessment instrument, given the intended purpose and context. Regarding intended purpose, researchers and clinicians should carefully reflect on what frailty assessment aims to accomplish and whether the measures included are appropriate to meet those goals. Studies intending to measure frailty for risk stratification may consider a number of the available instruments; however, some instruments would be less useful for etiologic investigations of frailty (Xue & Varadhan, 2014), especially those that include measures of disability and comorbidity (Table 9-1). Consensus efforts have found support for considering disability—notably, as a distinct entity from frailty (Rodriguez-Manas et al., 2013).

As described earlier, theories of frailty provide a conceptual basis for selecting specific measures to assess frailty (Bortz, 2002; Buchner & Wagner, 1992; Ferrucci et al., 2005; Fried et al., 2001; Rockwood & Mitnitski, 2007; Varadhan, Seplaki, et al., 2008) and then validating them so as to demonstrate that the chosen measures accurately assess the concept ("construct") that the theory defines. While the literature indicates widespread recognition of the need for validation, most validation efforts implemented to evaluate frailty instruments have examined whether the instrument identifies older adults at elevated risk of adverse outcomes (evidencing predictive validity [Rockwood, 2005]) or whether a new or modified measure correlates considerably with assessment by an established instrument (evidencing concurrent validity).

TABLE 9-1 Domains Included in Highly Cited Frailty Instruments

Frailty Instrument	Physical Function?	Disability?	Physical Activity?	Cognition?	Comorbidity?	Weight Loss?	Other (e.g., Social, Sensory, Demographic)?
Physical Frailty	√	X	√	X	X	√	X
Phenotype Deficit Accumulation Index	√	√	X	√	√	X	√
Gill Frailty Measure	√	X	X	X	X	X	X
Frailty/Vigor Assessment	√	√	√	√	√	X	√
Clinical Frailty Scale	√	√	√	X	√	X	√
Brief Frailty Instrument	√	√	X	√	√	X	X
Vulnerable Elders Survey	√	√	X	X	X	X	√
FRAIL Scale	√	X	X	X	√	√	X
Winograd Screening Instrument	√	√	X	√	√	X	√
Total out of nine instruments	9	6	3	4	5	2	5

Reprinted from Ageing Res Rev. 26, Buta, B. J., Walston, J. D., Godino, J. G., et al. Frailty assessment instruments: Systematic characterization of the uses and contexts of highly cited instruments, pages 53-61. Copyright 2016, with permission from Elsevier.

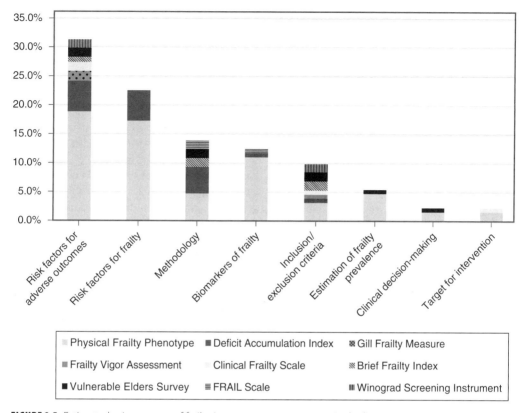

FIGURE 9-5 Estimated primary uses of frailty instruments per category in the literature, 1991–2013.

Data from Ageing Res Rev. 26, (Elsevier, 2016). Buta, B. J., Walston, J. D., Godino, J. G. et al. Frailty assessment instruments: Systematic characterization of the uses and contexts of highly cited instruments, Pages 53-61.

Two other aspects of validity, though not frequently assessed in frailty research, are important to establish whether a proposed measure accurately represents the concept it aims to assess. Content validity is achieved if the selected measures represent all the key aspects of the hypothesized frailty concept and exclude irrelevant aspects (DeVellis, 2012). For example, Fried and Walston's "cycle of frailty" conceptual framework provided the basis for studying the clinical manifestation of frailty through five indicators selected to represent key elements of the cycle: (1) weight loss, reflecting dysregulated nutrition; (2 and 3) exhaustion and low physical activity, reflecting energetic dysregulation; (4) weakness, reflecting degraded muscle; and (5) gait speed as an integrative measure (Fried et al., 2001).

By comparison, construct validity is achieved if the proposed measures manifest together (show internal construct validity), and relate to etiologic precursors and consequences (show external construct validity), as predicted by the theory delineating the frailty concept under study. For example, the PFP has been shown to have internal construct validity with respect to the hypothesized clinical presentation of frailty as a medical syndrome (Bandeen-Roche et al., 2006). It has been externally validated for its association with multisystem dysregulation as a hypothesized etiology (Fried et al., 2009). In summary, selected frailty measures should aim to match the core constructs of our current theoretical knowledge.

Instrument feasibility is another important consideration in research and clinical contexts. Frailty instruments range from single-measure assessments to an instrument with more than 92 measures. Such instruments may incorporate self-report items, objective measures, or a mixed approach. Considering this variation, in combination with real-world constraints such as limited time, funding, resources, and space, certain instruments may better suit specific clinic or research needs. For example, the Study of Osteoporotic Fractures Index has been investigated as a potentially more simple instrument than the PFP for defining frailty in a clinical setting (Ensrud et al., 2008).

Here we pause to reiterate that more research is needed to better understand the levels of agreement among frailty instruments. Although one instrument may be readily feasible in a clinical setting, we ideally must confirm that it delineates the same frail group, and meets the other tests of validity, when compared to a more rigorous instrument. Also, feasibility may be a matter of evolving perspective: Examples can be cited of measures that were once argued to be infeasible or difficult to collect but that are now routinely employed (e.g., C-reactive protein as an inflammatory risk predictor for cardiovascular disease [Pepys & Hirschfield, 2003]). If demonstrated to have clinical value or through technological advancement or policy mandates, frailty-related measures once viewed as impractical can become routine.

▶ Links Between Frailty and Geriatric Syndromes

Derived from the Greek roots *syn* (meaning "together") and *dromo* (meaning "a running"), the word *syndrome* in medical literature generally refers to "the aggregate of symptoms and signs associated with any morbid process, and constituting together the picture of the disease" (Flacker, 2003). Cushing's syndrome is a classic example of a medical syndrome:

It is a wide-ranging collection of signs and symptoms resulting from prolonged exposure to excessive cortisol—a unitary cause involving a single physiologic system (i.e., the hypothalamic–pituitary–adrenal axis). In contrast, a geriatric syndrome is typically assumed to result from accumulated impairments in multiple systems contributing to a particular outcome (e.g., incontinence). Using the term "syndrome" to describe geriatric conditions with a multifactorial etiology is, therefore, at odds with its original usage because "the outcome is a single phenomenology rather than a spectrum of symptoms and signs, and results from numerous rather than a single disruption" (Flacker, 2003).

In contrast, the physical frailty phenotype may be considered as a medical syndrome, such that labeling PFP as a geriatric syndrome risks misinforming research on biological links between frailty and geriatric syndromes. To formally evaluate the degree to which the frailty phenotype conforms to the definition of a medical syndrome, Bandeen-Roche et al. (2006) analyzed patterns of co-occurrence of the five frailty-defining criteria based on data from a combined sample of women aged 70-79 from the Women's Health and Aging Studies (WHAS) I and II. Patterns of criteria co-occurrence that would support the syndrome definition are (1) manifestation in a critical mass and (2) aggregation in a hierarchical order, as would occur in a cycle in which dysregulation in a sentinel system triggers a cascade of alterations across other systems. Propensity for criteria to co-occur in distinct subgroups would suggest the effects of distinct biologic processes rather than a syndrome. Using latent class analysis (LCA; Goodman, 1974), three population subsets (also termed "classes") were identified with similar profiles of frailty criteria co-occurrence; each criterion's prevalence increased progressively across the population subsets, indicating an increase in frailty severity. These findings supported the internal validity of the frailty criteria vis-à-vis stated theory characterizing frailty as a medical syndrome and provided justification for the current counting strategy for defining frailty categories (i.e., non-frail, pre-frail, frail). To further validate the theory of frailty as a medical syndrome, it would be important to replicate this analysis in men and other populations, and to make advances in research on the biology of frailty so as to shed light on the dimensionality of its etiology.

▶ Studies of Associations Between Geriatric Syndromes and Frailty

Frailty has been studied in connection with each of the discussed geriatric syndromes. Frailty and geriatric syndromes share the common risk factors of older age, functional impairments, and mobility limitations, as well as comorbidities, polypharmacy, and poor nutrition. Decreased strength and physical impairments may play a common role in the association of frailty with falls and incontinence, and frailty and delirium may be related through inflammatory and other biological pathways. Etiologic studies to elucidate these relationships are needed, and the possibility of bidirectional influence should be considered.

Multiple studies have reported the association between frailty and increased risk of falls in older women and men (Ensrud et al., 2009; Ensrud et al., 2007; Fried et al., 2001); this may be partially explained by the common risk factors contributing to muscle weakness and functional decline. Frail older adults with a history of falling are also significantly more likely to have a fear of falling when compared to robust fallers (Ni Mhaolain et al., 2012). Both frailty and falls are regarded as a "manifestation of complex system failure" (Nowak & Hubbard, 2009). A recent meta-analysis found

that frailty was a significant predictor of future falls in community-dwelling older adults, even with the use of differing frailty criteria (Kojima, 2015).

A strong correlation between urinary incontinence (UI) and frailty—assessed using four items: activities of daily living (ADLs), Mini-Mental State Examination (MMSE), hand grip strength, and self-reported health—was found among the very old (Berardelli et al., 2013). Talley and colleagues (2011) reviewed conservative interventions for UI among frail older adults (defined as adults 60 years and older with functional impairments, homebound, or requiring daily activity assistance); multicomponent behavioral interventions (risk assessment combined with pelvic muscle and bladder training) were recommended for frail older persons. Studies have suggested that incident incontinence is associated with risk for functional impairment, suggesting that incontinence may be an early marker of frailty onset (Miles et al., 2001; Wagg et al., 2015). A recent study found that combined urinary and fecal incontinence is associated with medical conditions such as limited mobility—a factor related to frailty (Matthews, 2014). Overall, incontinence is viewed as a frequent health problem in frail older adults, but the direction of this relationship remains to be determined (Gammack, 2004).

Several studies have explored the relationship between delirium and frailty in older patients, though the results have been mixed. One study found that frailty score (assessed using the frailty phenotype) was significantly associated with the development of postoperative delirium (Leung, Tsai, & Sands, 2011), while another study found that frailty (assessed using both the frailty phenotype and the Study of Osteoporotic Fractures index) was not an independent risk factor for delirium among older hospital patients (Joosten, Demuynck, Detroyer, & Milisen, 2014). Eeles and colleagues (2012) found that delirium was associated with higher levels of frailty (assessed using a deficit accumulation index). Quinlan and colleagues (2011) reviewed the potential intersections of frailty and delirium, and proposed a potential shared pathophysiology that includes inflammation, atherosclerosis, and chronic nutritional deficiencies.

In an effort to provide a theoretical framework unifying the concept of frailty and geriatric syndromes, Inouye et al. (2007) proposed a conceptual model that treats frailty as an intermediary outcome in the causal pathway from geriatric outcomes to distal outcomes including disability, dependence, nursing home admission, and death, while acknowledging the possibility that feedback relationships might exist between frailty and geriatric syndromes. It is commonly believed that geriatric syndromes share risk factors. For example, risk factors shared across all five geriatric syndromes reviewed by Inouye et al. (2007) (pressure ulcers, incontinence, falls, functional decline, and delirium) included older age, functional impairment, cognitive impairment, and impaired mobility, all of which are also known to be associated with frailty. Moreover, the shared risk factors raised the possibility of the existence of common pathophysiologic underpinnings shared by these geriatric syndromes, including inflammation (Walston et al., 2002; Walston, Xue, et al., 2006), hormonal dysfunction (Maggio et al., 2005), and interacting dysregulated systems (Fried et al., 2005).

▸ Physiologic Risk Factors for Frailty and Geriatric Syndromes

Frailty has been called "the overarching geriatric syndrome" due to the hypothesis that it may encompass or feedback upon other geriatric syndromes and their common risk factors (Inouye et al., 2007). Although the etiology of frailty is unknown, stress response systems have been hypothesized to play a role in its development (Walston, 2015). Proposed systems (and related biomarkers) include innate immune/

inflammatory factors (IL-6, C-reactive protein, tumor necrosis factor alpha, lipopolysaccharide stimulation, neopterin, white blood cells), the hypothalamic–pituitary–adrenal axis (cortisol, dehydroepiandrosterone-sulfate, urinary catechol), and the sympathetic nervous system (epinephrine/norepinephrine, heart rate variability). In this section, we review reported associations of physiologic risk factors with frailty and geriatric syndromes (falls, incontinence, delirium) (**FIGURE 9-6**).

Changes in the innate immune system, and related inflammatory responses, occur with aging and lead to elevated vulnerability to infection and disease among older adults (Weinberger & Grubeck-Loebenstein, 2009). Cross-sectional studies have consistently reported an association between inflammatory markers (IL-6, CRP) and frailty among older adults (Leng et al., 2007; Leng, Yang, & Walston, 2004; Walston, 2005). A recent longitudinal study of CRP and fibrinogen and incident frailty reported an association between elevated levels of these inflammatory markers and the onset of frailty among women, but not among men (Gale, Baylis, Cooper, & Sayer, 2013). The relationship between inflammation and falls has not been explicitly studied, though studies have shown associations between higher CRP levels and balance problems, as well as elevated CRP levels among those older adults with hip fracture (Lumbers, New, Gibson, & Murphy, 2001; Tudor-ache et al., 2015). There is limited evidence on the connection between inflammation and incontinence. Two studies have found a positive association between high serum CRP and overactive bladder, which is related to urge incontinence (Hsiao, Lin, & Kuo, 2012; Kupelian et al., 2012). Finally, studies have explored the relationship between inflammation and delirium in clinical patients; an association between preoperatively elevated markers (IL-6, CRP) and postoperative-onset delirium has been found in multiple studies (Capri et al., 2014; Pol et al., 2014; Vasunilashorn et al., 2015).

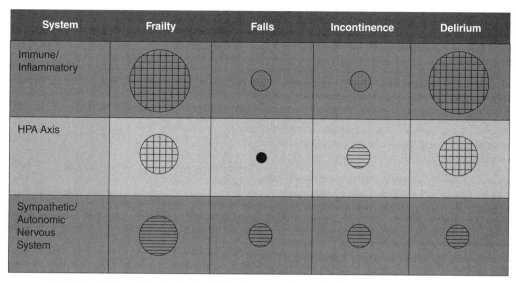

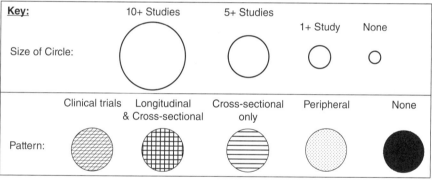

FIGURE 9-6 Physiologic systems and geriatric syndromes: studies to date.

Activation of the hypothalamic–pituitary–adrenal axis is a crucial feature of the acute stress response, but chronic activation and over-activation over time can result in detrimental health effects and contribute to allostatic load (Ferrari et al., 2001; McEwen, 1998). Cross-sectional studies have shown an association between blunted cortisol variation and increased frailty in older adults (Holanda et al., 2012; Johar et al., 2014; Varadhan, Walston, et al., 2008). Frail individuals had lower DHEA-S levels than their nonfrail counterparts cross-sectionally (Leng et al., 2004). Moreover, in a longitudinal study, lower DHEA-S levels were significantly associated

with increased risk of frailty at 10 years among older men and women (Baylis et al., 2013). No published evidence was found on the relationship between HPA-axis dysregulation and falls. There has been limited research on the relationship between HPA-axis markers and incontinence; in one study, no association was found between cortisol and urinary incontinence among women age 50–59 (Teleman, Persson, Mattiasson, & Samsioe, 2009). Regarding HPA-axis function and delirium, several studies have shown associations between elevated cortisol levels and postoperative delirium (Cerejeira, Batista, Nogueira, Vaz-Serra, & Mukaetova-Ladinska, 2013; Colkesen,

Giray, Ozenli, Sezgin, & Coskun, 2013; Mu et al., 2010). Additionally, cortisol and DHEA-S, studied as primary mediators of allostatic load, were found to be predictive of delirium incidence among hospitalized older adults (Rigney, 2010).

The sympathetic nervous system (SNS) plays the primary role in the stress response and in maintaining homeostasis as part of the autonomic nervous system (ANS). Parvaneh et al.'s 2015 systematic review summarized six observational studies on impaired cardiac ANS, including loss of complexity in heart rate dynamics and reduced heart rate variability, and frailty in older adults. Evidence of an association between frailty and impaired autonomic control was reported, though further research is needed to confirm this relationship (Parvaneh et al., 2015). Emerging but limited evidence supports a relationship between heart rate variability (HRV) and falls; studies on this association propose analyses of electrocardiograms to use HRV as a potential predictor of falls (Castaldo, Melillo, Izzo, De Luca, & Pecchia, 2016; Melillo, Jovic, De Luca, & Pecchia, 2015). The SNS plays a regulatory role in the lower urinary tract, which influences urge incontinence. A small number of studies have shown preliminary evidence of an association between impaired heart rate measures and urinary incontinence among women (Hubeaux, Deffieux, Ismael, Raibaut, & Amarenco, 2007; Kim et al., 2010; Miller, 2005). Very few studies have explored the relationship between SNS and delirium, with mixed results (Deiner, Lin, Bodansky, Silverstein, & Sano, 2014; Zaal, van der Kooi, van Schelven, Oey, & Slooter, 2015).

Overall, the stress response systems discussed here are associated with frailty, although the degrees of evidence supporting those relationships vary. For the other syndromes, the role of stress response systems appears to be mixed. More evidence is needed, especially from longitudinal studies of the relationship between dysregulated systems and the development of frailty and geriatric syndromes.

▶ Latest Findings from Frailty Research

Prevalence and Incidence of Frailty

A recent systematic review reported that frailty prevalence ranges from 4% to 59.1% in community-dwelling older adults (Collard, Boter, Schoevers, & Voshaar, 2012). The lack of standardization of frailty assessment can at least partially explain the wide-ranging estimates. Considerable variability in frailty prevalence has also been reported even when restricting the assessment to the use of the PFP, with estimates ranging from 4% to 17% (Collard et al., 2012). These studies employed diverse geographic catchment and sampling methods, which likely contributed to the variation observed.

A recent study using data from the baseline evaluation of the National Health and Aging Trends Study (NHATS) and the PFP assessment paradigm reported a nationally representative prevalence of 15.3% in the United States in 2011 (Bandeen-Roche et al., 2015). This study reported steep age-related increases in frailty prevalence (as one might expect), ranging from approximately 9% among 65- to 69-year-olds to 38% in persons 90 years of age or older. In the Cardiovascular Health Study (CHS), PFP prevalence increased from 3.9% in the 65–74 age group to 25% in the 85 and older group (Fried et al., 2001). In both of these studies, frailty prevalence was greater in women than men (17% versus 13% in NHATS and 8% versus 5% in CHS), which is consistent with other reports that women, while having longer life expectancy, are more likely to experience functional limitations and disabilities than men. Similar age trends and gender differences were reported by Collard et al. (2012). Similar studies have also found striking disparities in frailty prevalence by race, income, and geographic region.

African Americans were more likely to be frail than Caucasians in the NHATS (23% versus 14%), CHS (13% versus 6%; Hirsch et al., 2006), and WHAS (16% versus 10%; unpublished). The 1996 estimate of frailty among Mexican Americans from the Hispanic Established Populations for Epidemiologic Studies of the Elderly was 7.8%—a rate similar to that for Caucasians (Graham et al., 2009); in contrast, in NHATS, the prevalence for Hispanic Americans was considerably inflated (25%) as compared to Caucasians. Research to further elucidate and ameliorate these disparities is a high priority for the next generation of frailty scholarship.

The prevalence of PFP also varies internationally (**FIGURE 9-7**). For example, a survey of 7510 community-dwelling older adults in 10 European countries found that prevalence of frailty ranged from 5.8% in Switzerland to 27%

in Spain, with an overall prevalence of 17%; rates were higher in southern than in northern Europe, consistent with an unexplained north–south health risk gradient previously reported in the same population (Borsch-Supan et al., 2005; Santos-Eggimann, Cuenoud, Spagnoli, & Junod, 2009). The latest estimates of PFP from the European Project on Osteoarthritis (EPOSA), which was conducted in six European countries, ranged from 5.6% to 15.4%, exhibiting similar altitudinal gradients (Castell et al., 2015). The geographic variation in frailty prevalence among these European countries persisted after adjusting for age and gender, which led the authors to speculate that differences in cultural characteristics may influence the perception of health or interpretation of the frailty questions (Santos-Eggimann et al., 2009). Surveys conducted in Turkey (Eyigor et al., 2015) and Latin American countries

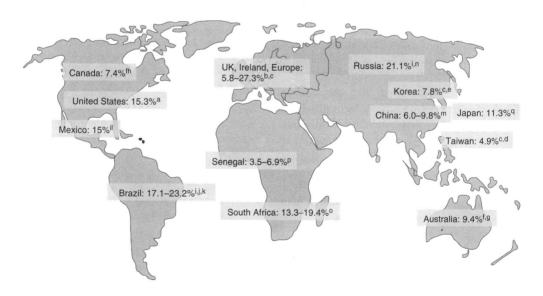

[a]Bandeen-Roche 2015; [b]Santos-Eggimann 2009; [c]Choi 2015; [d]Chen 2010; [e]Lee Y 2014; [f]Collard 2012; [g]Blyth 2008; [h]Wong 2010; [i]Nguyen 2015; [j]Alencar 2013; [k]Sousa 2012; [l]Castrejon-Perez 2012; [m]Lee JS 2014: [n]Gurina 2011; [o]Pathai 2013; [p]Cournil 2014; [q]Shimada 2013.

FIGURE 9-7 Estimated mean prevalence of frailty worldwide in population studies using the frailty phenotype.

Contributed by Xue, Q. L., Buta, B., Varadhan, R., Szanton, S. L., Chaves, P., Walston, J. D., Bandeen-Roche, K.

(Aguilar-Navarro, Amieva, Gutierrez-Robledo, & Avila-Funes, 2015; Alvarado, Zunzunegui, Beland, & Bamvita, 2008) consistently found a much higher prevalence of PFP in both men (21–35%) and women (30–48%) in these areas compared to their U.S. and European counterparts.

The annual incidence of PFP estimated from published reports ranges from 1.2% to 8.2% (Dalrymple et al., 2013; Gale, Cooper, & Sayer, 2014; Garcia-Esquinas, Guallar-Castillon, et al., 2016; Garcia-Esquinas, Rahi, et al., 2016; Gross et al., 2016; Kalyani et al., 2012; LaCroix et al., 2008; Lakey et al., 2012; Sandoval-Insausti et al., 2016; Woods et al., 2005; Xue, Bandeen-Roche, Varadhan, Zhou, & Fried, 2008). In the Seniors—ENRICA cohort from Spain, the incidence rate of PFP varied from 7.2% to 11.6% over 3.5 years (2.1–3.5% annually) depending on inclusion and exclusion criteria (Garcia-Esquinas, Guallar-Castillon, et al., 2016; Garcia-Esquinas, Rahi, et al., 2016; Sandoval-Insausti et al., 2016; Soler-Vila et al., 2016). Comparable incidence rates have been reported by the English Longitudinal Study of Ageing (ELSA) in England (10% over 4 years or 2.6% annually [Gale et al., 2014]), WHAS II (13% [Gross et al., 2016], 14% [Xue et al., 2008], 23.4% [Kalyani et al., 2012] over 6.8, 7.5, and 8.6 years, respectively, or 2.0%, 2.0%, and 3.1% annually), and the Cardiovascular Health Study (6.2% over 4 years or 1.6% annually [Dalrymple et al., 2013]) in the United States. In contrast, the estimates from the Three-City Bordeaux and the Aging Multidisciplinary Investigation Cohort were noticeably higher, with a 2-year incidence rate of 15.7% and 15.4% (or 8.2% and 8.0% annually), respectively (Garcia-Esquinas, Rahi, et al., 2016). The estimates from the Women's Health Initiative Study were 13.6–14.9% over 3 years (or 4.8–5.2% annually) (LaCroix et al., 2008; Lakey et al., 2012; Woods et al., 2005), which were higher than those from the WHAS, possibly due to the fact that the Rand-36 physical function scale score (less than 75) was used to define the weakness and slowness components in the PFP instead of the usual

performance-based measures of gait speed and grip strength. Women tend to have higher incidence of PFP than men. In the Seniors—ENRICA cohort, the incidence rate was 4.2% for men compared to 10.0% for women over 4 years (Soler-Vila et al., 2016); and it was 7.5% for men and 11.9% for women in ELSA (Gale et al., 2014). Incidence data for different racial/ethnic groups are scarce. In the WHI study, Woods et al. (2005) found that African Americans had less PFP incidence than whites after covariate adjustment.

Natural History of Manifestations of the Frailty Syndrome

Understanding points of onset of frailty is vital if at-risk individuals are to be identified and those components that are first affected are to be subjected to interventions early, when reversal may be most possible. Preclinical detection of early manifestations leading to frailty syndrome requires understanding the natural history of frailty development. We suggest two potential hypotheses as to the natural history of PFP initiation and progression: (1) that a cycle of frailty could be initiated via any of the clinical manifestations, which could then precipitate a "vicious cycle" culminating in an aggregate syndrome, and (2) that different initial manifestations may lead to differential rates of progression to frailty. Based on a 7.5-year longitudinal study of 420 WHAS II participants who were defined as nonfrail using the PFP at baseline, Xue, Bandeen-Roche, et al. (2008) found evidence of a partially hierarchical order in the onset of frailty manifestations over time. Although there was notable heterogeneity in the initial manifestations of frailty, weakness was the most common first manifestation, with the occurrence of weakness, slowness, and low physical activity preceding exhaustion and weight loss in 76% of the women who were nonfrail at baseline. The finding of heterogeneity in the initial criteria is consistent with the hypothesis that the cycle of frailty may be initiated by insults at many points in a hypothesized cycle of dysregulated energetics (Fried et al., 2001; Fried & Walston, 1998). Additionally, it was not the number of early manifestations (i.e., one or two) but rather the specific manifestations initially present that distinguished the risk and rate of onset of frailty. Specifically, women with weakness, exhaustion, or weight loss as initial presenting symptoms were 3–5 times more likely to become frail than were women without any criterion. In contrast, neither slow walking speed nor low activity as a first-occurring condition was predictive of frailty onset. It remains to be determined whether the different patterns of initial accumulation of frailty criteria represent different etiologic pathways with different rates of progression to frailty, either organ specific or representing systemic physiologic dysregulations of aging. Alternatively, some criterion measures may be more sensitive than others to changes associated with "normal aging"—for instance, performance-based as opposed to self-reported criteria.

That weakness should presage frailty onset is consistent with earlier reports that loss of muscle strength begins in midlife (Lindle et al., 1997; Nair, 1995; Viitasalo, Era, Leskinen, & Heikkinen, 1985). Decline in strength has been attributed to the loss of muscle mass and muscle quality referred to as sarcopenia, which results from anatomic and biochemical changes in the aging muscle (Kamel, 2003). The causal mechanisms underlying sarcopenia are many, including oxidative stress, dysregulation of inflammatory cytokines and hormones, malnutrition, physical inactivity, and muscle apoptosis (Dirks, Hofer, Marzetti, Pahor, & Leeuwenburgh, 2005; Marcell, 2003), all of which have been hypothesized to contribute to frailty through interactive pathways at multiple temporal and spatial scales (Fried et al., 2005).

Despite heterogeneous entry points into the cycle of frailty, 80% of transitions to frailty involved adding exhaustion or weight loss. This finding raises the possibility that decreased energy production or increased utilization, as in wasting conditions, may be involved in the threshold transition in a final common pathway toward frailty. The fact that 83% of such transitions had weight loss and exhaustion co-occurring with other manifestations is consistent with the reliability theory (Lloyd & Lipow, 1962), whereby an emergent aggregation of multiple frailty manifestations would result from depletion of system redundancy or compensatory mechanisms, such that any new deficit leads to failure of the whole organism (Amaral, Diaz-Guilera, Moreira, Goldberger, & Lipsitz, 2004; Bortz, 2002; Gavrilov & Gavrilova, 2001; Kitano, 2002). If so, early detection of subclinical changes or deficits at the molecular, cellular, and/or physiologic level would be key to preventing or delaying the development of frailty.

The clinical utility of these findings lies in the fact that weakness is the most common initial manifestation of the frailty phenotype. It has shown only moderate predictive validity for incident frailty; however, our conceptualization posits that the development of frailty is progressive and multisystemic, such that any one specific criterion alone, especially at an early stage in the process as in the case of weakness, may be neither sufficient nor specific for frailty prediction. Given that the criterion-defining thresholds for grip strength are known to be associated with meaningfully greater risk of adverse outcomes including disability and mortality (Rantanen et al., 2003), weakness may nevertheless be a clinically meaningful indicator of increasing vulnerability at a relatively early stage of the frailty process, when preventive interventions could be easiest to implement and theoretically most effective. Although the subsequent or "concurrent" onset of weight loss or exhaustion with the other criteria may better predict frailty onset, by the time someone experiences weight loss or exhaustion, it may be too late to implement frailty interventions. Therefore, consideration should be given to the possible tradeoff between risk prediction and potential benefits in deciding the proper timing and targets of interventions.

Despite rapidly growing interest and investment in frailty intervention research led mostly by European and Australian researchers (Hoogendijk et al., 2016; Rodríguez-Mañas et al., 2014; Subra et al., 2012; Tavassoli et al., 2014), significant challenges remain. First, the lack of standardization in frailty assessment continues to be the major barrier in interpreting and comparing intervention efficacy across studies. This problem is exemplified by the observation that only 32% of all studies have included an operational definition of frailty, and among these studies only 3 (6%) included a validated definition of frailty.

Second, early efforts largely focused on interventions targeting "frail" older adults and assessment of differential efficacy based on age, gender, residential setting, intervention modality, and outcome measures. Only recently has frailty assessment been formally incorporated into screening for study eligibility; likewise, frailty itself, rather its phenotypic components or risk factors, has only recently become the primary outcome of a study. The distinction between targeting frailty as a syndrome versus treating its components is important if we envision frailty not "as a collection of symptoms, but rather as a collection of indicators of an underlying syndrome" (Robertson, Savva, & Kenny, 2013). With this perspective, treating the indicators themselves is not equivalent to treating the underlying condition.

Third, the premise that exercise and nutritional interventions are effective ways to prevent or reverse the functional decline associated with the development of frailty is built upon indirect evidence, reflecting correlations of frailty with functional outcomes, rather than specific scientific theories underlying the biology of frailty. It remains to be determined whether direct targeting of functional impairments proximal to frailty onset, such as muscle weakness, is sufficient for addressing or alleviating the root cause(s) of frailty. While the urgency to act is understandable, a theory-driven approach targeting specific—or a network of—biological targets may prove to be a more fruitful approach in elucidating the underlying etiology of frailty.

▶ Current Issues and Challenges of Frailty Research

Clarifying Conceptualization and Measurement

The proliferation of frailty instruments documented earlier in the chapter has been described by some as an advantage, providing practitioners with an array of options for frailty assessment (Morley et al., 2013). However, such a proliferation also may have adverse consequences, because different frailty instruments identify different people. One study found that only 3.1% of participants classified as frail by one of three prominent methods were classified as frail by all three of these methods (Inouye et al., 207). This outcome reflects different conceptualizations of the entity (i.e., frailty) as well as different choices of frailty measures within entities (Theou & Rockwood, 2015; Xue, Tian, et al., 2016).

Among the dozens of extant frailty instruments, at least three major schools of thought have emerged regarding frailty conceptualization:

- Frailty as a disordered physiologic state driven by multifactorial dysregulation, which manifests as a medical syndrome of low energy, shrinking, weakness, and impaired motor functioning, and which results in vulnerability to adverse outcomes upon stressors (Fried et al., 2001)
- Frailty as a state of high risk for adverse outcomes, marked by a high burden of health and functional impairments (Rockwood, 2005)
- Frailty as a condition presaging disability and loss of functional independence (Vellas et al., 2013)

At the very least, differences in conceptualization must be recognized; they also should be documented through resource materials mapping instruments to concepts, so as to guide practitioners in tailoring their choice of measure to their purpose in assessment. Beyond this, some have suggested that the field should more strongly and explicitly distinguish disparate concepts that are currently subsumed under the single label of "frailty" (Walston & Bandeen-Roche, 2015). Clarity in conceptualization likely will be crucial if the goal is to elucidate mechanisms and physiologic etiology and, ultimately, to develop and appropriately target interventions to ameliorate frailty.

Proposed measures of frailty, whatever the conceptualization, must be evaluated for reliability and validated. Predictive validity has been the most widely used method for validating measures of frailty (Bouillon et al., 2013; de Vries et al., 2011); more widespread assessment of content validity, construct validity, and reliability of frailty measures is needed (Xue & Varadhan, 2014). In the rare instances in which construct validity has been assessed, the investigation typically has addressed "convergent" external validity, in which the researcher seeks to observe associations that are predicted by the underlying theory. "Divergent" external validity, in contrast, is established when associations that should not be present according to the theory are ruled out. For example, if one hypothesizes that frailty and comorbidity are distinct, it should be possible to identify determinants of comorbidity that are not determinants of frailty, or vice versa. To date, this aspect of validity has been understudied in research on frailty.

Moreover, given that frailty is theoretically defined as a clinically recognizable state of increased vulnerability, the validation of frailty measures needs to be broadened to include the evaluation of frailty as a potential marker of increased vulnerability to stressors (i.e., effect modification of stressor effects on subsequent health declines with greater frailty). One might study ability to cope with and recover from acute stressors (Fried et al., 2005; Varadhan, Seplaki, et al., 2008), including both external stressors whose occurrence can be taken to be approximately independent

of frailty (e.g., death of a spouse) and internal stressors whose occurrence may be spurred by frailty (e.g., hospitalization). Evidence supporting modification by frailty of the effects of a stressor on distal health outcomes would strengthen the internal construct validity of a frailty measure; to our knowledge, no population-based study has yet been conducted to provide this support. Such evidence also might promote greater public awareness of the needs of older adults experiencing acute stressors and help determine what their family and friends, care providers, and the society at large can do to minimize resulting harms. Overall, continuing efforts to determine that instruments are measuring their intended frailty-related constructs, and to tailor **measurement** methodology to match the clinical aims of frailty assessment, are essential to the field.

Frailty as a Multidimensional Construct: Physical and Cognitive Frailty

Frailty is widely perceived as a multidimensional concept and, therefore, as a construct that should incorporate multiple domains in a synthetic assessment in addition to physical frailty (Morley et al., 2013; Rodriguez-Manas et al., 2013). For example, recent consensus papers have suggested expanding the definition of frailty to include cognition (Gobbens, Luijkx, Wijnen-Sponselee, & Schols, 2010a; Rodriguez-Manas et al., 2013). In fact, nearly 50% of the frailty instruments in the literature include a measure of cognition (Sternberg et al., 2011).

The rationale for such inclusion is based on several factors. First, physical frailty and cognitive impairment often coexist in older adults (Subra et al., 2012). Second, inclusion of cognition in the operational definition of the PFP has been found to improve the predictive validity of the PFP for adverse aging outcomes (Avila-Funes et al., 2009). Third, physical frailty and cognitive impairments share multiple pathophysiologic mechanisms

(Halil, Kizilarslanoglu, Kuyumcu, Yesil, & Jentoft, 2015).

Those holding opposing views, however, have argued danger in selecting content domains of frailty assessment based solely on predictive validity, because optimization of predictive validity may erode accuracy for identifying the intended construct of frailty as a medical syndrome (Xue et al., 2015). It is true that whether a frailty phenotype meets the definition of a medical syndrome may not matter greatly for practitioners who seek to identify "vulnerable" (broadly defined) patients for the purpose of deciding what to do about aspects of their care other than frailty (e.g., decision-making regarding an elective surgery). In this case, an integrated frailty phenotype designed to comprehensively capture global vulnerability may be warranted. In contrast, if frailty is a target of intervention in its own right, construct validity becomes critical. For example, suppose that two individuals are both classified as frail, but one is cognitively frail and the other is physically frail. It does not require an astute clinician to realize that they are different: Their underlying biology may differ greatly, and they likely need to be managed differently. Therefore, because of the heterogeneity of "frail" older adults, we need assessment tools that are specific in the types of frailty they aim to identify (Xue & Varadhan, 2014).

In an attempt to explain heterogeneity in the etiologic pathways of cognitive aging, a consensus group organized by the International Academy of Nutrition and Aging (IANA) and the International Association of Gerontology and Geriatrics (IAGG) provided a first definition of "cognitive frailty" as "a heterogeneous clinical manifestation characterized by the simultaneous presence of both physical frailty and cognitive impairment" in the absence of "concurrent AD dementia or other dementia" (Kelaiditi et al., 2013). The goal is to identify a state of reduced cognitive reserve that is a reversible condition caused by physical frailty instead of pathological brain aging. The underlying rationale is that "the

cognitive impairment due to a physical condition would benefit from completely different interventions from the one caused by a neurodegenerative disorder" (Canevelli & Cesari, 2015). While there is growing interest in this novel concept, issues surrounding its operationalization and lack of epidemiological data on the natural history of its clinical manifestations have hampered its clinical and research implementation (Canevelli & Cesari, 2015).

To begin addressing these challenges we first need to obtain population-representative prevalence estimates of physical frailty and cognitive impairments and compare the demographic and health characteristics of people by patterns of separate and joint occurrence. If patterns of co-occurrence in frailty and cognitive impairment are associated with different disease characteristics and health events, these two conditions, although sometimes co-occurring, may have distinct etiologic components. Second, we need a theoretical framework for evaluating physical frailty and cognitive impairment comprehensively but distinctly. For example, one approach to disentangle the influence of neurodegenerative etiology on physical frailty and cognitive decline seeks to exclude prevalent and incident dementia cases from validation analysis of the joint phenotype; in doing so, we aim to identify the systemic physiologic vulnerability contributing to both physical frailty and cognitive decline other than disease-specific manifestations. The resulting improved measurement specificity may be critical for intervention targeting. Third, we need to generate empirical evidence regarding the clinical utility of considering frailty and cognitive impairments separately versus jointly for predicting adverse aging outcomes. Finally, it is necessary to go beyond the evaluation of predictive validity to also consider the internal construct validity of a combined frailty and cognitive impairment phenotype. Collectively, the findings from these next steps should help delineate the interconnections between the different hypothesized domains of frailty, and buttress or refute an integrated frailty phenotype from both construct validity and clinical utility perspectives. A multidisciplinary approach to studying frailty is likely needed to strengthen these efforts (Karunananthan, Wolfson, Bergman, Béland, & Hogan, 2009).

Physiotypes of Frailty

To date, research on frailty assessment has largely focused on the development of phenotypes summarizing the clinical manifestation of the condition. However, for research on etiology or the development of interventions, ascertainment of the physiologic underpinnings or manifestation arguably is more relevant. We refer to measures targeted to such ascertainment as "physiotypes."

One promising direction for the development of physiotypes can be inferred from the generally accepted theory that frailty is a state of increased vulnerability that arises from decline in physiologic reserve, and results in diminished capacity to cope with everyday or acute stressors. This culminating outcome of impaired coping highlights that frailty is an inherently dynamic concept that may be best assessed through measurement of dynamic physiologic response to stressors (Varadhan, Seplaki, et al., 2008). Work to pioneer such measurement was carried out in subsets of participants in the Women's Health and Aging Study II. Kalyani and colleagues (2012) reported on a study in which standard oral glucose tolerance tests (OGTTs) were administered in the home. Serum samples were collected after a 12-hour fast and at 30, 60, 120, and 180 minutes following oral glucose administration. Trajectories of serum glucose and insulin were then compared for nonfrail, frail, and pre-frail (an intermediate state) women as identified by the PFP. Whereas the three groups of women were found to have similar baseline levels of glucose and insulin, the frail women had a larger peak response to glucose administration and a slower return toward initial status, compared to the nonfrail and

pre-frail women. This finding supports a linkage between altered glucose–insulin dynamics and frailty. Other substudies evaluated physiologic response to exercise, ACTH stimulation, cognitive testing, and influenza vaccine (Yao et al., 2011). Although the dynamic testing paradigm is effort intensive in older adults, it offers intriguing possibilities for increasing our knowledge of the etiology of frailty.

Even considering only static measures, there may be room for physiotypes to improve frailty measurement. Serum-based measures of inflammation (Leng, Xue, Tian, Fried, & Walston, 2005; Walston et al., 2002), nutrition (Bartali et al., 2005; Michelon et al., 2006; Semba et al., 2006), endocrine functioning (Cappola, Xue, & Fried, 2009), and stress response (Varadhan, Seplaki, et al., 2008) have been shown to be strongly associated with clinical phenotypes of frailty. The systems they reflect have been hypothesized as key in the development of frailty; therefore, it may be that the measures can be combined into a useful physiotype of frailty. Such physiotypes, reflecting processes more proximal to the etiologic drivers of frailty than clinical phenotypes, may provide superior targets of intervention. They also may prove effective as biomarkers to predict the onset of clinically observable frailty or to identify which patients are likely to respond to treatment. Mitochondrial and cellular discoveries now being developed mainly in animal models offer additional possibilities as elements of a frailty physiotype.

Frailty, Stress, and Compensation

According to the person–environment fit theory (Wallace & Bergeman, 1997), compensation or adaptation is a major outcome of stress arising from a misfit between the person and the environment, particularly when the environment does not provide adequate resources to meet the person's needs. Given that decreased reserve and diminished resistance to stressors are hallmarks of frailty, behavioral adaptations in response to intrinsic personal limitations or extrinsic environmental hazards may provide a previously undiscovered window into late-life vulnerability. In particular, by optimizing the person–environment fit, this approach may create new avenues for preserving function and, in turn, preventing or delaying the onset of overt frailty and disability.

Compensation—and behavioral adaptation in particular—has been studied extensively in the context of recognizing and delaying the near onset of functional disability. For disability prevention, the ability to detect incremental changes representing preclinical or subclinical stages of disability is of paramount importance. During this intermediate stage, some people choose to compensate for underlying functional decrements by adopting a modified routine of daily life (e.g., reduced frequency of walking for exercise). Epidemiological studies have demonstrated that such use of compensations is a useful marker of impending functional transition to mobility difficulty (Kuchel, 2009). In addition, these adaptations may help maintain functioning either within a normal range or at a compromised but self-satisfactory level without perceived dependency (Fried, Bandeen-Roche, Chaves, & Johnson, 2000; Fried & Guralnik, 1997).

One example of a behavioral adaptation that has been linked to frailty is life space—a measure of spatial mobility, defined as the size of the spatial area a person purposely moves through in his or her daily life, as well as the frequency of travel within a specific time frame (Baker, Bodner, & Allman, 2003; May, Nayak, & Isaacs, 1985). Xue, Fried, et al. (2008) analyzed the 3-year cumulative incidence of frailty using the PFP in relation to baseline life-space constriction among 599 community-dwelling women age 65 years or older who were not frail at baseline. Their findings suggest that constriction of life space may be a marker of declines in physiologic reserve. They also indicate that constriction of life space itself could lead to decreased physical activity and social engagement, accelerated deconditioning, and exacerbated decline in physiologic

reserve, directly contributing—as these processes progress—to the development of the frailty syndrome. It is also intriguing that difficulty with mobility, instrumental activities of daily living (IADL), and ADL tasks alone did not necessarily lead to a reduction in life space in Xue et al.'s study. In fact, 97% of the participants in their study cohort had already reported mobility disability at baseline. Such discordance between functional capacity and actual performance has been reported in a number of other studies (Cambois, Robine, & Romieu, 2005; Glass, 1998; Jette, 1994). This discrepancy could be explained by the employment of compensatory strategies (e.g., walking cane, social support) that minimize the impact of disability and thereby preserve life-space mobility.

The myriad ways in which older adults compensate can support their functioning, as evidenced by the life space example, or they can be maladaptive. For example, as older adults shrink in height, they may climb on top of kitchen counters to reach a top shelf. Because this behavior increases the individual's fall risk, it is maladaptive. Using the framework of person–environment fit, it is important to consider both the person and the environment to improve adaptation of older adults. In that example, if kitchen cabinets can be lowered, the older adult would no longer need to put himself or herself at risk to reach kitchen items.

Most interventions for disabled older adults have focused on the adult exclusively (Beswick et al., 2008; Daniels, van Rossum, de Witte, Kempen, & van den Heuvel, 2008). Some community interventions have focused on the home environment exclusively, such as giving out grab bars or raised toilet seats. Few studies have systematically targeted both modifiable intrinsic (person-based) and extrinsic (environmental-based) risk factors, even though disability results from the combination and complex interaction of these factors. It is important to intervene with both the person and the environment because multiple overlapping and interacting factors of resilience (e.g., biological, individual, community) exist; when more levels of factors are targeted with interventions, improvement in resilience is more likely to be long-lasting (as posited in the society-to-cells resilience framework [Szanton & Gill, 2010]). Applying this understanding to older individuals, it becomes clear that interventions that can involve not only the whole individual, but also that person's biology or family or built environment, may create better compensation than interventions that address only a coping strategy, for example.

To test this hypothesis, Szanton and Gill (2010) developed CAPABLE, a program that provides time-limited nurse, occupational therapist (OT), and handyman services to functionally impaired community-dwelling older adults to improve their specific limitations in daily function (see **PEARL 9-4**). CAPABLE was adapted from the ABLE program designed by Gitlin, Winter, et al. (2006) to modify behavioral and environmental contributors to functional difficulties. ABLE, which cost only $1222 per participant in 2006 (Jutkowitz, Gitlin, Pizzi, Lee, & Dennis, 2012), improved self-care outcomes for intervention recipients and delayed mortality. At $13,179 per additional year of life saved, ABLE would be judged extremely cost-effective by most criteria (Gitlin et al., 2009; Gitlin, Hauck, et al., 2006; Gitlin, Winter, et al., 2006). The CAPABLE intervention differs from the ABLE program in that it adds a nurse to the team, along with an OT and a physical therapist to address pain, depression, polypharmacy, and primary care provider communication; a

---

PEARL 9-4 CAPABLE Intervention

The CAPABLE intervention is informed by theory and evidence-based practices. It involves 10 or fewer home sessions, each 60-90 minutes in duration, over a 4-month period. It draws upon clinical approaches to enhance uptake and adoption of intervention strategies by study participants, such as patient-centered care and motivational interviewing (Prochaska, 1997; Reuben, 2007; Richards, 2007; Von Korff, 1997).

Each intervention participant receives every component of the intervention (i.e., assessment, education, interactive problem solving), but interventionists clinically tailor content to each participant's risk profile and goals. Key staff include the following personnel:

- *Occupational therapist (OT):* In the first two home sessions, the OT meets with the participant to help identify and prioritize problematic functional areas. The OT observes the participant's performance, evaluating it for safety, efficiency, difficulty, and presence of environmental barriers and supports. The OT assesses the home for basic safety issues that support or undermine participant function, such as poorly lit entrances, cracked concrete stairs, and unstable or unsafe flooring. The OT and the participant discuss possible environmental modifications and assistive devices, which the OT synthesizes into a work order for the handyman that is prioritized based on the participant's functional goals.
- *Registered nurse (RN):* The four RN visits start one month after the first OT visit. The RN works on functional goals, focusing on helping the participant identify whether and how pain, depression, strength and balance, medication management, and ability to communicate with the primary care provider impact daily function. The RN helps the participant identify and prioritize goals. In subsequent visits, the RN and the participant work on the goals, review the participant's effective strategies, and help generalize them to future challenges.
- *Handyman:* The handyman assesses requirements for the work order and then returns within a few weeks to complete the work order. These modifications may include a railing on each side of the stairs, grab bars in the shower, and repairing broken flooring. The home modification budget is up to $1300 per household (Szanton et al., 2011).

handyman to repair the home; and provision of assistive devices (e.g., grab bars, raised toilet seats). Preliminary data provided by a pilot trial of 40 older adults with ADL disability (Szanton et al., 2011) and a Centers for Medicaid and Medicare Services (CMS) trial suggest that CAPABLE improves ADL activities and quality of life (Szanton et al., 2011; Szanton et al., 2015). An expanded trial to formally evaluate the CAPABLE program was funded by both the CMS and the National Institutes of Health in 2012 (Szanton et al., 2014) and is in its final stage of data collection.

The CAPABLE program was built on the premise that if we address intrinsic (e.g., pain, depression) and extrinsic factors (e.g., unsafe stairs) that provide more environmental control, people will experience less environmental stress and can practice their mobility tasks to become stronger, which may then improve their functional status. For example, an older adult living in a house with a shaky banister and a hole in the floor by the door may minimize the number of times that he or she goes upstairs or outside, leading to a vicious cycle of decreased activity that decreases muscle strength and confers higher risk for further disability. Fixing the banister and the holes may enable the participant to practice new exercises taught by the nurse, prepare more food, and reverse this cycle.

Ultimately, however, the ability for older adults to effectively compensate may be a function of both person-environment fitness and individual's reserve. Therefore, addressing individual symptoms such as pain and environmental hazards alone may not be sufficient to break the vicious cycle if, for example, the person's physiologic reserve has fallen below a critical level and the individual has become too frail to rebound. Thus, it may be the interplay of functional limitations, environmental press, and functional reserve that determines actual performance in real life. This interaction may also explain the discordance between reserve-driven functional capacity and physical disability found in the life space study.

Future studies of differential effectiveness of interventions such as CAPABLE by frailty status are needed to explicate the role that reserve and resilience play in disability prevention and intervention.

▸ Summary

Encouraged by the significant progress made on frailty research over the last two decades, there is a growing sense of urgency in translating frailty research into clinical practice. While it is a noble goal worth fighting for in the face of the "silver tsunami," many questions remain to be answered. For example:

- What is the precise meaning of the word "frailty"?
- How is it different from normal aging?
- Is there one frailty with a unifactorial or multifactorial etiology, or are there multiple frailty phenotypes with different etiologies and/or natural histories?
- Which information can frailty assessment provide above and beyond information already available in a clinical setting (e.g., disease diagnoses) to help inform clinical decision making?

As first steps toward answering these questions, we need to tailor measurement methodologies to match both the clinical aims of frailty assessment and the underlying theories of frailty development. Development of experimental, measurement, and analytic techniques to identify and quantify multisystem and multilevel (molecular, cellular, and physiologic) vulnerabilities, such as poor responses to stressors, is also needed. Outcome evaluation of frailty interventions should be extended beyond clinical signs and symptoms to assess biological parameters of system integrity.

Ultimately, the real and meaningful advances in research on frailty, and on aging more broadly, are the ones that will make the saying "70 is the new 60" come closer to reality.

▶ Conclusion and Future Directions

To speed the design and development of effective frailty surveillance and intervention strategies, and then to translate them into the routine clinical management of frail older adults, frailty research needs to refine and standardize measurements. It also needs to make advances in three other major areas: (1) design of an integrative approach for etiologic research, (2) development of methodologies to evaluate interventions targeting multisystem dysregulation, and (3) implementation of frailty assessment in clinical settings. For elucidating the etiology of frailty, an integrated approach is important because the physiologic changes underlying frailty may occur in parallel across multiple systems/pathways. Perhaps the aggregate loss of redundancy resulting from decrements in multiple systems constitutes what is thought of as loss of reserves with aging, leading to increased vulnerability to stressors and the development of the clinical phenotype of frailty. Consistent with this hypothesis, analyses from the Women's Health and Aging Study have shown that the presence of multiple hormone deficiencies, including lower levels of testosterone, DHEA-S, and IGF-1, when considered in aggregate, was a strong and independent predictor of frailty and mortality, whereas deficiency in any of these hormones alone was not (Cappola, O'Meara, et al., 2009; Fried et al., 2009). An increasing body of evidence also details interactions of signaling pathways beyond the endocrine system to include additional networks—notably inflammation—in predicting adverse health outcomes in older adults (Cappola et al., 2003). If the multiplicity of systems affected is the issue in the etiology of frailty, then repletion or treatment of one system might not be effective in itself to produce clinical benefits.

While tremendous progress has been made in the last decade in the study of frailty etiology, the studies conducted so far have two major limitations. First, most have utilized cross-sectional and correlative designs. As a result, causal relationships cannot be stated with assurance. Moreover, the underlying individual-level aging-related physiologic changes have not been well characterized. In fact, increasing evidence suggests that trajectories of change should illustrate the concept of resilience as a dynamic process—that is, stability in levels over time suggests robustness, whereas significant changes or fluctuations suggest metabolic disruption (Cappola, O'Meara, et al., 2009). The individual trajectories, therefore, may be better predictors of frailty than a snapshot of a biomediator's level at a single point in time (Xue, Beamer, Chaves, Guralnik, & Fried, 2010; Xue et al., 2015; Xue, Walston, Fried, & Beamer, 2011).

As a second major limitation, previous studies have focused largely on the influence of a single physiologic system/signaling pathway on frailty. Patterns of accumulation of individual-level changes across multiple physiologic systems have not been studied. Joint analysis of multisystem trajectories of change, as well as their patterns of accumulation with aging, will not only generate new insights into possible etiologic mechanisms and pathways, but also help identify tipping points for the development of frailty, so as to better inform the choices and timing of interventions to most effectively prevent frailty in older adults. To test hypotheses related to multisystem decline with aging, we would need multisystem data collected prospectively over the lifespan. While collecting such data in humans is labor intensive and may be cost prohibitive, animal models with diverse genetic backgrounds suitable for the study of complex disease risks and aging are good alternatives to at least offer proof of concept and generate or refine hypotheses that can then be tested in humans. For example, the rat model of low versus high intrinsic aerobic exercise capacity developed by researchers at the University of Michigan could be a good candidate for such use (Koch & Britton, 2001; Xue, Yang, et al., 2016).

Successful delineation of the pathways by which multiple physiologic systems interact to regulate health in older age, and the subsequent design and evaluation of interventions to address dysregulation, depends on our ability to overcome significant methodological challenges. First, the development of a physiotype of frailty would require a validated approach to measure multisystem dysregulation from a set of biomediators selected a priori to represent, for example, the sentinel physiologic systems governing the stress response dynamics. Latent variable analysis provides an advantageous modeling framework for incorporating theories and accounting for measurement imperfection (i.e., measurement error) to achieve the desired end. The validation of the resulting physiotype, however, presents considerable challenges in the absence of a gold standard for frailty identification. An approach iterating physiotype definition and identification of etiologic factors underlying the physiotype may be needed.

Second, to build useful evidence on etiologic pathways and intervention effects, causal effects must be distinguished from associations. The definition of "causality" in the biological context presents challenges—at least, the complexity and tightness of linkages between physiologic regulators render unrealistic a potential outcomes framework in which one aspect of the physiology is varied while keeping other features constant.

Third, although randomized controlled trials remain the gold standard for causal inference, longitudinal epidemiological cohorts represent rich data resources that should be utilized to inform the design of future frailty intervention trials. Studies providing both clinical and biological data include the Women's Health and Aging Study I and II, the Cardiovascular Health Study, the Baltimore Longitudinal Study of Aging, and the InChianti Study. Data collected in such studies can inform estimation of screening yield, selection of biomediators for physiotype development and validation, sample size calculation, and rationalization of study eligibility

criteria for optimal targeting. To avoid conclusions that reflect spurious associations rather than biological mechanisms, however, proper modeling of major time-independent and time-dependent confounding factors will be required (Holland, 1986; Robins, Greenland, & Hu, 1999; Rubin, 1974).

Finally, studies of older adults are often compromised by missing data due to participants' illness or competing risk events (e.g., death) (Varadhan, Xue, & Bandeen-Roche, 2014), and treatment noncompliance (Gruenewald et al., 2016; Jo, Ginexi, & Ialongo, 2010). This is particularly likely in persons who are frail. More sophisticated statistical models such as the semi-competing risk model to account for competing mortality (Varadhan et al., 2014) and the Complier Average Causal Effect model for treatment noncompliance (Gruenewald et al., 2016; Jo et al., 2010) need to be applied to maximize validity and precision in analyzing such data.

On the front lines of clinical translation, a number of challenges remain, including the consideration of clinical feasibility in assessing frailty while maintaining the validity of the construct. For example, theory-based operational definitions, such as the PFP, include performance-based measures that are not standard in clinical practice, while short self-report frailty questionnaires may not accurately identify frail patients. There is also uncertainty as to whether frailty assessment should be standardized for all clinical care settings, or if it should be tailored to each application. Specific treatment options for frailty, with consideration to a given clinical population, need to be developed. The current incorporation of frailty into clinical settings is largely based on observational findings; clinical trial evidence is needed. Future studies are also needed to independently validate frailty measures in different specialties, so as to better understand the feasibility and predictive ability of frailty for risk stratification for treatments and procedures. Finally, the identification of clinical and laboratory biomarkers to diagnose frailty and to guide the development and targeting of preventive strategies should be explored (Walston et al., 2006).

References

Abellan van Kan, G., Rolland, Y., Bergman, H., Morley, J. E., Kritchevsky, S. B., & Vellas, B. (2008). The I.A.N.A Task Force on frailty assessment of older people in clinical practice. *Journal of Nutrition, Health & Aging, 12*(1), 29-37.

Abellan van Kan, G., Rolland, Y. M., Morley, J. E., & Vellas, B. (2008). Frailty: Toward a clinical definition. *Journal of the American Medical Directors Association, 9*(2), 71-72.

Aguilar-Navarro, S. G., Amieva, H., Gutierrez-Robledo, L. M., & Avila-Funes, J. A. (2015). Frailty among Mexican community-dwelling elderly: A story told 11 years later. *The Mexican Health and Aging Study. Salud publica de Mexico, 57*(suppl 1), S62-S69.

Akki, A. Y. H., Gupta, A., Chacko, V. P., Yano, T., Leppo, M. K., Steenbergen, C.,... Weiss, R. G. (2014). Skeletal muscle ATP kinetics are impaired in frail mice. *Age (Dordrecht), 36*(1), 21-30.

Alencar, M. A., Figueiredo, L. C., & Dias, R. C. (2013). Frailty and cognitive impairment among community-dwelling elderly. *Arqivos de Neuro-Psiquiatria, 71*(6), 362-367.

Alvarado, B. E., Zunzunegui, M. V., Beland, F., & Bamvita, J. M. (2008). Life course social and health conditions linked to frailty in Latin American older men and women. *Journal of Gerontology, 63*(12), 1399-1406.

Amaral, L. A., Diaz-Guilera, A., Moreira, A. A., Goldberger, A. L., & Lipsitz, L. A. (2004). Emergence of complex dynamics in a simple model of signaling networks. *Proceedings of the National Academy of Sciences USA, 101*(44), 15551-15555.

Avila-Funes, J. A., Amieva, H., Barberger-Gateau, P., Le Goff, M., Raoux, N., Ritchie, K.,... Dartigues, J. F. (2009). Cognitive impairment improves the predictive validity of the phenotype of frailty for adverse health outcomes: The three-city study. *Journal of the American Geriatrics Society, 57*(3), 453-461.

Baker, P. S., Bodner, E. V., & Allman, R. M. (2003). Measuring life-space mobility in community-dwelling older adults. *Journal of the American Geriatrics Society, 51*(11), 1610-1614.

Bandeen-Roche, K., Seplaki, C. L., Huang, J., Buta, B., Kalyani, R. R., Varadhan, R.,... Kasper, J. D. (2015). Frailty in older adults: A nationally representative profile in the United States. *Journals of Gerontology Series A: Biological Sciences and Medical Sciences, 70*(11), 1427-1434.

Bandeen-Roche, K., Xue, Q. L., Ferrucci, L., Walston, J., Guralnik, J. M., Chaves, P.,... Fried, L. P. (2006). Phenotype of frailty: Characterization in the Women's Health and Aging Studies. *Journals of Gerontology Series A: Biological Sciences and Medical Sciences, 61*(3), 262-266.

Bartali, B., Frongillo, E. A., Bandinelli, S., Lauretani, F., Semba, R. D., Fried, L. P., & Ferrucci, L. (2005). Deficient nutrient intake is an essential component of frailty in older persons. *Journal of the American Geriatrics Society, 53*(4), S177-S177.

Baylis, D., Bartlett, D. B., Syddall, H. E., Ntani, G., Gale, C. R., Cooper, C.,... Sayer, A. A. (2013). Immune-endocrine biomarkers as predictors of frailty and mortality: A 10-year longitudinal study in community-dwelling older people. *Age (Dordrecht), 35*(3), 963-971.

Berardelli, M., De Rango, F., Morelli, M., Corsonello, A., Mazzei, B., Mari, V.,... Passarino, G. (2013). Urinary incontinence in the elderly and in the oldest old: Correlation with frailty and mortality. *Rejuvenation Research, 16*(3), 206-211.

Bergman, H., Ferrucci, L., Guralnik, J., Hogan, D. B., Hummel, S., Karunananthan, S., & Wolfson, C. (2007). Frailty: An emerging research and clinical paradigm: Issues and controversies. *Journals of Gerontology Series A: Biological Sciences and Medical Sciences, 62*(7), 731-737.

Beswick, A. D., Rees, K., Dieppe, P., Ayis, S., Gooberman-Hill, R., Horwood, J., & Ebrahim, S. (2008). Complex interventions to improve physical function and maintain independent living in elderly people: A systematic review and meta-analysis. *Lancet, 371*(9614), 725-735.

Blyth, F. M., Cumming, R. G., Creasey, H., Handelsman, D. J., Le Couteur, D. G., Naganathan, V.,... Waite, L. M. (2008). Pain, frailty and comorbidity on older men: The CHAMP study. *Pain, 140*(1), 224-230.

Borsch-Supan, A., Brugiavini, A., Jurges, H., Mackenbach, J., Sirgrist, J., & Weber, G. (2005). *First results from the Survey of Health, Ageing and Retirement in Europe.* Mannheim, Germany: Mannheim Research Institute for the Economics of Aging.

Bortz, W. M., 2nd. (1993). The physics of frailty. *Journal of the American Geriatrics Society, 41*(9), 1004-1008.

Bortz, W. M. (2002). A conceptual framework of frailty: A review. *Journals of Gerontology Series A: Biological Sciences and Medical Sciences, 57*(5), M283-M288.

Bouillon, K., Kivimaki, M., Hamer, M., Sabia, S., Fransson, E. I., Singh-Manoux, A.,... Batty, G. D. (2013). Measures of frailty in population-based studies: An overview. *BMC Geriatrics, 13*, 64.

Buchner, D. M., & Wagner, E. H. (1992). Preventing frail health. *Clinics in Geriatric Medicine, 8*(1), 1-17.

Buta, B. J., Walston, J. D., Godino, J. G., Park, M., Kalyani, R. R., Xue, Q. L.,... Varadhan, R. (2016). Frailty assessment instruments: Systematic characterization of the uses and contexts of highly cited instruments. *Ageing Research Reviews, 26*, 53-61.

Cambois, E., Robine, J. M., & Romieu, I. (2005). The influence of functional limitations and various demographic factors on self-reported activity restriction at older ages. *Disability Rehabilitation, 27*(15), 871-883.

Campbell, A. J., Borrie, M. J., & Spears, G. F. (1989). Risk factors for falls in a community-based prospective study of people 70 years and older. *Journal of Gerontology, 44*(4), M112-M117.

Campbell, A. J., & Robertson, M. C. (2006). Implementation of multifactorial interventions for fall and fracture prevention. *Age and Ageing, 35*(suppl 2), ii60-ii64.

Canevelli, M., & Cesari, M. (2015). Cognitive frailty: What is still missing? *Journal of Nutrition Health & Aging, 19*(3), 273-275.

Cappola, A. R., O'Meara, E. S., Guo, W., Bartz, T. M., Fried, L. P., & Newman, A. B. (2009). Trajectories of dehydroepiandrosterone sulfate predict mortality in older adults: The Cardiovascular Health Study. *Journal of Gerontology, 64*(12), 1268-1274.

Cappola, A. R., Xue, Q. L., Ferrucci, L., Guralnik, J. M., Volpato, S., & Fried, L. P. (2003). Insulin-like growth factor I and interleukin-6 contribute synergistically to disability and mortality in older women. *Journal of Clinical Endocrinology and Metabolism, 88*(5), 2019-2025.

Cappola, A. R., Xue, Q. L., & Fried, L. P. (2009). Multiple hormonal deficiencies in anabolic hormones are found in frail older women: The Women's Health and Aging Studies. *Journals of Gerontology Series A: Biological Sciences and Medical Sciences, 64*(2): 243-248.

Capri, M., Yani, S. L., Chattat, R., Fortuna, D., Bucci, L., Lanzarini, C.,... Franceschi, C. (2014). Pre-operative, high-IL-6 blood level is a risk factor of post-operative delirium onset in old patients. *Frontiers in Endocrinology, 5*, 173.

Castaldo, R., Melillo, P., Izzo, R., De Luca, N., & Pecchia, L. (2016). Fall prediction in hypertensive patients via short-term HRV analysis. *IEEE Journal of Biomedical and Health Informatics.* Retrieved from http://ieeexplore.ieee.org/document/7436766/

Castell, M. V., van der Pas, S., Otero, A., Siviero, P., Dennison, E., Denkinger, M.,... Deeg, D. (2015). Osteoarthritis and frailty in elderly individuals across six European countries: Results from the European Project on OSteoArthritis (EPOSA). *BMC Musculoskeletal Disease, 16*, 359.

Castrejon-Perez, R. C., Borges-Yanez, S. A., Gutierrez-Robledo, L. M., & Avila-Funes, J. A. (2012). Oral health conditions and frailty in Mexican community-dwelling elderly: A cross sectional analysis. *BMC Public Health, 12*, 773.

Cerejeira, J., Batista, P., Nogueira, V., Vaz-Serra, A., & Mukaetova-Ladinska, E. B. (2013). The stress response to surgery and postoperative delirium: Evidence of hypothalamic-pituitary-adrenal axis hyperresponsiveness and decreased suppression of the GH/IGF-1 axis. *Journal of Geriatric Psychiatry and Neurology, 26*(3), 185-194.

Chen, C. Y., Chen, L. J., & Lue, B. H. (2010). The prevalence of subjective frailty and factors associated with frailty in Taiwan. *Archives of Gerontology and Geriatrics, 50*(suppl 1), S43-S47.

Choi, J., Kim, S., & Won, C. W. (2015). Global prevalence of physical frailty by Fried's criteria in community-dwelling elderly with national population-based surveys. *Journal of the American Medical Directors Association, 16*(7), 548-550.

Clegg, A., Siddiqi, N., Heaven, A., Young, J., & Holt, R. (2014). Interventions for preventing delirium in older people in institutional long-term care. *Cochrane Database of Systematic Reviews, 1*, CD009537.

Colkesen, Y., Giray, S., Ozenli, Y., Sezgin, N., & Coskun, I. (2013). Relation of serum cortisol to delirium occurring after acute coronary syndromes. *American Journal of Emergency Medicine, 31*(1), 161-165.

Collard, R. M., Boter, H., Schoevers, R. A., & Oude Voshaar, R. C. (2012). Prevalence of frailty in community-dwelling older persons: A systematic review. *Journal of the American Geriatrics Society, 60*(8), 1487-1492.

Collier, R. (2012). Hospital-induced delirium hits hard. *Canadian Medical Association Journal, 184*(1), 23-24.

Cournil, A., & Diouf, A.; Groupe d'étude de la cohorte ANRS 1215. (2014). Bone aging and frailty syndrome after 10 years of ARV treatment in Senegal. *Bulletin de la Société de pathologie exotique, 107*(4), 238-240.

Crimmins, E. M., & Beltran-Sanchez, H. (2011). Mortality and morbidity trends: Is there compression of morbidity? *Journals of Gerontology Series B: Psychological Sciences and Social Sciences, 66*(1), 75-86.

Dalrymple, L. S., Katz, R., Rifkin, D. E., Siscovick, D., Newman, A. B., Fried, L. F.,... Shlipak, M. G. (2013). Kidney function and prevalent and incident frailty. *Clinical Journal of the American Society of Nephrology, 8*(12), 2091-2099.

Daniels, R., van Rossum, E., de Witte, L., Kempen, G. I., & van den Heuvel, W. (2008). Interventions to prevent disability in frail community-dwelling elderly: A systematic review. *BMC Health Services Research, 8*, 278.

Davis, D. H., Kreisel, S. H., Muniz Terrera, G., Hall, A. J., Morandi, A., Boustani, M.,... Brayne, C. (2013). The epidemiology of delirium: Challenges and opportunities for population studies. *American Journal of Geriatric Psychiatry, 21*(12), 1173-1189.

Deiner, S., Lin, H. M., Bodansky, D., Silverstein, J., & Sano, M. (2014). Do stress markers and anesthetic technique predict delirium in the elderly? *Dementia and Geriatric Cognitive Disorders, 38*(5-6), 366-374.

de Lange, E., Verhaak, P. F., & van der Meer, K. (2013). Prevalence, presentation and prognosis of delirium in older people in the population, at home and in long term care: A review. *International Journal of Geriatric Psychiatry, 28*(2), 127–134.

DeVellis, R. F. (2012). *Scale development: Theory and applications* (3rd ed.). Thousand Oaks, CA: Sage.

de Vries, N. M., Staal, J. B., van Ravensberg, C. D., Hobbelen, J. S. M., Rikkert, M., & Nijhuis-van der Sanden, M. W. G. (2011). Outcome instruments to measure frailty: A systematic review. *Ageing Research Reviews, 10*(1), 104–114.

Dirks, A. J., Hofer, T., Marzetti, E., Pahor, M., & Leeuwenburgh, C. (2006). Mitochondrial DNA mutations, energy metabolism and apoptosis in aging muscle. *Ageing Research Reviews, 5*(2), 179–195.

Eeles, E. M., White, S. V., O'Mahony, S. M., Bayer, A. J., & Hubbard, R. E. (2012). The impact of frailty and delirium on mortality in older inpatients. *Age and Ageing, 41*(3), 412–416.

Ensrud, K. E., Ewing, S. K., Cawthon, P. M., Fink, H. A., Taylor, B. C., Cauley, J. A.,… Orwoll, E. S. (2009). A comparison of frailty indexes for the prediction of falls, disability, fractures, and mortality in older men. *Journal of the American Geriatrics Society, 57*(3), 492–498. doi: 10.1111/j.1532-5415.2009.02137.x

Ensrud, K. E., Ewing, S. K., Taylor, B. C., Fink, H. A., Stone, K. L., Cauley, J. A.,… Cawthon, P. M. (2007). Frailty and risk of falls, fracture, and mortality in older women: The Study of Osteoporotic Fractures. *Journal of Gerontology, 62*(7), 744–751.

Ensrud, K. E., Ewing, S. K., Taylor, B. C., Fink, H. A., Cawthon, P. M., Stone, K. L.,… Cummings, S. R. (2008). Comparison of 2 frailty indexes for prediction of falls, disability, fractures, and death in older women. *Archives of Internal Medicine, 168*(4), 382–389.

Eyigor, S., Kutsal, Y. G., Duran, E., Huner, B., Paker, N., Durmus, B.,… Ceceli, E. (2015). Frailty prevalence and related factors in the older adult: FrailTURK Project. *Age, 37*(3), 9791.

Ferrari, E., Cravello, L., Muzzoni, B., Casarotti, D., Paltro, M., Solerte, S. B.,… Magri, F. (2001). Age-related changes of the hypothalamic–pituitary–adrenal axis: Pathophysiological correlates. *European Journal of Endocrinology, 144*(4), 319–329.

Ferrucci, L., Windham, B. G., & Fried, L. P. (2005). Frailty in older persons. *Genus, 61*, 39–53.

Flacker, J. M. (2003). What is a geriatric syndrome anyway? *Journal of the American Geriatrics Society, 51*(4), 574–576.

Flaherty, J. H. (2011). The evaluation and management of delirium among older persons. *Medical Clinics of North America, 95*(3), 555–577, xi.

Flaherty, J. H., Gonzales, J. P., & Dong, B. (2011). Antipsychotics in the treatment of delirium in older hospitalized adults: A systematic review. *Journal of the American Geriatrics Society, 59*(suppl 2), S269–S276.

Fried, L. P. (1992). Conference on the Physiologic Basis of Frailty. April 28, 1992, Baltimore, MD. Introduction. *Aging (Milano), 4*(3), 251–252.

Fried, L. P., Bandeen-Roche, K., Chaves, P. H., & Johnson, B. A. (2000). Preclinical mobility disability predicts incident mobility disability in older women. *Journal of Gerontology, 55*(1), M43–N52.

Fried, L. P., Ferrucci, L., Darer, J., Williamson, J. D., & Anderson, G. (2004). Untangling the concepts of disability, frailty, and comorbidity: Implications for improved targeting and care. *Journal of Gerontology, 59*(3), 255–263.

Fried, L. P., & Guralnik, J. M. (1997). Disability in older adults: Evidence regarding significance, etiology, and risk. *Journal of the American Geriatrics Society, 45*(1), 92–100.

Fried, L. P., Hadley, E. C., Walston, J., Newman, A. B., Guralnik, J. M., Studenski, S.,… Ferrucci, L. (2005). From bedside to bench: Research agenda for frailty. *Science of Aging Knowledge Environment, 2005*(31), 24.

Fried, L. P., Tangen, C. M., Walston, J., Newman, A. B., Hirsch, C., Gottdiener, J.,… McBurnie, M. A. (2001). Frailty in older adults: Evidence for a phenotype. *Journals of Gerontology Series A: Biological Sciences and Medical Sciences, 56*(3), M146–M156.

Fried, L. P., & Walston, J. (1998). Frailty and failure to thrive. In W. R. Hazzard, J. P. Blass, W. H. Ettinger, Jr., J. B. Halter, & J. Ouslander (Eds.), *Principles of geriatric medicine and gerontology* (Vol. 4, pp. 1387–1402). New York, NY: McGraw-Hill.

Fried, L. P., Xue, Q. L., Cappola, A. R., Ferrucci, L., Chaves, P., Varadhan, R.,… Bandeen-Roche, K. (2009). Nonlinear multisystem physiological dysregulation associated with frailty in older women: Implications for etiology and treatment. *Journal of Gerontology, 64*(10), 1049–1057. doi: 10.1093/gerona/glp076

Fries, J. F. (1980). Aging, natural death, and the compression of morbidity. *New England Journal of Medicine, 303*(3), 130–135.

Gale, C. R., Baylis, D., Cooper, C., & Sayer, A. A. (2013). Inflammatory markers and incident frailty in men and women: The English Longitudinal Study of Ageing. *Age (Dordrecht), 35*(6), 2493–2501.

Gale, C. R., Cooper, C., & Sayer, A. A. (2014). Framingham cardiovascular disease risk scores and incident frailty: The English Longitudinal Study of Ageing. *Age (Dordrecht), 36*(4), 9692.

Gammack, J. K. (2004). Urinary incontinence in the frail elder. *Clinics in Geriatric Medicine, 20*(3), 453–466, vi.

Garcia-Esquinas, E., Guallar-Castillon, P., Carnicero, J. A., Buno, A., Garcia-Garcia, F. J., Rodriguez-Manas, L., & Rodriguez-Artalejo, F. (2016). Serum uric acid concentrations and risk of frailty in older adults. *Experimental Gerontology, 82*, 160–165. doi: 10.1016/j.exger.2016.07.002

Garcia-Esquinas, E., Rahi, B., Peres, K., Colpo, M., Dartigues, J. F., Bandinelli, S.,... Rodriguez-Artalejo, F. (2016). Consumption of fruit and vegetables and risk of frailty: A dose-response analysis of 3 prospective cohorts of community-dwelling older adults. *American Journal of Clinical Nutrition, 104*(1), 132-142.

Gavrilov, L. A., & Gavrilova, N. S. (2001). The reliability theory of aging and longevity. *Journal of Theoretical Biology, 213*(4), 527-545.

Gibson, W., Athanasopoulos, A., Goldman, H., Madersbacher, H., Newman, D., Spinks, J.,... Wagg, A. (2014). Are we shortchanging frail older people when it comes to the pharmacological treatment of urgency urinary incontinence? *International Journal of Clinical Practice, 68*(9), 1165-1173.

Gill, T. M., Baker, D. I., Gottschalk, M., Peduzzi, P. N., Allore, H., & Byers, A. (2002). A program to prevent functional decline in physically frail, elderly persons who live at home. *New England Journal of Medicine, 347*(14), 1068-1074.

Gillespie, L. D., Robertson, M. C., Gillespie, W. J., Sherrington, C., Gates, S., Clemson, L. M., & Lamb, S. E. (2012). Interventions for preventing falls in older people living in the community. *Cochrane Database of Systematic Reviews, 9*, CD007146. doi: 10.1002/14651858.CD007146.pub3

Gitlin, L. N., Hauck, W. W., Dennis, M. P., Winter, L., Hodgson, N., & Schinfeld, S. (2009). Long-term effect on mortality of a home intervention that reduces functional difficulties in older adults: Results from a randomized trial. *Journal of the American Geriatrics Society, 57*(3), 476-481.

Gitlin, L. N., Hauck, W. W., Winter, L., Dennis, M. P., & Schulz, R. (2006). Effect of an in-home occupational and physical therapy intervention on reducing mortality in functionally vulnerable older people: Preliminary findings. *Journal of the American Geriatrics Society, 54*(6), 950-955.

Gitlin, L. N., Winter, L., Dennis, M. P., Corcoran, M., Schinfeld, S., & Hauck, W. W. (2006). A randomized trial of a multicomponent home intervention to reduce functional difficulties in older adults. *Journal of the American Geriatrics Society, 54*(5), 809-816.

Glass, T. A. (1998). Conjugating the "tenses" of function: Discordance among hypothetical, experimental, and enacted function in older adults. *Gerontologist, 38*(1), 101-112.

Gobbens, R. J., Luijkx, K. G., Wijnen-Sponselee, M. T., & Schols, J. M. (2010a). Toward a conceptual definition of frail community dwelling older people. *Nursing Outlook, 58*(2), 76-86.

Gobbens, R. J. J., Luijkx, K. G., Wijnen-Sponselee, M. T., & Schols, J. M. G. A. (2010b). Towards an integral conceptual model of frailty. *Journal of Nutrition Health & Aging, 14*(3), 175-181.

Goodman, L. A. (1974). Exploratory latent structure analysis using both identifiable and unidentifiable models. *Biometrika, 61*(2), 215-231.

Gorina, Y., Schappert, S., Bercovitz, A., Elgaddal, N., & Kramarow, E. (2014). Prevalence of incontinence among older Americans. *Vital & Health Statistics: Series 3, Analytical and Epidemiological Studies (U.S. Department of Health and Human Services, Public Health Service, National Center for Health Statistics), 36*, 1-33.

Graham, J. E., Snih, S. A., Berges, I. M., Ray, L. A., Markides, K. S., & Ottenbacher, K. J. (2009). Frailty and 10-year mortality in community-living Mexican American older adults. *Gerontology, 55*(6), 644-651.

Gross, A. L., Xue, Q. L., Bandeen-Roche, K., Fried, L. P., Varadhan, R., McAdams-DeMarco, M. A.,... Carlson, M. C. (2016). Declines and impairment in executive function predict onset of physical frailty. *Journal of Gerontology Series A, Biological Sciences and Medical Sciences, 71*(12), 1624-1630.

Gruenewald, T. L., Tanner, E. K., Fried, L. P., Carlson, M. C., Xue, Q. L., Parisi, J. M.,... Seeman, T. E. (2016). The Baltimore Experience Corps Trial: Enhancing generativity via intergenerational activity engagement in later life. *Journal of Gerontology Series B: Psychological Sciences and Social Sciences, 71*(4), 661-670.

Gurina, N. A., & Degryse, J. M. (2011). A roadmap of aging in Russia: The prevalence of frailty in community-dwelling older adults in the St. Petersburg district: The "Crystal" study. *Journal of the American Geriatrics Society, 59*(6), 980-988.

Halil, M., Kizilarslanoglu, M. C., Kuyumcu, M. E., Yesil, Y., & Jentoft, A. J. C. (2015). Cognitive aspects of frailty: Mechanisms behind the link between frailty and cognitive impairment. *Journal of Nutrition Health & Aging, 19*(3), 276-283.

Hirsch, C., Anderson, M. L., Newman, A., Kop, W., Jackson, S., Gottdiener, J.,... Fried, L. P. (2006). The association of race with frailty: The Cardiovascular Health Study. *Annals of Epidemiology, 16*(7), 545-553.

Hogan, D. B., MacKnight, C., & Bergman, H. (2003). Models, definitions, and criteria of frailty. *Aging Clinical and Experimental Research, 15*(3 suppl), 1-29.

Holanda, C. M., Guerra, R. O., Nobrega, P. V., Costa, H. F., Piuvezam, M. R., & Maciel, A. C. (2012). Salivary cortisol and frailty syndrome in elderly residents of long-stay institutions: A cross-sectional study. *Archives of Gerontology and Geriatrics, 54*(2), e146-e151.

Holland, P. W. (1986). Statistics and Causal Inference. *Journal of the American Statistical Association, 81*(396), 945-960.

Holland, P. W. (1986). Statistics and Causal Inference—Rejoinder. *Journal of the American Statistical Association, 81*(396), 968-970.

Hoogendijk, E. O., van der Horst, H. E., van de Ven, P. M., Twisk, J. W., Deeg, D. J., Frijters, D. H.,... van Hout,

H. P. (2016). Effectiveness of a geriatric care model for frail older adults in primary care: Results from a stepped wedge cluster randomized trial. *European Journal of Internal Medicine, 28*, 43-51.

Hsiao, S. M., Lin, H. H., & Kuo, H. C. (2012). The role of serum C-reactive protein in women with lower urinary tract symptoms. *International Urogynecology Journal, 23*(7), 935-940.

Hubeaux, K., Deffieux, X., Ismael, S. S., Raibaut, P., & Amarenco, G. (2007). Autonomic nervous system activity during bladder filling assessed by heart rate variability analysis in women with idiopathic overactive bladder syndrome or stress urinary incontinence. *Journal of Urology, 178*(6), 2483-2487.

Inouye, S. K. (2006). Delirium in older persons. *New England Journal of Medicine, 354*(11), 1157-1165.

Inouye, S. K., Studenski, S., Tinetti, M. E., & Kuchel, G. A. (2007). Geriatric syndromes: Clinical, research, and policy implications of a core geriatric concept. *Journal of the American Geriatrics Society, 55*(5), 780-791.

Inouye, S. K., Westendorp, R.G., & Saczynski, J. S. (2014). Delirium in elderly people. *Lancet, 383*(9920), 911-922.

Jette, A. M. (1994). How measurement techniques influence estimates of disability in older populations. *Social Science and Medicine, 38*(7), 937-942.

Jo, B., Ginexi, E. M., & Ialongo, N. S. (2010). Handling missing data in randomized experiments with noncompliance. *Prevention Science, 11*(4), 384-396.

Johar, H., Emeny, R. T., Bidlingmaier, M., Reincke, M., Thorand, B., Peters, A.,… Ladwig, K. H. (2014). Blunted diurnal cortisol pattern is associated with frailty: A cross-sectional study of 745 participants aged 65 to 90 years. *Journal of Clinical Endocrinology and Metabolism, 99*(3), E464-E468.

Joosten, E., Demuynck, M., Detroyer, E., & Milisen, K. (2014). Prevalence of frailty and its ability to predict in hospital delirium, falls, and 6-month mortality in hospitalized older patients. *BMC Geriatrics, 14*, 1.

Jutkowitz, E., Gitlin, L. N., Pizzi, L. T., Lee, E., & Dennis, M. P. (2012). Cost effectiveness of a home-based intervention that helps functionally vulnerable older adults age in place at home. *Journal of Aging Research, 2012*, 680265.

Kalyani, R. R., Tian, J., Xue, Q. L., Walston, J., Cappola, A. R., Fried, L. P.,… Blaum, C. S. (2012). Hyperglycemia and incidence of frailty and lower extremity mobility limitations in older women. *Journal of the American Geriatrics Society, 60*(9), 1701-1707.

Kalyani, R. R., Varadhan, R., Weiss, C. O., Fried, L. P., & Cappola, A. R. (2012). Frailty status and altered glucose-insulin dynamics. *Journals of Gerontology Series A: Biological Sciences and Medical Sciences, 67*(12), 1300-1306.

Kamel, H. K. (2003). Sarcopenia and aging. *Nutrition Reviews, 61*(5), 157-167.

Kaminskyy, V. O., & Zhivotovsky, B. (2014). Free radicals in cross talk between autophagy and apoptosis. *Antioxidants & Redox Signaling, 21*(1), 86-102.

Karunananthan, S., Wolfson, C., Bergman, H., Béland, F., & Hogan, D. B. (2009). A multidisciplinary systematic literature review on frailty: Overview of the methodology used by the Canadian Initiative on Frailty and Aging. *BMC Medical Research Methodologies, 9*, 68.

Kelaiditi, E., Cesari, M., Canevelli, M., van Kan, G. A., Ousset, P. J., Gillette-Guyonnet, S.,… Vellas, B. (2013). Cognitive frailty: Rationale and definition from an (I.A.N.A./I.A.G.G.) international consensus group. *Journal of Nutrition, Health & Aging, 17*(9), 726-734.

Kim, J. C., Joo, K. J., Kim, J. T., Choi, J. B., Cho, D. S., & Won, Y. Y. (2010). Alteration of autonomic function in female urinary incontinence. *International Neurourology Journal, 14*(4), 232-237.

Kitano, H. (2002). Systems biology: A brief overview. *Science, 295*(5560), 1662-1664.

Ko, F., Yu, Q. L., Xue, Q. L., Yao, W. L., Brayton, C., Yang, H.,… Walston, J. (2012). Inflammation and mortality in a frail mouse model. *Age, 34*(3), 705-715.

Koch, L. G., & Britton, S. L. (2001). Artificial selection for intrinsic aerobic endurance running capacity in rats. *Physiological Genomics, 5*(1), 45-52.

Kojima, G. (2015). Frailty as a predictor of future falls among community-dwelling older people: A systematic review and meta-analysis. *Journal of the American Medical Directors Association, 16*(12), 1027-1033.

Kuchel, G. (2009). Aging and homeostatic regulation. In J. B. Halter, M. E. Tinnetti, S. Studenski, K. P. High, & S. Asthana (Eds.), *Hazzard's geriatric medicine and gerontology* (6th ed.). New York, NY: McGraw-Hill. Retrieved from http://accessmedicine.mhmedical.com/content.aspx?bookid=371&Sectionid=41587663

Kupelian, V., Rosen, R. C., Roehrborn, C. G., Tyagi, P., Chancellor, M. B., & McKinlay, J. B. (2012). Association of overactive bladder and C-reactive protein levels: Results from the Boston Area Community Health (BACH) survey. *BJU International, 110*(3), 401-407.

LaCroix, A. Z., Gray, S. L., Aragaki, A., Cochrane, B. B., Newman, A. B., Kooperberg, C.L.,… Woods, N. F. (2008). Statin use and incident frailty in women aged 65 years or older: Prospective findings from the Women's Health Initiative Observational Study. *Journal of Gerontology, 63*(4), 369-375.

Lakey, S. L., LaCroix, A. Z., Gray, S. L., Borson, S., Williams, C. D., Calhoun, D.,… Woods, N. F. (2012). Antidepressant use, depressive symptoms, and incident frailty in women aged 65 and older from the Women's Health Initiative Observational Study. *Journal of the American Geriatrics Society, 60*(5), 854-861.

Lee, J. S., Leung, J., Kwok, T., & Woo, J. (2014). Transitions in frailty states among community-living older adults and their associated factors. *Journal of the American Medical Directors Association, 15*(4), 281-286.

Lee, Y., Han, E. S., Ryu, M., Cho, Y., & Chae, S. (2014). Frailty and body mass index as predictors of 3-year mortality in older adults living in the community. *Gerontology, 60*(6), 475-482.

Leng, S. X., Cappola, A. R., Andersen, R. E., Blackman, M. R., Koenig, K., Blair, M., & Walston, J. D. (2004). Serum levels of insulin-like growth factor-I (IGF-I) and dehydroepiandrosterone sulfate (DHEA-S), and their relationships with serum interleukin-6, in the geriatric syndrome of frailty. *Aging Clinical and Experimental Research, 16*(2), 153-157.

Leng, S., Xue, Q., Tian, J., Fried, L., & Walston, J. (2005). Elevated IL-6 levels are associated with frailty in community-dwelling older women. *Gerontologist, 45,* 247-247.

Leng, S. X., Xue, Q. L., Tian, J., Walston, J. D., & Fried, L. P. (2007). Inflammation and frailty in older women. *Journal of the American Geriatrics Society, 55*(6), 864-871.

Leng, S. X., Yang, H., & Walston, J. D. (2004). Decreased cell proliferation and altered cytokine production in frail older adults. *Aging Clinical and Experimental Research, 16*(3), 249-252.

Leslie, D. L., & Inouye, S. K. (2011). The importance of delirium: Economic and societal costs. *Journal of the American Geriatrics Society, 59*(suppl 2), S241-S243.

Leung, J. M., Tsai, T. L., & Sands, L. P. (2011). Brief report: Preoperative frailty in older surgical patients is associated with early postoperative delirium. *Anesthesia and Analgesia, 112*(5), 1199-1201.

Levy, R., & Muller, N. (2006). Urinary incontinence: Economic burden and new choices in pharmaceutical treatment. *Advances in Therapy, 23*(4), 556-573.

Lindle, R. S., Metter, E. J., Lynch, N. A., Fleg, J. L., Fozard, J. L., Tobin, J.,... Hurley, B. F. (1997). Age and gender comparisons of muscle strength in 654 women and men aged 20-93 yr. *Journal of Applied Physiology, 83*(5), 1581-1587.

Lipsitz, L. A. (2002). Dynamics of stability: The physiologic basis of functional health and frailty. *Journals of Gerontology Series A: Biological Sciences and Medical Sciences, 57*(3), B115-B125.

Lipsitz, L. A. (2004). Physiological complexity, aging, and the path to frailty. *Science of Aging Knowledge Environment, 2004*(16), e16.

Lloyd, D. K., & Lipow, M. (1962). *Reliability: Management, methods, and mathematics.* Englewood Cliffs, NJ: Prentice-Hall.

Lumbers, M., New, S. A., Gibson, S., & Murphy, M. C. (2001). Nutritional status in elderly female hip fracture patients: Comparison with an age-matched home living group attending day centres. *British Journal of Nutrition, 85*(6), 733-740.

Maggio, M., Cappola, A. R., Ceda, G. P., Basaria, S., Chia, C. W., Valenti, G., & Ferrucci, L. (2005). The

hormonal pathway to frailty in older men. *Journal of Endocrinological Investigation, 28*(11 suppl proc), 15-19.

Manal, B., Suzana, S., & Singh, D. K. (2015). Nutrition and frailty: A review of clinical intervention studies. *Journal of Frailty & Aging, 4*(2), 100-106.

Marcell, T. J. (2003). Sarcopenia: Causes, consequences, and preventions. *Journals of Gerontology Series A: Biological Sciences and Medical Sciences, 58*(10), 911-916.

Markland, A. D., Richter, H. E., Fwu, C. W., Eggers, P., & Kusek, J. W. (2011). Prevalence and trends of urinary incontinence in adults in the United States, 2001 to 2008. *Journal of Urology, 186*(2), 589-593.

Martin, F. C. (2011). Falls risk factors: Assessment and management to prevent falls and fractures. *Canadian Journal on Aging, 30*(1), 33-44.

Matthews, C. A. (2014). Risk factors for urinary, fecal, or double incontinence in women. *Current Opinion in Obstetrics & Gynecology, 26*(5), 393-397.

May, D., Nayak, U. S., & Isaacs, B. (1985). The life-space diary: A measure of mobility in old people at home. *International Rehabilitation Medicine, 7*(4), 182-186.

McEwen, B. S. (1998). Stress, adaptation, and disease: Allostasis and allostatic load. *Annals of the New York Academy of Sciences, 840,* 33-44.

Melillo, P., Jovic, A., De Luca, N., & Pecchia, L. (2015). Automatic classifier based on heart rate variability to identify fallers among hypertensive subjects. *Healthcare Technology Letters, 2*(4), 89-94.

Michelon, E., Blaum, C., Semba, R. D., Xue, Q. L., Ricks, M. O., & Fried, L. P. (2006). Vitamin and carotenoid status in older women: Associations with the frailty syndrome. *Journal of Gerontology, 61*(6), 600-607.

Miles, T. P., Palmer, R. F., Espino, D. V., Mouton, C. P., Lichtenstein, M. J., & Markides, K. S. (2001). New-onset incontinence and markers of frailty: Data from the Hispanic Established Populations for Epidemiologic Studies of the Elderly. *Journal of Gerontology, 56*(1), M19-M24.

Miller, K. L. (2005). Stress urinary incontinence in women: Review and update on neurological control. *Journal of Women's Health, 14*(7), 595-608.

Minassian, V. A., Drutz, H. P., & Al-Badr, A. (2003). Urinary incontinence as a worldwide problem. *International Journal of Gynaecology and Obstetrics, 82*(3), 327-338.

Mitnitski, A. B., Mogilner, A. J., & Rockwood, K. (2001). Accumulation of deficits as a proxy measure of aging. *Scientific World Journal, 1,* 323-336.

Mitnitski, A. B., Song, X., & Rockwood, K. (2004). The estimation of relative fitness and frailty in community-dwelling older adults using self-report data. *Journal of Gerontology, 59*(6), M627-M632.

Morley, J. E. (2004). A brief history of geriatrics. *Journals of Gerontology Series A: Biological Sciences and Medical Sciences, 59*(11), 1132-1152.

Morley, J. E., Vellas, B., van Kan, G. A., Anker, S. D., Bauer, J. M., Bernabei, R.,… Walston, J. (2013). Frailty consensus: A call to action. *Journal of the American Medical Directors Association, 14*(6), 392-397.

Mu, D. L., Wang, D. X., Li, L. H., Shan, G. J., Li, J., Yu, Q. J., & Shi, C. X. (2010). High serum cortisol level is associated with increased risk of delirium after coronary artery bypass graft surgery: A prospective cohort study. *Critical Care, 14*(6), R238.

Nair, K. S. (1995). Muscle protein-turnover: Methodological issues and the effect of aging. *Journals of Gerontology Series A: Biological Sciences and Medical Sciences, 50*, 107-112.

Newman, A. B., Gottdiener, J. S., McBurnie, M. A., Hirsch, C. H., Kop, W. J., Tracy, R.,… Fried, L. P. (2001). Associations of subclinical cardiovascular disease with frailty. *Journals of Gerontology Series A: Biological Sciences and Medical Sciences, 56*(3), M158-M166.

Ni Mhaolain, A. M., Fan, C. W., Romero-Ortuno, R., Cogan, L., Cunningham, C., Lawlor, B., & Kenny, R. A. (2012). Depression: A modifiable factor in fearful older fallers transitioning to frailty? *International Journal of Geriatric Psychiatry, 27*(7), 727-733.

Nowak, A., & Hubbard, R. E. (2009). Falls and frailty: Lessons from complex systems. *Journal of the Royal Society of Medicine, 102*(3), 98-102.

Nykänen, I. R. T., Sulkava, R., & Hartikainen, S. (2014). Effects of individual dietary counseling as part of a comprehensive geriatric assessment (CGA) on nutritional status: A population-based intervention study. *Journal of Nutrition, Health & Aging, 18*(1), 54-58.

Panel on Prevention of Falls in Older Persons, American Geriatrics Society/British Geriatrics Society. (2011). Summary of the updated American Geriatrics Society/British Geriatrics Society clinical practice guideline for prevention of falls in older persons. *Journal of the American Geriatrics Society, 59*(1), 148-157.

Parvaneh, S., Howe, C. L., Toosizadeh, N., Honarvar, B., Slepian, M. J., Fain, M.,… Najafi, B. (2015). Regulation of cardiac autonomic nervous system control across frailty statuses: A systematic review. *Gerontology, 62*(1), 3-15.

Pathai, S., Weiss, H. A., Cook, C., Wood, R., Bekker, L. G., & Lawn, S. D. (2013). Frailty in HIV-infected adults in South Africa. *Journal of Acquired Immune Deficiency Syndromes, 62*(1), 43-51.

Pepys, M. B., & Hirschfield, G. M. (2003). C-reactive protein: A critical update. *Journal of Clinical Investigation, 111*(12), 1805-1812.

Pol, R. A., van Leeuwen, B. L., Izaks, G. J., Reijnen, M. M., Visser, L., Tielliu, I. F., & Zeebregts, C. J. (2014). C-reactive protein predicts postoperative delirium following vascular surgery. *Annals of Vascular Surgery, 28*(8), 1923-1930.

Prochaska, J. O., & Velicer, W. F. (1997). The transtheoretical model of health behavior change. *American Journal of Health Promotion, 12*, 38-48.

Quinlan, N., Marcantonio, E. R., Inouye, S. K., Gill, T. M., Kamholz, B., & Rudolph, J. L. (2011). Vulnerability: The crossroads of frailty and delirium. *Journal of the American Geriatrics Society, 59*(suppl 2), S262-S268.

Rantanen, T., Volpato, S., Ferrucci, L., Heikkinen, E., Fried, L. P., & Guralnik, J. M. (2003). Handgrip strength and cause-specific and total mortality in older disabled women: Exploring the mechanism. *Journal of the American Geriatrics Society, 51*(5), 636-641.

Reuben, D. B. (2007). Better care for older people with chronic diseases: An emerging vision. *Journal of the American Medical Association, 298*, 2673-2674.

Richards, K. C., Enderlin, C. A., Beck, C., McSweeney, J. D., Jones, T. C., & Roberson, P. K. 2007. Tailored biobehavioral interventions: A literature review and synthesis. *Research in Theory of Nursing Practice, 21*, 271-285.

Rigney, T. (2010). Allostatic load and delirium in the hospitalized older adult. *Nursing Research, 59*(5), 322-330.

Robertson, D. A., Savva, G. M., & Kenny, R. A. (2013). Frailty and cognitive impairment: A review of the evidence and causal mechanisms. *Ageing Research Reviews, 12*(4), 840-851.

Robins, J. M., Greenland, S., & Hu, F-C. Estimation of the causal effect of a time-varying exposure on the marginal mean of a repeated binary outcome. (1999). *Journal of The American Statistical Association, 94*, 687–700.

Rockwood, K. (2005). What would make a definition of frailty successful? *Age and Ageing, 34*(5), 432-434.

Rockwood, K., Andrew, M., & Mitnitski, A. (2007). A comparison of two approaches to measuring frailty in elderly people. *Journals of Gerontology Series A: Biological Sciences and Medical Sciences, 62*(7), 738-743.

Rockwood, K., & Mitnitski, A. (2007). Frailty in relation to the accumulation of deficits. *Journal of Gerontology, 62*(7), 722-727.

Rockwood, K., Mitnitski, A., Song, X., Steen, B., & Skoog, I. (2006). Long-term risks of death and institutionalization of elderly people in relation to deficit accumulation at age 70. *Journal of the American Geriatrics Society, 54*(6), 975-979.

Rockwood, K., Song, X., MacKnight, C., Bergman, H., Hogan, D. B., McDowell, I., & Mitnitski, A. (2005). A global clinical measure of fitness and frailty in elderly people. *Canadian Medical Association Journal, 173*(5), 489-495.

Rockwood, K., Stadnyk, K., MacKnight, C., McDowell, I., Hebert, R., & Hogan, D. B. (1999). A brief clinical instrument to classify frailty in elderly people. *Lancet, 353*(9148), 205-206.

Rodríguez-Mañas, L., Bayer, A. J., Kelly, M., Zeyfang, A, Izquierdo, M., Laosa, O.,… Cook, J. (2014). An evaluation of the effectiveness of a multi-modal intervention in frail and pre-frail older people with type 2 diabetes: The MID-Frail study: Study protocol for a randomised controlled trial. *Trials, 15*(34), 1-9.

Rodriguez-Manas, L., Feart, C., Mann, G., Vina, J., Chatterji, S., Chodzko-Zajko, W.,... Vega, E. (2013). Searching for an operational definition of frailty: A Delphi method based consensus statement. The Frailty Operative Definition-Consensus Conference Project. *Journals of Gerontology Series A: Biological Sciences and Medical Sciences, 68*(1), 62-67.

Rubenstein, L. Z. (2006). Falls in older people: Epidemiology, risk factors and strategies for prevention. *Age and Ageing, 35*(suppl 2), ii37-ii41.

Rubenstein, L. Z., & Josephson, K. R. (2002). The epidemiology of falls and syncope. *Clinics in Geriatric Medicine, 18*(2), 141-158.

Rubin, D. B. (1974). Estimating causal effects of treatments in randomized and nonrandomized studies. *Journal of Educational Psychology, 66*(5), 688–701.

Saliba, D., Elliott, M., Rubenstein, L. Z., Solomon, D. H., Young, R. T., Kamberg, C. J.,... Wenger, N. S. (2001). The Vulnerable Elders Survey: A tool for identifying vulnerable older people in the community. *Journal of the American Geriatrics Society, 49*(12), 1691-1699.

Sandoval-Insausti, H., Perez-Tasigchana, R. F., Lopez-Garcia, E., Garcia-Esquinas, E., Rodriguez-Artalejo, F., & Guallar-Castillon, P. (2016). Macronutrients intake and incident frailty in older adults: A prospective cohort study. *Journal of Gerontology, 71*(10), 1329–1334.

Santos-Eggimann, B., Cuenoud, P., Spagnoli, J., & Junod, J. (2009). Prevalence of frailty in middle-aged and older community-dwelling Europeans living in 10 countries. *Journal of Gerontology, 64*(6), 675-681.

Semba, R. D., Bartali, B., Zhou, J., Blaum, C., Ko, C. W., & Fried, L. P. (2006). Low serum micronutrient concentrations predict frailty among older women living in the community. *Journals of Gerontology Series A: Biological Sciences and Medical Sciences, 61*(6), 594-599.

Sepehri, A., Beggs, T., Hassan, A., Rigatto, C., Shaw-Daigle, C., Tangri, N., & Arora, R. C. (2014). The impact of frailty on outcomes after cardiac surgery: A systematic review. *Journal of Thoracic and Cardiovascular Surgery, 148*(6), 3110-3117.

Shimada, H., Doi, T., Yoshida, D., Tsutsumimoto, K., Anan, Y., Uemura, K.,... Suzuki, T. (2013). Combined prevalence of frailty and mild cognitive impairment in a population of elderly Japanese people. *Journal of the American Medical Directors Association, 14*(7), 518-524.

Shubert, T. E., Smith, M. L., Prizer, L. P., & Ory, M. G. (2014). Complexities of fall prevention in clinical settings: A commentary. *Gerontologist, 54*(4), 550-558.

Siddiqi, N., House, A. O., & Holmes, J. D. (2006). Occurrence and outcome of delirium in medical in-patients: A systematic literature review. *Age and Ageing, 35*(4), 350-364.

Sleet, D. A., Moffett, D. B., & Stevens, J. (2008). CDC's research portfolio in older adult fall prevention: A review of progress, 1985-2005, and future research directions. *Journal of Safety Research, 39*(3), 259-267.

Soler-Vila, H., Garcia-Esquinas, E., Leon-Munoz, L. M., Lopez-Garcia, E., Banegas, J. R., & Rodriguez-Artalejo, F. (2016). Contribution of health behaviours and clinical factors to socioeconomic differences in frailty among older adults. *Journal of Epidemiology and Community Health, 70*(4), 354-360.

Soriano, T. A., DeCherrie, L. V., & Thomas, D. C. (2007). Falls in the community-dwelling older adult: A review for primary-care providers. *Clinical Interventions in Aging, 2*(4), 545-554.

Sousa, A. C., Maciel, Á. C., & Guerra, R. O. (2012). Frailty syndrome and associated factors in community-dwelling elderly in Northeast Brazil. *Archives of Gerontology and Geriatrics, 54*(2), e95-e101.

Speechley, M., & Tinetti, M. (1991). Falls and injuries in frail and vigorous community elderly persons. *Journal of the American Geriatrics Society, 39*(1), 46-52.

Sternberg, S. A., Wershof Schwartz, A., Karunananthan, S., Bergman, H., & Mark Clarfield, A. (2011). The identification of frailty: A systematic literature review. *Journal of the American Geriatrics Society, 59*(11), 2129-2138.

Stevens, J. A., Corso, P. S., Finkelstein, E. A., & Miller, T. R. (2006). The costs of fatal and non-fatal falls among older adults. *Injury Prevention, 12*(5), 290-295.

Subra, J., Gillette-Guyonnet, S., Cesari, M., Oustric, S., Vellas, B., & Platform, T. (2012). The integration of frailty into clinical practice: Preliminary results from the Gerontopole. *Journal of Nutrition, Health & Aging, 16*(8), 714-720.

Szanton, S. L., & Gill, J. M. (2010). Facilitating resilience using a society-to-cells framework: A theory of nursing essentials applied to research and practice. *Advances in Nursing Science, 33*(4), 329-343.

Szanton, S. L., Thorpe, R. J., Boyd, C., Tanner, E. K., Leff, B., Agree, E.,... Gitlin, L. N. (2011). Community aging in place, advancing better living for elders: A bio-behavioral–environmental intervention to improve function and health-related quality of life in disabled older adults. *Journal of the American Geriatrics Society, 59*(12), 2314-2320.

Szanton, S. L., Wolff, J. L., Leff, B., Roberts, L., Thorpe, R. J., Tanner, E. K.,... Gitlin, L. N. (2015). Preliminary data from community aging in place, advancing better living for elders, a patient-directed, team-based intervention to improve physical function and decrease nursing home utilization: The first 100 individuals to complete a Centers for Medicare and Medicaid Services Innovation Project. *Journal of the American Geriatrics Society, 63*(2), 371-374.

Szanton, S. L., Wolff, J. W., Leff, B., Thorpe, R. J., Tanner, E. K., Boyd, C.,... Gitlin, L. N. (2014). CAPABLE trial: A randomized controlled trial of nurse, occupational therapist and handyman to reduce disability among older adults: rationale and design. *Contemporary Clinical Trials, 38*(1), 102-112.

Talley, K. M., Wyman, J. F., & Shamliyan, T. A. (2011). State of the science: Conservative interventions for urinary incontinence in frail community-dwelling older adults. *Nursing Outlook, 59*(4), 215-220.

Tavassoli, N., Guyonnet, S., Abellan van Kan, G., Sourdet, S., Krams, T., Soto, M. E., Vellas, B. (2014). Description of 1,108 older patients referred by their physician to the "Geriatric Frailty Clinic (G.F.C) for Assessment of Frailty and Prevention of Disability" at the Gerontopole. *Journal of Nutrition, Health & Aging, 18*(5), 457-464.

Tchkonia, T., Von Zglinicki, T., Van Deursen, J., Lustgarten, J., Scrable, H., Khosla, S.,... Kirkland, J. L. (2010). Fat tissue, aging, and cellular senescence. *Aging Cell, 9*(5), 667-684.

Teleman, P. M., Persson, J., Mattiasson, A., & Samsioe, G. (2009). The relation between urinary incontinence and steroid hormone levels in perimenopausal women: A report from the Women's Health in the Lund Area (WHILA) study. *Acta Obstetrica et Gynecologica Scandinavica, 88*(8), 927-932.

Theou, O., & Rockwood, K. (2015). Comparison and clinical applications of the frailty phenotype and frailty index approaches. *Interdisciplinary Topics in Gerontology and Geriatrics, 41*, 74-84.

Tudorache, E., Oancea, C., Avram, C., Fira-Mladinescu, O., Petrescu, L., & Timar, B. (2015). Balance impairment and systemic inflammation in chronic obstructive pulmonary disease. *International Journal of Chronic Obstructive Pulmonary Disease, 10*, 1847-1852.

Varadhan, R., Chaves, P. H., Lipsitz, L. A., Stein, P. K., Tian, J., Windham, B. G.,... Fried, L. P. (2009). Frailty and impaired cardiac autonomic control: New insights from principal components aggregation of traditional heart rate variability indices. *Journal of Gerontology, 64*(6), 682-687.

Varadhan, R., Seplaki, C. L., Xue, Q. L., Bandeen-Roche, K., & Fried, L. P. (2008). Stimulus-response paradigm for characterizing the loss of resilience in homeostatic regulation associated with frailty. *Mechanisms of Ageing and Development, 129*(11), 666-670.

Varadhan, R., Walston, J., Cappola, A. R., Carlson, M. C., Wand, G. S., & Fried, L. P. (2008). Higher levels and blunted diurnal variation of cortisol in frail older women. *Journal of Gerontology, 63*(2), 190-195.

Varadhan, R., Xue, Q. L., & Bandeen-Roche, K. (2014). Semicompeting risks in aging research: Methods, issues and needs. *Lifetime Data Analysis, 20*(4), 538-562.

Vasunilashorn, S. M., Ngo. L., Inouye, S. K., Libermann, T. A., Jones, R. N., Alsop, D. C.,... Marcantonio, E. R. (2015). Cytokines and postoperative delirium in older patients undergoing major elective surgery. *Journal of Gerontology, 70*(10), 1289-1295.

Vellas, B., Balardy, L., Gillette-Guyonnet, S., Abellan van Kan, G., Ghisolfi-Marque, A., Subra, J.,... Cesari, M. (2013). Looking for frailty in community-dwelling older persons: The Gerontopole Frailty Screening Tool (GFST). *Journal of Nutrition, Health & Aging, 17*(7), 629-631.

Viitasalo, J. T., Era, P., Leskinen, A. L., & Heikkinen, E. (1985). Muscular strength profiles and anthropometry in random samples of men aged 31-35, 51-55 and 71-75 years. *Ergonomics, 28*(11), 1563-1574.

Von Korff, M., Gruman, J., Schaefer, J., Curry, S. J., & Wagner, E. H. (1997). Collaborative management of chronic illness. *Annals of Internal Medicine, 127*, 1097-1102.

Wagg, A., Gibson, W., Ostaszkiewicz, J., Johnson, T., 3rd, Markland, A., Palmer, M. H.,... Kirschner-Hermanns, R. (2015). Urinary incontinence in frail elderly persons: Report from the 5th International Consultation on Incontinence. *Neurourology and Urodynamics, 34*(5), 398-406.

Wallace, K. A., & Bergeman, C. S. (1997). Control and the elderly: "Goodness-of-fit." *International Journal of Aging and Human Development, 45*(4), 323-339.

Walston, J. D. (2005). Biological markers and the molecular biology of frailty. In J. R. Carey, J.-M. Robine, J.-P. Michel, & Y. Christen (Eds.), *Longevity and frailty* (pp. 83-90). Berlin, Germany: Springer-Verlag.

Walston, J. D. (2015). Connecting age-related biological decline to frailty and late-life vulnerability. *Nestle Nutrition Institute Workshop Series, 83*, 1-10.

Walston, J. D., & Bandeen-Roche, K. (2015). Frailty: A tale of two concepts. *BMC Medicine, 13*, 185.

Walston, J., Fedarko, N., Yang, H., Leng, S., Beamer, B., Espinoza, S.,... Becker, K. (2008). The physical and biological characterization of a frail mouse model. *Journal of Gerontology Series A, Biological Sciences and Medical Sciences, 63*(4), 391-398.

Walston, J., Hadley, E. C., Ferrucci, L., Guralnik, J. M., Newman, A. B., Studenski, S. A.,... Fried, L. P. (2006). Research agenda for frailty in older adults: Toward a better understanding of physiology and etiology: Summary from the American Geriatrics Society/ National Institute on Aging Research Conference on Frailty in Older Adults. *Journal of the American Geriatrics Society, 54*(6), 991-1001.

Walston, J., McBurnie, M. A., Newman, A., Tracy, R. P., Kop, W. J., Hirsch, C. H.,... Fried, L. P. (2002). Frailty and activation of the inflammation and coagulation systems with and without clinical comorbidities: Results from the Cardiovascular Health Study. *Archives of Internal Medicine, 162*(20), 2333-2341.

Walston, J., Xue, Q., Semba, R. D., Ferrucci, L., Cappola, A. R., Ricks, M.,... Fried, L. P. (2006). Serum antioxidants, inflammation, and total mortality in older women. *American Journal of Epidemiology, 163*(1), 18–26.

Weinberger, B., & Grubeck-Loebenstein, B. (2009). Immunology and aging. In J. O. Halter, M. E. Tinetti, S. Studenski, K. P. High, & S. Asthana (Eds.), *Hazzard's geriatric medicine and gerontology* (6th ed.). New York, NY: McGraw-Hill. Retrieved from http://accessmedicine.mhmedical.com/content.aspx?bookid=371&Sectionid=41587606

Winograd, C. H., Gerety, M. B., Chung, M., Goldstein, M. K., Dominguez, F. Jr., & Vallone, R. (1991). Screening for frailty: Criteria and predictors of outcomes. *Journal of the American Geriatrics Society, 39*(8), 778–784.

Wong, C. H., Weiss, D., Sourial, N., Karunananthan, S., Quail, J. M., Wolfson, C., & Bergman, H. (2010). Frailty and its association with disability and comorbidity in a community-dwelling sample of seniors in Montreal: A cross-sectional study. *Aging clinical and experimental research, 22*(1), 54–62.

Woods, N. F., LaCroix, A. Z., Gray, S. L., Aragaki, A., Cochrane, B. B., Brunner, R. L.,… Newman, A. B. (2005). Frailty: Emergence and consequences in women aged 65 and older in the Women's Health Initiative observational study. *Journal of the American Geriatrics Society, 53*(8), 1321–1330.

World Health Organization (WHO). (2007). WHO global report on falls prevention in older age. Retrieved from http://www.who.int/violence_injury_prevention/publications/other_injury/falls_prevention.pdf?ua=1

World Health Organization (WHO). (2015). *World report on ageing and health: Summary.* Geneva, Switzerland: Author.

Xue, Q. L., Bandeen-Roche, K., Varadhan, R., Zhou, J., & Fried, L. P. (2008). Initial manifestations of frailty criteria and the development of frailty phenotype in the Women's Health and Aging Study II. *Journal of Gerontology, 63*(9), 984–990.

Xue, Q. L., Beamer, B. A., Chaves, P. H. M., Guralnik, J. M., & Fried, L. P. (2010). Heterogeneity in rate of decline in grip, hip, and knee strength and the risk of all-cause mortality: The Women's Health and Aging Study II. *Journal of the American Geriatrics Society, 58*(11), 2076–2084.

Xue, Q. L., Fried, L. P., Glass, T. A., Laffan, A., & Chaves, P. H. M. (2008). Life-space constriction, development of frailty, and the competing risk of mortality. *American Journal of Epidemiology, 167*(2), 240–248.

Xue, Q. L., Guralnik, J. M., Beamer, B. A., Fried, L. P., & Chaves, P. H. M. (2015). Monitoring 6-month trajectory of grip strength improves the prediction of long-term change in grip strength in disabled older women. *Journals of Gerontology Series A: Biological Sciences and Medical Sciences, 70*(3), 365–371.

Xue, Q. L., Tian, J., Fried, L. P., Kalyani, R. R., Varadhan, R., Walston, J. D., & Bandeen-Roche, K. (2016). Physical frailty assessment in older women: Can simplification be achieved without loss of syndrome measurement validity? *American Journal of Epidemiology, 183*(11), 1037–1044.

Xue, Q. L., & Varadhan, R. (2014). What is missing in the validation of frailty instruments? *Journal of the American Medical Directors Association, 15*(2), 141–142.

Xue, Q. L., Walston, J., Fried, L. P., & Beamer, B. (2011). Prediction of the risk of falling, physical disability, and frailty by rate of decline in grip strength. *Archives of Internal Medicine, 171*(12), 1119–1121.

Xue, Q. L., Yang, H., Li, H. F., Abadir, P. M., Burks, T. N., Koch, L. G.,… Leng, S. X. (2016). Rapamycin increases grip strength and attenuates age-related decline in maximal running distance in old low capacity runner rats. *Aging, 8*(4), 769–776.

Yao, X., Hamilton, R. G., Weng, N. P., Xue, Q. L., Bream, J. H., Li, H.,… Leng, S. X. (2011). Frailty is associated with impairment of vaccine-induced antibody response and increase in post-vaccination influenza infection in community-dwelling older adults. *Vaccine, 29*(31), 5015–5021.

Zaal, I. J., van der Kooi, A. W., van Schelven, L. J., Oey, P. L., & Slooter, A. J. (2015). Heart rate variability in intensive care unit patients with delirium. *Journal of Neuropsychiatry and Clinical Neurosciences, 27*(2), e112–e116.

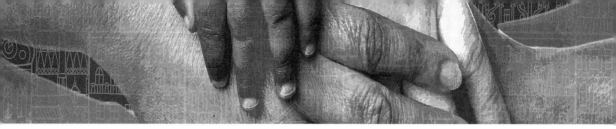

CHAPTER 10

Aging and Falls

Wenjun Li

ABSTRACT

Falls are common in older age. Globally, falls are the leading cause of unintentional injuries, and a major unintentional injury-related cause of disability-adjusted life-years lost and fatality annually. The annual death rate of unintentional falls has been steadily increasing in recent decades. Fall injuries result in significant economic burdens to the injured individuals, their families, and society. As the population ages rapidly, the economic burden due to falls will likely continue to increase. Falls prevention is a national priority in many countries, including the United States and many European countries. Effective prevention is necessary not only to improve health, quality of life, independent living, and longevity of older adults, but also to curb the rising healthcare costs attributable to elderly falls. This chapter provides an overview of the causes, consequences, and prevention of unintentional falls. It also discusses sex, racial/ethnic, and broader geographic variations in falls and fall injuries. The discussions focus on heterogeneity in people who fall, their risk factors, the influences of time and space use on falls (i.e., human–environment interactions), and differential consequences of falling. The chapter shows the eminent need for individualized fall risk assessment and prevention strategies and related technological innovations, and advocates for a paradigm shift in future falls prevention research.

KEYWORDS

falls	physical limitations	prevention
fall injury	home environment	technology
heterogeneity	neighborhood environment	

▶ Introduction

Falls are common among older adults (persons age 65 and older). Approximately 30% of community-dwelling older adults and 50% of nursing home residents fall each year (Berg, Alessio, Mills, & Tong, 1997; Campbell et al., 1990; Tinetti, 2003). A fall is typically defined as a person unintentionally coming to rest on the ground or other lower level not as a result of a major intrinsic event (e.g., heart attack, stroke, seizure) or an overwhelming external hazard (e.g., hit by a vehicle or large object). Based on the purpose of research and the varied focuses of intervention strategies, falls can be classified by location, activity, causes, and consequences.

Globally, falls are the leading cause of unintentional injuries (Global Burden of Disease Study, 2015), and a major unintentional injury-related cause of disability-adjusted life-years lost and fatality annually (Chandran, Hyder, & Peek-Asa, 2010; Krug, Sharma, & Lozano, 2000). Various studies showed that 10% to 30% of falls result in injuries requiring medical attention (Alexander, Rivara, & Wolf, 1992; CDC, 2008; Rubenstein & Josephson, 2002; Schwartz, Capezuti, & Grisso, 2001; Tinetti, 2003; Tinetti, Speechley, & Ginter, 1988). Falls are the leading cause of injury-related deaths (Murphy, 2000), nonfatal injuries (CDC, 2016), and hospital admissions among older adults in the United States (Alexander et al., 1992). According to the Centers for Disease Control and Prevention (CDC), the annual death rate of unintentional falls has been steadily increasing since 1994. In the past two decades, the rate increased more than 2.6-fold, rising from 22.1 per 100,000 older adults in 1994 to 58.5 per 100,000 older adults in 2014 (CDC, 2016).

Falls and fall injuries have a major negative impact on older adults' health and quality of life (Gill, Desai, Gahbauer, Holford, & Williams, 2001; Tinetti & Williams, 1997, 1998). Fall injuries may result in functional loss, bodily pain, hospitalization, prolonged bed rest, decreases in mobility, loss of independence, and poor mental health. More than 90% of hip fractures in older Americans result from a fall. Even when no physical injury occurs, falls can result in the "post-fall syndrome" (Howland, Lachman, Peterson, Cote, Kasten, & Jette, 1998; Murphy & Isaacs, 1982) or fear of falling (Tinetti & Speechley, 1989; Vellas, Cayla, Bocquet, de Pemille, & Albarede, 1987). Fear of falling can become a significant barrier to physical activity (Tinetti, Mendes de Leon, Doucette, & Baker, 1994; Wijlhuizen, de Jong, & Hopman-Rock, 2006), leading to decreased independence and mobility (Nevitt, Cummings, & Hudes, 1991; Northridge, Nevitt, Kelsey, & Link, 1995; Tinetti et al., 1988), increased social isolation (Howland et al., 1993), depression and anxiety (Arfken, Lach, Birge, & Miller, 1994), and premature admission to nursing homes (Cumming, Salkeld, Thomas, & Szonyi, 2000; Mendes de Leon, Seeman, Baker, Richardson, & Tinetti, 1996; Vellas et al., 1987).

Fall injuries result in significant economic burden (Carroll, Slattum, & Cox, 2005; Stevens, Corso, Finkelstein, & Miller, 2006). An analysis of the 1997 Medical Expenditure Panel Survey estimated that fall-related medical conditions in community-dwelling older adults cost $8 billion per year (Carroll et al., 2005). Fall injuries are among the 20 most expensive medical conditions (Carroll et al., 2005). The average hospital cost for a **fall injury** was $35,000 in 2006 (Stevens et al., 2006). The total direct cost of all fall injuries exceeded $19 billion in 2000 (Stevens et al., 2006). The combined cost (medical and work loss) increased to nearly $32 billion in 2010. The CDC predicts that the cost of fall-related injuries will reach $44 billion by 2020 (Englander, Hodson, & Terregrossa, 1996). The National Electronic Injury Surveillance System-All Injury Program recently reported a steadily increasing trend in rates of fall injury-related emergency department (ED) visits and hospitalizations among U.S. older adults

(Orces & Alamgir, 2014). As the country's population ages rapidly, the escalation of economic burden due to falls will likely continue.

Falls **prevention** is a national priority in the United States (*Healthy People 2020* Objectives IVP-23.2 and OA-11). Effective prevention is necessary not only to improve health, quality of life, independent living, and longevity of older adults, but also to curb the rising healthcare costs attributable to elderly falls. A better understanding of the epidemiology of falls is critical to design, implementation, and evaluation of falls prevention programs.

▶ Heterogeneity and Classification of Falls

Falls are highly heterogeneous with respect to personal sociodemographic, health condition, **physical limitations**, lifestyle factors, living arrangements, environmental conditions, causes and consequences, and location and activity at the time of falling (Kelsey, Procter-Gray, Hannan, & Li, 2012; Li et al., 2014). Depending on the specific purpose of the research or the focus of intervention strategies, falls can be classified by causes (e.g., environmental versus nonenvironmental), location (e.g., indoor versus outdoor), activity (e.g., walking versus vigorous activity versus other activity related), and consequences (e.g., injurious versus non-injurious).

First, falls can be classified as environmental versus non-environmental. For example, an environmental fall is defined as a fall precipitated by an environmental factor such as an uneven surface and tripping or slipping on an object outdoors or a loose rug at home (Northridge et al., 1995; Li et al., 2006). Home hazards are associated with increased risk for falls among vigorous older adults (Northridge et al., 1995). Most outdoor falls (more than 73%) are precipitated by environmental factors (Li et al., 2006). A nonenvironmental fall is defined as a fall that does not involve an environmental factor, but rather an intrinsic event such as tiredness and sudden sickness.

For research into consequences of and environmental hazards for fall injuries, fall events can be classified as injurious falls and non-injurious falls. Injurious falls include falls that result in a soft-tissue injury to any body part or a fracture of any bone (Kelsey, Berry, et al., 2010; Li et al., 2006; Li et al., 2014). In recent years, more than 20% of elderly falls have resulted in an injury or discomfort that required medical attention. However, the proportion of injurious falls increases with age, and is higher among frail older adults.

Circumstances and consequences of falling vary substantially by location and activity at the time of falling (Duckham et al., 2013; Kelsey, Berry, et al., 2010; Li et al., 2014). Rates and determinants of indoor and outdoor falls and outdoor walking differ substantially by sex, suggesting the need for gender-specific interventions (Duckham et al., 2013). Location- and activity-specific fall rates are influenced by personal characteristics, neighborhood perception, access to neighborhood resources, and neighborhood conditions (Li et al., 2014).

In research into place-specific fall risks, fall events can be classified as indoors versus outdoors (Connell & Wolf, 1997; Gill, Williams, & Tinetti, 2000; Northridge, Nevitt, & Kelsey, 1996; Northridge et al., 1995; Sattin, Rodriguez, & DeVito, 1998; Tinetti & Williams, 1997); or as outdoors (outside a building or in a parking garage) versus outside the home but indoors (in a building other than the subject's own home, excluding parking garages), versus in the home (inside the residence of the subject, including hallways of apartment buildings). The more frequent occurrence of outdoor falls compared to indoor falls among community-dwelling elderly is a common phenomenon across geographic regions (Bath & Morgan, 1999; Bergland, Jarnlo, & Laake, 2003; Bergland, Pettersen, & Laake, 1998; Li et al., 2006; Weinberg & Strain, 1995; Yasumura, Haga, & Niino, 1996).

The circumstances and consequences of location-specific falls differ substantially (Duckham et al., 2013; Kelsey, Berry, et al., 2010; Li et al., 2014). Outdoor and indoor falls have different pathways (O'Loughlin, Boivin, Robitaille, & Suissa, 1994) and consequences (Graafmans, Ooms, Bezemer, Bouter, & Lips, 1996; Kelsey, Berry, et al., 2010) and, therefore, should be treated as separate outcomes (Bath & Morgan, 1999; Kelsey, Berry, et al., 2010). Risk factor profiles for outdoor and indoor falls differ significantly as well (Bath & Morgan, 1999; Graafmans et al., 1996; Kelsey, Berry, et al., 2010; Li et al., 2006; Li et al., 2014; O'Loughlin et al., 1994). Outdoor falls are associated with compromised health status in active people, whereas indoor falls are associated with frailty (Bath & Morgan, 1999; Bergland et al., 1998). Thus, the distinction between outdoor and indoor falls may be critical in understanding location- and activity-related risks for falls, since many vigorous and possibly higher-risk activities (e.g., recreational walking, shopping) are performed outdoors. Current research on falls focuses mostly on intrinsic personal factors and the **home environment** (Connell & Wolf, 1997; Gill et al., 2000; Gillespie et al., 2005; McClure et al., 2005; Northridge et al., 1996; Northridge et al., 1995; Sattin et al., 1998; Schwartz et al., 2001; Tinetti & Williams, 1997). Current prevention approaches emphasize individual behavioral change or adaptation to existing conditions and modification of the home (American Geriatrics Society, British Geriatrics Society, & American Academy of Orthopedic Surgeons Panel on Falls Prevention, 2001; Gillespie et al., 2005; McClure et al., 2005; Myers, Young, & Langlois, 1996). Only in recent years has research been undertaken on the relationship between risk for falls and characteristics of the outdoor environment.

Contemporary studies attempt to better understand the risk factors for falls in different kinds of outdoor places. In these studies, outdoor falls are further classified as on or in (1) sidewalks, (2) streets, (3) curbs, (4) gardens or yards, (5) stairs or steps, (6) parks or recreation places, (7) parking garages or parking lots, and (8) other outdoor places (Kelsey, Berry, et al., 2010; Li et al., 2006; Lie et al., 2014). Outdoor falls are also classified as within or outside the subject's neighborhood, which help identify the associations of mobility patterns with risk for falling.

To understand the activity-related risk factors for falls, falls can be classified according to activity at the time of fall: (1) walking on level ground; (2) engaging in vigorous activity; (3) walking up or down stairs; (4) stepping on or off a curb; (5) getting into or out of a motor vehicle; (4) doing household chores; (5) bathing; (6) getting into or out of a chair, sofa, or bed; or using the toilet; (7) sitting or lying; or (8) others. Injurious potential of falls vary by activity type at the time of falling. The highest risk for a fall injury occurs when an older adult is walking up or down stairs, engaging in modest to vigorous activities, or carrying a heavy load (Li et al., 2014). For frail older adults, bathing and getting into or out of bed are associated with fall risks.

In summary, the substantial **heterogeneity** in risk factors, circumstances, and consequences of falls indicate the need for multilevel, multifactorial, and individualized falls interventions. Future falls research should attempt to better understand the inter-relationships among personal health, social, behavioral, home, and neighborhood

---

PEARL 10-1 Future Approaches to Falls Prevention

Future falls research should attempt to better understand the inter-relationships among personal health, social, behavioral, home, and neighborhood environmental risk factors. A better understanding of the influences of person–environment interactions, such as time and space use, on fall risks may lead to new, more effective approaches to falls prevention among older adults.

environmental risk factors. A better understanding of the influences of person–environment interactions, such as time and space use, on fall risks may lead to new, more effective approaches to falls prevention among older adults.

▶ Measurement Methods

Falls are usually tracked by self-report at a specific time interval or a period in the immediate past. In large surveillance studies or clinical practice, older adults are often queried about any number of falls in the past 3, 6, or 12 months. Such queries are often repeated at each follow-up or clinical visit to track longitudinal changes in fall risks.

In more rigorous research, falls are often tracked using a monthly falls calendar. This fall calendar is usually printed on a modest-size postcard in large font. An older adult participant is instructed to check the box corresponding to an "F" for a *fall* or an "N" for *no fall* on a daily basis (Tinetti, Liu, & Claus, 1993). At the end of each month, each participant mails his or her calendar to a dedicated research staff. Depending on the nature of the research project or intervention program, additional questions can be included on the falls calendar to measure dynamic changes in behaviors and fall risks, such as the severity of pain, change in mobility, any hospitalization or major medical or life event, use of assistive devices at home or when going outdoors in the past month, change in home settings, or travel out of town. Postcards received are logged in a longitudinal tracking database. If a fall is indicated on the calendar, the participant will be queried by telephone or in person regarding the place, possible causes, circumstances and consequences of the fall(s).

Questions concerning place of fall may include whether the subject was inside her or his own home, inside someone else's home, inside a public building, inside other places, or outdoors. For indoor falls, the elder may be queried about whether the fall occurred in the kitchen, bathroom, living room, dining room, bedroom, washing room, stairs or steps, or garage. For outdoor falls, the elder may be queried about whether the fall occurred on the sidewalk or walkway, street, curb, or stairs or steps; or in an outdoor park or recreation place, a parking garage/lot, or somewhere else.

Further, information on circumstances may include the following items: (1) distance to home or locale visited when the fall took place; (2) activity engaged in when the fall took place; (3) whether the person slipped or tripped on something; (4) whether the surface was wet or dry, or snowy/icy; (5) whether the fall was thought to have occurred because of a health or medical problem; (6) whether the lighting was adequate; (7) whether the person was knocked down by someone or something; and (8) whether and which type of assistive device was being used at the time of the fall.

Information on consequences of falls includes whether the fall resulted in any soft-tissue injury, dislocated joint, other types of bone or joint injury, or fracture of a bone, and whether the injury required medical attention or hospitalization.

In large-scale observational and evaluation studies, the falls calendar approach is often impractical. Measurement of falls relies on recall of any or number of falls in the past 3, 6, or 12 months, and querying the details of the most recent fall. Information to be gathered is similar to that collected via a monthly falls calendar, but with substantially less details.

Large-scale fall injury research and program evaluation also rely heavily on hospital administration and insurance claims databases. For example, national and state emergency room visits, hospitalization databases, and Medicare claims databases are routinely used to track trends in incidence, fatalities, and medical expenditures associated with falls (CDC, 2007).

▶ Personal Risk Factors

The pathways that lead to falls are complex and multifactorial (Gill et al., 2000; Hill, Schwarz, Flicker, & Carroll, 1999; Northridge et al., 1996; Rubenstein, 2006; Rubenstein & Josephson, 2006; Schwartz et al., 1999; Tromp, Smit, Deeg, Bouter, & Lips, 1998). A large number of individual-level risk factors for falls have been associated with falls in the literature. Several cohort studies have evaluated risk for falls and noted that elders—especially those with comorbidities—are at increased risk (Bath & Morgan, 1999; O'Loughlin et al., 1994). Individual-level risk factors for falls and fall-related injuries have been summarized in several comprehensive reviews and various falls prevention guidelines (American Geriatrics Society et al., 2001; Ganz, Bao, Shekelle, & Rubenstein, 2007; Myers et al., 1996; Rubenstein, 2006; Rubenstein & Josephson, 2002, 2006; Schwartz et al., 2001).

Briefly, higher risk for falls among older people is associated strongly with the following factors:

- Older age
- Female gender
- History of falls in the past 3 months or year
- Functional impairments (e.g., limitations in activities of daily living [ADLs], use of assistive devices at home and when going outdoors)
- Abnormalities in gait and balance (e.g., walking speed, postural sway, impaired reflexes)
- Lower-extremity disability and weakness
- Musculoskeletal and neuromuscular disorders (e.g., reduced muscle strength and foot disorders, grip strength [Sayer et al., 2006])
- Sensory impairment (e.g., poor vision and distant visual acuity [Elliott, 2014], poor lower-extremity sensory perception)
- Cognitive impairment and depression
- Chronic illnesses (e.g., Parkinson's disease, neuromuscular disease, stroke, urinary incontinence, arthritis, low back pain, knee pain)
- Body mass index (obesity, especially osteosarcopenic [Hita-Contreras, Martinez-Amat, Cruz-Diaz, & Perez-Lopez, 2015] and dynapenic obesity [Scott et al., 2014])
- Medication use (e.g., number and type of medications used; hypnotics, sedatives, antipsychotics, antidepressants [Global Burden of Disease Study, 2015], anticoagulants, and anticholinergics [Chandran et al., 2010])

Modest elevation of risk for falls is associated with arthritis, acute illness, mental health, and psychosocial factors (e.g., depression, anxiety, resilience, and falls efficacy [Tinetti, Richman, & Powell, 1990]). An association between poor early growth and falls in older men, likely mediated through sarcopenia, has also been reported (Sayer et al., 2006).

Higher fall risks have also been associated with a number of personal socioeconomic and lifestyle factors (Kelsey, Berry, et al., 2010; Kelsey, Procter-Gray, Hannan, et al., 2012; Li et al., 2014). Relevant socioeconomic and demographic factors include race and ethnicity, less education, poverty, lower income, living in poor housing conditions, and living alone. Older people receiving in-home informal care may be subject to increased risk of falls possibly in part due to the caregivers having greater burdens of care and depression (Meyer et al., 2012). A number of lifestyle factors may contribute to higher fall risks, including alcohol and substance use, both high and low levels of physical activity (Kelsey, Berry, et al., 2010; Li et al., 2006), utilitarian and recreational walking (Li et al., 2014), wearing of bifocal or trifocal eyeglasses, and wearing certain types of potentially hazardous footwear (Kelsey, Procter-Gray, et al., 2010; Menz, Morris, & Lord, 2006; Sherrington & Menz, 2003).

▶ Environmental Risk Factors

Older adults are vulnerable to environmental hazards, and the risk of falling may be increased by exposure to such hazards and by a reduced capacity to respond to the consequent challenge to balance (Keegan et al., 2004; King & Tinetti, 1995; Northridge et al., 1996). As many as half of falls in the elderly are precipitated by environmental factors (Bath & Morgan, 1999; Northridge et al., 1995). Among outdoor falls, nearly three-fourths are precipitated by one or more environmental factors (Li et al., 2006).

Risk factors related to the home environment have been the subject of many studies (Brooke-Wavell, Perrett, Howarth, & Haslam, 2002; Connell, 1996; Connell & Wolf, 1997; Josephson, Fabacher, & Rubenstein, 1991; Rubenstein, 1997, 1999). Evidence is inconsistent, but home environmental factors—such as poor lighting, clutter, lack of stair railings, loose rugs or other tripping hazards, lack of grab bars in the bathroom, and frictional variations between shoes and floor coverings—may be modestly associated with falls among healthy elderly individuals (Brooke-Wavell et al., 2002; Connell, 1996; Connell & Wolf, 1997; Marshall et al., 2005; Northridge et al., 1995; Northridge et al., 1996; Schwartz et al., 2001). Frail elders are more than twice as likely as vigorous elders to fall, and living with more home hazards appears to be related to a greater risk for falls among vigorous (but not frail) elders (Northridge et al., 1995).

The impact of the **neighborhood environment** on risk for falls remains under studied. Until recent years, the outdoor neighborhood environment had not been a focus of research on falls, and none of the previous cohort studies of falls in the elderly has addressed the potential contribution of the neighborhood physical and socioeconomic environment to the risk of falls. Several recent studies have associated a number

PEARL 10-2 Future Areas of Research, #1

Among the areas for improvement in falls research, a particular knowledge gap is the inadequate understanding of an older adult's utilization of neighborhood resources, such as frequency, location, and determinants of space and time use for physical activity and their relationship to falls.

of neighborhood socioeconomic status (SES) and built environmental factors with risk for falling among the elderly (Li et al., 2014).

Neighborhood SES influences physical activity (PA) and risk for falls. Neighborhood SES (Estabrooks, Lee, & Gyurcsik, 2003; Fisher, Li, Michael, & Cleveland, 2004; Giles-Corti & Donovan, 2002; Li, Fisher, Bauman, et al., 2005; Li, Fisher, & Brownson, 2005), social disorganization (Glass, Rasmussen, & Schwartz, 2006; Lee & Cubbin, 2002; Lee, Reese-Smith, Regan, Booth, & Howard, 2003), and safety (CDC, 1999; Kimsey, Ham, & Macera, 2001) are predictive of residents' PA. Adults living in lower-SES neighborhoods have less PA (Giles-Corti & Donovan, 2002; Lee & Cubbin, 2002; Lynch et al., 1998; Yen & Kaplan, 1998) than persons with similar attributes living in higher-SES neighborhoods. A recent study by Li et al. (2014) found that neighborhood SES indicators are associated with frequency of utilitarian versus recreational walking,

PEARL 10-3 Future Areas of Research, #2

The age-dependent changes in fall rates have not been rigorously examined. Because older adults' location and time of indoor and outdoor activities change with age, it is important to investigate whether and how accelerations of fall rates may differ according to location and activity of falling.

and with rates of indoor and outdoor falls. In this study, falls on sidewalks and streets were more likely to result in an injury than were falls in recreational areas. Utilitarian-only walkers tended to live in neighborhoods with the lowest neighborhood SES and had the highest rate of outdoor falls despite walking 14 and 25 fewer blocks per week compared to the recreational-only and dual walkers, respectively (Li et al., 2014).

The effect of neighborhood SES on PA and falls may in part be explained by the associations between neighborhood SES and availability and quality of neighborhood resources (Larson, Story, & Nelson, 2009; Li et al., 2014). Neighborhood SES indicators, which serve as markers of community public financial and planning resources, may predict the availability, design features, and maintenance of neighborhood resources that are important to residents' daily life, such as sidewalks and outdoor parks or recreational places. Neighborhoods with lower SES may have poorer walkability and safety—factors that increase the rate of outdoor falls among the elderly residents. Studies have reported that poorer neighborhoods tend to have fewer resources for PA and generally poorer walkability and safety (Estabrooks et al., 2003; Lee et al., 2003). Thus, it is important to consider neighborhood SES when analyzing the relationships between PA and risk for falls.

Many studies have examined the impact of the outdoor physical environment on health outcomes known to be associated with falls in community-dwelling elderly persons, such as functional loss (Balfour & Kaplan, 2002; Glass & Balfour, 2003; Halpern, 1995) and impaired mobility (Patla & Shumway-Cook, 1999; Shumway-Cook, 2003, 2005). The physical environment mediates the relationship between functional limitations related to walking and the development of mobility disability (Patla & Shumway-Cook, 1999; Shumway-Cook, 2003). Critical environmental determinants of mobility of the elderly include distance to destinations (e.g., grocery stores, pharmacies, parks, or recreational places), temporal characteristics (e.g., weather, season), ambient conditions (e.g., light and weather conditions), terrain characteristics, physical load (e.g., whether carrying objects), attentional demands, postural transitions, and density (e.g., number of people and objects in immediate environment) (Patla & Shumway-Cook, 1999; Shumway-Cook, 2002, 2003, 2005). Because these factors are associated with fall risks, the influences of the neighborhood physical environment on these health outcomes and health behaviors may also directly or indirectly affect fall risks.

Neighborhood physical environmental factors, both natural and built, have been associated with adult PA (Ball, Bauman, Leslie, & Owen, 2001; Booth, Owen, Bauman, Clavisi, & Leslie, 2000; Brownson et al., 2000; CDC, 1996; Humpel, Owen, & Leslie, 2002; King et al., 2000; Reis et al., 2004; Sallis, Bauman, & Pratt, 1998; Sallis et al., 1990; Sallis, Kraft, & Linton, 2002; van Lenthe, Brug, & Mackenbach, 2005; Zabina, Blanton, Macera, & Pratt, 1998; Zlot, Librett, Buchner, & Schmid, 2006), including weather and seasonality (Ma et al., 2006; Matthews et al., 2001), rurality (CDC, 1998; Reis et al., 2004; Zabina et al., 1998), low population density in suburbs and motor vehicle dependency (Frank, 2000; Healthy People 2010, 2001; Lopez-Zetina, Lee, & Friis, 2006; Pendola & Gen, 2006), traffic volume and safety (McGinn, Evenson, Herring, Huston, & Rodriguez, 2007; Ogilvie, Mitchell, Mutrie, Petticrew, & Platt, 2008), proximity to shops and healthcare facilities (Ogilvie et al., 2008), lack of access to fitness facilities (Blanchard et al., 2005), poor land-use mix and lower "walkability" (Newman & Kenworth, 1991; Saelens, Sallis, Black, & Chen, 2003), availability and conditions of sidewalks or walkways in neighborhoods (Cervero & Duncan, 2003; Frank, Schmid, Sallis, Chapman, & Saelens, 2005), and limited access to public parks and recreational areas (Hanibuchi, Kawachi, Nakaya, Hirai, & Kondo, 2011; Shores, West, Theriault, & Davison, 2009; Weiss et al., 2011). Ability to make utilitarian walking trips from home and perception of favorable neighborhood conditions are associated with increased PA levels (King et al., 2003). However, a considerable number of studies found no (Humpel et al., 2002; McCormack et al., 2004; Owen, Humpel, Leslie, Bauman, & Sallis, 2004) or very weak associations between environmental factors and PA (Lindsey, Han, Wilson, & Yang, 2006; Norman et al., 2006). Innovative studies with enriched prospective data are needed to reconcile these inconsistencies.

Among the areas for improvement, a particular knowledge gap is the inadequate understanding of older adults' utilization of neighborhood resources such as frequency, location, and determinants of space and time use for PA and their relationship to falls. Older adults have more physical limitations and no longer routinely travel outside their neighborhoods to work. Therefore, their daily living, health, and well-being depend more on neighborhood resources in close proximity to their homes. Compromised mobility, reduced income, and decreased ability to drive limit their use of fitness facilities and recreational areas distant from home. A good pedestrian network and public parks that provide walking opportunities near home are crucial resources for them to remain active and socially connected. However, in low-density, small, rural neighborhoods, access to these critical resources is limited in most, if not all, of these aspects. The impacts of this limited access on health and health behaviors are likely additive. When these barriers accumulate to a certain threshold, prevention of falls is difficult to achieve.

▶ Increasing Falls Risks with Advancing Age

Numerous studies have shown that the overall fall rate accelerates with advancing age. The most common explanation for this trend attributes the acceleration to worsening of health conditions, declines in functioning, and increases in frailty that are naturally associated with aging. However, this explanation contradicts the data in the literature: Age remains a very strong predictor of falls and fall injuries even after adjustment of data for a large number of these covariables. The age-dependent changes in fall rates have not been rigorously examined to date. Because older adults' location and time of indoor and outdoor activities change with age, it is important in investigate whether and how accelerations of fall rates may differ according to location and activity of falling. A better understanding of the relative contributions of outdoor and indoor falls to the overall rates of falls may have important implications for future clinical practice and public health prevention.

Analysis of the Mobilize Boston Study cohort of 765 community-dwelling older adults found remarkably different age-dependent trends in indoor and outdoor fall rates (**FIGURE 10-1**; unpublished data). Indoor fall rates increased with age, and the rate of increase was robust to covariate adjustment. However, outdoor fall rates decreased with age, and the trend of decrease diminished after adjusting for a set of covariables. In addition, the ratio of indoor to outdoor fall rates increased steadily over age, rising progressive from about 1 fall per 100,000 before age 80, to more than 1.5 fall per 100,000 at age 85, and 3 falls per 100,000 after age 90 (**FIGURE 10-2**). Covariate-adjustment slightly reduced this age trend, but did not change the general trend.

Known age-related predictors for falls can explain the age trend in the rate of outdoor falls, but not the rate of indoor falls. It is evident that age-related acceleration of the overall fall rate is primarily due to the increased rate of indoor falls. In addition, in the Boston data, the outdoor fall rate was higher than the indoor fall rate before approximately age 76. After age 76, the indoor fall rate was higher than the outdoor fall rate. These data also suggest that outdoor falls are more likely to result in an injury than indoor falls in the middle age group (75-84 years). Future studies should assess the injurious potential of falls by place and activity of falling in relation to advancing age.

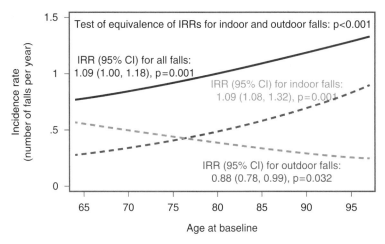

FIGURE 10-1 Annualized incidence rates and incidence rate ratios (IRR) by 5-year increase in baseline age.

▶ Sex Differences in Indoor and Outdoor Falls

Substantial sex differences exist in risk factors, circumstances, and consequences of falling indoors and outdoors, and identified behavioral factors that are particularly important to older men and women (Duckham et al., 2013). Women have lower rates of outdoor falls overall, in locations of recreation, during vigorous activity, and on snowy or icy surfaces compared to men. Women and men do not differ significantly in their rates of falls outdoors on sidewalks, streets, and curbs,

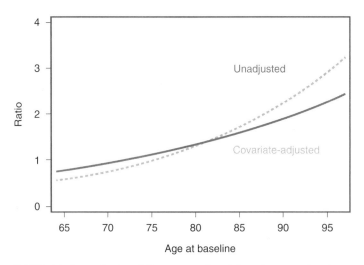

FIGURE 10-2 Ratio of indoor fall rate to outdoor fall rate by age at baseline.

and during walking. Compared to men, women have greater fall rates in the kitchen and while performing household activities.

While the injurious outdoor fall rates are equivalent in both sexes, women's overall rate of injurious indoor falls is nearly twice that of men's, seven times that in the kitchen, close to twice that in their own home, and nearly five times that in another residential home or more than twice that in other buildings. As shown in **FIGURE 10-3**, in unpublished data from the Mobilize Boston Study, older women had a much higher proportion of injurious falls across the three age groups—both indoor and outdoor falls. Outdoor falls are more likely to result in an injury than indoor falls in older age groups (75-84 years and 85 and older), especially among older men. In this age group, many older persons remain active but their health condition deteriorates quickly.

Because of the large sex differences in mobility patterns, circumstances, and injury potential when older adults fall indoors and outdoors, sex-specific prevention strategies are

> **PEARL 10-4** Sex-Specific Fall Prevention Strategies
>
> Because of the large sex differences in mobility patterns, circumstances, and injury potential when older adults fall indoors and outdoors, sex-specific prevention strategies are needed to meet the particular needs of older men and women.

needed to meet the particular needs of older men and women.

▶ Racial Differences in Activity Patterns and Fall Risks

Studies have reported notable racial differences in fall rates, which may be attributable to racial differences in individual- as well as

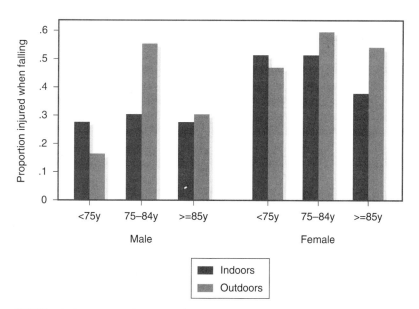

FIGURE 10-3 Proportion of persons who are injured when falling by place of falling, sex, and age group.

community-level risk factors (Bhalla et al., 2009; Bhalla, Harrison, Shahraz, & Fingerhut, 2010; Bikbov, Perico, & Remuzzi, 2014; Chandran et al., 2010). In data from the Mobilize Boston Study (Bhalla et al., 2009), compared to blacks, whites had an approximately 1.8 times higher rate of any fall, a 1.8 times higher outdoor fall rate, a 1.4 times higher indoor fall rate, and a 1.8 times higher injurious fall rate. With the exception of injurious falls, the higher fall rates in whites than blacks were substantially attenuated with adjustment for personal risk factors and neighborhood characteristics.

A nationally representative longitudinal survey of 7609 community-dwelling participants in the National Health and Aging Trends Study reported that the annual incidence rates of any fall and recurrent falls were 34% and 16%, respectively, in whites compared to 27% and 12% in blacks (Bhalla et al., 2010). Overall, blacks had 30% and 40% lower risk of reporting any fall and recurrent falls, respectively. This difference in risk was not explained by known risk factors measured by the study, including physical performance, mobility disability, physical activity, and likelihood of living alone. An analysis of data from the Health and Retirement Study from 2000 to 2010 ($n = 10,484$) reported lower risk for any fall and lower number of falls among African Americans compared to non-Hispanic whites. Latinos did not differ from non-Hispanic whites in the likelihood or number of falls. The reasons for this lower risk for falls and fall injuries among blacks remain to be rigorously examined.

▶ Geographic Variations in Fall Rates

Rates of falls, fall injuries, and fatalities vary substantially across geographic regions and countries. Several studies have examined geographic variations in burden of fall injuries both globally and nationally (Bikbov et al.,

2014; Global Burden of Disease Study, 2015; World Health Organization [WHO], 2008). The percentage of older adults who fell each year ranged from 6% to 31% in China (Li, Jiao, & Shi, 2006; Liang, Liu, & Weng, 2004; Meng & Yang, 2002), 20% in Japan (Yoshida & Kim, 2006), 22% in Barbados, 34% in Chile (Reyes-Ortiz, Al Snih, & Markides, 2005), and 30% in the United States (Crews, Chou, Stevens, & Saaddine, 2016). Among unintentional injury deaths, proportions related to falls ranged from 10% in low- and middle-income countries to 22% in high-income countries (Chandran et al., 2010).

In the United States, according to the CDC's most recent fall injury surveillance data, national average fall mortality rate was 58 deaths per 100,000 older adults in 2014. However, state-level rates of unintentional fall deaths varied nearly 6-fold, ranging from 23 (Alabama) to 131 (Vermont) per 100,000 older adults (CDC, 2007). A number of states had fall death rates more than twice that of the national average rate, including Minnesota (120), Wisconsin (125), and Vermont (131). These high-rate states appear to have higher proportions of rural white populations. However, the reasons for such large state-level variations remain to be investigated.

At a more granular level, large variations in indoor and outdoor fall rates were observed among neighborhoods in the Boston, Massachusetts, area. In the Mobilize Boston Study of 765 community-dwelling older adults, covariate-adjusted annualized outdoor fall rates ranged from 13 to 37 while annualized indoor fall rates ranged from 26 to 58 per 100 person-years (**FIGURE 10-4**). Further, covariate-adjusted ratios of indoor to outdoor fall rates ranged from 0.9 to 2.3. These large neighborhood-level variations in indoor and outdoor fall rates persisted after adjustment for a comprehensive list of personal risk factors. The analysis showed that variations in indoor fall rates were very likely due to differences in participants' fall risk factors. However, the variations in outdoor fall rates were unlikely to be attributable to disparities in personal risk factors.

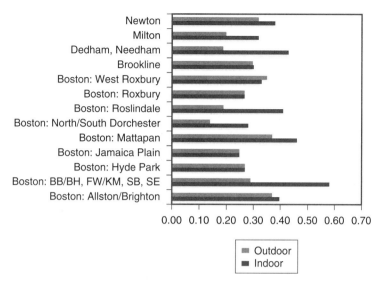

FIGURE 10-4 Covariate-adjusted indoor and outdoor fall rates among Boston neighborhoods.

Most of the studies carried out in the past have been limited to documenting prevalence or incidence rates of fall injuries or fatalities among all age groups. International comparative studies on the causes, circumstances, and treatment or prevention of elderly falls and fall injuries are greatly needed. A good understanding of the causes of the geographic variations may inform future falls prevention programs that address the specific needs of geographic regions with the greatest burden of fall-related death rates. Future studies should attempt to characterize the patterns and identify causes of the geographic variations in fall rates at various geographic scales. Along this line of research, it is important to examine community-level sociodemographic and built environmental factors.

▶ Nutrition and Falls

Good nutrition and healthy eating have a very important role in the etiology and prevention of falls. Poorer diets, such as those characterized by inadequate intake of dietary protein, mono-unsaturated fatty acids (MUFAs), vitamin D, and fruits and vegetables, have been associated with many fall risk factors, including incident frailty (Garcia-Esquinas et al., 2016; Sandoval-Insausti et al., 2016); greater loss of cognitive and physical functions; loss of mobility (Milaneschi et al., 2011); obesity; metabolic diseases; unintentional loss of weight (Lana,

PEARL 10-5 International Studies of Fall Epidemiology

Most of the studies carried out in the past have been limited to documenting prevalence or incidence rates of fall injuries or fatalities among all age groups. International comparative studies on the causes, circumstances, and treatment or prevention of elderly falls and fall injuries are greatly needed.

Rodriguez-Artalejo, & Lopez-Garcia, 2015; Leon-Munoz, Garcia-Esquinas, Lopez-Garcia, Banegas, & Rodriguez-Artalejo, 2015); slow walking speed (Lana et al., 2015; Leon-Munoz et al., 2015); loss of muscle mass, strength, and coordination; and health of bones and joints. Higher dietary fiber intake has been associated with better physical performance measures, including gait speed, 6-minute walk distance, timed up and go, and hand grip strength in Taiwanese older men and women (Wu et al., 2013).

Several dietary patterns have been associated with frailty and fall risks. In a prospective cohort study of 1872 community-dwelling older adults, a prudent dietary pattern, characterized by high intake of olive oil and vegetables, had an inverse dose–response relationship with the risk of frailty. In contrast, a Westernized pattern, with a high intake of refined bread, whole dairy products, and red and processed meat, as well as low consumption of fruits and vegetables, was associated with several components of frailty, including slow walking speed and unintentional weight loss (Leon-Munoz et al., 2015). A population-based 4-year longitudinal follow-up study of 877 Japanese older adults showed that a mainly meat diet was associated with reduced risk of fall-related fracture, whereas a mainly vegetarian diet was associated with increased risk for fall-related fracture (Monma et al., 2010). Because older people have lower rates of protein synthesis and whole-body proteolysis in response to an anabolic stimulus (food or resistance exercise), consuming a protein-rich diet is important to maintaining skeletal muscle mass and strength in older age.

Dietary interventions and micronutrient supplementation may reduce the risk of falling in middle-aged and older adults. The Women's Health Initiative Dietary Modification Trial, which followed 48,835 postmenopausal women age 50–79 years for an average of 8.1 years, reported that a low-fat and increased fruit, vegetable, and grain diet intervention modestly reduced the risk of multiple falls and slightly lowered hip bone mineral density among these women (McTiernan et al., 2009). A recent randomized intervention study of 210 malnourished older adults (age 60 or older) who were newly admitted to an acute hospital demonstrated that a short-term nutritional intervention consisting of oral nutritional supplements and calcium–vitamin D supplementation decreased fall rates by 59% (hazard ratio = 0.41; 95% confidence interval [CI] = 0.19–0.86) (Neelemaat et al., 2012). A meta-analysis published in 2009 showed that supplemental vitamin D in a dose of 700–1000 IU/day reduced the risk of falling among older individuals by 19% (Bischoff-Ferrari et al., 2009). An adequate weight-loss diet and good nutritional intake, with an appropriate amount of vitamin D and the right protein-to-carbohydrates ratio, may help reduce osteosarcopenic obesity and, therefore, fall risk (Hita-Contreras et al., 2015). A review of randomized trials suggested that consumption of 1.0 to 1.3 g/kg/day dietary protein combined with twice-weekly progressive resistance exercise reduces age-related muscle mass loss (Nowson & O'Connell, 2015). Tailored nutritional guidance with home visits over the course of one year may increase protein intake, improve health-related quality of life, and prevent falls among persons with Alzheimer's disease who are living with a spouse (Suominen et al., 2015).

Because poor diets are common in older adults and largely modifiable, investigation of the roles of dietary intake and micronutrient supplementation in falls and fall injuries is critical to effective falls prevention. The efforts

---

PEARL 10-6 Diet and Falls Prevention

Because poor diets are common in older adults and largely modifiable, investigation of the roles of dietary intake and micronutrient supplementation in falls and fall injuries is critical to effective falls prevention.

in nutrition research related to falls have been making steady progress in the past decade, and greater advancement in this area of research is anticipated.

▶ Physical Activity and Falls

Adequate levels of physical activity are critical to the prevention of both fall injuries and chronic diseases (Diabetes Prevention Program Research Group, 2000; Mozaffarian, Fried, Burke, Fitzpatrick, & Siscovick, 2004; Siscovick et al., 1997), and to the maintenance of good health and independent living among older adults (Bath & Morgan, 1998; Miller et al., 2000). On the one hand, walking—the most common type of PA among older adults (Rafferty, Reeves, McGee, & Pivarnik, 2002; Yusuf et al., 1996)—has been associated with lower risk for mortality (Hakim et al., 1998; Rockhill et al., 2001), coronary heart disease (Hakim et al., 1999; LaCroix, Leveille, Hecht, Grothaus, & Wagner, 1996; Lee, Rexrode, Cook, & Manson, 2001; Manson et al., 1999), diabetes (Hu et al., 1999), hip fracture (Cummings et al., 1995; Feskanich, Willett, & Colditz, 2002), and depression (Fukukawa et al., 2004); it has also been linked to better ability to maintain functional capacity (Simonsick, Guralnik, Volpato, Balfour, & Fried, 2005), better cognitive function (Weuve et al., 2004), and more social involvement (Leyden, 2003). On the other hand, PA has been implicated in the etiology of falls (Myers et al., 1996; O'Loughlin et al., 1994; O'Loughlin, Robitaille, Boivin, & Suissa, 1993). Serious fall injury has been associated with both relatively high (Kelsey, Browner, Seeley, Nevitt, & Cummings, 1992; Sorock et al., 1988) and low (O'Loughlin et al., 1993; Province et al., 1995) levels of PA, while diversity of activity has been found to be protective from fall injuries (O'Loughlin et al., 1994; O'Loughlin et al., 1993).

Active older persons are more likely to maintain the balance, flexibility, reflexes,

muscle strength, coordination, and reaction time required to successfully counteract the postural imbalance that leads to falls. However, engaging in frequent or high-level PA increases exposure to hazardous situations and the opportunity to fall. Physically active elders are three times more likely to fall outdoors than inactive elders, and elders afraid of falling tend to reduce their PA to prevent outdoor falls (Wijlhuizen et al., 2006). Thus, PA is important in fall risk analysis (Rubenstein et al., 2000; Wijlhuizen et al., 2006). During the promotion of PA among older adults, the fall risks associated with modest and rigorous activities should be carefully considered, and participants should be made aware of these risks.

▶ Prevention Strategies

Falls prevention is a national priority. Falls are preventable through proper medical treatment, behavioral changes, and modification of home and outdoor environments as suggested by the systematic reviews and existing evidence-based clinical guidelines for the screening and management of falls (Kelly, Phillips, Cain, Polissar, & Kelly, 2002; Kosse, Brands, Bauer, Hortobagyi, & Lamoth, 2013; Michael, Lin, et al., 2010; Michael, Whitlock, et al., 2010; Northridge et al., 1995; Panel on Prevention of Falls in Older Persons, 2011). Effective prevention approaches, which can reduce frequency and injurious potential of falls, include but are not limited to the following measures:

- Screening and monitoring of fall risks and risk factors, such as medication review and modification and falls risk assessment by a healthcare professional
- Exercise and strength training, such as muscle strengthening and balance retraining (e.g., Matter of Balance [Cumming et al., 2008; Kosse et al., 2013; Zijlstra et al., 2009]); Tai Chi (Li et al., 2005); multifaceted podiatry including foot and ankle exercises; multicomponent group or

home-based exercise; and modest physical activity and regular walking
- Protein-rich diet; nutrition and dietary supplements, such as supplementation of vitamin D in people with lower levels (Bischoff-Ferrari et al., 2009; Bischoff-Ferrari et al., 2004; Michael, Whitlock, et al., 2010; Murad et al., 2011); and oral supplementation of protein, calcium, and vitamin D in malnourished older adults (Neelemaat et al., 2012)
- Treatment of fall-related chronic conditions, such as low blood pressure
- Effective pain management
- Improving medication adherence
- Treatment of correctable visual impairment (e.g., cataract surgery [Elliott, 2014]) and wearing proper eyeglasses (e.g., single lens versus multifocal)
- Prescription and proper use of assistive devices among those with physical and sensory impairment
- Wearing proper footwear (e.g., anti-slip shoes)
- Home safety inspection and modification
- Application of prevention technologies in hospitals, nursing homes, and long-term care facilities
- Multifactorial interventions (Kelly et al., 2002)

Because the risk of falling among elders is influenced by multiple and multilevel risk factors (Rubenstein, 2006; Tinetti, 2003; Tinetti et al., 1988), contemporary prevention has moved toward comprehensive, multilevel, and multifaceted strategies. Prevention efforts involve not only geriatric care and clinical interventions that focus on individuals, but also public health initiatives to identify high-risk subpopulations and locales, establish health policies and legislation to support prevention efforts, create and maintain safer home and neighborhood environments, promote individuals' behavioral and lifestyle adaptation to adverse health conditions and living arrangements, train healthcare providers on evidence-based prevention strategies, and raise awareness and uptake of fall risks and evidence-based prevention strategies among older adults, care providers, family members, and communities. Several national and international guidelines for the prevention of falls in older adults have been published to inform prevention practice in community and nursing home settings, including the guideline by American and British Geriatrics Societies (American Geriatrics Society et al., 2001; Krug et al., 2000), and the clinical guidance statement of the Academy of Geriatric Physical Therapy of the American Physical Therapy Association (Sayer et al., 2006). The CDC has also published the STEADI Tool Kit for falls prevention (Casilari, Luque, & Moron, 2015; Habib et al., 2014; Schwickert et al., 2013).

Studies including clinical trials suggest that multifactorial interventions are likely most effective in preventing falls (American Geriatrics Society et al., 2001; Gillespie et al., 2009; Tinetti & Kumar, 2010). Interventions with multifactorial assessment and management may reduce falls by 30% to 40%, and most of these interventions begin with identifying people at high risk of falls (Chang et al., 2004). However, due to limited visit time and lack of both user-friendly tools and easy-to-understand individual-specific data, fall screening and assessment are often overlooked in physicians' offices when older adults present with multiple chronic conditions. Implementation of falls prevention guidelines, including regular screening, remains a grossly understudied area. Expanded and in-depth research into these issues may

PEARL 10-7 Future Areas of Research, #3

Implementation of falls prevention guidelines, including regular screening, remains a grossly understudied area. Expanded and in-depth research into these issues may substantially improve falls prevention practice in the future.

substantially improve falls prevention practice in the future.

▶ Fall Prevention Technologies

New methods and technologies for fall prevention continue to be developed and tested. An emerging field is the development of wearable devices for falls detection (Kosse et al., 2013; Schwickert et al., 2013), including use of smartphones (Casilari et al., 2015; Habib et al., 2014). In the past two decades, various technological approaches and types of sensors have been explored. Evidence has yet to be accumulated to show whether such devices can be effectively applied in real-world settings, and whether they actually contribute to reduction of fall injuries.

In one type of **technology,** lightweight, credit card–sized, water- and shock-proof wearable sensors are attached to an older person's thigh or foot (Kelly et al., 2002; Widder, 1985). Nurses and patients are alerted when the patient assumes a weight-bearing position (Kelly et al., 2002) or shifts the leg from the horizontal to an angle smaller than 45 degrees (Widder, 1985). Such alarms seem to be effective in reducing fall rates in both hospital and nursing home settings. Future research is expected to improve such sensors and assess whether they can be used to reduce falls in ambulatory settings.

Efforts have also been made to integrate fall detection through the various types of devices. Researchers in the field have called for a worldwide research group consensus to address fundamental issues such as incident verification, establishment of guidelines for fall reporting, and development of a common definition of "fall." Closer collaboration among engineering researchers, geriatricians, and falls epidemiologists is needed to move the field forward (Schwickert et al., 2013). High-quality, multicenter randomized trials using wearable

---

PEARL 10-8 Technology and Falls Prevention

Technology development for investigating etiology of falls and preventing fall injuries is expected to advance rapidly, riding on the waves of growth of computing technologies—in particular, digital health. In the near future, wearable sensors will be developed to collect an older adult's behavioral and health data, with these data then being used to provide real-time or near real-time falls and fall injury risk assessments and to deliver individualized feedback for falls prevention. This emerging field may help shift the paradigm of current falls epidemiology and prevention research.

---

or nonwearable fall detection and prevention sensor systems will be necessary to gather evidence on the practical value of these sensors. Future studies are recommended to develop sensor systems applicable in a large variety of circumstances, both indoors and outdoors; better predictive algorithms that consider the individual's fall risk and the underlying processes; and greater user-friendliness (Kosse et al., 2013).

▶ Conclusion and Future Directions

In the past several decades, significant advancements have been made in falls epidemiology and prevention research. A large number of personal and environmental risk factors have been identified. Various effective intervention approaches have been created, tested, and implemented in practice, among which, multifactorial and multilevel interventions are gaining momentum. Nevertheless, despite these advancements, the escalating rates of falls and fall injuries among older adults continue to challenge practitioners in the field to develop more effective, inexpensive, and easy-to-implement intervention approaches. To facilitate the creation of such prevention approaches, future research may benefit from consideration of recent advancements, current methodological limitations, and critical gaps identified in the past decade.

First, the heterogeneity of falls is now well recognized with respect to characteristics of the faller, causes, circumstances, and consequences of falls. Future efforts should further examine the heterogeneity associated with falls by properly defining falls outcomes by location, activity, and consequences of falling; specific fall outcomes may also vary by older adults' health conditions and behavioral phenotypes. For example, the clear separation of indoor versus outdoor falls led to identification of differential sets of risk factors for indoor and outdoor falls, and distinct groups of indoor versus outdoor fallers (Kelsey, Procter-Gray, Berry, et al., 2012; Kelsey, Procter-Gray, Hannan, et al., 2012; Li et al., 2006; Li et al., 2014), which has very important implications for prevention practice (Kelsey, Procter-Gray, Berry, et al., 2012).

Second, most studies to date have quantified fall risks based on calendar time. A paradigm shift is necessary in falls epidemiology research. Future studies of location and activity-specific fall risks should account for not only calendar time at risk, but also the actual amount of time older adults spend in various places and activities. Because an individual's risk is determined by risk per unit exposure time (rate) multiplied by time exposed to a hazard, the misuse of calendar time as exposure time is a barrier to achieving a better understanding of activity and location-specific falls (Li et al., 2014). Location- and activity-specific exposure time, instead of calendar time, should be used for falls risk assessment. Future studies should create innovative and cost-effective approaches to overcome this methodological barrier.

Third, the existing literature suggests that the injurious potential of falls increases with age and likely varies by location and activity of falls. However, no study has rigorously examined this issue. Future studies should assess the injurious potential of falls by place and activity of falling in relation to advancing age.

Fourth, large geographic variations in rates of falls, fall injuries, and fall deaths have been noted. However, few efforts have been made to understand the patterns and causes of such geographic or regional differences. International comparative studies, especially those focusing on geographic differences in causes, circumstances, and risk factors, may shed new light on future falls epidemiology and prevention. In addition, because most of the studies on falls and PA of older adults have been conducted in urban neighborhoods, little is known about falls epidemiology in rural settings. Future studies on rural–urban differences in falls and fall injuries may shed light on sociodemographic and environmental determinants of falls, identify high-risk locales for targeted interventions, and support optimal resource allocation.

Fifth, very few studies have accurately measured space and time use in older adults. The lack of information regarding timing, duration, types, and locations of outdoor activities and falls hinders the development of individualized strategies for promoting active aging and falls prevention that are suitable for older adults living in settings other than urban neighborhoods. Future studies should shift this paradigm by introducing new methods for quantifying older adults' time and space use, place- and activity-specific fall risks, and rural–urban and racial differences in these behavioral phenotypes.

Sixth, technology development for investigating the etiology of falls and preventing fall injuries is expected to advance rapidly as computing technologies (e.g., digital health) likewise advance. In the near future, wearable sensors will be developed to collect an older adult's behavioral and health data, and with these data then being used to provide immediate assessment of falls and fall injury risk as well as individualized feedback for falls prevention. This emerging field may help shift the paradigm of current falls epidemiology and prevention research.

Finally, improved methodologies, rich detailed behavioral phenotype data, and contemporary informatics technology will make it possible to build predictive models to accurately quantify an older adult's falls risk, not only overall, but also in a location-, time-, activity-, and consequence-specific manner. Such highly individualized risk prevention can support more effective, targeted falls prevention. It is not difficult to envision that an era of "precision" falls prevention is coming.

References

Alexander, B. H., Rivara, F. P., & Wolf, M. E. (1992). The cost and frequency of hospitalization for fall related injuries in older adults. *American Journal of Public Health, 82*, 1020-1023.

American Geriatrics Society, British Geriatrics Society, & American Academy of Orthopedic Surgeons Panel on Falls Prevention. (2001). Guideline for the prevention of falls in older persons. *Journal of American Geriatrics Society, 49*, 664-672.

Arfken, C. L., Lach, H. W., Birge, S. J., & Miller, J. P. (1994). The prevalence and correlates of fear of falling in elderly persons living in the community. *American Journal of Public Health, 84*(4), 565-570.

Balfour, J. L., & Kaplan, G. A. (2002). Neighborhood environment and loss of physical function in older adults: Evidence from the Alameda County Study. *American Journal of Epidemiology, 155*(6), 507-515.

Ball, K., Bauman, A., Leslie, E., & Owen, N. (2001). Perceived environmental aesthetics and convenience and company are associated with walking for exercise among Australian adults. *Preventive Medicine, 33*(5), 434-440.

Bath, P. A., & Morgan, K. (1998). Customary physical activity and physical health outcomes in later life. *Age and Ageing, 27*(suppl 3), 29-34.

Bath, P. A., & Morgan, K. (1999). Differential risk factor profiles for indoor and outdoor falls in older people living at home in Nottingham, UK. *European Journal of Epidemiology, 15*(1), 65-73.

Berg, W. P., Alessio, H. M., Mills, E. M., & Tong, C. (1997). Circumstances and consequences of falls in independent community-dwelling older adults. *Age and Ageing, 26*(4), 261-268.

Bergland, A., Jarnlo, G. B., & Laake, K. (2003). Predictors of falls in the elderly by location. *Aging Clinical and Experimental Research, 15*(1), 43-50.

Bergland, A., Pettersen, A. M., & Laake, K. (1998). Falls reported among elderly Norwegians living at home. *Physiotherapy Research International, 3*(3), 164-174.

Bhalla, K., Harrison, J., Abraham, J., Borse, N. N., Lyons, R., Boufous, S.,… Aharonson-Daniel, L. (2009). Data sources for improving estimates of the global burden of injuries: Call for contributors. *PLoS Medicine, 6*(1), e1.

Bhalla, K., Harrison, J. E., Shahraz, S., & Fingerhut, L. A. (2010). Availability and quality of cause-of-death data for estimating the global burden of injuries. *Bulletin of the World Health Organization, 88*(11), 831-838C.

Bikbov, B, Perico, N., & Remuzzi, G. (2014). Mortality landscape in the global burden of diseases, injuries and risk factors study. *European Journal of Internal Medicine, 25*(1), 1-5.

Bischoff-Ferrari, H. A., Dawson-Hughes, B., Staehelin, H. B., Orav, J. E., Stuck, A. E., Theiler, R.,… Henschkowski, J. (2009). Fall prevention with supplemental and active forms of vitamin D: A meta-analysis of randomised controlled trials. *BMJ, 339*, b3692.

Bischoff-Ferrari, H. A., Dawson-Hughes, B., Willett, W. C., Staehelin, H. B., Bazemore, M. G., & Wong, J. B. (2004). Effect of vitamin D on falls: A meta-analysis. *Journal of the American Medical Association, 291*(16), 1999-2006.

Blanchard, C. M., McGannon, K. R., Spence, J. C., Rhodes, R. E., Nehl, E., Baker, F., & Bostwick, J. (2005). Social ecological correlates of physical activity in normal weight, overweight, and obese individuals. *International Journal of Obesity (London), 29*(6), 720-726.

Booth, M. L., Owen, N., Bauman, A., Clavisi, O., & Leslie, E. (2000). Social-cognitive and perceived environment influences associated with physical activity in older Australians. *Preventive Medicine, 31*(1), 15-22.

Brooke-Wavell, K., Perrett, L. K., Howarth, P. A., & Haslam, R. A. (2002). Influence of the visual environment on the postural stability in healthy older women. *Gerontology, 48*(5), 293-297.

Brownson, R. C., Housemann, R. A., Brown, D. R., Jackson-Thompson, J., King, A. C., Malone, B. R., & Sallis, J. F. (2000). Promoting physical activity in rural communities: Walking trail access, use, and effects. *American Journal of Preventive Medicine, 18*(3), 235-241.

Campbell, A. J., Borrie, M. J., Spears, G. F., Jackson, S. L., Brown, J. S., & Fitzgerald, J. L. (1990). Circumstances and consequences of falls experienced by a community population 70 years and over during a prospective study. *Age and Ageing, 19*(2), 136-141.

Carroll, N. V., Slattum, P. W., & Cox, F. M. (2005). The cost of falls among the community-dwelling elderly. *Journal of Managed Care Pharmacy, 11*(4), 307-316.

Casilari, E., Luque, R., & Moron, M. J. (2015). Analysis of Android device-based solutions for fall detection. *Sensors, 15*(8), 17827-17894.

Centers for Disease Control and Prevention (CDC). (1996). Neighborhood safety and the prevalence of physical inactivity-selected states. *Morbidity and Mortality Weekly Report, 48,* 143-146.

Centers for Disease Control and Prevention (CDC). (1998). Self-reported physical inactivity by degree of urbanization—United States, 1996. *Morbidity and Mortality Weekly Report, 47*(50), 1097-1100.

Centers for Disease Control and Prevention (CDC). (1999). Neighborhood safety and the prevalence of physical inactivity—selected states, 1996. *Morbidity and Mortality Weekly Report, 48*(7), 143-146.

Centers for Disease Control and Prevention (CDC). (2007). Web-based Injury Statistics Query and Reporting System (WISQARS). Retrieved from http://www.cdc.gov/injury/wisqars/index.html#

Centers for Disease Control and Prevention (CDC). (2008). Self-reported falls and fall-related injuries among persons ages >=65 years—United States, 2006. *Morbidity and Mortality Weekly Report, 57*(9), 225-229.

Centers for Disease Control and Prevention (CDC). (2016). Web-based Injury Statistics Query and Reporting System (WISQARS). Retrieved from http://www.cdc.gov/injury/wisqars/fatal.html

Cervero, R., & Duncan, M. (2003). Walking, bicycling, and urban landscapes: Evidence from the San Francisco Bay Area. *American Journal of Public Health, 93*(9), 1478-1483.

Chandran, A., Hyder, A. A., & Peek-Asa, C. (2010). The global burden of unintentional injuries and an agenda for progress. *Epidemiologic Reviews, 32,* 110-120.

Chang, J. T., Morton, S. C., Rubenstein, L. Z., Mojica, W. A., Maglione, M., Suttorp, M. J.,... Shekelle, P. G. (2004). Interventions for the prevention of falls in older adults: Systematic review and meta-analysis of randomised clinical trials. *BMJ, 328*(7441), 680.

Connell, B. R. (1996). Role of the environment in falls prevention. *Clinical Geriatric Medicine, 12*(4), 859-880.

Connell, B. R., & Wolf, S. L. (1997). Environmental and behavioral circumstances associated with falls at home among healthy elderly individuals. Atlanta FICSIT Group. *Archives of Physical Medicine and Rehabilitation, 78*(2), 179-186.

Crews, J. E., Chou, C. F., Stevens, J. A., & Saaddine, J. B. (2016). Falls among persons aged >= 65 years with and without severe vision impairment—United States, 2014. *Morbidity and Mortality Weekly Report, 65*(17), 433-437.

Cumming, R. G., Salkeld, G., Thomas, M., & Szonyi, G. (2000). Prospective study of the impact of fear of falling on activities of daily living, SF-36 scores, and nursing home admission. *Journal of Gerontology, Series A: Biological Sciences and Medical Sciences, 55*(5), M299-M305.

Cumming, R. G., Sherrington, C., Lord, S. R., Simpson, J. M., Vogler, C., Cameron, I. D., & Naganathan, V. (2008). Cluster randomised trial of a targeted multifactorial intervention to prevent falls among older people in hospital. *BMJ, 336*(7647), 758-760.

Cummings, S. R., Nevitt, M. C., Browner, W. S., Stone, K., Fox, K. M., Ensrud, K. E.,... Vogt, T. M. (1995). Risk factors for hip fracture in white women. Study of Osteoporotic Fractures Research Group. *New England Journal of Medicine, 332*(12), 767-773.

Diabetes Prevention Program Research Group. (2000). The Diabetes Prevention Program: Baseline characteristics of the randomized cohort. *Diabetes Care, 23*(11), 1619-1629.

Duckham, R. L., Procter-Gray, E., Hannan, M. T., Leveille, S. G., Lipsitz, L. A., & Li, W. (2013). Sex differences in circumstances and consequences of outdoor and indoor falls in older adults in the Mobilize Boston cohort study. *BMC Geriatrics, 13,* 133.

Elliott, D. B. (2014). The Glenn A. Fry Award lecture 2013: Blurred vision, spectacle correction, and falls in older adults. *Optometry and Vision Science, 91*(6), 593-601.

Englander, F., Hodson, T. J., & Terregrossa, R. A. (1996). Economic dimensions of slip and fall injuries. *Journal of Forensic Science, 41*(5), 733-746.

Estabrooks, P. A., Lee, R. E., & Gyurcsik, N. C. (2003). Resources for physical activity participation: Does availability and accessibility differ by neighborhood socioeconomic status? *Annals of Behavioral Medicine, 25*(2), 100-104.

Feskanich, D., Willett, W., & Colditz, G. (2002). Walking and leisure-time activity and risk of hip fracture in postmenopausal women. *Journal of the American Medical Association, 288*(18), 2300-2306.

Fisher, K. J., Li, F., Michael, Y., & Cleveland, M. (2004). Neighborhood-level influences on physical activity among older adults: A multilevel analysis. *Journal of Aging and Physical Activity, 12*(1), 45-63.

Frank, L. D. (2000). Land use and transportation interaction: Implications on public health and quality of life. *Journal of Planning Education and Research, 20*(1), 6-22.

Frank, L. D., Schmid, T. L., Sallis, J. F., Chapman, J., & Saelens, B. E. (2005). Linking objectively measured physical activity with objectively measured urban form: Findings from SMARTRAQ. *American Journal of Preventive Medicine, 28*(2 suppl 2), 117-125.

Fukukawa, Y., Nakashima, C., Tsuboi, S., Kozakai, R., Doyo, W., Niino, N.,... Shimokata, H. (2004). Age differences in the effect of physical activity on depressive symptoms. *Psychology and Aging, 19*(2), 346-351.

Ganz, D. A., Bao, Y., Shekelle, P. G., & Rubenstein, L. Z. (2007). Will my patient fall? *Journal of the American Medical Association, 297*(1), 77-86.

Garcia-Esquinas, E., Rahi, B., Peres, K., Colpo, M., Dartigues, J. F., Bandinelli, S.,... Rodríguez-Artalejo, F. (2016). Consumption of fruit and vegetables and risk of frailty: A dose-response analysis of 3 prospective cohorts of community-dwelling older adults. *American Journal of Clinical Nutrition, 104*(1), 132-142.

Giles-Corti, B., & Donovan, R. J. (2002). Socioeconomic status differences in recreational physical activity levels and real and perceived access to a supportive physical environment. *Preventive Medicine, 35*(6), 601-611.

Gill, T. M., Desai, M. M., Gahbauer, E. A., Holford, T. R., & Williams, C. S. (2001). Restricted activity among community-living older persons: Incidence, precipitants, and health care utilization. *Annals of Internal Medicine, 135*(5), 313-321.

Gill, T. M., Williams, C. S., & Tinetti, M. E. (2000). Environmental hazards and the risk of nonsyncopal falls in the homes of community-living older persons. *Medical Care, 38*(12), 1174-1183.

Gillespie, L. D., Gillespie, W. J., Robertson, M. C., Lamb, S. E., Cumming, R. G., & Rowe, B. H. (2005 February 23). Interventions for preventing falls in elderly people. *Cochrane Database of Systematic Reviews, 2,* CD000340.

Gillespie, L. D., Robertson, M. C., Gillespie, W. J., Lamb, S. E., Gates, S., Cumming, R. G., & Rowe, B. H. (2009). Interventions for preventing falls in older people living in the community. *Cochrane Database of Systematic Reviews, 2,* CD007146.

Glass, T. A., & Balfour, J. L. (2003). Neighborhoods, aging and functional limitations. In I. Kawachi & L. F. Berkman (Eds.), *Neighborhoods and health* (pp. 303-334). New York, NY: Oxford University Press.

Glass, T. A., Rasmussen, M. D., & Schwartz, B. S. (2006). Neighborhoods and obesity in older adults: The Baltimore Memory Study. *American Journal of Preventive Medicine, 31*(6), 455-463.

Global Burden of Disease Study. (2015). Global, regional, and national incidence, prevalence, and years lived with disability for 301 acute and chronic diseases and injuries in 188 countries, 1990-2013: A systematic analysis for the Global Burden of Disease Study 2013. *Lancet, 386*(9995), 743-800.

Graafmans, W. C., Ooms, M. E., Bezemer, P. D., Bouter, L. M., & Lips, P. (1996). Different risk profiles for hip fractures and distal forearm fractures: A prospective study. *Osteoporosis International, 6*(6), 427-431.

Habib, M. A., Mohktar, M. S., Kamaruzzaman, S. B., Lim, K. S., Pin, T. M., & Ibrahim, F. (2014). Smartphone-based solutions for fall detection and prevention: Challenges and open issues. *Sensors, 14*(4), 7181-7208.

Hakim, A. A., Curb, J. D., Petrovitch, H., Rodriguez, B. L., Yano, K., Ross, G. W.,... Abbott, R. D. (1999). Effects of walking on coronary heart disease in elderly men: The Honolulu Heart Program. *Circulation, 100*(1), 9-13.

Hakim, A. A., Petrovitch, H., Burchfiel, C. M., Ross, G. W., Rodriguez, B. L., White, L. R.,... Abbott, R. D. (1998). Effects of walking on mortality among nonsmoking retired men. *New England Journal of Medicine, 338*(2), 94-99.

Halpern, D. (1995). *Mental health and the built environment: More than bricks and mortar?* London, UK: Taylor & Francis.

Hanibuchi, T., Kawachi, I., Nakaya, T., Hirai, H., & Kondo, K. (2011). Neighborhood built environment and physical activity of Japanese older adults: Results from the Aichi Gerontological Evaluation Study (AGES). *BMC Public Health, 11*(1), 657.

Healthy People 2010. (2001). *Understanding and improving health.* Washington, DC: U.S. Department of Health and Human Services.

Hill, K., Schwarz, J., Flicker, L., & Carroll, S. (1999). Falls among healthy, community-dwelling, older women: A prospective study of frequency, circumstances, consequences and prediction accuracy. *Australia and New Zealand Journal of Public Health, 23*(1), 41-48.

Hita-Contreras, F., Martinez-Amat, A., Cruz-Diaz, D., & Perez-Lopez, F. R. (2015). Osteosarcopenic obesity and fall prevention strategies. *Maturitas, 80*(2), 126-132.

Howland, J., Lachman, M. E., Peterson, E. W., Cote, J., Kasten, L., & Jette, A. (1998). Covariates of fear of falling and associated activity curtailment. *Gerontologist, 38*(5), 549-555.

Howland, J., Peterson, E. W., Levin, W. C., Fried, L., Pordon, D., & Bak, S. (1993). Fear of falling among the community-dwelling elderly. *Journal of Aging and Health, 5*(2), 229-243.

Hu, F. B., Sigal, R. J., Rich-Edwards, J. W., Colditz, G. A., Solomon, C. G., Willett, W. C.,... Manson, J. E. (1999). Walking compared with vigorous physical activity and risk of type 2 diabetes in women: A prospective study. *Journal of the American Medical Association, 282*(15), 1433-1439.

Humpel, N., Owen, N., & Leslie, E. (2002). Environmental factors associated with adults' participation in physical activity: A review. *American Journal of Preventive Medicine, 22*(3), 188-199.

Josephson, K. R., Fabacher, D. A., & Rubenstein, L. Z. (1991). Home safety and fall prevention. *Clinical Geriatric Medicine, 7*(4), 707-731.

Keegan, T. H., Kelsey, J. L., King, A. C., Quesenberry, C. P., Jr., & Sidney, S. (2004). Characteristics of fallers who fracture at the foot, distal forearm, proximal humerus, pelvis, and shaft of the tibia/fibula compared with fallers who do not fracture. *American Journal of Epidemiology, 159*(2), 192-203.

Kelly, K. E., Phillips, C. L., Cain, K. C., Polissar, N. L., & Kelly, P. B. (2002). Evaluation of a nonintrusive monitor to reduce falls in nursing home patients. *Journal of the American Medical Directors Association, 3*(6), 377-382.

Kelsey, J. L., Berry, S. D., Procter-Gray, E., Quach, L., Nguyen, U. S., Li, W.,... Hannan, M. T. (2010). Indoor and outdoor falls in older adults are different: The maintenance of balance, independent living, intellect, and zest in the Elderly of Boston Study. *Journal of the American Geriatrics Society, 58*(11), 2135-2141.

Kelsey, J. L., Browner, W. S., Seeley, D. G., Nevitt, M. C., & Cummings, S. R. (1992). Risk factors for fractures of the distal forearm and proximal humerus. The Study of Osteoporotic Fractures Research Group. *American Journal of Epidemiology, 135*(5), 477–489.

Kelsey, J. L., Procter-Gray, E., Berry, S. D., Hannan, M. T., Kiel, D. P., Lipsitz, L. A., & Li, W. (2012). Reevaluating the implications of recurrent falls in older adults: Location changes the inference. *Journal of the American Geriatrics Society, 60*(3), 517–524.

Kelsey, J. L., Procter-Gray, E., Hannan, M. T., & Li, W. (2012). Heterogeneity of falls among older adults: Implications for public health prevention. *American Journal of Public Health, 102*(11), 2149–2156.

Kelsey, J. L., Procter-Gray, E., Nguyen, U. S., Li, W., Kiel, D. P., & Hannan, M. T. (2010). Footwear and falls in the home among older individuals in the Mobilize Boston Study. *Footwear Science, 2*(3), 123–129.

Kimsey, C. D., Jr., Ham, S. A., & Macera, C. A. F. (2001). Neighborhood safety and the prevalence of physical activity. *Medicine & Science in Sports & Exercise, 33*(5), S237.

King, A. C., Castro, C., Wilcox, S., Eyler, A. A., Sallis, J. F., & Brownson, R. C. (2000). Personal and environmental factors associated with physical inactivity among different racial–ethnic groups of U.S. middle-aged and older-aged women. *Health and Psychology, 19*(4), 354–364.

King, M. B., & Tinetti, M. E. (1995). Falls in community-dwelling older persons. *Journal of the American Geriatrics Society, 43*(10), 1146–1454.

King, W. C., Brach, J. S., Belle, S., Killingsworth, R., Fenton, M., & Kriska, A. M. (2003). The relationship between convenience of destinations and walking levels in older women. *American Journal of Health Promotion, 18*(1), 74–82.

Kosse, N. M., Brands, K., Bauer, J. M., Hortobagyi, T., & Lamoth, C. J. C. (2013). Sensor technologies aiming at fall prevention in institutionalized old adults: A synthesis of current knowledge. *International Journal of Medical Informatics, 82*(9), 743–752.

Krug, E. G., Sharma, G. K., & Lozano, R. (2000). The global burden of injuries. *American Journal of Public Health, 90*(4), 523–526.

LaCroix, A. Z., Leveille, S. G., Hecht, J. A., Grothaus, L. C., & Wagner, E. H. (1996). Does walking decrease the risk of cardiovascular disease hospitalizations and death in older adults? *Journal of the American Geriatrics Society, 44*(2), 113–120.

Lana, A., Rodriguez-Artalejo, F., & Lopez-Garcia, E. (2015). Dairy consumption and risk of frailty in older adults: A prospective cohort study. *Journal of the American Geriatrics Society, 63*(9), 1852–1860.

Larson, N. I., Story, M. T., & Nelson, M, C. (2009). Neighborhood environments: Disparities in access to healthy foods in the U.S. *American Journal of Preventive Medicine, 36*(1), 74–81.

Lee, I. M., Rexrode, K. M., Cook, N. R., Manson, J. E., & Buring, J. E. (2001). Physical activity and coronary heart disease in women: Is "no pain, no gain" passé? *Journal of the American Medical Association, 285*(11), 1447–1454.

Lee, R. E., & Cubbin, C. (2002). Neighborhood context and youth cardiovascular health behaviors. *American Journal of Public Health, 92*(3), 428–436.

Lee, R. E., Reese-Smith, J., Regan, G., Booth, K., & Howard, H. (2003). Applying GIS technology to assess the obesogenic structure of neighborhoods surrounding public housing developments. *Medicine & Science in Sports & Exercise, 35*(5), S65.

Leon-Munoz, L. M., Garcia-Esquinas, E., Lopez-Garcia, E., Banegas, J. R., & Rodriguez-Artalejo, F. (2015). Major dietary patterns and risk of frailty in older adults: A prospective cohort study. *BMC Medicine, 13*, 11.

Leyden, K. M. (2003). Social capital and the built environment: The importance of walkable neighborhoods. *American Journal of Public Health, 93*(9), 1546–1551.

Li, F., Fisher, K. J., Bauman, A., Ory, M. G., Chodzko-Zajko, W., Harmer, P.,… Cleveland, M. (2005). Neighborhood influences on physical activity in middle-aged and older adults: A multilevel perspective. *Journal of Aging and Physical Activity, 13*(1), 87–114.

Li, F., Fisher, K. J., & Brownson, R. C. (2005). A multilevel analysis of change in neighborhood walking activity in older adults. *Journal of Aging and Physical Activity, 13*, 145–159.

Li, F., Harmer, P., Fisher, K. J., McAuley, E., Chaumeton. N., Eckstrom. E., & Wilson, N. L. (2005). Tai Chi and fall reductions in older adults: A randomized controlled trial. *Journal of Gerontology, Series A: Biological Sciences and Medical Sciences, 60*(2), 187–194.

Li, G., Jiao, S., & Shi, Y. (2006). The incidence status on injury of the community-dwelling elderly in Beijing. *Chinese Journal of Preventive Medicine, 40*(1), 37.

Li, W., Keegan, T. H., Sternfeld, B., Sidney, S., Quesenberry, C. P., Jr., & Kelsey, J. L. (2006). Outdoor falls among middle-aged and older adults: A neglected public health problem. *American Journal of Public Health, 96*(7), 1192–1200.

Li, W., Procter-Gray, E., Lipsitz, L. A., Leveille, S. G., Hackman, H., Biondolillo, M., & Hannan, M. T. (2014). Utilitarian walking, neighborhood environment, and risk of outdoor falls among older adults. *American Journal of Public Health, 104*(9), e30–e37.

Liang, W., Liu, Y., & Weng, X. (2004). An epidemiological study on injury of the community-dwelling elderly in Beijing. *Chinese Journal of Disease Control and Prevention, 8*(6), 489–492.

Lindsey, G., Han, Y., Wilson, J., & Yang, J. (2006). Neighborhood correlates of urban trail use. *Journal of Physical Activity and Health, 3*(suppl 1), S139–S157.

Lopez-Zetina, J., Lee, H., & Friis, R. (2006). The link between obesity and the built environment: Evidence from an ecological analysis of obesity and vehicle miles of travel in California. *Health and Place, 12*(4), 656-664.

Lynch, J. W., Kaplan, G. A., Pamuk, E. R., Cohen, R. D., Heck, K. E., Balfour, J. L., & Yen, I. H. (1998). Income inequality and mortality in metropolitan areas of the United States. *American Journal of Public Health, 88*(7), 1074-1080.

Ma, Y., Olendzki, B. C., Li, W., Hafner, A. R., Chiriboga, D., Hebert, J. R.,… Ockene, I. S. (2006). Seasonal variation in food intake, physical activity, and body weight in a predominantly overweight population. *European Journal of Clinical Nutrition, 60*(4), 519-528.

Manson, J. E., Hu, F. B., Rich-Edwards, J. W., Colditz, G. A., Stampfer, M. J., Willett, W. C.,… Hennekens, C. H. (1999). A prospective study of walking as compared with vigorous exercise in the prevention of coronary heart disease in women. *New England Journal of Medicine, 341*(9), 650-658.

Marshall, S. W., Runyan, C. W., Yang, J., Coyne-Beasley, T., Waller, A. E., Johnson, R. M., & Perkis, D. (2005). Prevalence of selected risk and protective factors for falls in the home. *American Journal of Preventive Medicine, 28*(1), 95-101.

Matthews, C. E., Hebert, J. R., Freedson, P. S., Stanek, E. J. 3rd, Merriam, P. A., Ebbeling, C. B., & Ockene, I. S. (2001). Sources of variance in daily physical activity levels in the seasonal variation of blood cholesterol study. *American Journal of Epidemiology, 153*(10), 987-995.

McClure, R., Turner, C., Peel, N., Spinks, A., Eakin, E., & Hughes, K. (2005). Population-based interventions for the prevention of fall-related injuries in older people. *Cochrane Database of Systematic Reviews, 1*, CD004441.

McCormack, G., Giles-Corti, B., Lange, A., Smith, T., Martin, K., & Pikora, T. J. (2004). An update of recent evidence of the relationship between objective and self-report measures of the physical environment and physical activity behaviours. *Journal of Science and Medicine in Sport/Sports Medicine Australia, 7*(1 suppl), 81-92.

McGinn, A. P., Evenson, K. R., Herring, A. H., Huston, S. L., & Rodriguez, D. A. (2007). Exploring associations between physical activity and perceived and objective measures of the built environment. *Journal of Urban Health: Bulletin of the New York Academy of Medicine, 84*(2), 162-184.

McTiernan, A., Wactawski-Wende, J., Wu, L., Rodabough, R. J., Watts, N. B., Tylavsky, F.,… Jackson, R. (2009). Low-fat, increased fruit, vegetable, and grain dietary pattern, fractures, and bone mineral density: The Women's Health Initiative Dietary Modification Trial. *American Journal of Clinical Nutrition, 89*(6), 1864-1876.

Mendes de Leon, C. F., Seeman, T. E., Baker, D. I., Richardson, E. D., & Tinetti, M. E. (1996). Self-efficacy, physical decline, and change in functioning in community-living elders: A prospective study. *Journal of Gerontology, Series B: Psychological Sciences and Social Sciences, 51*(4), S183-S190.

Meng, W., & Yang, L. (2002). Analysis of risk factors for elderly falls. *Chinese Journal of Behavioral Medical Science, 11*(6), 697-699.

Menz, H. B., Morris, M. E., & Lord, S. R. (2006). Footwear characteristics and risk of indoor and outdoor falls in older people. *Gerontology, 52*(3), 174-180.

Meyer, C., Dow, B., Bilney, B. E., Moore, K. J., Bingham, A. L., & Hill, K. D. (2012). Falls in older people receiving in-home informal care across Victoria: Influence on care recipients and caregivers. *Australasian Journal on Ageing, 31*(1), 6-12.

Michael, Y. L., Lin, J. S., Whitlock, E. P., Gold, R., Fu, R., O'Connor, E. A.,… Lutz, K. W. (2010, December). *Interventions to prevent falls in older adults: An updated systematic review.* Report No.: 11-05150-EF-1. Rockville, MD: Agency for Healthcare Research and Quality.

Michael, Y. L., Whitlock, E. P., Lin, J. S., Fu, R., O'Connor, E. A., & Gold, R.; U.S. Preventive Services Task Force. (2010). Primary care-relevant interventions to prevent falling in older adults: A systematic evidence review for the U.S. Preventive Services Task Force. *Annals of Internal Medicine, 153*(12), 815-825.

Milaneschi, Y., Bandinelli, S., Corsi, A. M., Lauretani, F., Paolisso, G., Dominguez, L. J.,… Ferrucci, L. (2011). Mediterranean diet and mobility decline in older persons. *Experimental Gerontology, 46*(4), 303-308.

Miller, M. E., Rejeski, W. J., Reboussin, B. A., Ten Have, T. R., & Ettinger, W. H. (2000). Physical activity, functional limitations, and disability in older adults. *Journal of the American Geriatrics Society, 48*(10), 1264-1272.

Monma, Y., Niu, K., Iwasaki, K., Tomita, N., Nakaya, N., Hozawa, A.,… Tsuji, I. (2010). Dietary patterns associated with fall-related fracture in elderly Japanese: A population based prospective study. *BMC Geriatrics, 10*, 31.

Mozaffarian, D., Fried, L. P., Burke, G. L., Fitzpatrick, A., & Siscovick, D. S. (2004). Lifestyles of older adults: Can we influence cardiovascular risk in older adults? *American Journal of Geriatric Cardiology, 13*(3), 153-160.

Murad, M. H., Elamin, K. B., Abu Elnour, N. O., Elamin, M. B., Alkatib, A. A., Fatourechi, M. M.,… Montori, V. M. (2011). Clinical review: The effect of vitamin D on falls: A systematic review and meta-analysis. *Journal of Clinical Endocrinology and Metabolism, 96*(10), 2997-3006.

Murphy, J., & Isaacs, B. (1982). The post-fall syndrome: A study of 36 elderly patients. *Gerontology, 28*(4), 265-270.

Murphy, S. L. (2000). Deaths: Final data for 1998. *National Vital Statistics Report, 48*(11), 1-105.

Myers, A. H., Young, Y., & Langlois, J. A. (1996). Prevention of falls in the elderly. *Bone, 18*(1 suppl), 87S-101S.

Neelemaat, F., Lips, P., Bosmans, J. E., Thijs, A., Seidell, J. C., & van Bokhorst-de van der Schueren, M. A. (2012). Short-term oral nutritional intervention with protein and vitamin D decreases falls in malnourished older adults. *Journal of the American Geriatrics Society, 60*(4), 691-699.

Nevitt, M. C., Cummings, S. R., & Hudes, E. S. (1991). Risk factors for injurious falls: A prospective study. *Journal of Gerontology, 46*(5), M164-M170.

Newman, P. W., & Kenworth, J. R. (1991). Transport and urban form in thirty-two of the world's principal cities. *Transportation Review, 11*, 149-272.

Norman, G. J., Nutter, S. K., Ryan, S., Sallis, J. F., Calfas, K. J., & Patrick, K. (2006). Community design and access to recreational facilities as correlates of adolescent physical activity and body mass index. *Journal of Physical Activity and Health, 3*(suppl 1), S55-S76.

Northridge, M. E., Nevitt, M. C., & Kelsey, J. L. (1996). Non-syncopal falls in the elderly in relation to home environments. *Osteoporosis International, 6*(3), 249-255.

Northridge, M. E., Nevitt, M. C., Kelsey, J. L., & Link, B. (1995). Home hazards and falls in the elderly: The role of health and functional status. *American Journal of Public Health, 85*(4), 509-515.

Nowson, C., & O'Connell, S. (2015). Protein requirements and recommendations for older people: A review. *Nutrients, 7*(8), 6874-6899.

Ogilvie, D., Mitchell, R., Mutrie, N., Petticrew, M., & Platt, S. (2008). Perceived characteristics of the environment associated with active travel: Development and testing of a new scale. *International Journal of Behavioral Nutrition and Physical Activity, 5*, 32.

O'Loughlin, J. L., Boivin, J. F., Robitaille, Y., & Suissa, S. (1994). Falls among the elderly: Distinguishing indoor and outdoor risk factors in Canada. *Journal of Epidemiology and Community Health, 48*(5), 488-489.

O'Loughlin, J. L., Robitaille, Y., Boivin, J. F., & Suissa, S. (1993). Incidence of and risk factors for falls and injurious falls among the community-dwelling elderly. *American Journal of Epidemiology, 137*(3), 342-354.

Orces, C. H., & Alamgir, H. (2014). Trends in fall-related injuries among older adults treated in emergency departments in the USA. *Injury Prevention, 20*(6), 421-423.

Owen, N., Humpel, N., Leslie, E., Bauman, A., & Sallis, J. F. (2004). Understanding environmental influences on walking; Review and research agenda. *American Journal of Preventive Medicine, 27*(1), 67-76.

Panel on Prevention of Falls in Older Persons, American Geriatrics Society & British Geriatrics Society. (2011). Summary of the Updated American Geriatrics Society/British Geriatrics Society clinical practice guideline for prevention of falls in older persons. *Journal of the American Geriatrics Society, 59*(1), 148-157.

Patla, A. E., & Shumway-Cook, A. (1999). Dimensions of mobility: Defining the complexity and difficulty associated with community mobility. *Journal of Aging and Physical Activity, 7*, 7-19.

Pendola, R., & Gen, S. (2007). BMI, auto use, and the urban environment in San Francisco. *Health and Place, 13*(2), 551-556.

Province, M. A., Hadley, E. C., Hornbrook, M. C., Lipsitz, L. A., Miller, J. P., Mulrow, C. D.,… Wolf, S. L. (1995). The effects of exercise on falls in elderly patients: A preplanned meta-analysis of the FICSIT Trials (Frailty and Injuries: Cooperative Studies of Intervention Techniques). *Journal of the American Medical Association, 273*(17), 1341-1347.

Rafferty, A. P., Reeves, M. J., McGee, H. B., & Pivarnik, J. M. (2002). Physical activity patterns among walkers and compliance with public health recommendations. *Medicine & Science in Sports & Exercise, 34*(8), 1255-1261.

Reis, J. P., Bowles, H. R., Ainsworth, B. E., Dubose, K. D., Smith, S., & Laditka, J. N. (2004). Nonoccupational physical activity by degree of urbanization and U.S. geographic region. *Medicine & Science in Sports & Exercise, 36*(12), 2093-2098.

Reyes-Ortiz, C. A., Al Snih, S., & Markides, K. S. (2005). Falls among elderly persons in Latin America and the Caribbean and among elderly Mexican-Americans. *Revista Panamericana de Salud Pública, 17*(5-6), 362-369.

Rockhill, B., Willett, W. C., Manson, J. E., Leitzmann, M. F., Stampfer, M. J., Hunter, D. J., & Colditz, G. A. (2001). Physical activity and mortality: A prospective study among women. *American Journal of Public Health, 91*(4), 578-583.

Rubenstein, L. Z. (1997). Preventing falls in the nursing home. *Journal of the American Medical Association, 278*(7), 595-596.

Rubenstein, L. Z. (1999). The importance of including the home environment in assessment of frail older persons. *Journal of the American Geriatrics Society, 47*(1), 111-112.

Rubenstein, L. Z. (2006). Falls in older people: Epidemiology, risk factors and strategies for prevention. *Age and Ageing, 35*(suppl 2), ii37-ii41.

Rubenstein, L. Z., & Josephson, K. R. (2002). The epidemiology of falls and syncope. *Clinical Geriatric Medicine, 18*(2), 141-158.

Rubenstein, L. Z., & Josephson, K. R. (2006). Falls and their prevention in elderly people: What does the evidence show? *Medical Clinics of North America, 90*(5), 807-824.

Rubenstein, L. Z., Josephson, K. R., Trueblood, P. R., Loy, S., Harker, J. O., Pietruszka, F. M., & Robbins, A. S. (2000). Effects of a group exercise program on strength, mobility, and falls among fall-prone elderly men. *Journal of Gerontology, Series A: Biological Sciences and Medical Sciences, 55*(6), M317-M321.

Saelens, B. E., Sallis, J. F., Black, J. B., & Chen, D. (2003). Neighborhood-based differences in physical activity: An environment scale evaluation. *American Journal of Public Health, 93*(9), 1552-1558.

Sallis, J. F., Bauman, A., & Pratt, M. (1998). Environmental and policy interventions to promote physical activity. *American Journal of Preventive Medicine, 15*(4), 379-397.

Sallis, J. F., Hovell, M. F., Hofstetter, C. R., Elder, J. P., Hackley, M., Caspersen, C. J., & Powell, K. E. (1990). Distance between homes and exercise facilities related to frequency of exercise among San Diego residents. *Public Health Reports, 105*(2), 179-185.

Sallis, J. F., Kraft, K., & Linton, L S. (2002). How the environment shapes physical activity: A transdisciplinary research agenda. *American Journal of Preventive Medicine, 22*(3), 208.

Sandoval-Insausti, H., Perez-Tasigchana, R. F., Lopez-Garcia, E., Garcia-Esquinas, E., Rodriguez-Artalejo, F., & Guallar-Castillon, P. (2016). Macronutrients intake and incident frailty in older adults: A prospective cohort study. *Journal of Gerontology, Series A: Biological Sciences and Medical Sciences, 71*(10), 1329-1334.

Sattin, R. W., Rodriguez, J. G., DeVito, C. A., & Wingo, P. A. (1998). Home environmental hazards and the risk of fall injury events among community-dwelling older persons: Study to Assess Falls Among the Elderly (SAFE) Group. *Journal of the American Geriatrics Society, 46*(6), 669-676.

Sayer, A. A., Syddall, H. E., Martin, H. J., Dennison, E. M., Anderson, F. H., & Cooper, C. (2006). Falls, sarcopenia, and growth in early life: Findings from the Hertfordshire cohort study. *American Journal of Epidemiology, 164*(7), 665-671.

Schwartz, A. V., Capezuti, E., & Grisso, J. A. (2001). Falls as risk factors for fractures. In R. Marcus, D. Feldman, & J. Kelsey (Eds.), *Osteoporosis* (2nd ed., pp. 795-807). San Diego, CA: Academic Press.

Schwartz, A. V., Villa, M. L., Prill, M., Kelsey, J. A., Galinus, J. A., Delay, R. R.,... Kelsey, J. L. (1999). Falls in older Mexican-American women. *Journal of the American Geriatrics Society, 47*(11), 1371-1378.

Schwickert, L., Becker, C., Lindemann. U., Maréchal, C., Bourke, A., Chiari, L.,... Klenk, J. (2013). Fall detection with body-worn sensors: A systematic review. *Zeitschrift Fur Gerontologie Und Geriatrie, 46*(8), 706-719.

Scott, D., Sanders, K. M., Aitken, D., Hayes, A., Ebeling, P. R., & Jones, G. (2014). Sarcopenic obesity and dynapenic obesity: 5-year associations with falls risk in middle-aged and older adults. *Obesity (Silver Spring), 22*(6), 1568-1574.

Sherrington, C., & Menz, H. B. (2003). An evaluation of footwear worn at the time of fall-related hip fracture. *Age and Ageing, 32*(3), 310-314.

Shores, K. A., West, S. T., Theriault, D. S., & Davison, E. A. (2009). Extra-individual correlates of physical activity attainment in rural older adults. *Journal of Rural Health, 25*(2), 211-218.

Shumway-Cook, A., Patla, A. E., Stewart, A., Ferrucci, L., Ciol, M. A., & Guralnik, J. M. (2002). Environmental demands associated with community mobility in older adults with and without mobility disabilities. *Physical Therapy, 82*(7), 670-681.

Shumway-Cook, A., Patla, A., Stewart, A., Ferrucci, L., Ciol, M. A., & Guralnik, J. M. (2003). Environmental components of mobility disability in community-living older persons. *Journal of the American Geriatrics Society, 51*(3), 393-398.

Shumway-Cook, A., Patla, A., Stewart, A., Ferrucci, L., Ciol, M. A., & Guralnik, J. M. (2005). Assessing environmentally determined mobility disability: Self-report versus observed community mobility. *Journal of the American Geriatrics Society, 53*(4), 700-704.

Simonsick, E. M., Guralnik, J. M., Volpato, S., Balfour, J., & Fried, L. P. (2005). Just get out the door! Importance of walking outside the home for maintaining mobility: Findings from the Women's Health and Aging Study. *Journal of the American Geriatrics Society, 53*(2), 198-203.

Siscovick, D. S., Fried, L., Mittelmark, M., Rutan, G., Bild, D., & O'Leary, D. H. (1997). Exercise intensity and subclinical cardiovascular disease in the elderly: The Cardiovascular Health Study. *American Journal of Epidemiology, 145*(11), 977-986.

Sorock, G. S., Bush, T. L., Golden, A. L., Fried, L. P., Breuer, B., & Hale, W. E. (1988). Physical activity and fracture risk in a free-living elderly cohort. *Journal of Gerontology, 43*(5), M134-M139.

Stevens, J. A., Corso, P. S., Finkelstein, E. A., & Miller, T. R. (2006). The costs of fatal and non-fatal falls among older adults. *Injury Prevention, 12*(5), 290-295.

Suominen, M. H., Puranen, T. M., Jyvakorpi, S. K., Eloniemi-Sulkava, U., Kautiainen. H., Siljamäki-Ojansuu, U., & Pitkala, K. H. (2015). Nutritional guidance improves nutrient intake and quality of life, and may prevent falls in aged persons with Alzheimer disease living with a spouse (NuAD Trial). *Journal of Nutrition, Health, and Aging, 19*(9), 901-907.

Tinetti, M. E. (2003). Clinical practice: Preventing falls in elderly persons. *New England Journal of Medicine, 348*(1), 42-49.

Tinetti, M. E., & Kumar, C. (2010). The patient who falls: "It's always a trade-off." *Journal of the American Medical Association, 303*(3), 258-266.

Tinetti, M. E., Liu, W. L., & Claus, E. B. (1993). Predictors and prognosis of inability to get up after falls among elderly persons. *Journal of the American Medical Association, 269*(1), 65-70.

Tinetti, M. E., Mendes de Leon, C. F., Doucette, J. T., & Baker, D. I. (1994). Fear of falling and fall-related efficacy in relationship to functioning among community-living elders. *Journal of Gerontology, 49*(3), M140-M147.

Tinetti, M. E., Richman, D., & Powell, L. (1990). Falls efficacy as a measure of fear of falling. *Journal of Gerontology, 45*(6), P239-P243.

Tinetti, M. E., & Speechley, M. (1989). Prevention of falls among the elderly. *New England Journal of Medicine, 320*(16), 1055-1059.

Tinetti, M. E., Speechley, M., & Ginter, S. F. (1988). Risk factors for falls among elderly persons living in the community. *New England Journal of Medicine, 319*, 1701-1707.

Tinetti, M. E., & Williams, C. S. (1997). Falls, injuries due to falls, and the risk of admission to a nursing home. *New England Journal of Medicine, 337*(18), 1279-1284.

Tinetti, M. E., & Williams, C. S. (1998). The effect of falls and fall injuries on functioning in community-dwelling older persons. *Journal of Gerontology, Series A: Biological Sciences and Medical Sciences, 53*(2), M112-M119.

Tromp, A. M., Smit, J. H., Deeg, D. J., Bouter, L. M., & Lips, P. (1998). Predictors for falls and fractures in the Longitudinal Aging Study Amsterdam. *Journal of Bone Mineral Research, 13*(12), 1932-1939.

van Lenthe, F. J., Brug, J., & Mackenbach, J. P. (2005). Neighbourhood inequalities in physical inactivity: The role of neighbourhood attractiveness, proximity to local facilities and safety in the Netherlands. *Social Science & Medicine, 60*(4), 763-775.

Vellas, B., Cayla, F., Bocquet, H., de Pemille, F., & Albarede, J. L. (1987). Prospective study of restriction of activity in old people after falls. *Age and Ageing, 16*(3), 189-193.

Weinberg, L. E., & Strain, L. A. (1995). Community-dwelling older adults' attributions about falls. *Archives of Physical Medicine and Rehabilitation, 76*(10), 955-960.

Weiss. C. C., Purciel, M., Bader, M., Quinn, J. W., Lovasi, G., Neckerman, K. M., & Rundle, A. G. (2011). Reconsidering access: Park facilities and neighborhood disamenities in New York City. *Journal of Urban Health: Bulletin of the New York Academy of Medicine, 88*(2), 297-310.

Weuve, J., Kang, J. H., Manson, J. E., Breteler, M. M., Ware, J. H., & Grodstein, F. (2004). Physical activity, including walking, and cognitive function in older women. *Journal of the American Medical Association, 292*(12), 1454-1461.

Widder, B. (1985). A new device to decrease falls. *Geriatric Nursing, 6*(5), 287-288.

Wijlhuizen, G. J., de Jong, R., & Hopman-Rock, M. (2007). Older persons afraid of falling reduce physical activity to prevent outdoor falls. *Preventive Medicine, 44*(3), 260-264.

World Health Organization (WHO), Ageing and Life Course, Family and Community Health. (2008). *WHO global report on falls prevention in older age.* Geneva, Switzerland: Author.

Wu, I. C., Chang, H. Y., Hsu, C. C., Chiu, Y. F., Yu, S. H., Tsai, Y. F.,... Hsiung, C. A. (2013). Association between dietary fiber intake and physical performance in older adults: A nationwide study in Taiwan. *PLoS One, 8*(11), e80209.

Yasumura, S., Haga, H., & Niino, N. (1996). Circumstances of injurious falls leading to medical care among elderly people living in a rural community. *Archives of Gerontology and Geriatrics, 23*(2), 95-109.

Yen, I. H., & Kaplan, G. A. (1998). Poverty area residence and changes in physical activity level: Evidence from the Alameda County Study. *American Journal of Public Health, 88*(11), 1709-1712.

Yoshida, H., & Kim, H. (2006). Frequency of falls and their prevention. *Clinical Calcium, 16*(9), 1444-1450.

Yusuf, H. R., Croft, J. B., Giles, W. H., Anda, R. F., Casper, M. L., Caspersen, C. J., & Jones, D. A. (1996). Leisure-time physical activity among older adults. United States, 1990. *Archives of Internal Medicine, 156*(12), 1321-1326.

Zabina, H. Y., Blanton, C. J., Macera, C. A., & Pratt, M. F. (1998). Physical inactivity in relation to degree of urbanization and geographic region. *Medicine & Science in Sports & Exercise, 30*(5), S201.

Zijlstra, G. A., van Haastregt, J. C., Ambergen, T., van Rossum, E., van Eijk, J. T., Tennstedt, S. L., & Kempen, G. I. (2009). Effects of a multicomponent cognitive behavioral group intervention on fear of falling and activity avoidance in community-dwelling older adults: Results of a randomized controlled trial. *Journal of the American Geriatrics Society, 57*(11), 2020-2028.

Zlot, A. I., Librett, J., Buchner, D., & Schmid, T. (2006). Environmental, transportation, social and time barriers to physical activity. *Journal of Physical Activity and Health, 3*, 15-21.

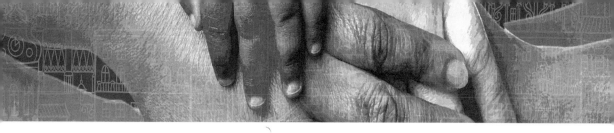

CHAPTER 11

Motor Vehicle Crashes and Other Traffic-Related Causes of Injury and Death in Older Populations

Richard A. Marottoli and **Desmond O'Neill**

ABSTRACT

Transportation is essential for out-of-home mobility and social engagement. However, transportation in all its forms poses potential risks, particularly as one ages. Walking, cycling, getting into or out of a car, driving, or riding as a passenger in a car or bus all carry some potential risk. This chapter reviews what these risks are, where they originate, and what can potentially be done to lessen them.

KEYWORDS

aging   motor vehicle crashes

▶ Introduction

As populations around the world age, more people will engage with the traffic environment at advancing ages. Due to widely ingrained ageism and the challenges of linking gerontology, traffic medicine, and public health (O'Neill, 2012), an undue focus has been placed on the potential impact of age-related disease, disability, and medications that might increase older adults' risk for crashes and other adverse driving events or lead them to stop driving. In fact, older drivers are a group with a good—and ever improving—crash record (Cicchino & McCartt, 2014). Rather than driving itself, the greatest risks to older people in traffic arise from pedestrian and bicyclist injuries, non-collision injuries in public transport, and single pedestrian crashes (O'Neill, 2012). The greater fragility of these older car occupants also increases their risk of injury and death from crashes compared to younger age groups (Polders et al., 2015). This confluence of demographics and disability has led to apocalyptic predictions and misplaced concern about the public health and safety implications of a growing older driver population. In practice, at least thus far, this has not been the case—which in turn suggests that academic and policy efforts should focus on the real issues underlying fatalities and injuries among older people in the traffic environment, which have been poorly addressed up to this point (Marin-Lamellet & Haustein, 2015). These issues, and the factors contributing to them, are the subject of this chapter.

▶ Why Crashes?

We begin with a discussion of the choice of primary outcome for many investigations related to older adults and traffic—namely, **motor vehicle crashes.** A range of potential adverse driving events could be considered, such as moving violations, near misses, or episodes of getting lost. However, from a public health and safety perspective, the desire to minimize fatal and injurious crashes is paramount. Fortunately, these events are relatively rare occurrences. From a public health and safety perspective, this is a good thing. From a measurement perspective, however, it means that the outcome of interest is difficult to detect. This often leads to the use of large population-based data sets so as to obtain a sufficient sample size to detect and study the outcome. Unfortunately, such large data sets often lack detailed information on the health and function of drivers, making it difficult to identify potential risk factors. Consequently, investigators have often turned to smaller data sets that offer richer, more detailed data on participants—but this choice of data source either limits the number of independent variables that can be assessed or necessitates the use of proxy outcomes, such as on-road driving performance. The rationale for the latter choice is that driving performance is the "gold standard" by which driving licenses are issued or revoked in most jurisdictions. Nevertheless, the content of these evaluations and their scoring criteria can vary considerably. Thus, when considering driving, the primary focus of discussion in this chapter is crashes.

Because crash data are lacking in certain topic areas and because a discussion of crash risk is often interwoven with changes in driving patterns and cessation, we will touch on these topics as well. Even limiting the discussion to crashes poses some difficulty and forces some choices. Crashes range in severity and consequences from fatal at one extreme, to those that result in injury or necessitate hospitalization, to those that result in only property damage, to those involving only a minor dent or scrape or no visible damage at all at the other extreme.

Similarly, crash ascertainment methods may vary, from events that are reported to licensing or traffic safety agencies to self-reported events. The criteria for agency-reported events vary by jurisdiction, but often require a crash of sufficient magnitude/severity to result in injury to the driver or occupant or a certain level of property damage. Self-reported events rely on the willingness and ability of the reporter to disclose the event, but can capture more minor events that do not reach the threshold for agency reporting, which may be valuable if such events are harbingers of subsequent, more serious crashes. Considerable debate in the literature has arisen regarding the advantages and disadvantages of each of these detection approaches (Marottoli, Coney, & Tinetti, 1997, 2003; Roberts, Vingilis, Wilk, & Seeley, 2008). The issue of concern here is to make the reader aware of the need to understand the choices made in a particular study and the tradeoffs involved in interpreting the findings.

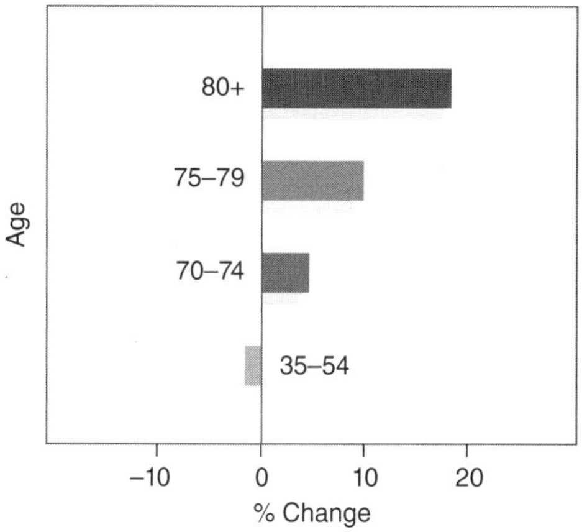

FIGURE 11-1 Percent change in licensure rates in the Unites States by driver age, 1997–2008.

Modified from: Insurance Institute for Highway Safety Highway Loss Data Institute. (2016). Older drivers' crash rates decline unexpectedly. Status Report, 45 (6).

▶ Driving Demographics

The population of most countries is **aging,** leading to an increasing number of older drivers and users of other forms of transportation. In the United States from 1997 to 2008, while the number of drivers aged 35–54 years decreased slightly, there was considerable growth in the number of drivers aged 70 and older, and in particular those aged 80 and older (**FIGURE 11-1**; Insurance Institute for Highway Safety, 2010). In addition to the growing number of older drivers, those drivers are driving more frequently and for more miles than earlier cohorts did (Mizenko, Tefft, Arnold, & Grabowski, 2014). Specifically, data from the 2009 National Household Travel Survey indicated that drivers aged 65 years and older were driving more miles and taking more trips than their counterparts in 1990 (Rosenbloom & Santos, 2014).

While this growth is often considered in safety terms and viewed as a potential negative, it also brings tremendous opportunities: marketing new vehicles, safety features, and technologies; training individuals how to appropriately utilize these features and

technologies; and developing better ways to connect people with other transportation options to facilitate their eventual transition from driving, while maintaining their out-of-home mobility and social engagement.

▶ Crash and Injury Risk

How one views the crash risk of older drivers depends on one's perspective. The absolute risk of crashes decreases with advancing age. The previous emphasis on exposure (typically miles/kilometers driven), which suggested crash risk increases with advancing age (**FIGURES 11-2** and **11-3**; Evans, 1988; Williams & Carsten, 1989) is now generally understood as an artifact of low mileage, as this relationship disappears when statistical adjustments are made (Langford, Methorst, & Hakamies-Blomqvist, 2006). The paradox of fewer crashes and more deaths and serious injuries is largely due to the intersection of increased fragility (older drivers are at 2 to 4 times the risk of injury, hospitalization, or death in a crash of similar magnitude

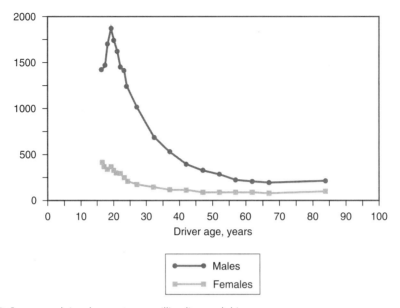

FIGURE 11-2 Severe crash involvements per million licensed drivers.

Reprinted from: McGwin, J. G., & Brown, D. B. (1999). Characteristics of traffic crashes among young, middle-aged, and older drivers. Accident Analysis & Prevention, 31(3), 181–198. Reprinted with permission from Elsevier.

compared to middle-aged [35-54 years old] drivers [Barancik et al., 1986; Fife, Barancik, & Chatterjee, 1984; Li, Braver, & Chen, 2003]) with a traffic system and automotive safety features that have not sufficiently adapted to this fragility. Motor vehicle crashes are the leading cause of injurious death for individuals aged 65 to 74 years and the second leading

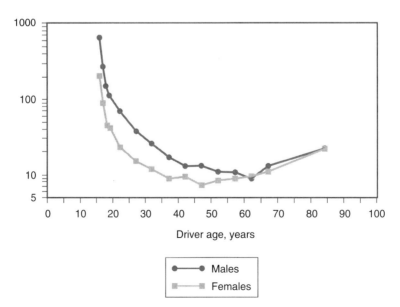

FIGURE 11-3 Severe crash involvements per unit distance of travel.

Reprinted from: McGwin, J. G., & Brown, D. B. (1999). Characteristics of traffic crashes among young, middle-aged, and older drivers. Accident Analysis & Prevention, 31(3), 181–198. Reprinted with permission from Elsevier.

cause for individuals aged 75 to 84 years (Dellinger & Stevens, 2006).

Some encouraging signs do appear when one considers recent temporal trends. Data from the National Highway Traffic Safety Administration (NHTSA) demonstrate an overall decline in traffic fatalities from 2003 to 2012 (**FIGURE 11-4**; NHTSA National Center for Statistics and Analysis, 2014). Perhaps more surprisingly to non-gerontologists, the magnitude of decline among individuals aged

65 years and older was greater with advancing age (**FIGURE 11-5**; NHTSA National Center for Statistics and Analysis, 2014). (Note that these trends are not entirely monotonic, with periodic plateaus or increases for a given group, but the overall trends are downward.) Analyses by the Insurance Institute for Highway Safety have demonstrated that from 1997 to 2008 these downward trends did, indeed, increase with advancing age and were more pronounced than the decreases for drivers aged 35-54

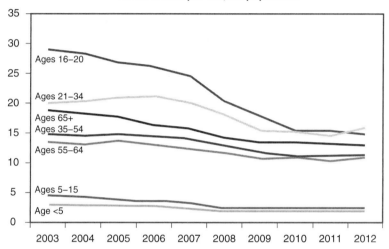

FIGURE 11-4 Motor vehicle traffic fatality rates by age group, 2003–2012.

Reproduced from: NHTSA National Center for Statistics and Analysis 2014 (revised).

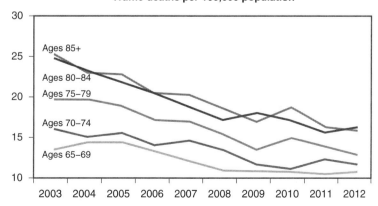

FIGURE 11-5 Motor vehicle traffic fatality rates among older populations by age group, 2003–2012.

Reproduced from: NHTSA National Center for Statistics and Analysis 2014 (revised).

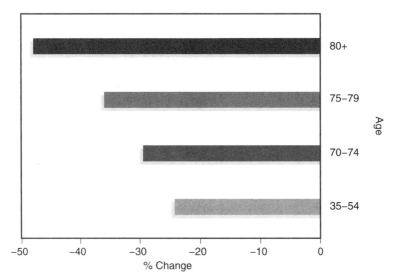

FIGURE 11-6 Percent change in fatal crashes per 100,000 licensed drivers, by driver age, 1997–2008.

Modified from: Cheung, L., McCartt, A.T. (2011). Declines in fatal crashes of older drivers: Changes in crash risk and survivability. Accident Analysis and Prevention, 43, 666-674.

years (**FIGURE 11-6**; Cheung & McCartt, 2011). Cicchino and McCartt (2014) extended these analyses with updated data through 2012 and found that although the differences among age groups leveled off, there was a continued downward trend in crashes and fatalities. The reasons for these trends are now being explored, but they likely reflect a combination of healthier drivers, safer vehicles, safer roadways, and enhanced emergency responses. In summary, these findings suggest that although the number of older drivers is increasing, this growth may be offset by fewer crashes and lower crash fatality rates, dampening the potential public health and safety concerns that the demographic trends might otherwise imply.

▶ Exposure

On the surface, one might anticipate a linear relationship between exposure and crash risk: The more you drive, the greater your likelihood of being in a crash. The actual relationship is more complicated. At high mileages, crash risk tends to flatten out, in part because to achieve high mileage a person is more likely to drive a greater proportion of those miles on limited-access highways, which in general are quite safe despite their higher speeds of vehicle travel because vehicles are traveling in the same direction and are often separated from oncoming traffic. In contrast, very low-mileage drivers (particularly those traveling less than 3000 km [1800 miles] per year) are at increased risk of crashes. There are a number of likely explanations for this relationship, including the fact that for low-mileage drivers a greater proportion of miles driven are likely to be near home and, therefore, involve intersections and interaction with cross traffic in areas where crashes involving older drivers are more likely to occur. Also, low-mileage drivers may have more health problems that contribute to their decision to drive less often, yet increase their risk of crashes and other adverse driving events (Griffin, 2004; Keall & Firth, 2004, 2006; Langford et al., 2006; Lyman, McGwin, & Sims, 2001; Mayhew, Simpson, & Ferguson, 2006). Common older-driver errors resulting in crashes include inadequate surveillance and misjudging gaps or speed of other vehicles, particularly when making left turns at intersections (Cicchino & McCartt, 2015).

▶ Risk Factors

Gender

There has not been a clear association of gender with crash occurrence or fatality risk if analyses are adjusted for driving exposure (Evans, 1988). Women may be more likely to limit or stop driving sooner than men, which, along with their greater longevity, may contribute to more years for women past driving retirement (Anstey, Windsor, Luszcz, & Andrew, 2006; Dit Asse, Fabrigoule, Helmer, Laumon, & Lafort, 2014; Foley, Heimovitz, Guralnik, & Brock, 2002; Mezuk & Rebok, 2008). While some have viewed this pattern as women stopping prematurely, it may reflect better judgment or greater awareness of capabilities and limitations. While women drive in fewer risky situations, they appear equally confident as men in situations where both drive (Marottoli & Richardson, 1998). Societal perceptions of older drivers, however, may have a greater effect on women, suggesting possible avenues for intervention, such as enhancing women's views of their abilities in relation to other drivers (Levy, Ng, Myers, & Marottoli, 2013).

Medical Conditions

A range of medical conditions may contribute to increased crash risk, although the contribution is generally considered to be modest, and may be more prominent among younger than older drivers in contact with the healthcare system (Redelmeier, Yarnell, Thiruchelvam, & Tibshirani, 2012). A detailed review of this literature is beyond the scope of this chapter. The interested reader is referred to recent detailed reviews (Charlton et al., 2010; Dobbs, 2005; Staplin, Lococco, Martell, & Stutts, 2012), as well as to the guidelines for older drivers that are issued by professional societies and licensing agencies in a number of countries and are updated and revised regularly (American Geriatrics Society & Pomidor, 2015, Austroads, 2012; Canadian Medical Association,

2012; Drivers Medical Group DVLA, 2014; Road Safety Authority, 2014). In general, problematic medical conditions for driving include conditions that affect sensory input, cognition, consciousness, flexibility, speed of movement, or delivery of oxygen to the brain. In addition, a range of potentially driving-impairing (PDI) medications can affect driving safety, most of which are directly or indirectly psychoactive (Hetland & Carr, 2014; LeRoy & Morse, 2008).

Functional Impairments

Impairments in functional abilities relevant to the driving task, such as vision, cognition, and physical ability, may increase with advancing age or due to an underlying medical condition. While the distinction between the underlying medical condition and its functional manifestations may be difficult to discern at times, there are plausible clinical reasons for doing so, as both offer potential avenues for interventions that may provide synergistic benefits.

A number of visual functions, including acuity, visual fields, and contrast sensitivity, may have particular relevance to the driving task (Owsley & McGwin, 2010). Although visual acuity alone is only weakly associated with crashes, one study found that testing for all three of these elements provided the best prediction of crash risk (Decina & Staplin, 1993).

With regard to cognition, global cognitive measures are relatively poor predictors of crashes. Joseph et al. (2014) found no association between Mini-Mental State Exam (MMSE) scores and crashes that were self-reported or resulted in a hospitalization. While the sample size in their study was large, the participants were relatively young, adjustment for driving exposure was limited, and low cognitive test scores and crashes were infrequent.

Despite the weak association of global cognitive measures and crash risk, it is likely that the more cognitively impaired a person is, the greater the likelihood of a crash. Determining a particular threshold for impairment beyond which continued driving is too risky has proved difficult, however, in part because of variability in capabilities at different levels of cognitive impairment, the limited ability of global measures to assess relevant cognitive domains in sufficient detail to gauge risk, and a lack of data on crashes in dementia-affected populations (Man-Son-Hing, Marshall, Molnar, & Wilson, 2007). Given that global measures are widely used in clinical practice, efforts have been made to determine a threshold by consensus (Johanssen & Lundberg, 1997). Alternatively, meta-analyses and systematic reviews of available evidence have identified and rated potential risk factors in cognitively impaired drivers, primarily for impaired driving performance (Carr & Ott, 2010; Iverson et al., 2010; Reger et al., 2004).

In the realm of physical ability, flexibility and speed of movement have been associated with impaired driving performance (Marottoli et al., 1994; Marottoli et al., 1998). A recent systematic review and meta-analysis found an association of falls with crash risk, which may be a direct effect or in part due to shared risk factors (Scott et al., 2016).

For unprotected road users, significant age-related disability may hinder their ability to enter the traffic system. The car is the most common and useful form of gerotechnology, extending the ability to travel when travel as a pedestrian or through public transport is no longer possible (Hjorthol, Levin, & Sirén, 2010). When older adults are pedestrians, functional impairments affect their ability to travel with ease and security, although there is evidence that, akin to the compensatory strategies adopted by older drivers, such pedestrians have insight into their vulnerability (Rosenbloom, Sapir-Lavid, & Perlman, 2016) and behave more prudently when crossing the road (Dommes, Granie, Cloutier, Coquelet, & Huguenin-Richard, 2015).

The risk of fatality and injury to older bicyclists increases quite dramatically with age, almost certainly related to fragility and a traffic environment that does not cater adequately to vulnerable road users (Edwards & Mason,

> **PEARL 11-1** Technology and Mobility
>
> New technologies are proliferating and may enhance the safety and mobility of older persons, but only if the needs of older persons are considered in those technologies' development, and only if older adults have adequate access to them and appropriate training in their use.

2014; Johan de Hartog, Boogaard, Nijland, & Hoek, 2010). The same is true for older motorcyclists (Beck, Dellinger, & O'Neil, 2007).

▶ Interventions

An earlier focus on identification of medical fitness to drive at license renewal and during clinical encounters is maturing into a recognition of the need to tackle a broad of range of issues relating to older people in the traffic milieu, particularly in higher-income areas of the world.

In any systems approach, there are four key elements: (1) infrastructure interventions, (2) education and training, (3) licensing and enforcement, and (4) vehicle and intelligent transportation system technologies. A substantial challenge is the inclusion of sectors that have traditionally had little engagement with traffic medicine or understanding of their role. For example, the education of medical students in traffic medicine is deficient (Hawley, Galbraith, & deSouza, 2008), and in many jurisdictions physicians have low awareness of guidelines on medical fitness to drive (Jang et al., 2007). The implementation of training and education programs can be effective (Kahvedzic, McFadden, Cummins, Carr, & O'Neill, 2015) but needs wider implementation across the healthcare sector in most countries, just as expertise in gerontologic issues relating to older drivers needs to be diffused throughout law enforcement systems (Hill, Rybar, Stowe, & Jahns, 2016).

PEARL 11-2 Older Drivers and Safety

Older road users are quite safe overall, but fragility and health conditions place some of them at increased risk for adverse events and injuries. A growing number of interventions may help to lower this risk.

Key elements are the age-attuning of the traffic environment, including highway redesign for cars (Classen et al., 2007), reconfiguring the traffic environment for vulnerable road users (pedestrians [OECD International Transport Forum, 2012], bicyclists, motorcyclists [Haworth & Schulze, 1996] and users of public transport [O'Neill, 2015]), and review of automotive safety features for both occupants and other road users (Simms & O'Neill, 2005). These changes need to be evidence based: A 2015 analysis of serious older-driver crashes suggested countermeasures that simplify or remove the need to make turns across traffic, such as roundabouts, protected signals when crossing traffic, and diverging diamond intersection designs, could decrease the frequency of inadequate surveillance and gap or speed misjudgment errors. In addition, the authors of this study suggested that vehicle-to-vehicle and vehicle-to-infrastructure communications may help protect older drivers from these errors (Cicchino & McCartt, 2015).

With due attention to these broader themes, the identification of medical conditions and functional impairments that contribute to increased crash risk has led to the development of interventions that attempt to lower this risk, and that provide insight and inspiration regarding how age-attuning traffic safety for older people can be fostered in other elements of the traffic system. For example, cataracts have been shown to affect driving performance, crash risk, and driving safety; cataract repair consequently has been shown to restore driving frequency, improve driving performance, and decrease crash risk (Owsley et al., 2002). Decreases in information processing speed have been associated with poor driving performance and crash risk, while interventions to enhance processing speed have been shown to improve driving performance, decrease crash risk, and delay the time to driving cessation (Ball, Edwards, Ross, & McGwin, 2010; Edwards, Delahunt, & Mahncke, 2009; Roenker, Cissell, Ball, Wadley, & Edwards, 2003). Interventions to enhance flexibility and speed of movement have been associated with maintained driving performance (Marottoli, Allore, et al., 2007).

Other interventions have focused on the driving task itself in an effort to enhance driving performance. While classroom-based instruction has yielded mixed effects (Bedard, Isherwood, Moore, Gibbons, & Lindstrom, 2004; Janke, 1984; McKnight et al., 1982; Nasvadi & Varik, 2007), studies combining classroom and on-road instruction have found a positive effect on driving performance (Bedard et al., 2008; Marottoli, Ness, et al., 2007).

Another line of education-based interventions has focused on raising driver awareness of functional limits/capabilities (Eby, Molnar, Shope, Vivoda, & Fordyce, 2003; Owsley, Stalvey, & Phillips, 2003), raising caregiver or clinician awareness of how to address the issue (Meuser, Carr, Irmiter, Schwartz, & Ulfarsson, 2010; Stern et al., 2008), and helping drivers adjust to the effects of driving cessation (Liddle et al., 2014).

While many of these studies are limited in scope or choice of outcome, they are encouraging in several respects. They cast the issue in a more positive light than it is often viewed. Rather than focusing on whether someone should stop driving or lose his or her license, it may eventually be possible to emphasize ways to improve underlying functional capabilities or driving performance to enhance and prolong safe driving. This may allow for more clinical discussion on the topic and serve as an entry to discussion about transportation goals and ways to eventually meet those goals if the older adult is no longer able to drive.

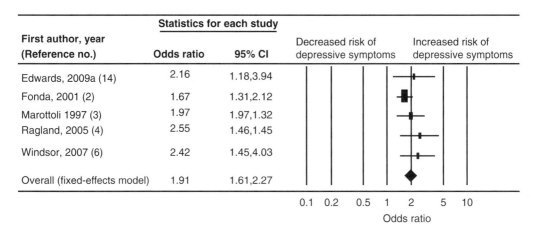

	Statistics for each study			
First author, year (Reference no.)	**Odds ratio**	**95% CI**	Decreased risk of depressive symptoms	Increased risk of depressive symptoms
Edwards, 2009a (14)	2.16	1.18,3.94		
Fonda, 2001 (2)	1.67	1.31,2.12		
Marottoli 1997 (3)	1.97	1.97,1.32		
Ragland, 2005 (4)	2.55	1.46,1.45		
Windsor, 2007 (6)	2.42	1.45,4.03		
Overall (fixed-effects model)	1.91	1.61,2.27		

FIGURE 11-7 Effect for the association of driving cessation with depressive symptoms.

Reproduced from: Chihuri, S., Mielenz, T.J., DiMaggio, C.J., Betz, M.E., DiGiuseppi, C., Jones, V.C., et al. (2016). Driving cessation and health outcomes in older adults. Journal of the American Geriatrics Society, 64(2), 332-341.

Another intriguing feature of some of these interventions is the prospect of additional or ancillary benefits besides the effects on driving-related outcomes. For instance, in the ACTIVE trial, in addition to benefits in driving performance, crash risk, and driving duration, cognitive training enhanced the participants' ability to perform activities of daily living (Ball, Edwards, & Ross, 2007). On a smaller scale, a physical conditioning program to enhance flexibility and speed of movement not only maintained driving performance, but also found a 50% reduction in falls, though this result did not achieve statistical significance because of the small sample size and short study duration (Marottoli, Allore, et al., 2007). Nevertheless, these kinds of additional benefits may facilitate the eventual implementation and dissemination of such interventions by broadening their applicability.

factors contributing to the decision to stop driving: advanced age, female gender, health difficulties (particularly visual and neurologic disorders), cost, and the availability of transportation options (Anstey et al., 2006; Dit Asse et al., 2014; Freeman, Munoz, Turano, & West, 2005; Marottoli & Drickamer, 1993). That these decisions are not made lightly is understandable given the potential consequences of driving cessation, including increased depressive symptoms, decreased out-of-home activity participation, and decreased social interaction (Fonda, Wallace, & Herzog, 2001; Freeman et al., 2005; Marottoli et al., 1997b; Marottoli et al., 2000; Mezuk & Rebok, 2008; Ragland, Satariano, & MacLeod, 2005). A recent systematic review and meta-analysis found a remarkably consistent magnitude of effect for the association of driving cessation with depressive symptoms (**FIGURE 11-7**; Chihuri et al., 2016).

▶ Driving Cessation and Its Effects

The decision to stop driving is seldom made lightly, particularly in countries where other forms of transportation are less available. A number of studies have demonstrated similar

▶ Transitioning from Driving

Because of these concerns, recent decades have seen a growing awareness of the need to take a more holistic view and focus on transportation needs—not just driving needs—and the living environment (Lynott, McAuley, & McCutcheon, 2009; Satariano et al., 2012). This approach entails considering that as people limit or stop driving, something must fill the void to allow them to remain active and socially engaged. Numerous sources of transportation exist to help bridge this gap, but challenges remain in making these services available, affordable, accessible, acceptable, and adaptable (Beverly Foundation, 2011). Much more needs to be done in incorporating new technologies and ride-sharing services to meet the transportation needs of older individuals who choose to drive less or not at all.

▶ Pedestrians

Moving from the car to other forms of transportation is not without safety risk. Dellinger et al. (2008) demonstrated the potential dangers of getting into or out of a vehicle. When they are pedestrians, older individuals face a number of safety risks, such as the availability and condition of sidewalks and potential fall/trip hazards. In some cases, the timing of signal lights at crosswalks may not adequately accommodate the gait speed limitation of older pedestrians (Langlois et al., 1997). Cognitive, sensory, and physical factors may not only affect crash risk, but also alter older pedestrians' ability to safely navigate their environment (Tournier, Dommes, & Cavallo, 2016).

▶ Noncollision Injuries in Public Transport

A range of options may be available for reducing noncollision injuries in public transport modalities. Driver education may be one fruitful avenue that can be exploited to reduce noncollision bus injuries (Broome, Worrall, Fleming, & Boldy, 2011) as well as the barriers to public transport use by older people, though

this potential is not always widely recognized. The recent Attaining Energy-Efficient Mobility in an Ageing Society (AENEAS) project handbook for training bus drivers to serve older passengers makes only one small reference to careful acceleration in its 58 pages (AENEAS Consortium, 2010). Driver education is just one aspect of safety, as pointed out in a study of bus and taxi drivers driving wheelchair users: It is clear that driver "errors" are probably markers of system failures, especially deficient safety culture in traffic organizations (Wretstrand, Petzall, Bylund, & Falkmer, 2010).

Given that accelerations quickly followed by harsh decelerations are frequent events for urban buses and are likely to result in more severe injuries in the event of loss of balance for a standing occupant, Palacio et al. (2009) suggest that driver training should be expanded to include mandatory viewing of videos based on multibody occupant simulations of noncollision crash scenarios, thereby demonstrating the influence of driving patterns on standing occupant balance loss and subsequent injury risk. Some indication of factors that might be important arise from the study of Strathman et al. (2010). An increased frequency of noncollision injuries is associated with less experience (the expected incident frequency for an operator with, for example, 20 years of service is nearly 24% lower than that for an operator with 10 years of service), absenteeism, overtime hours driving, female gender (possibly a reporting issue), part-time work, late departures, and lift usage (suggesting a link with more disabled passengers).

In addition, the development of protocols to ensure that older passengers are seated before the bus moves to the greatest extent possible, and to ensure that they can make their way to the exit while the bus is stationary rather than still moving, would be helpful. Likewise, passengers should be discouraged from standing in the aisles (to prevent leg injury risk from contact with the stiff seat frames) and immediately behind the stairwell (to prevent head contact with the stairwell wall). They should instead stand in a dedicated area opposite the stairwell.

The current design of bus entrances and exits often fails to meet the needs of an older population. Björnstig et al. (2005) point out that even coaches and buses "adapted" for the disabled have a step height that substantially exceeds the step height recommended for older people in housing. Moreover, the lifespan of these vehicles means that this discrepancy will remain in the Swedish transport system (and presumably many other European systems) for many years to come (Björnstig et al., 2005).

In terms of physical design within the bus for prevention and reduction of primary and secondary injuries, Palacio et al. (2009) offer the following recommendations:

- Dedicated standing areas opposite the stairwell and roof-mounted vertical handholds should be included. Padding in these areas is important as well.
- Horizontal metal seat handles should be replaced with vertical ones hung from the roof of the bus (but low enough for shorter people to reach).
- Less stiff rubber flooring should be considered.

▶ **Conclusion and Future Directions**

The vast majority of older persons are able to safely drive, walk, cycle, or ride in vehicles. However, as individuals age, increasing fragility and the sequellae of certain diseases, functional impairments, and medications place some of them at increased risk for adverse events and injury in those different transportation modes. Fortunately, an increasing range of interventions are becoming available to enhance the health and function of older transportation users, as well as to make their vehicles and environments safer and more accommodating—not only for them, but for

all transportation users. In the future, we will need to determine the effects of these interventions on a broader range of outcomes and in different groups of individuals.

We also need more information on changes that are occurring in middle/lower-income countries with respect to older drivers and transportation users and the particular challenges that these countries face in implementing programs. Examples of "best practices" regarding possible solutions to these challenges will be needed as well.

Another area where more information is needed is the rapidly changing field of vehicle technology, ranging from in-vehicle technologies, to driverless cars, to ride services. We will need to ensure that the needs of older individuals are considered when these technologies are developed and tested, and that older individuals have sufficient access to beneficial technologies and are appropriately trained in their use.

References

AENEAS Consortium. (2010). *Serving older passengers: Training manual for bus drivers.* Salzburg, Austria: Salzburg AG für Energie.

American Geriatrics Society & Pomidor, A. (2015). *Clinicians guide to assessing and counseling older drivers* (3rd ed.). Report No. DOT HS 812 228. Washington, DC: National Highway Traffic Safety Administration.

Anstey, K. J., Windsor, T. D., Luszcz, M. A., & Andrew, G. R. (2006). Predicting driving cessation over 5 years in older adults: Psychological well-being and cognitive competence are stronger predictors than physical health. *Journal of the American Geriatrics Society, 54,* 121–126.

Austroads. (2012). *Assessing fitness to drive for commercial and private vehicle drivers: Medical standards for licensing and clinical management guidelines.* Sydney, Australia: Author.

Ball, K., Edwards, J. D., & Ross, L. A. (2007). The impact of speed of processing training on cognitive and everyday functions. *Journal of Gerontology: Series B, 62B,* 19–31.

Ball, K., Edwards, J. D., Ross, L. A, & McGwin, G. Jr. (2010). Cognitive training decreases motor vehicle collision involvement of older drivers. *Journal of the American Geriatrics Society, 58,* 2107–2113.

Barancik, J. I., Chatterjee, B. F., Greene-Cradden, Y. C., Michenzi, E. M., Kramer, C. F., Thode, H. C., & Fife, D. (1986). Motor vehicle trauma in northeastern Ohio. I: Incidence and outcome by age, sex, and road-use category. *American Journal of Epidemiology, 123,* 846–861.

Beck, L. F., Dellinger, A. M., & O'Neil, M. E. (2007). Motor vehicle crash injury rates by mode of travel, United States: Using exposure-based methods to quantify differences. *American Journal of Epidemiology, 166*(2), 212–218.

Bedard, M., Isherwood, J., Moore, E., Gibbons, C., & Lindstrom, W. (2004). Evaluation of a re-training program for older drivers. *Canadian Journal of Public Health, 95*(4), 295–298.

Bedard, M., Porter, M., Marshall, S., Isherwood, I., Riendeau, J., Weaver, B., et al. (2008). The combination of two training approaches to improve older adults driving safety. *Traffic Injury Prevention, 9,* 70–76.

Beverly Foundation. (2011). *Supplemental transportation programs for seniors.* Washington, DC: AAA Foundation for Traffic Safety.

Björnstig, U., Albertsson, P., Björnstig, J., Bylund, P. O., Falkmer, T., & Petzäll, J. (2005). Injury events among bus and coach occupants: Non-crash injuries as important as crash injuries. *IATSS Research, 29*(1), 79–87.

Broome, K., Worrall, L. E., Fleming, J. M., & Boldy, D. P. (2011). Identifying age-friendly behaviours for bus driver age-awareness training. *Canadian Journal of Occupational Therapy, 78*(2), 118–126.

Canadian Medical Association. (2012). *CMA driver's guide: Determining medical fitness to operate motor vehicles* (8th ed.). Ottawa, Ontario: Canadian Medical Association.

Carr, D. B., & Ott, B. R. (2010). The older adult driver with cognitive impairment: It's a very frustrating life. *Journal of the American Medical Association, 303,* 1632–1641.

Charlton, J., Koppel, S., Odell, M., Devlin, A., Langford, J., O'Hare, M.,… Scully, M. (2010). *Influence of chronic illness on crash involvement of motor vehicle drivers.* Report No. 300. Victoria, Australia: Monash University Accident Research Centre.

Cheung, L., & McCartt, A. T. (2011). Declines in fatal crashes of older drivers: Changes in crash risk and survivability. *Accident Analysis and Prevention, 43,* 666–674.

Chihuri, S., Mielenz, T. J., DiMaggio, C. J., Betz, M. E., DiGiuseppi, C., Jones, V. C., & Li, G. (2016). Driving cessation and health outcomes in older adults. *Journal of the American Geriatrics Society, 64,* 332–341.

Cicchino, J. B., & McCartt, A. T. (2014). Trends in older driver crash involvement rates and survivability in the United States: An update. *Accident Analysis and Prevention, 72,* 44–54.

Cicchino, J. B., & McCartt, A. T. (2015). Critical older driver errors in a national sample of serious U.S. crashes. *Accident Analysis and Prevention, 80,* 211–219.

Classen, S., Shechtman, O., Stephens, B., Davis, E., Justiss, M., Bendixen, R.,… Mann, W. (2007). The impact of roadway intersection design on driving performance of young and senior adults. *Traffic Injury Prevention, 8*(1), 69–79.

Decina, L. E., & Staplin, L. (1993). Retrospective evaluation of alternative vision screening criteria for older and younger drivers. *Accident Analysis and Prevention, 25*(3), 267–275.

Dellinger, A. M., Boyd, R. M., & Haileyesus, T. (2008). Fall injuries in older adults from an unusual source: Entering and exiting a vehicle. *Journal of the American Geriatrics Society, 56*(4), 609–614.

Dellinger, A. M., & Stevens, J. A. (2006). The injury problem among older adults: Mortality, morbidity, and costs. *Journal of Safety Research, 37*(5), 519–522.

Dit Asse, L. M., Fabrigoule, C., Helmer, C., Laumon, B., & Lafort, S. (2014). Automobile driving in older adults: Factors affecting driving restriction in men and women. *Journal of the American Geriatrics Society, 62,* 2071–2078.

Dobbs, B. M. (2005). *Medical conditions and driving: A review of the literature.* DOT HS 809.690. Washington, DC: U.S. Department of Transportation.

Dommes, A., Granie, M. A., Cloutier, M. S., Coquelet, C., & Huguenin-Richard, F. (2015). Red light violations by adult pedestrians and other safety-related behaviors at signalized crosswalks. *Accident Analysis and Prevention, 80,* 67–75.

Drivers Medical Group DVLA. (2014). *For medical practitioners: At a glance guide to the current medical standards of fitness to drive.* Swansea, UK: Driver & Vehicle Licensing Agency.

Eby, D. W., Molnar, L. J., Shope, J. T., Vivoda, J. M., & Fordyce, T. A. (2003). Improving older driver knowledge and self-awareness through self-assessment: The Driving Decisions Workbook. *Journal of Safety Research, 34,* 371–381.

Edwards, J. E., Delahunt, P. B., & Mahncke, H. M. (2009). Cognitive speed of processing training delays driving cessation. *Journal of Gerontology: Medical Sciences, 64A,* 1262–1267.

Edwards, R. D., & Mason, C. N. (2014). Spinning the wheels and rolling the dice: Life-cycle risks and benefits of bicycle commuting in the U.S. *Preventive Medicine, 64,* 8–13.

Evans, L. (1988). Older driver involvement in fatal and severe traffic crashes. *Journal of Gerontology: Social Sciences, 43,* S186–S193.

Fife, D., Barancik, J. I., & Chatterjee, B. F. (1984). Northeastern Ohio trauma study: II. Injury rates by age, sex, and cause. *American Journal of Public Health, 74,* 473–478.

Foley, D., Heimovitz, H., Guralnik, J., & Brock, D. (2002). Driving life expectancy of persons aged 70 years and older in the United States. *American Journal of Public Health*, 92(8), 1284–1289.

Fonda, S. J., Wallace, R. B., & Herzog, A. R. (2001). Changes in driving patterns and worsening depressive symptoms among older adults. *Journal of Gerontology: Social Sciences*, 56B, S343–S351.

Freeman, E. E., Gange, S. J., Munoz, B., & West, S. K. (2006). Driving status and risk of entry into long term care in older adults. *American Journal of Public Health*, 96 (7), 1254–1259.

Freeman, E. E., Munoz, B., Turano, K. A., & West, S. K. (2005). Measures of visual function and time to driving cessation in older adults. *Optometry and Vision Science*, 82(8), 765–773.

Griffin, L. I. (2004). *Older driver involvement in injury crashes in Texas 1975–1999*. Washington, DC: AAA Foundation for Traffic Safety.

Hawley, C. A., Galbraith, N. D., & deSouza, V. A. (2008). Medical education on fitness to drive: A survey of all UK medical schools. *Postgraduate Medical Journal*, 84(998), 635–638.

Haworth, N. L., & Schulze, M. T. (1996). *Motorcycle crash counter measures: Literature review and implementation workshop*. Report No. 87. Victoria, Australia: Monash University Accident Research Centre.

Hetland, A., & Carr, D. B. (2014). Medications and impaired driving. *Annals of Pharmacotherapy*, 48, 494–506.

Hill, L. L., Rybar, J., Stowe, J., & Jahns, J. (2016). Development of a curriculum and roadside screening tool for law enforcement identification of medical impairment in aging drivers. *Injury Epidemiology*, 3, 13.

Hjorthol, R. J., Levin, L. & Sirén, A. (2010). Mobility in different generations of older persons: The development of daily travel in different cohorts in Denmark, Norway and Sweden. *Journal of Transport Geography*, 18(5), 624–633.

Insurance Institute for Highway Safety, Highway Loss Data Institute. (2016). Older drivers' crash rates decline unexpectedly. *Status Report*, 45(6).

Iverson, D. J., Groneth, G. S., Reger, M. A., Classen, S., Dubinsky, R., & Rizzo, M. (2010). Practice parameter update: Evaluation and management of driving risk in dementia. *Neurology*, 74, 1316–1324.

Jang, R. W., Man-Son-Hing, M., Molnar, F. J., Hogan, D. B., Marshall, S. C., Auger, J.,… Naglie, G. (2007). Family physicians' attitudes and practices regarding assessments of medical fitness to drive in older persons. *Journal of General Internal Medicine*, 22(4), 531–543.

Janke, M. (1984). The mature driver improvement program in California. *Transportation Research Record*, 1438, 77–83.

Johan de Hartog, J., Boogaard, H., Nijland, H., & Hoek, G. (2010). Do the health benefits of cycling outweigh the risks? *Environmental Health Perspectives*, 118(8), 1109–1116.

Johansson, K., & Lundberg, C. (1997). The 1994 International Consensus Conference on Dementia and Driving: a brief report. *Alzheimer's Disease and Associated Disorders*, 11, 62–69.

Joseph, P. G., O'Donnell, M. J., Teo, K. K., Gao, P., Anderson, C., Probstfield, J. L.,… Yusuf, S. (2014). The Mini-Mental State Examination, clinical factors, and motor vehicle crash risk. *Journal of the American Geriatrics Society*, 62, 1419–1426.

Kahvedzic, A., McFadden, R., Cummins, G., Carr, D., & O'Neill, D. (2015). Impact of new guidelines and educational program on awareness of medical fitness to drive among general practitioners in Ireland. *Traffic Injury Prevention*, 16(6), 593–598.

Keall, M. D., & Frith, W. J. (2004). Older driver crash rates in relation to type and quantity of travel. *Traffic Injury Prevention*, 5(1), 26–36.

Keall, M. D., & Frith, W. J. (2006). Characteristics and risks of drivers with low annual distance driven. *Traffic Injury Prevention*, 7(3), 248–255.

Langford, J., Methorst, R., & Hakamies-Blomqvist, L. (2006). Older drivers do not have a high crash risk: A replication of low mileage bias. *Accident Analysis and Prevention*, 38, 574–578.

Langlois, J. A., Keyl, P. M., Guralnik, J. M., Foley, D. J., Marottoli, R. A., & Wallace, R. B. (1997). Characteristics of older pedestrians who have difficulty crossing the street. *American Journal of Public Health*, 87(3), 393–397.

Leroy, A. A., & Morse, M. L. (2008). *Multiple medications and vehicle crashes: Analysis of databases*. Report No. DOT HS 810 858. Washington, DC: National Highway Traffic Safety Administration.

Levy, B. R., Ng, R., Myers, L. M., & Marottoli, R. A. (2013). A psychological predictor of elders' driving performance: Social comparisons on the road. *Journal of Applied Social Psychology*, 43, 556–561.

Li, G., Braver, E. R., & Chen, L. (2003). Fragility versus excessive crash involvement as determinants of high death rates per vehicle-mile of travel among older drivers. *Accident Analysis and Prevention*, 35, 227–235.

Liddle, J., Haynes, M., Pachana, N. A., Mitchell, G., McKenna, K., & Gustafsson, L. (2014). Effect of a group intervention to promote older adults' adjustment to driving cessation on community mobility: A randomized controlled trial. *Gerontologist*, 54, 409–422.

Lyman, J. M., McGwin, G., & Sims, R. V. (2001). Factors related to driving difficulty and habits in older drivers. *Accident Analysis and Prevention*, 33(3), 413–421.

Lynott, J., McAuley, W. J., & McCutcheon, M. (2009). Getting out and about: The relationship between urban form and senior travel patterns. *Journal of Housing for the Elderly*, *23*, 390–402.

Man-Son-Hing, M., Marshall, S. C., Molnar, F. J., & Wilson, K. G. (2007). Systematic review of driving risk and the efficacy of compensatory strategies in persons with dementia. *Journal of the American Geriatrics Society*, *55*, 878–884.

Marin-Lamellet, C., & Haustein, S. (2015). Managing the safe mobility of older road users: How to cope with their diversity? *Journal of Transport and Health*, *2*(1), 22–31.

Marottoli, R. A., Allore, H., Araujo, K. L., Iannone, L. P., Acampora, D., Gottschalk, M.,… Peduzzi, P. (2007). A randomized trial of a physical conditioning program to enhance the driving performance of older persons. *Journal of General Internal Medicine*, *22*, 590–597.

Marottoli, R. A., Cooney, L. M., & Tinetti, M.E. (1997). Self-report versus state records for identifying crashes among older drivers. *Journal of Gerontology: Medical Sciences*, *52A*(3), M184–M187.

Marottoli, R. A., & Drickamer, M. A. (1993). Psychomotor mobility and the elderly driver. *Clinics in Geriatric Medicine*, *9*, 403–411.

Marottoli, R. A., Mendes de Leon, C. F., Glass, T. A., Williams, C. S., Cooney, L. M., & Berkman, L. F. (2000). Consequences of driving cessation: Decreased out-of-home activity levels. *Journal of Gerontology: Social Sciences*, *55B*, S334–S340.

Marottoli, R. A., Mendes de Leon, C. F., Glass, T. A., Williams, C. S., Cooney, L. M., Berkman, L. F., et al. (1997b). Driving cessation and increased depressive symptoms: Prospective evidence from the New Haven EPESE. *Journal of the American Geriatrics Society*, *45*, 202–206.

Marottoli, R. A., Ness, P. H., Araujo, K. L., Iannone, L. P., Acampora, D., Charpentier, P., & Peduzzi, P. (2007). A randomized trial of an education program to enhance older driver performance. *Journal of Gerontology, Serices A: Biological Sciences and Medical Sciences*, *62*(10), 1113–1119.

Marottoli, R. A., & Richardson, E. D. (1998). Confidence in and self-rating of driving ability among older drivers. *Accident Analysis and Prevention*, *30*(3), 331–336.

Marottoli, R. A., Richardson, E. D., Stowe, M. H., Miller, E. G., Brass, L. M., Cooney, L. M., Jr., & Tinetti, M. E. (1998). Development of a test battery to identify older drivers at risk for self-reported adverse driving events. *Journal of the American Geriatrics Society*, *46*, 562–568.

Marottoli, R. A., Wagner, D. R., Cooney, L. M., & Tinetti, M. E. (1994). Predictors of crashes and moving violations among elderly drivers. *Annals of Internal Medicine*, *121*, 842–846.

Mayhew, D. R., Simpson, H. M., & Ferguson, S. A. (2006). Collisions involving senior drivers: High-risk conditions and locations. *Traffic Injury Prevention*, *7*(2), 117–124.

McKnight, A. J., Simone, G., & Weldman, J. (1982). *Elderly driver retraining.* Report DOT HS-806 336. Washington, DC: National Highway Traffic Safety Administration.

Meuser, T. M., Carr, D. B., Irmiter, C., Schwartz, J. G., & Ulfarsson, G. F. (2010). The American Medical Association older driver curriculum for health professionals: Changes in trainee confidence, attitudes, and practice behavior. *Gerontology & Geriatrics Education*, *31*, 290–309.

Mezuk, B., & Rebok, G. W. (2008). Social integration and social support among older adults following driving cessation. *Journal of Gerontology: Social Sciences*, *63B*(S), S298–S303.

Mizenko, A. J., Tefft, B. C., Arnold, L. S., & Grabowski, J. (2014). *Older American drivers and traffic safety culture: A LongROAD study.* Washington, DC: AAA Foundation for Traffic Safety.

Nasvadi, G. E., & Vavrik, J. (2007). Crash risk of older drivers after attending a mature driver education program. *Accident Analysis and Prevention*, *39*(6),1073–1079.

NHTSA National Center for Statistics and Analysis. (2014). *Traffic safety facts: Older population.* DOT HS 812 005. Washington, DC: National Highway Traffic Safety Administration.

OECD International Transport Forum. (2012). *Pedestrian safety, urban space and health.* Paris, France: International Transport Forum, Organization for Economic Cooperation and Development.

O'Neill, D. (2012). More mad and more wise. *Accident Analysis and Prevention*, *49*, 263–265.

O'Neill, D. (2015). Transport, driving and ageing. *Reviews in Clinical Gerontology*, *25*(2), 147–158.

Owsley, C., & McGwin, G. (2010). Vision and driving. *Vision Research*, *50*, 2348–2361.

Owsley, C., McGwin, G., Sloane, M., Wells, J., Stalvey, B. T., & Gauthreaux, S. (2002). Impact of cataract surgery on motor vehicle crash involvement by older adults. *Journal of the American Medical Association*, *288*, 841–849.

Owsley, C., Stalvey, B. T., & Phillips, J. M. (2003). The efficacy of an educational intervention in promoting self-regulation among high risk-older drivers. *Accident Analysis and Prevention*, *35*, 393–400.

Palacio, A., Tamburro, G., O'Neill, D., & Simms, C. K. (2009). Non-collision injuries in urban buses—strategies for prevention. *Accident Analysis and Prevention*, *41*(1), 1–9.

Polders, E., Brijs, T., Vlahogianni, E., Papadimitriou, E., Yannis, G., & Leopold, F. (2015). *ElderSafe: Risks and countermeasures for road traffic of the elderly in Europe.* Brussels, Belgium: European Commission, Directorate-General for Mobility and Transport (DG-MOVE).

Ragland, D. R., Satariano, W. A., & MacLeod, K. E. (2005). Driving cessation and increased depressive symptoms. *Journal of Gerontology: Medical Sciences*, *60*(3), 399–403.

Redelmeier, D. A., Yarnell, C. J., Thiruchelvam, D., & Tibshirani, R. J. (2012). Physicians' warnings for unfit drivers and the risk of trauma from road crashes. *New England Journal of Medicine*, *367*(13), 1228–1236.

Reger, M. A., Welsh, R. K., Watson, G., Cholerton, B., Baker, L. D., & Craft, S. (2004). The relationship between neuropsychological functioning and driving ability in dementia: A meta-analysis. *Neuropsychology*, *18*(1), 85–93.

Road Safety Authority. (2014). *Medical fitness to drive guidelines* (3rd ed.). Dublin, Ireland: Author.

Roberts, S. E., Vingilis, E., Wilk, P., & Seeley, J. (2008). A comparison of self-reported motor vehicle collision injuries compared with official collision data: An analysis of age and sex trends using the Canadian National Population Health Survey and Transport Canada data. *Accident Analysis and Prevention*, *40*, 559–566.

Roenker, D. L., Cissell, G. M., Ball, K. K., Wadley, V. G., & Edwards, J. D. (2003). Speed-of-processing and driving simulator training result in improved driving performance. *Human Factors*, *45*, 218–233.

Rosenbloom, S., & Santos, R. (2014). *Understanding older drivers: An examination of medical conditions, medication use, and travel behavior*. Washington, DC: AAA Foundation for Traffic Safety.

Rosenbloom, T., Sapir-Lavid, Y., & Perlman, A. (2016). Risk factors in road crossing among elderly pedestrians and readiness to adopt safe behavior in socio-economic comparison. *Accident Analysis and Prevention*, *93*, 23–31.

Satariano, W. A., Guralnik, J. M., Jackson, R. J., Marottoli, R. A., Phelan, E. A., & Prohaska, T. R. (2012). Mobility and aging: New directions for public health. *American Journal of Public Health*, *102*(8), 1508–1515.

Scott, K. A., Rogers, E., Betz, M. E., Hoffecker, L., Li, G., & DiGiuseppi, C. (2016). *Association between falls and driving outcomes in older adults: A systematic review and meta-analysis*. Washington, DC: AAA Foundation for Traffic Safety.

Simms, C., & O'Neill, D. (2005). Sports utility vehicles and older pedestrians. *BMJ*, *331*(7520), 787–788.

Staplin, L., Lococco, K. H., Martell, C., & Stutts, J. (2012). *Taxonomy of older driver behaviors and crash risk*. DOT HS 811 468A. Washington, DC: National Highway Traffic Safety Administration.

Stern, R. A., D'Ambrosio, L. A., Mohyde, M., Carruth, A., Tracton-Bishop, B., Hunter, J. C.,… Coughlin, J. F. (2008). At the crossroads: Development and evaluation of a dementia caregiver group intervention to assist in driving cessation. *Gerontology and Geriatrics Education*, *29*, 363–382.

Strathman, J. G., Wachana, P., & Callas, S. (2010). Analysis of bus collision and non-collision incidents using transit ITS and other archived operations data. *Journal of Safety Research*, *41*(2), 137–144.

Tournier, I., Dommes, A., & Cavallo, V. (2016). Review of safety and mobility issues among older pedestrians. *Accident Analysis and Prevention*, *91*, 24–35.

Williams, A. F., & Carsten, O. (1989). Driver age and crash involvement. *American Journal of Public Health*, *79*, 326–327.

Wretstrand, A., Petzall, J., Bylund, P. O., & Falkmer, T. (2010). Reducing non-collision injuries in transportation services by enhanced safety culture. *Medical Engineering and Physics*, *32*(3), 254–262.

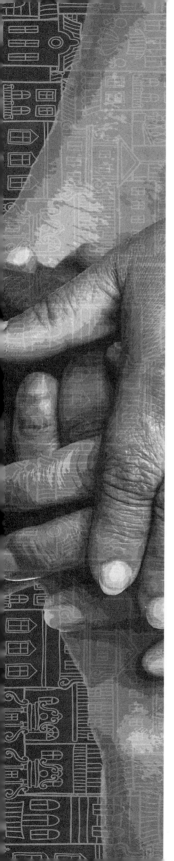

SECTION III

Conduct and Analysis

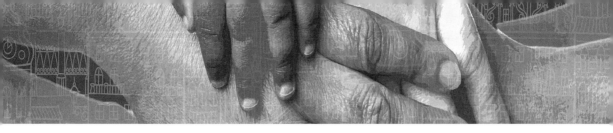

CHAPTER 12

Conducting International Epidemiological Studies of Aging

Afshin Vafaei, Nadia Minicuci, and **Maria Victoria Zunzunegui**

ABSTRACT

The objectives of this chapter are threefold: (1) to present the rationale for conducting international epidemiological studies and to explore the contribution of international epidemiological research to understanding human aging, (2) to describe the main objectives and design features of the most important current international epidemiological studies of aging, and (3) to provide practical suggestions for designing and conducting international epidemiological studies of aging, to discuss the main threats to their validity and ways to prevent them, and to consider ethical aspects specific to the conduct of international health research.

We conclude that the value of multicenter international population aging research depends on (1) the use of a single evidence-based conceptual framework in all sites, a life course perspective, valid designs, and measurement methods; (2) the ability for transferring knowledge to change local social structures, behaviors, and professional practices; and (3) research capacity building and the sustainability of collaborative research.

KEYWORDS

aging	longitudinal studies	international
epidemiological research	research capacity building	global health
surveys	knowledge transfer	

▶ Introduction

Population **aging** is a global phenomenon. It is expected that by 2050, the proportion of the world's population older than 60 years will reach 22%, double the proportion of approximately 11% in 2000. Translating that percentage into absolute numbers, there will be approximately 2 billion older adults by the middle of the 21st century (United Nations, 2009).

Globally, people older than age 60 years are the fastest-growing age group, and it is projected that by 2025 individuals age 65 and older will account for 10.4% of the world's population. Although the more developed regions will experience greater overall aging over that period, meaning that they will have a high percentage of older individuals (20.8%) as part of their total populations, less developed regions will also have to contend with larger shares of their populations consisting of older adults—specifically, an estimated 8.4% of their total populations (Rowland, 2012, pp. 7–8).

The two main reasons for this drastic demographic change are longer life expectancy and declining fertility rates. Both are a direct function of improvements in living conditions and, to a lesser extent, enhanced public health and medical care (Link & Phelan, 2002; McKeown, 1979).

Aging-related health issues such as mobility disability and cognition impairment are complex processes, and are best described through an ecological-social perspective (Bronfenbrenner, 1979; Krieger, 2001). This perspective is currently the dominant approach in epidemiological studies of aging and remains the most appropriate strategy for simultaneous consideration of multiple individual, cultural, social, economic, and physical contextual factors. Older adults have greater exposure to their immediate social and physical surroundings due to the longer duration they spend close to their place of residence as a result of age-related limitations in life space (Simon, Walsh, Regnier, & Krauss, 1992); hence, the vast majority of their environmental exposure takes place in their residential neighborhoods

(Windley & Scheidt, 2015). At the same time, upstream factors—culture, political and economic systems, and health and social welfare systems—are also important determinants of older adults' physical and mental health (World Health Organization [WHO], 2015). All of the aforementioned factors vary across countries and regions; thus, to provide a realistic picture of age-related issues and for a scientific study of aging, we need to obtain population samples from regions and countries with different cultural and socioeconomic backgrounds.

There is no shortage of epidemiological studies of aging, but most research of this kind has been conducted in developed countries, especially in Western Europe and North America. Studies from other regions are mostly conducted within a single country; **international** studies that include regions from very different geographical and cultural contexts are truly scarce.

This chapter has the following objectives:

■ To present the rationale for conducting international epidemiological studies and to explore the contributions of international **epidemiological research** to understanding human aging
■ To describe the main objectives and design features of the most important current international epidemiological studies of aging
■ To provide practical suggestions for designing and conducting international epidemiological studies of aging, to discuss the main threats to their validity and ways to prevent them from coming to fruition, and to consider ethical aspects specific to the conduct of international health research

▶ Rationale

Why Should We Conduct International Studies?

In terms of absolute numbers, the majority of older adults live in middle- and lower-income countries (MLICs), where living conditions differ greatly from those found in high-income countries. Compared to their counterparts in high-income countries, older adults in MLICs experience different and often more adverse life course conditions and generally are exposed to the ill effects of hostile environmental and social factors such as lack of access to clean water, food insecurity, conflicts and wars, and social, economic, and gender inequalities. Cross-sectional **surveys** and longitudinal international studies are needed to address these issues. Well-designed surveys with a focus on current health status and needs of older adults would be useful in devising health services policies and public health planning; however, cross-sectional data inherently are not able to establish causality and fail to describe the whole picture of the trajectory of health changes in older adults.

Longitudinal international studies should be conducted to describe these aging processes under different life course conditions. Such studies should also assess whether research findings from high-income countries are universal and applicable to populations in which aging happens in very diverse social, economic, and physical environments.

A wealth of scientific literature is available today through the Internet. However, studies conducted in different settings and by different research groups, despite having similar research questions, might adopt different measurement and analytic procedures. Although each of the individual studies might be valid on its own, the process of comparing and pooling their findings can lead to unreliable results due to the often substantial methodological inconsistencies in their conduct.

Multimorbidity—defined as the co-occurrence of at least two chronic conditions—is observed in two thirds of older adults (Marengoni et al., 2011). On a worldwide basis, this prevalence is expected to increase as the human population age. Some sources have suggested that patterns of multimorbidity vary across different countries. For example, using several international aging databases, Garin et al.

(2016) performed exploratory factor analyses to examine patterns of multimorbidity in various countries. They found very specific patterns of "metabolic-respiratory" multimorbidity in Russia and Finland, whereas the dominant pattern for other countries was "cardio-respiratory" multimorbidity. The only way to evaluate these important population health patterns is to perform international studies.

What Are the Contributions of International Studies to Science?

Life course studies suggest that the way populations and individuals age depends on the physical and social context where they live. To date, most aging studies have been conducted in high-income countries in Western Europe, North America, Japan, Australia, or New Zealand. Considering the life course perspective, would it be valid to extend the aging process–related information obtained from these studies to middle-income countries such as Brazil, India, and Russia or to other low-income countries with rapidly aging populations? Is it reasonable to suggest that social and physical environmental exposures during the life course are so different that population studies findings from wealthy countries would not be valid for populations in more deprived settings? What about those areas of the world (e.g., sub-Saharan Africa) where life expectancy is lower than 60 years of age—is there really an "aging process" in effect in these regions? Is it even possible to study "aging" in countries that have not yet entered into the epidemiological transition? Well-designed and well-conducted longitudinal international studies can provide evidence to answer these scientific questions.

In addition to differential "aging processes" being noted in different parts of the world, "age-related health issues" may potentially vary across societies. Older adults in developed countries are more likely to suffer from chronic and degenerative conditions such as coronary heart diseases, osteoarthritis, and Alzheimer's disease; in contrast, in less developed regions, complications from nutritional deficits and infectious diseases (e.g., malaria) remain major population health concerns. International epidemiological studies can evaluate different age-related health issues across societies, address each issue accordingly, and suggest appropriate region-specific social and health policies.

Studying international populations of older adults within a single platform also provides very specific methodological advantages in terms of the measurement of variables and analysis approaches. First, use of international data collected via the same measurement approaches expands the range of values for exposures and health outcomes. As an illustration, consider the associations between inflammation and physical function. In an international study, the distribution of inflammation biomarkers will cover a wide range, since the mean of those distributions will vary from a higher end in LMICs to a lower end in high-income countries. The same is true for physical function, for which values will be lower in LMICs and higher in high-income countries. This widening of the range of distributions allows for examination of the associations of interest along a complete range of plausible biological values. Benefits include increased power of the statistical models and reduced risk that selection bias will be introduced by examining truncated samples of exposures and outcomes that include mostly less-exposed persons and those with better health outcomes.

Second, wide ranges for social factors allow testing for the heterogeneity of associations between exposures and health outcomes according to social and cultural characteristics (i.e., testing for interaction effects of specific social factors such as social networks, social support, and multigenerational households).

Third, access to international data at different measurement levels provides opportunities to examine cross-level interactions between individual-level variables such as social networks, neighborhood-level variables such as social capital, and country-level factors such as economic security through old age pensions. People live in hierarchical aggregate levels that are nested within each other, ranging from small geographical areas such as neighborhoods up to larger contexts of states and countries. According to ecological-social models (Bronfenbrenner, 1979; Krieger, 2001), the specific impact of each aggregate level should be recognized. Adopting multistage sampling design allows for collection of pertinent data at all levels. Multilevel analysis—a sophisticated data analysis procedure that is now feasible to perform with most standard statistical packages—can simultaneously estimate independent effects of variables at each level and test for interactions between the contextual and individual characteristics to further explore the etiology of age-related health processes.

▶ Design Features of Current Epidemiological Studies in Aging

There are few ongoing international studies on aging. Most of these studies are designed explicitly to answer specific research questions through panel surveys or longitudinal designs. Examples of questions that can be explored and answered by international studies include:

- How does exposure to domestic violence throughout the life course increase the risk of poor health and function in the old age?
- How does reproductive history influence physical and cognitive function in old age?
- How do gender roles, norms, and identities influence health behaviors and mobility?

- What are the effects of social networks and social support on adverse health outcomes in old age?
- How do "neighborhoods" affect the health and functioning of older adults? Do the "neighborhood effects" on the physical and cognitive function of older populations vary across geographical and cultural settings?
- What is "normal aging"? Does the weakness associated with aging have the same definition everywhere? For instance, are cut-off points for muscle weakness universal?
- How does reproductive history in women affect their physical function in old age?
- How is healthcare access related to diagnosis and control of chronic diseases across different healthcare systems?
- How are socioeconomic inequalities related to medical drug prescriptions across different healthcare systems?

No single study could possibly answer all of these questions. Instead, different types of studies might be performed to address them. In this section, we present four examples of international studies. The first two are examples of "general health" population health studies, which cover a wide range of mostly chronic and common health issues; the next two are examples of international aging studies with a focus on a "single condition." This section concludes with a description of a post hoc harmonization study, SAGE+, which is a very good example of how results obtained from different studies conducted in different settings can be compared and how valid conclusions can be derived.

Survey of Health, Ageing, and Retirement

The Survey of Health, Ageing, and Retirement (SHARE; http://www.share-project.org/) is a multidisciplinary and cross-national panel database of health, socioeconomic status, and social and family networks microdata from approximately 110,000 individuals aged 50 or older from 20 European countries[1] from Scandinavia to the Mediterranean and Israel. Since its inception in 2004, five data collection waves have been implemented. The fieldwork of the latest wave of SHARE was completed in November 2013.

The design of SHARE reflects Europe's cultural and institutional diversity. The study's focus is those social, economic, and demographic conditions throughout the life course that have an impact on quality of life and general well-being of older populations; however, general information about health status and health behavior is also available. Although some more specific measurements such as "grip strength" are conducted as part of SHARE, physical performance tests needed for valid measurement of mobility status are very limited. At the time of this text's writing, blood and saliva samples results were not available. SHARE follows a dynamic approach and includes new participant countries and adds more variables in each wave. For example, new items on social exclusion and new modules on early childhood conditions and computer utilization at work were added to the latest wave of 2013.

World Health Organization's Study on Global Ageing and Adult Health

WHO's Study on Global Ageing and Adult Health (SAGE; http://www.who.int/healthinfo /sage/en) is a longitudinal panel study conducted in China, Ghana, India, Mexico, Russian Federation, and South Africa on nationally representative samples of the population aged 50 years and older and with a smaller cohort

---

1. Austria, Belgium, Czech Republic, Denmark, Estonia, France, Germany, Greece, Hungary, Ireland, Israel, Italy, Luxemburg, the Netherlands, Poland, Portugal, Slovenia, Spain, Sweden, and Switzerland.

of respondents aged 18–49 for comparison purposes. SAGE was developed by WHO's Evidence, Measurement, and Analysis unit as part of an ongoing program of work to compile comprehensive longitudinal information on the health and well-being of adult populations and the aging process.

During 2002–2004, WHO coordinated the World Health Survey (WHS), a health interview survey in 70 countries of adults aged 18 years or older, including the six SAGE countries. The WHS samples were drawn from a current national sampling frame using a stratified, multistage cluster design. Pooling the data from the six SAGE countries resulted in 18,883 respondents aged 50 and older and 44,554 respondents aged 18–49 years; this sample is referred to as SAGE Wave 0.

SAGE Wave 1 was carried out during 2007–2010; China used a new sampling frame for Wave 1 and South Africa decided not to follow up Wave 0 respondents for Wave 1. Households were classified into one of two mutually exclusive categories: (1) all persons aged 50 years and older were selected from households classified as "50+ households"; and (2) one person aged 18–49 years was selected from a household classified as an "18–49 household." Wave 1 included 34,124 respondents aged 50 and older and 8340 respondents aged 18–49 years; interviews were completed either with a computer-aided personal interview (CAPI) or using paper and pencil. Wave 2 data collection (2014–2015) has been completed in all six countries and data quality control is now being performed. Wave 3 will be implemented in the near future.

In the SAGE program, household-level analysis weights and person-level analysis weights have been calculated for each country, which include sample selection and a post stratification factor. The focus of SAGE is on health and health-related outcomes and their determinants, with an explicit aim to enhance cross-population comparability especially in lower- and middle-income countries. Standardized survey instruments, methods, interviewer training, and translation protocols are used across all SAGE countries.

SAGE modules involve a "household questionnaire" consisting of a household roster and modules about the dwelling, income, transfers in and out of the household, assets, and expenditures; an "individual questionnaire" with modules on health and its determinants, disability, work history, risk factors, chronic conditions, caregiving, subjective well-being, healthcare utilization, and health systems responsiveness; a "proxy questionnaire" about health, functioning, chronic conditions, and healthcare utilization; and a "verbal autopsy module questionnaire" to ascertain the probable cause of death for deaths in the household in the 24 months prior to the interview or between interview waves. In addition, SAGE Wave 1 included anthropometric measurements, blood pressure measures and a blood sample via finger prick, and performance tests including near and distant vision, a timed 4-m walk, grip strength, lung function, and cognition. SAGE also includes two substudies: (1) SAGE-INDEPTH, which is a network of local longitudinal demographic surveillance studies in 19 countries in Africa, Asia, America, and Oceania and (2) SAGE-HIV (Kowal et al., 2012).

The 10/66 Dementia Research Group

The 10/66 Dementia Research Group (http://www.alz.co.uk/1066/) is a collective of 30 research groups in 20 countries in Latin America, the Caribbean, India, Russia, China, and Southeast Asia carrying out population-based research on dementia, noncommunicable diseases, and aging in low- and middle-income countries. This research project is notable because of its population-based approach and its exclusive focus on low- and middle-income countries. The title of the study comes from two statistical facts: Two-thirds (66%) of all people with dementia live in low- and middle-income countries, but only 10% or less of population-based research studies are being carried out in those regions.

The main objectives of the 10/66 Dementia Research Group's study were to estimate the annual incidence rates of dementia and its subtypes by age group, education, and center, as well as to investigate risk factors for incident dementia, particularly cardiovascular and nutritional risk factors. This focused and well-designed study had two main phases: a prevalence phase (in 2006–2007) and an incidence phase (2.5–3 years later). One notable strength of this study was the development and validation of a novel approach for diagnosing dementia (the 10/66 Dementia Diagnosis) that addresses difficulties in making diagnoses among older people with little or no education. This feat was achieved in the pilot phase of the study.

To address the issue of caregiver burden in countries with resource-limited healthcare systems, a randomized controlled trial of a caregiver education and training intervention was also conducted in Russia, India, Venezuela, Peru, Dominican Republic, and China.

The work of the 10/66 Dementia Research Group is a good example of an international population-based epidemiological study with a focus on a single condition. As conceptualized by the researchers, studying risk factors for dementia in developing low- and middle-income countries will help in planning future targeted prevention strategies in these regions, as well as possibly provide new insights into risk factors that were not apparent from research that was limited to populations in developed countries with higher socioeconomic status (SES), and in the case of some northern European countries, with fairly homogenous lifestyles and predominately Caucasian populations.

International Mobility in Aging Study

International Mobility in Aging Study (IMIAS) is a prospective cohort study of community-dwelling older adults between 64 and 75 years of age conducted in five locations: Kingston (Ontario, Canada), Saint-Hyacinthe (Quebec, Canada), Tirana (Albania), Manizales (Colombia), and Natal (Brazil) (Zunzunegui et al., 2015). To the best of our knowledge, this is the only study comparing aging both in high-income (Canada) and middle-income countries (Albania, Brazil, Colombia). The conceptual base of IMIAS is grounded on ecological-social and life course perspectives and is similar to that employed by the 10/66 Dementia Research Group; that is, IMIAS follows a single condition focus and collects data on all aspects and risk factors predicting mobility disability. Explaining the variations in mobility disability rates between men and women constitutes the main objective of the study. Four main factors have been hypothesized to explain the gender gap in mobility: lifetime exposures to domestic violence, poverty, social isolation, and physical inactivity. In addition, women's reproductive history—in particular, adolescent childbirth—is hypothesized to impact physical function and mobility in old age through multiple social and biological mechanisms. Including five samples from older adults of four countries with different socioeconomic, built-environment, and cultural characteristics enables the researchers to also study the possible interaction effects of these factors on the occurrence of mobility disability. This longitudinal study was funded by the Canadian Institutes of Health Research for three waves during a six-year period; data collection for waves 1 and 2 was completed in 2012 and 2014, respectively, and the 2016 wave is ongoing. Data are collected by personal interviews conducted at homes. The questionnaire includes socioeconomic conditions, social integration, neighborhood characteristics, chronic health conditions, and behaviors. Levels of cognition, vision acuity, height, weight, and physical performance status are evaluated via standard tools. Blood samples were collected at baseline and analyzed for metabolic and inflammatory biomarkers. Saliva samples to assess cortisol diurnal variation were also collected in a subsample.

Before implementation of the main study, pilot studies were conducted in Quebec (Canada), Brazil, and Colombia to validate the measurement tools in local languages and with diverse populations (Freire, Guerra, Alvarado, Guralnik, & Zunzunegui, 2012; Gomez, Zunzunegui, Lord, Alavarado, & Garcia, 2013; Vafaei et al., 2014).

SAGE-Plus: A Post Hoc Harmonization Study

The availability of studies with similar methodologies and with comparable constructs and variables is critical to address questions related to postulated variations in population health within and across countries. Some studies have used similar methodologies and span a range of low-, middle-, and high-income countries; have large sample sizes; and include topics from health-related domains such as healthcare utilization and expenditures, well-being, social networks, and quality of life. In contrast, studies that use an ex-ante harmonization approach to allow valid comparisons across populations remain limited. COURAGE (Collaborative Research on Ageing in Europe) in Europe—a study carried out in Finland, Poland, and Spain (Leonardi et al., 2014)—and the Survey on Health, Well-Being, and Aging in Latin America and the Caribbean (Albala et al., 2005) are two rare examples. Few papers, however, have addressed the issue of the ex-post harmonization of aging studies. One of the first attempts to harmonize **longitudinal studies** on aging was made by Minicuci et al. (2003) using data from five European countries (Finland, Italy, the Netherlands, Spain, Sweden) and Israel.

The main goal of the ex-post harmonization process is to create a database that conceptually includes the same domains with the same measurement units, thereby allowing cross-country comparisons based on either cultural issues or regional policies and, most likely, both. This database may provide sorely needed information for developing public policy and highlights intervention areas where each country could improve its own situation by borrowing from other countries' health policies.

SAGE-Plus (SAGE+) is part of WHO's Study on Global Ageing and Adult Health (SAGE) effort to improve measurement strategies and comparability across large aging-related studies. SAGE+ includes SAGE, the English Longitudinal Study on Aging, (ELSA), the U.S.-based Health and Retirement Study (HRS), and the Survey of Health, Ageing, and Retirement in Europe (SHARE). Each of these individual studies is longitudinal in nature, and SAGE+ generates a harmonized secondary data resource that is available for cross-national and cross-study analyses.

Baseline SAGE+ includes 77,287 adults aged 50 years and older from SAGE, Wave 0 (2004, $n = 18,886$); ELSA, Wave 2 (2004, $n = 9181$); HRS, Wave 7 (2004, $n = 19,303$); and SHARE, Wave 1 (2004, $n = 29,917$). Follow-up SAGE+ includes 123,128 adults aged 50 years and older from SAGE, Wave 1 (2010, $n = 35,145$); ELSA, Wave 5 (2010, $n = 10,095$); HRS, Wave 10 (2010, $n = 21,034$); and SHARE, Wave 4 (2010, $n = 56,854$).

The process of harmonizing variables across this range of surveys was built upon established procedures. The first step included documenting the study design and the variables collected for each study; the second step determined the harmonizable domains and the group of core variables targeted for the domains; the third step addressed data processing, where harmonizable variables were constructed either with precisely common variables that made the pooling quite straightforward or with heterogeneous variables that required decisions for their definition and categorization; and the last step assessed data quality using statistical indicators.

Harmonized variables have been categorized into nine domains:

- Sociodemographic and economic: sex, age, marital status, living arrangements, educational level, occupation, and age at retirement.
- Health states describing physical functioning: activities of daily living (ADLs), instrumental activities of daily living (IADLs), mobility (described as functioning in a number of ADL/IADL-type questions), near vision, distance vision, hearing, and pain.
- Overall self-reported of health and mental state: self-reported health, cognition /memory, depression, sleep, and loneliness.
- Health examinations: blood pressure measures.
- Physical and mental performance tests: normal-pace walking test, rapid-pace walking test, grip strength, cognition /memory tests.
- Risk factors: body mass index, tobacco consumption, alcohol consumption, and physical activity.
- Chronic conditions: self-reported chronic conditions and disease treatments.
- Social network: social network index.
- Subjective well-being: Quality of life, life satisfaction, and well-being.

A main strength of harmonized data sets is the large sample size achieved and the increased power that allows for more robust and reliable analyses. However, when interpreting ex-post harmonization findings for the purpose of cross-country comparisons, the different response rates should be taken into account. Observed differences in self-reported health status are also difficult to interpret because this measurement may reflect social and cultural biases and the availability and accessibility of health services, which differs for high-income countries versus low- and middle-income countries. However, self-rated

health remains a valid measure of physical function and health within populations (Perez-Zepeda et al., 2016).

▶ Design Features of Epidemiological Aging Studies

In this section, after a short review of the main design features of epidemiological studies on aging, we will explore some of the specific issues related to international studies.

Types of Epidemiological Studies of Aging

On a broad scale, epidemiological studies may be classified into two main groups: experimental studies and observational studies. Due to ethical and feasibility issues, experimental studies or randomized controlled trials are rarely used in population health research.

The main types of observational studies include cross-sectional, case-control, and cohort studies. In cross-sectional studies, all variables are collected at the same time, mostly via survey methodologies. Cross-sectional studies are relatively inexpensive and easy to perform, and usually researchers have the opportunity to collect data from a large sample of population. Data from cross-sectional aging studies provide invaluable information about prevalence of and burdens imposed by diseases, diseases' distribution according to socioeconomic factors, and their associations with health behaviors, all of which can be used to assess needs for health and social services and to guide health policy. The main weakness of cross-sectional studies stems from their inability to establish causality due to lack of a temporal sequence in data collection.

A case-control design is a very efficient approach for studying rare outcomes and disease outbreaks. Since most health issues in older adults are chronic, degenerative, and common, however, case-control studies are seldom suitable for population aging studies.

Longitudinal studies have the best design features for examining the human aging process. In longitudinal studies, a group of people (a cohort) are followed for a period of time and changes in their health status are evaluated longitudinally. In theory, the optimal situation for aging research is to follow a "birth cohort," assessing the members of this group throughout their lives at prescheduled intervals. While this is the best way to obtain the whole picture of the impact of all life course adversities on health, in practice it is seldom possible. Instead, most aging studies employ a short-term longitudinal design, particularly when the objective is to look at a specific disease that biologically can develop in that time period. For example, IMIAS examines the mobility and physical function trajectories of men and women recruited from five populations of community-dwelling 65- to 75-year-old adults followed for four years—a period in which, according to the literature (Zunzunegui, Nunez, Durban, Garcia de Yebenes, & Otero, 2006), the mobility status of this age group changes substantially. Most recent population aging studies have also sought to collect retrospective information on early life, since it is now generally accepted that health and function in old age are determined by early-life conditions and then modified by socioeconomic status and health behaviors during adolescence and adulthood. Adverse early-life experiences have been classified into two major groups: economic adversities (e.g., poverty, hunger, parental unemployment) and social adversities (e.g., being physically abused, witnessing family violence, and being in a family with alcohol or illegal drugs abuse). Early-life adversities have been shown to affect levels of inflammation (Li et al., 2015) and are associated with poor physical function (Sousa et al., 2014) in old age.

General Features of a Proper Cohort Study for International Aging Research

Population

Choosing and recruiting the most appropriate populations for a cohort study is the most crucial, yet most challenging initial step of such an investigation. If research questions must be examined in a full range of exposures and outcomes, or if the context (either the physical environment or cultural characteristics) seems to be an important factor affecting the relationship of interest, then different settings should be considered for data collection. For example, if researchers are interested in studying the pattern of diabetes development in older adults, they must recognize that dietary behaviors are important determinants of diabetes and that the diet is a function of both SES and culture; thus, to provide a wide range of all exposures, samples from different cultures are needed. The challenge probably will be finding research institutes that are willing to participate in countries with those cultures.

Sampling

The process of sampling—including development of the sampling frame, sample selection strategies, and sample size calculation—is the same for international aging studies as for other epidemiological studies. Details of these procedures are beyond the scope of this text, but can be found in most standard epidemiology textbooks. Representativeness of samples means that the study sample correctly demonstrates the basic characteristics of the base population to which results are intended to be inferred. Researchers need to define those base populations at the local (city), region, or country level. To obtain a truly representative sample, the best strategy is to perform a multistage sampling scheme with proper weights from an available list of individuals within a population (Statistics Canada, 2003). However, sampling lists are sometimes not available to researchers due to restrictions imposed by local ethics review boards and because of a lack of census-level data in some international settings.

Follow-up

Length of follow-up, the required numbers of follow-ups, and follow-up intervals all depend on the natural history of the outcome of interest and should be established while planning the study design. As a general rule, the follow-up time should be long enough to allow for measurable changes to occur in the health status of healthy individuals. Relevant literature needs to be consulted to understand the natural history of the disease of interest as well as to select reasonable values for the rates of the study exposure(s) and outcome(s). The required sample size can be calculated using this information under several assumptions.

Data Collection Procedures

The key issue in data collection in international studies is consistency across research sites. Providing instructive procedure manuals in local languages, training field staff at the beginning and during field work, and monitoring the collected data are needed to ensure high-quality data are obtained. Performing pilot studies to validate instruments across societies and to assess acceptability of measurement tools can help to identify potential problems and facilitate troubleshooting before the main study begins. These efforts will increase the validity and efficiency of the study.

Choice of Measures: Reliability and Validity Considerations

Measurement strategies should be inexpensive, easy to understand, and feasible to perform. Assessment of the inter-rater reliability or across-sites reliability of the measures, preferably via pilot studies, merits consideration. Most measurement tools and scales are typically validated during the initial stages of scale development; however, because validity is a context-related attribute, measures need to be validated in the language and context where the research will be conducted, independent of the original validation studies (Streiner, 2014).

Consideration of the Context

Most health outcomes depend on the physical and social environment, or the context, where the population resides. Context may refer either to the residential place, such as a neighborhood, or to the wider physical and social environment. The etiologies of most age-related health issues are best described by hierarchical ecological-social models in which "context" plays a crucial role at different levels.

Ethical Issues

Collaborations among researchers from different countries with different types of research facilities, capabilities, and histories bring up new ethical issues. Researchers from high-income countries can facilitate capacity building in research methods for other researchers by keeping those partners informed about all aspects of the study. Interviewers and researchers are required to respect the human rights of all participating subjects and to obtain their informed consent. Involvement of related ethics board committees for proper review of ethical issues should be considered at the design stage and may result in important modifications of the study protocols.

For instance, ethics requirements in Canada often limit the possibility of issuing direct invitations to participate in population research projects. That is, researchers can invite subjects to participate only through a third party—for instance, their primary care doctor. This particular requirement may affect the response rate of the study and introduce a potential selection bias, as the decision to participate in the study might be related to participants' exposure or outcome status, given that participants are already "patients." Such ethical considerations may extend to the period after conducting the research.

Analytic Strategies

Analysis of longitudinal data and evaluation of changes in the health status of individuals over time provide a better epidemiological understanding of the aging process. Statistical techniques that perform survival (time to event) analysis by estimating incidence rates suggest a higher level of evidence is achieved with etiology and mixed model analyses that account for within-individual correlations. However, these techniques are relatively complex and require advanced levels of statistical expertise to conduct. Plans for training of staff may need to be considered if these strategies will be employed.

Selection Bias

In longitudinal studies, selection bias may be introduced by low participation rates at the inception of the cohort and/or by high attrition during follow-up. This bias applies only when initial participation or attrition is associated with both the exposure *and* the outcome of the study. In contrast, if the probability of participation is not simultaneously associated with the exposure and the outcome under consideration, selection bias will *not* be possible. What makes the issue of selection bias in international studies more complex is the possibility that various sources for selection bias might exist in different research sites. Strategies to minimize selection bias should be adopted and implemented in both the design and data collection phases.

Specific (Practical) Aspects of Establishing, Managing, and Maintaining International Cohorts of Older Adults

This section focuses on specific logistic and practical aspects of the design and conduct of epidemiological studies in the context of international longitudinal research.

Establishment of the Cohorts

The first step in establishing a cohort for an epidemiological study to be carried out on an international scale is to identify local research teams with interests in both aging and population health research. Inviting additional experts from other disciplines that are directly or indirectly related to factors influencing aging for consultation will improve the quality of the research. For example, because knowing the health policies in effect at local levels will help the researchers better understand the trajectory of aging, consulting local health policy experts is a logical initial step. In addition, sources of local institutional support (e.g., universities and other academic centers, research institutions, local city governing bodies) need to be identified at each research site.

Before collecting data for the main study, researchers may need to perform some pilot studies to ensure the validity of scales in all study settings and to evaluate the feasibility of administering the questionnaires. Extra funding may be required for pilot studies.

In close collaboration with the other involved parties, to secure necessary funding and to clarify all steps of conducting the research, the principal investigator then writes a research protocol for the main study and applies for funding. Next administrative steps involve establishment of scientific and publication committees, preparing a board of international advisors, and signing agreements with local institutions to ensure a sustainable local support for the study at all centers.

Manuals of procedures and standardized questionnaires should be prepared in the local languages and validated via back-translation methodology by bilingual researchers. Local research staff should receive standard training in their native languages before data collection is undertaken in each wave, and regular quality control measures should be adopted during study data collection.

The required sample size should be precisely calculated according to the main outcome of the study. A too-small size may leave the study underpowered, whereas a too-large size might make it inefficient and unnecessarily expensive. In practice, different strategies may be adopted at different settings for sample size calculations.

Reasons that potential participants might refuse to participate in a health research study will vary at different locations. Therefore, recruitment strategies should be developed locally, while considering the cultural and socioeconomic setting, and methods to obtain a high response rate should be modified accordingly.

Cohort Maintenance

A major issue in longitudinal studies is loss to follow-up. For various reasons, participants may leave the study and decide not to participate in the next waves. Reasons for loss to follow-up in older adults include transfer to a nursing home, moving to another city to be closer to relatives, and health issues such as cognitive decline, health deterioration, and death. In the design stage, researchers should establish a system for tracking cohort dynamics. As a non-exhaustive list, we recommend the following steps: collecting next-of-kin information, accessing neighborhood clinic information, tracking home visits, and using electronic and postal mail to stay in touch with participants. In addition, planning and conducting knowledge transfer activities for the community from which participants come not only will keep local residents informed about the study, but also involve community organizations in the study and gain the support of local health professionals.

Long-Term Collaborative International Research and Research Capacity Building: Publication Policy

After completing a longitudinal study, there will be plenty of opportunities for producing science, presenting etiological results, and writing journal articles and reports. Local research teams are responsible for providing an environment fostering **research capacity building** at their local institutions and for ensuring that students at master's, doctoral, and post-doctoral levels will have opportunities for training and scientific exchange activities. A clear publication and authorship policy should be established for all scientific results obtained from the research according to the local ethical requirements and intellectual property laws.

Organizational Aspects, Interactions, and Communication

Managing international studies is not an easy task. People who work far from each other may easily lose interest in the collaborative work and shift their focus to their other responsibilities. The principal investigator(s) should establish a system for facilitating communication between researchers and team members. One effective strategy is to hold preplanned general meetings at regular intervals (at least yearly). Construction of a user-friendly website containing easy-to-access tabs for research results, information about research, the utilized methodology, and links to published papers will help in knowledge translation activities and help researchers stay in close touch with their partners.

Ethical Aspects of International Longitudinal Studies: Knowledge Transfer, Research Capacity Building, and Collaborative Research

Knowledge transfer activities and collaborative research pose important ethical challenges that need to be addressed in **global health** research. Issues related to governability and relationships of trust between researchers, community involvement, and participative research need to be considered in the planning and conducting phases of the research. This is particularly important in international research, which generally includes teams from low-, middle-, and high-income countries. Due to the historical and profound power imbalance among those countries, researchers from high-income countries have more financial and professional resources at their disposal than researchers from middle- and low-income countries. This inequality of resources with which to produce research often leads to a power imbalance among researchers on an international scale, which is particularly evident in the hegemonic position of North American science. In addition, high-income countries tend to act as "science vacuum-cleaners," absorbing scientists from medium- and low-income countries and stripping those countries of their "better brains," who might otherwise locally develop science and train younger individuals at local universities. International research teams should try to avoid this migration of scientists from the scientific South to the scientific North. Instead, they should aim to construct long-term cooperative relationships based on mutual trust, moving away from unethical competitiveness under conditions of imbalanced power and creating the conditions needed to develop locally relevant research.

Interpretation of the Results of International Studies: Special Methodological Issues and Lessons from Prior Studies

The main goal of epidemiological studies is to identify the etiologies behind the occurrence of health outcomes. Survival bias—a type of selection bias in which healthier individuals who are more resistant to life course adversities are more likely to reach older ages and, therefore, to be selected into aging studies—is an issue in all longitudinal aging studies, but its identification and interpretation is more complicated in international studies. People remaining in a cohort over time are increasingly the healthier people and those who have suffered fewer hazardous exposures. This bias tends to lead to underestimation of the strength of the associations between social and economic adversities over the life course and health status in old age.

Comparing the association between the APOE ε4 allele and Alzheimer's disease across two populations of older African American adults residing in Indianapolis, Indiana, and Nigeria, who participated in the Ibadan study

---

PEARL 12-1 International Research on Population Aging

International research on population aging is needed to increase our understanding of the aging process across different social and physical environments. Some international studies on aging are ongoing, and post-harmonization efforts have produced a database that includes data from high-, middle-, and low-income countries. International epidemiological researchers involved in such efforts need to consider specific challenges, such as sharing of a common conceptual framework, validity of measurement instruments, and ethical aspects involved in knowledge transfer, capacity building, and collaborative research.

Researchers involved in international epidemiological research should pursue research capacity building—that is, "a systematic, purposeful, and goal-oriented effort to strengthen human resources and infrastructure to enable local scientists and institutions to become independent and responsive to existing and emerging health needs and threats" (Pang et al., 2003). Capacity building at the individual level requires not just intensive training on scientific methods, but also career guidance and teaching and ethical principles for research and practice (Cottler, Zunt, Weiss, Kamal, & Vaddiparti, 2015). This kind of individual capacity building needs to be supported by institutional capacity building. Establishing an administrative foundation at the national level provides for both planning and sustainability, and offers opportunities to construct international collaborative research networks (Cash-Gibson, Guerra, & Salgado-de-Snyder, 2015).

(Oye, 2009), provides a good example of how survival bias might occur. The association between the APOE ε4 allele—a known and well-documented risk factor for Alzheimer's disease (Reitz et al., 2013)—was observed only in the United States (Hendrie et al., 2014). The failure to find this association in Nigeria can be explained by the potential existence of survival bias. According to the United Nations, life expectancy in Nigeria for persons born in 1950–1954 (first time it was estimated) was 34 years; it is reasonable to assume life expectancy was even lower for persons in 1940. Those people in Nigeria who lived until 60–70 years of age and were able to be part of the Ibadan study were more likely to be of higher socioeconomic status; to have better education, diet, and health behaviors; and to have fewer stressful life events. In summary, they likely represent a healthier cross section of the population and, therefore, were less likely to develop Alzheimer's disease anyway.

Another direct example of survival bias can be seen in the IMIAS cohorts. The life expectancy of the IMIAS Brazilian cohort (born in the years 1938–1947) located at Natal (northeast Brazil) was 34 years—almost 10 years less than Brazil's national-level life expectancy of 43 years for the same birth cohort. Life expectancy in Canada, another IMIAS site, was almost twice that for the Natal cohort: For those Canadians born between 1940 and 1942, life expectancy was 63 years for men and 66 years for women (Statistics Canada, 2003). Therefore, compared to Canadians, the Brazilian cohort of the IMIAS is composed of the most resilient members of this generation. The survival effect would explain the lack of significant associations between life course adversity and health and physical function outcomes in the Natal cohort, in contrast with the strong and significant associations found in the Canadian cohorts. As noted by Willson et al. (2007), despite the established fact that multiple dimensions of SES resources and lifetime economic history are related to health disparities as people age, researchers should

be cautious when interpreting data from people of old ages because of the disproportionate attrition and mortality of those with low SES.

Another methodological challenge is the presence of substantial differences in social and economic living conditions across settings. Socioeconomic factors are fundamental causes of health outcomes (Link & Phelan, 2002; Phelan, Link, & Tehranifar, 2010), and they need to be considered as background upstream factors driving the etiological process, and managed as potential confounders, effect modifiers, or mediators in etiological research. When interpreting the results of international studies, the impact of differential socioeconomic factors should be taken into account; however, the meaning of categories of socioeconomic indicators may be very different across societies. As an illustration, literacy level (being able to read and write) in some older adult cohorts is low. In northeastern Brazil, one of the settings of the IMIAS, the literacy level of the study cohort including people born between 1938 and 1947 was as low as 27%, almost 60% of the national level (for Brazil in that decade) of 43%. While comparing levels of health issues to educational levels for this population to the much better educated population of Canadians, the extreme categories of education may have very few observations, leading to a lack of precision in estimates of health outcomes for those participants at the extremes (i.e., illiteracy and university education).

▶ Conclusion and Future Directions

International aging researchers would be wise to keep these questions in mind while designing and conducting an aging research:

- What might be the most important global questions about health and function of older adults, and how they can be addressed by population health international research?

- How can international partners (academia and research institutions), international organizations (e.g., United Nations, WHO, International Labor Organization), and international donors and charities (e.g., Bill and Melinda Gates Foundation, nongovernmental associations such as Help Age) get involved in developing the research agenda on human aging in a constructive way?

- How can researchers mobilize local resources to encourage local health professionals and older adults to take part in the research and knowledge translation activities so that they can produce locally relevant research?

International researchers should jointly formulate and examine hypotheses that explore how the economic and social context influence the physical functioning and mental health of older populations. Organizing international workshops to design conceptual frameworks that integrate biological, economic, psychological, and social aspects of aging and facilitating consortia to fund such research projects in specific regions are two examples of these kinds of collaborations. Such broad approaches require an interdisciplinary approach. Nevertheless, because of lack of pertinent interest groups within funding agencies, interdisciplinary projects are less likely to get funded compared to more focused projects.

Some efforts are being made to pool international population-based data so that it will be available to interested researchers. One example is the Gateway to Global Aging Data (https://g2aging.org/index.php?section=homepage), a platform for population survey data on aging from around the world. This platform provides a digital library of searchable survey items that help researchers find comparable questions across surveys. Most countries contributing data to this project are high-income countries, but there are also data from middle-income countries such as Mexico, Indonesia, Costa Rica, and India. Another notable

platform is Maelstrom Research (https://www.maelstrom-research.org/), which has brought together an international team of epidemiologists, statisticians, and computer scientists to propose data harmonization tools and data sharing models. The ultimate goal is facilitation of collaborative epidemiological research.

In the following list, we provide a few examples of potential research projects that are feasible to conduct through international collaborations:

- Examination of pathways through which diseases result in disability using identical conceptual frameworks in different contexts.

- Establishment of evidence-based links between universal healthcare accessibility, universal old-age pensions, and opportunities for active aging by cross-country analyses, similar to what has been done in the SHARE study within European countries (Borsch-Supan et al., 2013).

- Collection of new data when needed to test new and innovative hypotheses in response to new challenges the populations face. Examples include studying the impact of climate change (e.g., nutritional changes imposed on older adults due to climate change; mortality related to heat waves in poor countries); emerging infectious diseases such as chikungunya, dengue fever, and Zika in Latin America; and financial fraud by banks and financial institutions geared toward misappropriating older adults' lifetime savings.

- Evaluation of the impact of social and economic interventions at local levels and in wider contexts on the health of older populations. For example, researchers might study the health benefits associated with improvements in social cohesion and personal safety as well as with decreased crime rates in neighborhoods.

- Evaluation of the rapid changes in the structure of modern societies and their potential effects on health status of older adults. Recent decades have witnessed events such as urbanization and migration that involve a large proportion of the population as well as very fast-paced changes in social constructs and values that happened within the lifespan of a single generation. Today's older adults have been brought up with different family values, more conservative gender roles, and less use of technology in their daily life. Although these social changes have happened all over the world, the degree of changes varies across countries. Exploration of the health attributes of these social changes is another international research opportunity.

▶ Summary

The value of a multicenter international population aging research study depends on several key aspects:

- The use of a single evidence-based conceptual framework at all sites
- A life course perspective
- A valid design and accurate measurement methods
- The ability to transfer knowledge so as to change social structures, behaviors, and professional practices
- Researchers' support for capacity building and ensuring the sustainability of collaborative research

Considering these issues as much as possible will encourage the development of a valid and reliable database for aging studies at the international level that can produce high-quality epidemiological evidence. This evidence will, in turn, guide health and social policies and ultimately improve the health of older adults. Since the public health burden associated with aging is expected to increase, improvements in the health of older adults can impact the well-being of the population at large.

References

Albala, C., Lebrao, M. L., Leon Diaz, E. M., Ham-Chande, R., Hennis, A. J., Palloni, A.,… Pratts, O. (2005). [The Health, Well-Being, and Aging ("SABE") survey: Methodology applied and profile of the study population]. *Revista Panamericana de Salud Públic*, *17*(5-6), 307-322.

Borsch-Supan, A., Brandt, M., Hunkler, C., Kneip, T., Korbmacher, J., Malter, F.,… Zuber, S. (2013). Data resource profile: The Survey of Health, Ageing and Retirement in Europe (SHARE). *International Journal of Epidemiology*, *42*(4), 992-1001.

Bronfenbrenner, U. (1979). *The ecology of human development: Experiments by nature and design.* Cambridge, MA: Harvard University Press.

Cash-Gibson, L., Guerra, G., & Salgado-de-Snyder, V. N. (2015). SDH-NET: A South–North–South collaboration to build sustainable research capacities on social determinants of health in low- and middle-income countries. *Health Research Policy and Systems*, *13*(45), 015-0048.

Cottler, L. B., Zunt, J., Weiss, B., Kamal, A. K., & Vaddiparti, K. (2015). Building global capacity for brain and nervous system disorders research. *Nature*, *527*(7578): S207-S213.

Freire, A. N., Guerra, R. O., Alvarado, B., Guralnik, J. M., & Zunzunegui, M. V. (2012). Validity and reliability of the short physical performance battery in two diverse older adult populations in Quebec and Brazil. *Journal of Aging and Health*, *24*(5), 863-878.

Garin, N., Koyanagi, A., Chatterji, S., Tyrovolas, S., Olaya, B., Leonardi, M.,… Haro, J. M. (2016). Global multimorbidity patterns: A cross-sectional, population-based, multi-country study. *Journal of Gerontology, Series A: Biological Sciences and Medical Sciences*, *71*(2), 205-214.

Gomez, F., Zunzunegui, M., Lord, C., Alvarado, B., & Garcia, A. (2013). Applicability of the MoCA-S test in populations with little education in Colombia. *International Journal of Geriatric Psychiatry*, *28*(8), 813-820.

Hendrie, H. C., Murrell, J., Baiyewu, O., Lane, K. A., Purnell, C., Ogunniyi, A.,… Gao, S. (2014). APOE epsilon4 and the risk for Alzheimer disease and cognitive decline in African Americans and Yoruba. *International Psychogeriatrics*, *26*(6), 977-985.

Kowal, P., Chatterji, S., Naidoo, N., Biritwum, R., Fan, W., Lopez Ridaura, R.,… Boerma, J. T. (2012). Data resource profile: The World Health Organization Study on global AGEing and adult health (SAGE). *International Journal of Epidemiology*, *41*(6), 1639-1649.

Krieger, N. (2001). Theories for social epidemiology in the 21st century: An ecosocial perspective. *International Journal of Epidemiology*, *30*(4), 668-677.

Leonardi, M., Chatterji, S., Koskinen, S., Ayuso-Mateos, J. L., Haro, J. M., Frisoni, G.,... Finocchiaro, C. (2014). Determinants of health and disability in ageing population: The COURAGE in Europe Project (collaborative research on ageing in Europe). *Clinical Psychology & Psychotherapy, 21*(3), 193-198.

Li, A., Tu, M. T., Sousa, A. C., Alvarado, B., Kone, G. K., Guralnik, J., & Zunzunegui, M. V. (2015). Early life adversity and C-reactive protein in diverse populations of older adults: A cross-sectional analysis from the International Mobility in Aging Study (IMIAS). *BMC Geriatrics, 15*(102), 015-0104.

Link, B. G., & Phelan, J. D. (2002). McKeown and the idea that social conditions are fundamental causes of disease. *American Journal of Public Health, 92*(5), 730-732.

Marengoni, A., Angleman, S., Melis, R., Mangialasche, F., Karp, A., Garmen, A.,... Fratiglioni, L. (2011). Aging with multimorbidity: A systematic review of the literature. *Ageing Research Reviews, 10*(4), 430-439.

McKeown, T. (1979). *The role of medicine: Dream, mirage, or nemesis?* Princeton, NJ: Princeton University Press.

Minicuci, N., Noale, M., Bardage, C., Blumstein, T., Deeg, D. J., Gindin, J.,... Maggi, S. (2003). Cross-national determinants of quality of life from six longitudinal studies on aging: The CLESA project. *Aging Clinical and Experimental Research, 15*(3), 187-202.

Oye, G. (2009). Ibadan Study of Ageing (ISA): Rationale and methods. Retrieved from http://apps.who.int /healthinfo/09_IbadanStudyAgeing_Gureje.pdf

Pang, T., Sadana, R., Hanney, S., Bhutta, Z. A., Hyder, A. A., & Simon, J. (2003). Knowledge for better health: A conceptual framework and foundation for health research systems. *Bulletin of the World Health Organization, 81*(11), 815-820.

Perez-Zepeda, M. U., Belanger, E., Zunzunegui, M. V., Phillips, S., Ylli, A., & Guralnik, J. (2016). Assessing the validity of self-rated health with the short physical performance battery: A cross-sectional analysis of the International Mobility in Aging Study. *PLoS One, 11*(4), e0153855.

Phelan, J. C., Link, B. G., & Tehranifar, P. (2010). Social conditions as fundamental causes of health inequalities: Theory, evidence, and policy implications. *Journal of Health and Social Behavior,51*(40), 0022146510383498.

Reitz, C., Jun, G., Naj, A., Rajbhandary, R., Vardarajan, B. N., Wang, L., S.,... Mayeux, R. (2013). Variants in the ATP-binding cassette transporter (ABCA7), apolipoprotein E4, and the risk of late-onset Alzheimer disease in African Americans. *Journal of the American Medical Association, 309*(14), 1483-1492.

Rowland, D. T. (2012). *Population aging: The transformation of societies.* The Netherlands: Springer.

Simon, S. L., Walsh, D. A., Regnier, V. A., & Krauss, I. K. (1992). Spatial cognition and neighborhood use: The relationship in older adults. *Psychology and Aging, 7*(3), 389-394.

Sousa, A. C., Guerra, R. O., Thanh Tu, M., Phillips, S. P., Guralnik, J. M., & Zunzunegui, M. V. (2014). Lifecourse adversity and physical performance across countries among men and women aged 65-74." *PLoS One, 9*(8), e102299.

Statistics Canada. (2003). *Survey methods and practices.* Catalogue no. 12-587-X. Ottawa, ON: Minister of Industry.

Statistics Canada. (2016). Life expectancy at birth, by sex, by province. Retrieved from http://www.statcan .gc.ca/tables-tableaux/sum-som/l01/cst01/health26-eng.htm

Streiner, D. L. (2014). *Health measurement scales.* Oxford, UK: Oxford University Press.

United Nations. (2009). *World population prospects: The 2008 revision population database.* New York, NY: Author.

Vafaei, A., Gomez, F., Zunzunegui, M. V., Guralnik, J., Curcio, C. L., Guerra, R., & Alvarado, B. E. (2014). Evaluation of the Late-Life Disability Instrument (LLDI) in low-income older populations. *Journal of Aging and Health, 26*(3), 495-515.

Willson, A. E, Shuey, K. M, & Elder, G. H., Jr. (2007). Cumulative advantage processes as mechanisms of inequality in life course health. *American Journal of Sociology,112*(6), 1886-1924.

Windley, P., & Scheidt, R. (2015). *Physical environments and aging: Critical contributions of M. Powell Lawton to theory and practice.* London, UK: Taylor & Francis.

World Health Organization (WHO). (2015). *World report on ageing and health* (pp. 7-18). Luxembourg, Luxembourg: Author.

Zunzunegui, M. V., Alvarado, B. E., Guerra, R., Gomez, J. F., Ylli, A., & Guralnik, J. M. (2015). The mobility gap between older men and women: The embodiment of gender. *Archives of Gerontology and Geriatrics, 61*(2), 140-148.

Zunzunegui, M. V., Nunez, O., Durban, M., Garcia de Yebenes, M. J., & Otero, A. (2006). Decreasing prevalence of disability in activities of daily living, functional limitations and poor self-rated health: A 6-year follow-up study in Spain. *Aging Clinical and Experimental Research, 18*(5), 352-358.

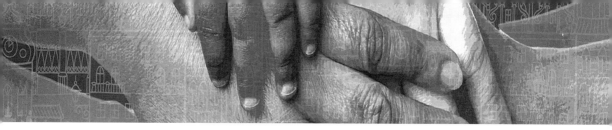

CHAPTER 13

Roadmap for Statistics in Aging Studies

Alan Hubbard

ABSTRACT

One of the main features of research in statistics of aging is that the effects of interest are almost always longitudinal ones. The result is that the most important methods used in this area of research are those that are most suitable for the study of changes over time. Examples of these methods include repeated measures, survival analysis, and multilevel models. It is clear that none of these methods is unique to the study of aging; thus, they can often be adopted and modified from other areas and strategies such as repeated measures, longitudinal data, survival analysis, statistics in epidemiology, causal inference, and multilevel models.

In this chapter, we provide a general roadmap of estimation in the context of aging research, as well as provide brief surveys of the topics listed previously. We emphasize how the researcher should choose the best approach that directly addresses the questions and study designs in aging research.

KEYWORDS

aging research	causal inference
estimation	longitudinal data

▶ Introduction

The main feature of the statistics of **aging research** is the centrality of time. Although study designs may differ, the effects of interest are almost always longitudinal ones. Thus, any education in the statistics of aging research will concentrate on methods suitable for the study of changes over time—for example, repeated measures, survival analysis, and multilevel models. In short, studying aging is studying a time-dependent process, and many issues—both subtle and technical—may arise in the analysis of a time-structured process. None of these methods is unique to the study of aging; thus, we can borrow from a large body of work on repeated measures, **longitudinal data,** survival analysis, statistics in epidemiology, **causal inference,** and multilevel models.

An exhaustive consideration of this extensive body of knowledge is not possible, and we will not try to achieve that feat in this chapter. Instead, we provide a general roadmap of **estimation** in the context of aging research, as well as provide brief surveys of the topics listed previously. Above all, we emphasize how the researcher should choose the best approach that directly addresses the question of interest, particularly for those questions and designs common in aging research.

FIGURE 13-1 shows the basic steps of any statistical estimation problem, via what has been referred to as the roadmap (Petersen & van der Laan, 2014; van der Laan & Rose, 2011). Although researchers conducting data analysis rarely go through these explicit steps, if the exercise is done rigorously, then one can

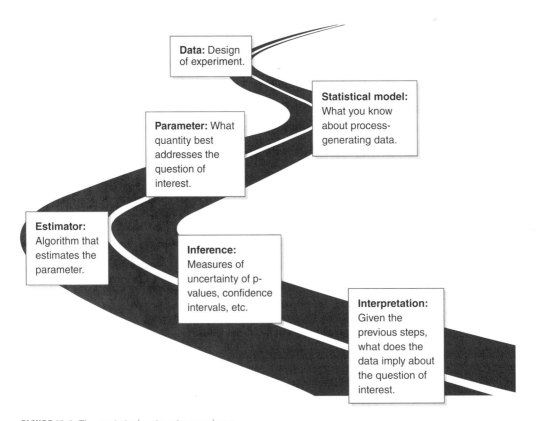

Data: Design of experiment.

Statistical model: What you know about process-generating data.

Parameter: What quantity best addresses the question of interest.

Estimator: Algorithm that estimates the parameter.

Inference: Measures of uncertainty of p-values, confidence intervals, etc.

Interpretation: Given the previous steps, what does the data imply about the question of interest.

FIGURE 13-1 The statistical estimation roadmap.

Data from: M. van der Laan and S. Rose, Targeted learning: causal inference for observational and experimental data. Springer, 2011. (and from) M. L. Petersen and M. J. van der Laan, "Causal models and learning from data: integrating causal modeling and statistical estimation," Epidemiology, vol. 25, no. 3, pp. 418–426, May 2014.

be confident of the inferences derived from such a process. We go in more detail about these steps in the discussion that follows.

▸ Data (and Notation)

Defining the data structure entails explicitly describing the experiment that produced the data so that a statistical model can be accurately proposed in the next step. Relevant questions include the following: What are the independent units? Are there missing values for some observations? Is the sample an unbiased representation of the target population, or was bias introduced by the design, such as probability-weighted sampling and case-control sampling? For example, suppose the design relies on a random sample of seniors between the ages of 60 and 80 years. In addition, there are three classes of variables: an exposure of interest (A), an outcome (Y), and a set of potential confounders (W). Also, we assume that the outcome, Y, is missing some observations in a random manner. To address this missing data structure in our notation, we introduce another variable, Δ, which is equal to 1 if the observation is not missing and equal to 0 if it is. Thus, we can represent our experiment as a series of independent and identically distributed draws from a random vector $O = (W, A, \Delta, \Delta^*Y)$, where Δ^*Y indicates that Y is observed only if $\Delta = 1$. Then, we can represent our data resulting from this experiment as O_1, O_2, ..., O_i, ..., O_n, where the subscript indexes the person, and we have a total of n subjects. A more complicated example might be that we randomly draw individuals from a population of age 60 and measure the same variables (W, A, Y) but both at entry into the study and again at every year for 20 years. Then, a single observation at a single year, t, is $O(t) = \{W(t), A(t), \Delta(t), \Delta(t)^*Y(t)\}$; all observations for a subject would be $O = (O(0), O(1), ..., O(20))$, and we can again represent our total study as a random draw of $O_1, O_2, ..., O_i, ..., O_n$ as described earlier. We can also incorporate other aspects,

such as biased sampling (i.e., any sampling process that does not result in something equivalent to a simple random sample of units, such as case-control or stratified sampling).

The notation is important because it allows the researcher to frame the study/experiment in a common language that everyone can immediately access. It then makes the remaining steps much more straightforward.

▸ Model

Causal Models

To make causal inferences regarding the results of an analysis, it is necessary to assert a so-called causal model. Suppose a general-population survey shows that people who exercise less, weigh more. There is no known direction of time for these data. Then the question becomes, "What came first—the increased weight or the reduced exercise?" If we have information outside the data that (strongly) suggests the direction of causality, then we might potentially interpret a resulting association estimate as reflecting the "causal" impact of such a variable. Otherwise, unless we have time-ordering information in the data (such as with a longitudinal study), then associations cannot distinguish whether more obese people exercise less because they find physical activity less rewarding, or whether a lack of exercise is actually the cause of weight gain. The causal model is a collection of hypothesized cause-effect relationships that the researcher can strongly assert from a priori knowledge—that is, from knowledge outside the data.

There are several ways to create a causal model, but we will stick with an intuitive form that shows which variables are related by causal arrows, using causal graphs (see Pearl, 2000, for a more thorough explanation). Consider **FIGURE 13-2**, which implies that the confounders W are not caused by anything (they are effectively randomized), A is affected by W, and Y is affected by both W and A. These

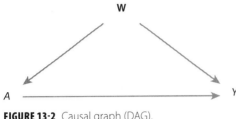

FIGURE 13-2 Causal graph (DAG).

Contributed by: Alan Hubbard.

variables are called nodes, the arrows are called pathways, and the resulting graphs are sometimes called directed acyclic (no circular paths) graphs (DAGs). In this case, if we are interested in the causal effect of A on Y, then W would be confounders (note that the nodes can imply more than one variable).

We can use this DAG to identify a parameter of interest from a theoretical experiment (intervention) on a node of this graph. For instance, we could ask what the outcomes would look like if we intervened on node A by setting this node to a single value (e.g., A = 0 could imply intervening by ensuring, in some theoretical experiment, that all subjects in a population are unexposed to a condition). We could label this outcome, Y_0. It is the outcome if, possibly counter to fact, a person was unexposed to the condition—hence the name of this outcome: counterfactual. Likewise, we could imagine the converse condition, in which all individuals in a population are exposed, or A is set to 1; through this theoretical experiment, we create outcome Y_1. In this case, we can define the counterfactual difference between these two as follows:

$$\text{ATE} = Y_1 - Y_0 \qquad \text{(Equation 13-1)}$$

where ATE is average treatment effect. Although we can never observe this quantity for any specific individual, we can use a DAG to justify estimating means of these counterfactuals, or a parameter like $E(Y_1 - Y_0)$. That is, although individual-level treatment or exposure effects can never be observed, we can estimate properties of these counterfactuals as averages across the individuals in the

population. We discuss this possibility in more detail later in this chapter, when we address parameters.

Statistical Models

Causal models are generally defined by a set of assumptions that cannot be tested by data—they can only be asserted. However, we can compare statistical models by examining how closely they fit our data. There is a long history of applied statisticians assuming some sort of relatively simple model, such as a linear regression model. These models are defined by a finite set of constants (parameters) and are referred to as parametric statistical models (in the linear model case, coefficients are an example of the parameters). The preponderance of statistical analyses involving aging research use such parametric models, particularly types of regression (e.g., linear, logistic, log-linear). There is rarely, if ever, theory to justify assuming such models, so the hope is they are useful approximations that yield information (and not misinformation) about the system being studied. Although we will focus on such models because they are the current standard of practice, the future holds promise for development of more widely available techniques that do not risk bias by making simplifying assumptions (e.g., van der Laan & Rose, 2011). In this case, the statistical model is typically semiparametric, which is a fancy way of saying it assumes almost nothing; for example, the regression of an outcome (e.g., cognitive function, depression, or falls) versus predictors can assume almost any shape and is not just linear in the covariates. Typically, theory provides little guidance about the form of the regression, so any specific form of parametric model assumption will no doubt introduce bias (see van der Laan, 2015, for a strong case against arbitrarily assumed parametric models). We note, however, that if we assume very little about the statistical model, then we often must use data-adaptive (machine learning) methods to fit the data (that is, we must "learn" the model from the data). It is relatively

PEARL 13-1 Counterfactuals

Most quantitative research in aging focuses on impacts of various factors on the trajectory of health and well-being as we age. In starker language, we want to assess the cause and the effect of potential interventions on these factors and their impact on health-status variables. Although well-meaning caveats exist about association not necessarily implying causation, the goals of such studies usually are to assess causality. To make this process more transparent, the idea of counterfactuals was introduced to define quantities (parameters) that have causal interpretations (Neyman, 1990; Rubin, 1974). Specifically, counterfactuals are theoretical outcome measurements under specific interventions.

As an example, define an outcome, Y (e.g., depression); a potential intervention variable, A (e.g., walking); and a set of pre-intervention variables, W (e.g., neighborhood walkability and lower-body strength), that are potentially related to Y. The counterfactual framework proceeds by considering a theoretical (and usually impossible) experiment in which we could assign a level of intervention to the population of interest, say $A = 0 \rightarrow$ no intervention, record the outcomes for all subjects, reset the clock and set $A = 1$ (intervention), and record the outcomes again. Thus, for each subject, we would have new data $X = (Y_0, Y_1, W)$; Y_0 is the outcome (possibly counter to fact—hence counterfactual) if the subject receives $A = 0$; and Y_1 is the outcome or counterfactual if $A = 1$. Now, we can define a causal parameter in this theoretical experiment, or $ATE = E(Y_1 - Y_0)$, where ATE is the average treatment effect. Thus, we define an explicit parameter of a theoretical data-generating distribution that defines a population causal effect—in this case, the mean difference of the outcome in the population if everyone receives the intervention versus no one does.

Given that some consensus can now be developed for defining causality in a statistical sense, the important work of the discipline of causal inference is to highlight the assumptions we need to make to assert that we can estimate these causal parameters from actual data, where, for instance, we observe the outcome for each subject under only one of the levels of A—that is, for data $O = (W, A, Y)$ (Pearl, 2000). In addition, much work has gone into development of estimators of causal parameters under these assumptions. Finally, the concept of counterfactuals provides a rigorous framework for understanding the importance of randomization in making strong statements about causality in studies of healthy aging research.

easy to derive uncertainty measures (standard errors, *p*-values, confidence intervals) when we assume a parametric model. However, the number of statisticians who have developed methodologies that can make rigorous inferences that provide useful estimates of the potential impacts of interventions is relatively small. Although such techniques are more widely available than a decade ago, particularly within statistical programming languages such as R (Ihaka & Gentleman, 1996), they are not commonly taught and their implementation usually requires advanced statistical knowledge. However, this situation is likely to change in the coming decade, and students should be aware that this is a rapidly developing time in statistics. Much as in the field of molecular

biology, introductory texts will have to be continually rewritten to match the pace of development of data science and statistics, and the informed user will have to be continually reeducated on these topics.

Mixed Models

One of the most commonly assumed models for longitudinal, repeated-measures data (that is, when following subjects over time and examining behavior and health as they age) is the so-called mixed model (Diggle, Heagerty, Liang, & Zeger, 2002; Hubbard et al., 2010). In this class of latent variable models, the variation observed in the outcome over time is explained by both fixed, measured factors and latent, unmeasured variables. Let Y_{ij} be the outcome for subject i at age j, $\mu(X_{ij}/\beta)$ be the average "response" of a person with the same covariates X_{ij} (also referred to as a regression function), β be a set of fixed coefficients, and $U_{ij}(\alpha_j, X_{ij})$ be an error term that is a function of an individual's random effects, α_j, and perhaps also a function of the covariates. The mean of the ith person in the jth age in this context can be written as follows:

$$E(Y_{ij} \mid X_{ij}, \alpha_i) = g[\mu(X_{ij} \mid \beta) + U_{ij}(\alpha_i, X_{ij})]$$

(Equation 13-2)

In this equation, g is the link function that depends on the regression—for example, linear: $g^{-1}(u) = u$, log: $g^{-1}(u) = \log(u)$, logistic: $g^{-1}(u) = \log[u/(1-u)])$, and $E\{U_{ij}(\alpha_i, X_{ij}) \mid X_{ij}\} = 0$, with the last being a sort of error term and sometimes called *random effects*. In this case, Y and X are measured variables and α is the latent variable. Thus, the variation in the outcome is explained by both of these factors.

Why is this model so commonly used for the sort of repeated-measures data associated with longitudinal studies of aging? **TABLE 13-1** (modified from Hubbard et al., 2010) contains some summary information on both the mixed model and generalized estimation equation (GEE; discussed later in this chapter) approaches; it accounts for the variation in the relationships of the explanatory variables and outcomes with age among different subjects. It parameterizes this variation via simple variance terms, and by doing so also implies models for the covariation of observations on the same subject. This approach has other virtues as well. However, one of the major pitfalls is that it assumes a model that is untestable by data—an infinite number of mixed models could equally fit the same data (this is technically called non-identifiability). Given that it is unlikely this model is ever true (it is too simple to be realistic in most situations), the interpretation of the estimates it returns can be complicated. Thus, the common use of this approach is typically justified more by precedent than by fundamental principles—a ubiquitous problem that plagues much of applied statistics.

Example

While we could look at any of the outcomes discussed in this book, we will consider the simple observational study of lung function as measured by forced expiratory volume at 1 second (FEV$_1$), a measure of lung function, versus age in a longitudinal study of 225 randomly selected 65-year-old subjects in the San Francisco Bay Area, California, from a large health system. The study follows these individuals for 5 years and measures their FEV$_1$ once a year, within a small window of time around the day of year they had their initial (baseline) measurement (see **TABLE 13-2** for a sampling of these data). In this case, we can plot a sampling of the data using a so-called spaghetti plot (**FIGURE 13-3**), where we can see the variability of FEV$_1$ at the beginning of the study (age = 65 years) and, to a less extent, variation in the trends among subjects versus age. Mixed models are used as a means to make mathematically explicit these sources of variation. We will start with a model that assumes that subjects enter the study at age 65 with different "characteristic" values of FEV$_1$, but have similar trends over time. Specifically, consider the following case:

$$E(Y_{ij} \mid X_{ij}, \alpha_i) = g[\mu(X_{ij} \mid \beta) + U_{ij}(\alpha_i, X_{ij})]$$

$$\beta_{0i} \sim N(0, \sigma^2_{\beta_0}), \; e_{ij} \sim N(0, \sigma^2_e) \quad \text{(Equation 13-3)}$$

where Y_{ij} is the jth measurement of $\log_e$ (FEV$_1$) − ($j = 1, \ldots, 5$; $i = 1, 2, \ldots, n = 225$) versus Age$_j$ (the age in years of any subject at the jth measurement), and $\beta_{0i} \sim N(0, \sigma^2_{\beta_0})$ means that the random intercept (one for each person), β_{0i}, is normally (very symmetrically) distributed with a mean of 0 and a variance of $\sigma^2_{\beta_0}$; anytime, in this context, one sees Greek symbols in an equation, it means that thing is

TABLE 13-1 Comparison of Mixed Model and Generalized Estimation Equation Approaches

	Mixed Model	GEE
Focus of interest	Variance components and regression coefficients	Regression coefficients
Parameter interpretation	Subject-specific	Population average
Linear (estimates equivalent)	Change in the mean outcome for a unit change in the associated subject explanatory variables, keeping the random effect (individual-level random effects) fixed	Change in the mean outcome for a unit change in the associated individual explanatory variable averaged across all of the individuals
Binary (estimates are *not* equivalent)	The log (OR) of an outcome for a unit change in the associated neighborhood exposure, keeping the neighborhood fixed; not identifiable in cross-sectional studies of neighborhoods without making additional assumptions about the random effects distribution	The log (OR) of an outcome for a unit change in the associated neighborhood exposure across all of the neighborhoods observed
Assumptions	Correctly specified error distribution	Number of neighborhoods sufficiently large for robust estimation of standard errors
Pitfalls	Standard error is not robust to model misspecification	With small number of subjects, standard error is not robust

Contributed by: Alan Hubbard.

an unknown constant (parameter). Similarly, e_{ij} (sometimes called residual error) is normally distributed with mean 0 and variance σ_e^2. Finally, this model implies that the observed distribution of all Y_{ij} measured on the same subject, $Y_i = (Y_{i1}, Y_{i2}, \ldots, Y_{i5})$, is multivariate normally distributed with a vector of population averages for overall subjects in the same age group, say Age_j, that is $\beta_0 + \beta_{0i} + \beta_1(Age_j - 65)$ for $Age_j = (65, 67, \ldots, 77)$, with variance of $\log(FEV_1)$ among individuals at the same

age Age_j being $\sigma_{\beta_0}^2 + \sigma_e^2$ and covariance of outcomes at different ages (Age_j and Age_k) $cov(Y_{ij}, Y_{ik}) = \sigma_{\beta_0}^2$, or the variance of FEV_1 at baseline. One can then expand this model to include variation in the intercepts among subjects in **Equation 13-2**:

$$Y_{ij} = \beta_0 + \beta_{0i} + (\beta_1 + \beta_{1i})(Age_j - 65) + e_{ij},$$

$$\beta_{0i} \sim N(0, \sigma_{\beta_0}^2), \beta_{1i} \sim N(0, \sigma_{\beta_1}^2), e_{ij} \sim N(0, \sigma_e^2),$$

$$cov(\beta_{0i}, \beta_{1i}) = \sigma_{\beta_0, \beta_1}$$

TABLE 13-2 Sample Observations from a Study on FEV_1 and Age		
Subject ID	**Age (years)**	**Y_{ij}**
1	65	3,510.67
1	68	2,450.801
1	71	1,749.994
1	74	1,344.912
1	77	1,011.441
2	65	2,575.949
2	68	1,959.096
2	71	1,560.348
2	74	1,073.209
2	77	817.4123
3	65	2,674.833
3	68	1,918.252

Contributed by: Alan Hubbard.

Because now the slope for a subject is random (every person has his or her own), this type of model is sometimes called a random coefficients model and can be generalized to both growth curve models and hierarchical random effects models. That is, the basic idea of mixed models generalizes to many different named subclasses. In any case, were such a model behind the generation of the FEV_1 data, we might expect the results to look like a more subtle form of the data in Figure 13-3. Note that there is variation both in FEV_1 at the starting times (some of which could be explain by β_{0i}, and some by e_{i0}) and in the trends by age.

We could imagine adding more complexity as well, such as more complicated patterns of FEV_1 with age, and in turn the possibility of more sources of covariation.

Thus, many different types of research with repeated measures on the same unit typically use variations of the latent variable models we discussed earlier. It is convenient for many applications, but researchers must be cautious: Strong assumptions are necessary to interpret the results without bias. We discuss another general approach later in this chapter that estimates very similar types of parameters (coefficients), but relies on fewer assumptions.

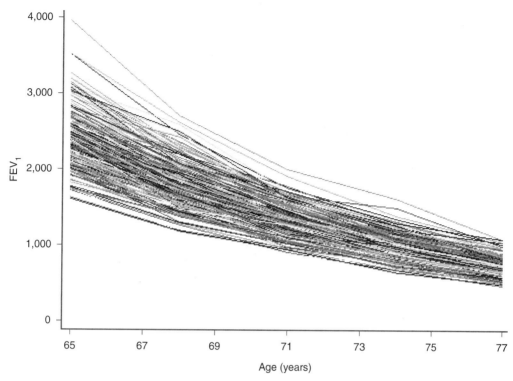

FIGURE 13-3 Spaghetti plot of FEV$_1$ versus age in years.
Contributed by: Alan Hubbard.

▶ Generalized Estimating Equations

Generalized estimating equations (GEE) are an estimating procedure, not a statistical model. GEEs estimate linear models similar to Equation 13-2, but rely on weaker assumptions when providing measures of uncertainty (i.e., standard errors). Basically, we can envision the GEE as a less ambitious approach, which we use when we want to estimate the average trend of subjects over time, but avoid estimating the distribution of those slopes and intercepts within the population (see Hubbard et al., 2010, for comparison and contrast of these approaches). In this case, we estimate the coefficient parameters alone (no variance terms). Thus, we would specify the following model in the FEV$_1$ case:

$$\mathrm{E}(Y_{ij} \mid \mathrm{Age}_j = a) = \beta_0 + \beta_1(a - 65)$$

$$\text{(Equation 13-4)}$$

where $a = (65, 67, \ldots, 77)$; we represent this set of means as blue dots on **FIGURE 13-4**. Thus, the statistical model in this case consists of only statements about the pattern of population means as a function of age; it says very little to nothing about how the FEV$_1$ values co-vary within the same subject. We will revisit these approaches when we discuss estimation later in this chapter.

▶ Semiparametric to Nonparametric Models

While the models described earlier represent a trend from making more assumptions about the data-generating mechanism (mixed

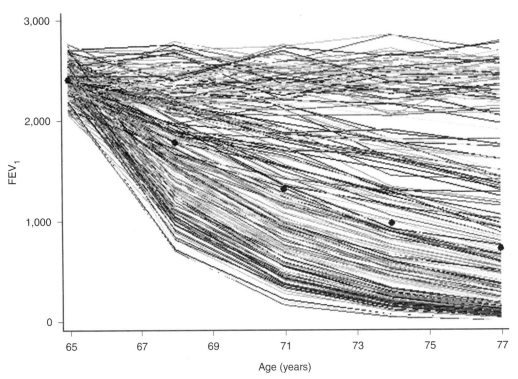

FIGURE 13-4 Spaghetti plot of data generated by random coefficients model. The black dots represent the average trend.

Contributed by: Alan Hubbard.

models) to fewer assumptions about that mechanism (GEE), we can also generalize GEE to make very few assumptions about the underlying statistical model. For instance, we could make **Equation 13-3** more flexible by allowing not just a linear relationship, but almost any functional form of the mean of log(FEV$_1$) versus age in years, or syntactically E(Y$_{ij}$|Age$_j$ = a) = m(a − 65), where m(.) remains unspecified (where a linear model is one of a nearly infinite number of possibilities, depending on how many levels of a exist). If there are only a few levels of a (e.g., age in the FEV$_1$ study), then a nonparametric model is simply one that has a different parameter for every level of a, or something like m(a − 65) = β$_a$. If there are many different levels of a in the population or if, in the limit, a is continuous so that there is a nearly infinite set of values, then a nonparametric model is typically not

practically estimable. In other words, if we need to estimate a different parameter for every a, and a has a huge number of levels, there simply will not be enough observations at the same a to ensure that the model has enough power to estimate the mean (say, via an average). Worse, there will always be values of a that exist in the target population, but will not be represented in the sample, so then many β$_a$ simply are not estimable. For these reasons, it is often more practical to invoke a semiparametric model.

It is more difficult to explicitly define a semiparametric model than a parametric or nonparametric model, though such a model clearly lies in between these two extremes. In short, with a semiparametric model we make assumptions about the distribution, but these assumptions do not limit the model to something that could be defined by a finite set of parameters.

In situations such as our study, where there are only two variables and we are interested in simple summaries, such as the mean, of one variable (FEV_1) among levels of another variable (age), then nonparametric models intersect with parametric models: A nonparametric model makes no assumptions, but still requires only a finite number of parameters to describe the relevant parts of the distribution. Formally, this case involves a nonparametric model, but there are only a small number of β_a necessary to define the whole curve of $m(a - 65)$ versus a; in the FEV_1 study, and there are five unique ages in our data set (65, 67, ..., 77), so a nonparametric model would require only seven parameters, $(\beta_{65}, \beta_{67}, ..., \beta_{77})$.

But now assume the study was more cross-sectional in nature and had randomly selected individuals at any possible age from 65 to 80, and say we wanted to define age to the nearest day. In this case, there are obviously a lot more ages and unless the sample size is huge (so-called Big Data), we can probably estimate the mean separately for each unique day. First, there will be ages now unrepresented at all in the data, and for those ages that are present, many might be represented by a single subject. Thus, a nonparametric (or sometimes called saturated) model would simply connect one observation to the next. Obviously, that would typically result in an impractically variable estimate of $m(a - 65)$. We can often reasonably invoke some assumptions in such a case and, therefore, define a semiparametric model. These assumptions could take the form of smoothness, where the precise functional form of $m(a - 65)$ can vary, but it cannot be "too volatile" (i.e., it cannot have too much up-and-down movement). Given we would expect the average FEV_1 to vary smoothly as a function of age, this is probably a reasonable assumption.

In any case, the definition of the model and the theory resulting from it become much more challenging when one goes from parametric models to semiparametric models. Nevertheless, there is rarely justification for using a parametric model, so the true model is typically a semiparametric model. Although the available techniques for estimating interesting quantities in such models (Robins & Rotnitzky, 1992; Rosenbaum & Rubin, 1983; van der Laan & Rose, 2011) are in their relative adolescence, with only relatively primitive software being currently available, an educated user will have to pay attention to developments in the next few years because user-friendly software will be maturing soon.

▶ Model Assumptions About Missing Data ("Missingness")

To interpret results accurately, we must also explicitly define models for design or nuisance features of the data, such as missing values on some variables. Suppose that FEV_1 measurements are sometimes missing for some ages for some subjects in our continuing example. A model describes which mechanism led to these missing values.

For instance, we might assume that the data are *missing completely at random* (MCAR), which means that whether an observation is missing is purely a coin flip. More formally, consider a new variable, $\Delta_{ij} = 1$ (observation not missing) or $= 0$ (observation missing). This now gives us a new data structure: $O_{ij} = \{Age_j, \Delta_{ij}, \Delta_{ij}*Y_{ij}\}$, $O_i = (0_{i1}, O_{i2}, ..., O_{i6})$, with $\Delta_{ij}*Y_{ij}$ indicating that we observed Y_{ij} only if $\Delta_{ij} = 1$. MCAR means $Y_i \perp \Delta_i$—that is, whether any observation is missing is independent of any of the outcomes.

This model makes fairly strong assumptions about the missing data ("missingness") but, in many practical situations, assuming complete independence can be a suspect decision. A bigger model would allow both independence and some structures for dependence; note, however, that *bigger* models make *fewer* assumptions. We could generalize this situation to allow for a relationship (statistical dependence) between the outcome level and the probability of a missed observation that is based on a variable that is always observed—a model referred to as *missing at random* (MAR).

As an example, consider that, on average, both FEV_1 decreases with age and the probability of a missing FEV_1 measurement increases over time. Thus, if we were interested in the mean FEV_1 as averaged with equal weight across these age groups, a simple average would be biased low (too few lower FEV_1 values). However, within each age category (each Age_j), the simple average of only those observations with non-missing values is not biased; that is, some observations might be missing, but it is still a representative sample, because the "missingness" is independent of FEV_1 within the age categories. Stated formally, MAR in this case is $Y_{ij} \perp \Delta_{ij} \mid Age_j$, so the "missingness" and outcome are independent conditionally on (or within strata defined by) age.

An even bigger model would be one in which data are *not missing at random* (NMAR)—where no conditional independence between "missingness" and the outcome exist, at least as stratified by the variables we always measure. This model means that we should go forward with our interpretation if we have a data-generating distribution model with no missing data (usually what is of interest), but we probably need to invoke stronger parametric assumptions to account for unmeasured sources of connection between the outcome and the random missing data process.

Typically, researchers make the assumption that their data are MAR. Thus, they assume there is some hope for properly adjusting the model for the "missingness" in a manner that will yield interpretable parameter estimates.

▶ Parameter of Interest

The parameter of interest is the constant or set of constants that the researcher would like 'to know to address the question of interest

with the data at hand. One way to formulate a parameter of interest is to say it is some function of either the data-generating distribution of the data you have or a distribution from a theoretical experiment. For instance, if our parameter of interest is the ATE as described earlier (**Equation 13-1**), then the theoretical experiment would be to observe the outcome for all units in the population of interest if everyone has an intervention (say, $A = 1$ resulting in Y_1), then to reset the clock and observe all the same people, under the same conditions with no intervention, $A = 0$, thereby generating counterfactual Y_0. When this approach is used, the ATE is just the average of difference of these two outcomes. However, that is typically not an experiment we can practically conduct.

Now consider a more practical experiment where we randomize the intervention or non-intervention to a randomly drawn subset of the target population (those about which we want to make inferences). We can certainly estimate the difference in mean outcomes for the two resulting groups, or $\Psi = E(Y \mid A = 1) - E(Y \mid A = 0)$ since that is accomplished just by a difference in the averages of Y in the two groups. However, if A is randomized, then it is independent of the prognosis of the individual (that is, both Y_0 and Y_1); also, if $A = a$ for an individual, then we observe the counterfactual Y_a for that individual, and we can write $E(Y \mid A = a) = E(Y_a \mid A = a) = E(Y_a)$. In other words, the parameter that we can estimate (a simple average of the outcome within a subgroup) is equal to the mean of the target population if everyone is given $A = a$. This process of showing that a parameter of interest can be estimated as a parameter of the actual data-generating distribution is called identifiability, and in the example it shows that we can identify the ATE by Ψ and, therefore, estimate the ATE by a simple difference of averages.

Next, consider a more complicated situation where the parameter of interest is still the ATE, but instead of randomizing A, we observe i.i.d. copies of O = (W, A, Y) according to the causal model in Figure 13-2. In other words, A is the intervention variable of interest, W are the potential confounders, and Y is the outcome. The question is whether we can still identify the ATE from this design. Given the causal model in Figure 13-2, we have that given W, A is independent of (Y_0, Y_1); this conditional independence assumption is also equivalent in this case to the assumption of no unmeasured confounders (there are no unmeasured variables that have an arrow into both A and Y). In this case, we can get the same result as obtained earlier by also conditioning on W, so E(Y|A = a,W) = E(Y_a|A = a,W) = E(Y_a|W); thus, given the assumptions, we can equate the mean of the outcome in subgroups where A = a and W are confounders, with the mean of the counterfactual Y_a (that is, the mean of an outcome in a theoretical experiment where everyone receives A = a) within subgroup W. We can get back to the marginal mean of the counterfactual Y_a by simply taking the average across all the subjects W, so now we get that E{E(Y|A = a,W)} = E{E(Y_a|W)} = EY_a. Finally, we can identify the parameter of the experiment where everyone gets the intervention (A = 1) versus no one gets it (A = 0) as follows:

$$ATE = E\{Y_1 - Y_0\} = E\{E(Y|A = 1, W)\}$$
$$- E\{E(Y|A = 0, W)\} \quad \text{(Equation 13-5)}$$

In words, the estimand (the value on the right side of **Equation 13-5**) is the difference from the predicted values of the mean of Y versus A and W, for every subject in the target population (every W) when we change A = 1 to A = 0. Thus, we can identify a "causal" quantity—that is, a parameter that quantifies the impacts of a theoretical experiment, based on the results of an observational study in which subjects are sampled and measured. We can also see that there is no obvious necessity to rely on a parametric model (like that in Equation 13-3)

to define an interesting parameter. For example, if we could estimate E(Y|A,W) in some other way (such as an automated machine learning algorithm), then we could estimate a very interesting parameter without resorting to classic statistical modeling approaches.

However, there is a connection between the estimand shown in Equation 13-5 and parameters typically returned in standard parametric regression. Consider the following model, not for the entire distribution of Y given A and W, but just for the mean of the outcome:

$$E(Y_{ij} | A_{ij}, W_{ij}) = \beta_0 + \beta_1 A_{ij} + \alpha_1 W_{1ij} +$$
$$\alpha_2 W_{2ij} + ... \quad \text{(Equation 13-6)}$$

To give **Equation 13-6** some context, consider another study of FEV_1 versus age. Instead of conducting a longitudinal study, however, the researchers simply select subjects from some frame (say, from a health insurance organization or neighborhood) where their age, A_{ij} is recorded and they are asked to come in for a lung function test (to measure Y = FEV_1). Because the researchers are worried that certain other factors might lead to a spurious association between the age at which the subjects are sampled and their FEV_1, they also collect what are considered potential confounding variables (the W_{kij}), such as ethnicity, smoking status, and so on. Also, assume that the data are generated by a causal model as represented in Figure 13-2. If Equation 13-6 is the actual (true) data-generating model, then the researchers can show, equivalent to Equation 13-5, that E($Y_{1ij} - Y_{0ij}|W_{ij}$) = E($Y_{ij}|A_{ij}$ = 1, W_{ij}) – E($Y_{ij}|A_{ij}$ = 0, W_{ij}) = β_1. So, the coefficient in this model (Equation 13-6) under assumptions has a causal interpretation. The implication of the model for the impact of age in this case is very, very strong: Specifically, the impact in no way depends on the characteristics of the individual, the W_{ij}; the model implies that the impact is always the same, β_1. The ATE will also be β_1, since it is just an average of this constant.

▶ Parameter Interpretation in Misspecified Models

A crucial question is how does one interpret an estimate of $\beta 1$ in the same circumstances but when—more plausibly—Equation 13-6 is not the true model (i.e., is misspecified)? Traditional statistical approaches have not developed a clear answer to this question, because there is in general no clear advice to give: The answer depends on how biased the model is. There has been a tradition of diagnostic work with regression to detect departures from the assumptions, but that development was at least partially based on the previous limitations of computing power and becomes unwieldy at higher dimensions. More fundamentally, this approach has been part of the model selection strategy (the researcher was not advised to simply give up if the diagnostics contradicted the initially assumed model), and the model selection strategy can impact the parameter that is ultimately chosen as the parameter of interest. Thus, the parameter of interest is not prespecified, but rather can be a consequence of going back and forth with the data to settle on a particular fit, which ultimately affects the choice of the parameter.

As a simple example, assume one intervention of interest A, one potential confounder W, and the following initial modeling assumption:

$$E(Y|A, W) = \beta_0 + \beta_1 A + \beta_2 W$$

In this case, the clear parameter of interest given the interest in the impact of intervention would be β_1, which is interpreted as the ATE for a unit increase in A, given that the assumptions for this model are correct. However, after some simple diagnostics, we notice that the trends for Y versus A appear quadratic rather than linear, so we expand the model to the following expression:

$$E(Y|A, W) = \beta_0 + \beta_1 A + \beta_2 W + \beta_3 A^2$$

Now, what is the parameter of interest? Since the impact of changing A (say, by one unit) differs at different starting points, reporting just one ATE is probably not enough. So, perhaps now we decide to report estimates of the parameters of a change in the mean given a change in A, keeping W fixed at an arbitrary constant, for several different starting values of A. Now the parameter of interest becomes $\beta_1 a + \beta_3 a^2$ for different values of a. That is, changing the model has now changed the parameter of interest. This problem just becomes more extreme as the number of patterns for A expands, and as the number of adjustment covariates grows. In this context, there is no theory that can provide convenient statistical inference (i.e., confidence intervals, p-values) if we honestly account for the fact that the selection of the parameter itself is random (different repeated experiments will produce variations in the model selected, resulting in variations in the parameters selected for reporting purposes).

Traditional approaches have advocated that we simply ignore this problem and treat the final model and the implied parameters of interest as prespecified. This strategy works if the same experiment (data collection, model fit, diagnostics, and refit) always produces the same final model. Of course, that is a huge assumption—especially given that, if this assumption is not true, interpretation of the results becomes problematic. Fortunately, new methods are available that leverage the enormous growth of computing power, by combining automated model selection (using machine learning [Hastie, Tibshirani, & Friedman, 2009]) and causal inference methods (targeted learning [van der Laan & Rose, 2011]; propensity score matching [Rosenbaum & Rubin,

1983]; and estimation equation approaches [van der Laan & Robins, 2002]).

▶ Estimation

Once we have made all of the previously mentioned decisions, the next choice is the estimator, or the algorithm we use to generate a parameter estimate. Sometimes, there is essentially a single choice. For instance, for mixed models, the estimator explicitly defines a likelihood; thus, maximum likelihood estimation is both the obvious choice and the approach that is almost ubiquitously used (in reality, even here there are some subchoices, such as restricted maximum likelihood [Laird & Ware, 1982]). For GEE, estimating equations are derived from the same equations used in maximum likelihood estimation, but in the case discussed earlier (Equation 13-3) they do not require us to specify exactly how the outcomes are related within a subject (Hubbard et al., 2010; Zeger, Liang, & Albert, 1988). For parameters in a semiparametric model, such as the ATE (Equation 13-5), several methods are available in various software platforms, including targeted maximum likelihood estimation (tmle [Gruber & van der Laan, 2012] and ltmle [Schwabb, van der Laan, & Petersen, 2014], which are packages in statistical software R [Ihaka & Gentleman, 1996]) and inverse probability weighted estimators (e.g., the *teffects* package in Stata [StataCorp, 2015]), among others.

How does one choose? What is the best estimator? And what do we mean by "best"? Given a prespecified parameter of interest, such as the ATE, "best" means that, within the true (honest) statistical model, we want a procedure that, as the sample size gets very big (or asymptotically), meets the following criteria:

- Respects the statistical model (i.e., includes only modeling assumptions that are well substantiated by background information).

- Has as little bias as possible (i.e., as the sample size goes to infinity, the estimator will return estimates that are negligibly close to the true value).

- Has as little variance as possible (i.e., in repeated experiments with the same sample size and design as the one generating the estimate, the variance of the estimate across these experiments will be as small as possible). Adding bias^2 + variance leads to the mean-squared error (MSE).
  - Estimators that are asymptotically unbiased and have the lowest variance are called *efficient estimators.*

- Returns estimates of the parameter of interest, whose distribution, if plotted as a histogram, is close to a normal (Gaussian) distribution.
  - This is the basis of most statistical inferences reported, and is typically an application of the central limit theorem (CLT). In its simplest form, the magic of the CLT is that, although the distribution of the original variable is neither normal nor symmetric (e.g., a binary variable), averages of these random variables are normally distributed as long as the sample size of the averages is large enough. This topic is covered in more detail in the next section.

Because the only statistical theory possible for many estimators is asymptotic theory (i.e., predicting the behavior of these estimators as the sample size gets very "big"), it plays a significant role in evaluating the relative merits of different estimators. Although we are entering the era of Big Data, so that the sizes of public health studies are growing and in some cases involving millions of observations, much of the research currently being conducted still comprises more modest sample sizes. For these studies, although the theoretical asymptotic performance is typically significant in deciding among competing estimators, it is only one set of relevant criteria, with the other being the finite sample performance. Examples of finite sample performance include the following criteria:

- The variability and bias in smaller samples. Certain estimators can be asymptotically optimal, but have poor finite sample performance.
  - Also, how universal is the performance across all possible data-generating models that are consistent with the background information (the statistical model)? If a model behaves well for only a very small subset of the possible models, then such an estimator carries too great a risk.
- Robustness, or sensitivity to outliers or contamination of a small fraction of data—that is, the sensitivity of the estimator to small changes in the data.
- A sampling distribution for the estimator that approaches normality in relatively small and smaller samples. Some estimators might have asymptotically normal distributions, but for smaller samples that have skewed or other non-normal distributions.
- Sufficient computation power to perform the estimation in a reasonable time and that is not greater than the available resources. If the researcher is forced to fit models on a relatively small device (say, a laptop with modest speed and memory), then some approaches/estimators will take a prohibitively long time to complete. This issue rarely is a compelling reason for choosing an estimator, given that even relatively modest machines can quickly (enough) accomplish the calculations for the most computational intensive approaches mentioned here.

As estimators become more automated, including performing the model selection that is required for the most data-adaptive (semiparametric) approaches, it is hoped that the choice of estimator will be made by the machines, not the users, as ultimately these are optimization problems that can be handled computationally. Until that day (which

lies not far in the future), researchers who are performing data analysis are well advised to consider the desirable characteristics cited in this section when choosing an approach.

▶ Measures of Uncertainty

A statistical analysis, to be complete, will usually involve both estimation and measures of uncertainty, where these combine to make up the concepts of statistical inference. Measures of uncertainty include standard error (the standard deviation of the sampling distribution of an estimator), α-level confidence intervals (random intervals generated with each experiment with the property that they include the population value of the target parameter $1 - \alpha$ proportion of the time), and p-values. We will concentrate on generating a standard error (SE), since the other quantities are usually just functions of the SE, the estimate, and the assumption that the sampling distribution of the estimator is normal (by an application of the central limit theorem). This SE can be calculated differently for the same estimator, depending on the statistical model.

▶ Parametric Models and Maximum Likelihood

If a model is assumed for distribution of the data collected on independent units and used to derive the estimates (i.e., maximum likelihood estimation [MLE]), then this likelihood can also be used to derive the standard errors for the relevant parameters. This process is sometimes referred to as maximum likelihood inference. Avoiding the technical details of how this happens, we can explain an equivalent way of deriving inferences that relies more on intuition, yet provides the necessary

TABLE 13-3 Results of Using MLE to Fit the Data in the FEV$_1$ Study

Mixed-effects ML regression					Number of obs (**5*n**) = 1125		
Group variable: id					Number of groups (**n**) = 225		
					Wald chi2(1) = 81119.86		
Log likelihood = 1351.5947					Prob > chi2 = 0.0000		

logy$_{ij}$ |	Coef.	Std. Err.	z	P>|z|	[95% Conf. Interval]	
$\hat{\beta}_1$ ageminus65 |	−.0997218	.0003501	−284.82	0.000	−.100408	−.0990355
$\hat{\beta}_0$ _cons |	7.811191	.0100982	773.52	0.000	7.791399	7.830983

Random-effects Parameters |	Estimate	Std. Err.	[95% Conf. Interval]	
id: Identity |				
$\hat{\sigma}\beta_0$ sd(_cons) |	.1464741	.0070651	.1332611	.1609971
$\hat{\sigma}_e$ sd(Residual) |	.049824	.0011744	.0475747	.0521797

Contributed by: Alan Hubbard.

insights; it is called the parametric bootstrap (Efron & Tibshirani, 1993).

The parametric bootstrap is a simulation-based method and works as follows:

1. MLE is applied to derive an estimate of the data-generating distribution, say P$_\theta$, where θ represents a vector of parameters that defines the distribution, such as coefficients and variance terms (e.g., the β's and σ's in Equation 13-3). Call the estimated distribution P$_{\theta n}$, where θ_n represents the MLE estimated parameters. **TABLE 13-3** shows an example of fitting the data using maximum likelihood/mixed models (StataCorp, 2015), so that the realizations of θ_n are the ($\hat{\beta}$, $\hat{\sigma}$) values as shown.

2. Generate a random sample "equivalent" to the original sample from P$_{\theta n}$. The equivalent will depend on the specific experimental design,

but we can base it on the FEV$_1$ study discussed earlier. In this study, FEV$_1$ was measured at each of seven unique ages, so we treat those ages as fixed for each randomly simulated individual. The possible output that we might get from this study is shown here. We mimic the data generated from Equation 13-3 but with estimated values θ_n = ($\hat{\beta}$, $\hat{\sigma}$) plugged into the equations (and using the results from Table 13-3) as follows:

a. Generate a random sample of size n (the original number of subjects in the study = 225) from a normal distribution with mean 0 and standard deviation $\hat{\sigma}\beta_0$ = 0.15. The results might look something like **FIGURE 13-5**. Assume that the current data consist of 225 rows with just one variable, β_{0i} and the associated id, which is just the row number: 1, 2, ..., $n = 225$. These represent the independent units in our study (the individuals).

b. Expand each of the rows 5 times. For each of the 5 rows per id, make an age variable that goes from 65 to 77 by increments of 2. Subtract 65 from this variable to make it equivalent to agemimus65 in Table 13-3. Now there are 225 * 5 = 1125 rows of data.

c. Generate for each row an independent random normal variable (representing the e_{ij} in Equation 13-3) of mean 0 and standard deviation $\hat{\sigma}_e = 0.050$.

d. Generate an outcome for each of the 5 rows ($j = 1, ..., 5$) for each of the 225 id's using the fitted equation $Y_{ij} = 7.81 + \beta_{0i} - 0.10$ (Age$_j$ – 65) + e_{ij}, so as to generate 1125 random Y_{ij} (log(FEV$_1$))

observations. The simulated data set now has the exact same structure as the original data used to generate Table 13-3.

3. Estimate the parameters of these randomly generated data using the same procedure used to get the original parameter estimates. Call these parameters $\theta_n^b = (\hat{\beta}^b, \hat{\sigma}^b)$, where b indexes the simulation (thus, for this first one, $b = 1$), and store them.

4. Repeat Steps 2 and 3 many (say, 1000) times so we now have 1000 repetitions of θ_n^b, $b = 1, ... , 1000$.

5. Derive the standard errors for each parameter as simply the square root of the sample variance. For example:

$$SE(\hat{\beta}_1) = \sqrt{\frac{1}{n-1}\sum_{b=1}^{1000}(\hat{\beta}_1^b - \hat{\beta}_1)^2}$$

In this case, the result would be very close to the standard error reported; for example

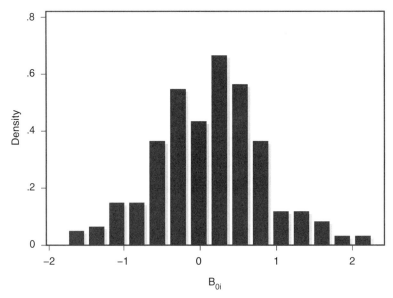

FIGURE 13-5 Histogram of 225 randomly generated β_{0i} values from an N(0, 211.9) distribution.

Contributed by: Alan Hubbard.

from Table 13-3, it would be 0.00035. The technical details of this step are not important, but the intuition is that the estimation uncertainty in this case is determined by assuming the estimation model was correctly specified. Not surprisingly, if that is the case, then this parametric bootstrap procedure, or the SE produced by the equivalent MLE, will be consistent (asymptotically unbiased). In contrast, if the model was not correctly specified, then it will generate a biased estimate of the SE for the parameter being estimated, which might have complexities of its own (if the model is misspecified, then the definition of the parameter itself can be challenging to determine).

We next discuss a closely related procedure that can generate consistent SEs for any algorithm used to produce estimates, regardless of model misspecification.

▶ Semiparametric Inferences

If we do not wish to rely on correct specification of the likelihood when deriving the inference, then we can use some methods that give consistent results when estimating the SE with few assumptions. We refer to these techniques in general as semiparametric inferential methods, and for our purposes they include methods that have been called nonparametric (implying no assumptions). As described earlier, the method used to understand semiparametric SEs is a bootstrap procedure, albeit the nonparametric version of this procedure (Efron & Tibshirani, 1993).

In this case, as opposed to using arbitrarily simulated data, we randomly sample data from the original sample. This process is sometimes referred to as drawing from the empirical distribution, which is just the distribution of the observations if we treated the sample as the target population. The theory justifying this approach might be complex, but can be summarized relatively simply (and tautologically): When sampling randomly from the empirical distribution (i.e., drawing independent units randomly with replacement from the sample) produces a sampling distribution of the estimator that is "close enough" to the true sampling distribution of the estimator when it is applied to repeated draws from the target population, then the bootstrap procedure works. The important point here is the intuition that this approach provides for making semiparametric inferences—namely, we can define the SE as the standard deviation of the estimates generated by the algorithm (the estimator) in repeated experiments in the target population. That is true even if that SE is for an estimator derived from an incorrectly specified model (e.g., MLE with a misspecified likelihood).

Some equivalent techniques are based not on resampling the data, but rather on using analytic methods to derive the SE. These methods are sometimes referred to as robust SEs because they are not sensitive to (they are robust to) assumptions of the estimator. In situations where the interpretation of the parameter estimate is not sensitive to the likelihood, then using a robust estimator of the SE presents few problems. For instance, if we are primarily interested in the estimate of β_1 in Equation 13-3, then even if we assume the likelihood as specified, the bias of the estimator is not affected by the parametric (normal) assumptions of the error terms or the precise mixed model. However, the MLE-based SE can be biased, so we get our cake (i.e., the estimate) and eat it, too (a consistent SE), if we rely on robust SEs. For situations where the interpretation is closely paired with the likelihood, we can still get a robust SE, but it is no longer clear what parameter is actually being estimated, given the model is likely to be misspecified. In some cases, the estimated parameter can be interpreted as the closest, for instance, linear approximation to the true model.

▶ Conclusion and Future Directions

The final step to make the whole process relevant to progress in aging research is the interpretation of the results, which is both tailored to the target audience and constrained by all that has come before. Given the assumptions of the causal and statistical models, given the original parameter of interest and the parameter ultimately estimated, and given the resulting estimate and the measures of uncertainty, which information is provided about the original goals of the analysis? If we believe that few arbitrary assumptions were required, if the estimator used is clearly the obvious choice, and if the resulting measures of uncertainty are small (such as a small confidence interval), then we can make very strong statements about the research question. A randomized clinical trial with very few missing data points might be such a place (which is why the Food and Drug Administration requires such studies to prove the safety and efficacy of interventions). In contrast, in an observational study where we are not confident of the causal model, where little is known to constrain the statistical model, and where there is significant measurement error, many missing data points, and consequently a quite large confidence interval for the parameter of interest, then obviously caution is warranted. The important point is to know the difference, to have thought clearly about the parameter of interest, to understand the sources of variability and bias and control for them as much as possible, and to have accurate measures of uncertainty. At least some of the current purported surfeit of misleading research findings (Ioannidis, 2008) could be ameliorated by more theoretically sound statistical analysis.

Currently, a wealth of new statistical methodologies and data science tools are being developed, though many of these are primarily accessible to experts in statistical computing and data science. Much of this work is open source and can be utilized by anyone with sufficient background in the relevant statistical packages, such as R (Ihaka & Gentleman, 1996). A large portion of this work deals with visualization and machine learning (Hastie et al., 2009). In addition, researchers are developing software that can utilize automated, data-adaptive methods for estimating causal parameters (e.g., van der Laan & Rose, 2011). While much of the current practice relies on the user having some background expertise—and certainly it is always wise to have some level of understanding of the tools being used—ultimately much of the inputs/decisions made in a data analysis will be automated and optimized, so the user can spend more time on the science and the questions of interest.

We hope this chapter serves as a general framework for statistical analysis, but we urge readers to do their best to keep abreast of developments. We have been in a stable period for a few decades, where many of the tools used in analysis of public health data and aging-related studies in particular are reasonably well understood and widely accepted as the standard of practice. As computers free users from some of the arbitrary assumptions that were necessary given the tools available, and as Big Data emerges as a more important contributor to aging research, practice will inevitably change. Even so, many of the fundamental principles presented herein will remain the same. Happy analyzing.

References

Diggle, P., Heagerty, P., Liang, K.-Y., & Zeger, S. (2002). *Analysis of longitudinal data*. Oxford, UK: Oxford University Press.

Efron, B., & Tibshirani, R. J. (1993). *An introduction to the bootstrap*. Boca Raton, FL: Chapman & Hall/CRC.

Gruber, S., & van der Laan, M. J. (2012). tmle: An R package for targeted maximum likelihood estimation. *Journal of Statistical Software, 51*(13), 1–35.

Hastie, T., Tibshirani, R., & Friedman, J. H. (2009). *The elements of statistical learning: Data mining, inference, and prediction* (2nd ed.). New York, NY: Springer-Verlag.

Hubbard, A. E., Ahern, J., Fleischer, N. L., van der Laan, M. J., Lippman, S. A., Jewell, N., Bruckner, T., &

Satariano, W. A. (2010). To GEE or not to GEE: Comparing population average and mixed models for estimating the associations between neighborhood risk factors and health. *Epidemiology*, *21*(4), 467.

Ihaka, R., & Gentleman, R. (1996). R: A Language for data analysis and graphics. *Journal of Computational and Graphical Statistics*, *5*(3), 299-314.

Ioannidis, J. P. A. (2008). Why most discovered true associations are inflated. *Epidemiology*, *19*(5), 640-648.

Laird, N. M., & Ware, J. H. (1982). Random-effects models for longitudinal data. *Biometrics*, 963–974.

Neyman, J. (1990). On the application of probability theory to agricultural experiments (1923). *Statistical Science 5*, 465–480.

Pearl, J. (2000). *Causality*. Cambridge, UK: Cambridge University Press.

Petersen, M. L., & van der Laan, M. J. (2014). Causal models and learning from data: Integrating causal modeling and statistical estimation. *Epidemiology*, *25*(3), 418-426.

Robins, J. M., & Rotnitzky, A. (1992). Recovery of information and adjustment for dependent censoring using surrogate markers. In *AIDS epidemiology*.

Rosenbaum, P. R., & Rubin, D. B. (1983). The central role of the propensity score in observational studies for causal effects. *Biometrika*, *70*, 41–55.

Rubin, D.B. (1974). Estimating causal effects of treatments in randomized and nonrandomized studies. *Journal of Educational Psychology*, *66*, 688–701.

Schwabb, J., van der Laan, M., & Petersen, M. (2014). ltmle: Longitudinal targeted maximum likelihood estimation. *R package version 0.9*. Retrieved from https://github.com/joshuaschwab/ltmle

StataCorp. (2015). *Stata Statistical Software: Release 14*. College Station, TX: Author.

van der Laan, M. (2015). Statistics as a science, not an art: The way to survive in data science, *Amstat News*, 29–30.

van der Laan, M. J., & Robins, J. M. (2002). *Unified methods for censored longitudinal data and causality*. New York, NY: Springer.

van der Laan, M., & Rose, S. (2011). *Targeted learning: Causal inference for observational and experimental data*. New York, NY: Springer.

Zeger, S. L., Liang, K.-Y., & Albert, P. S. (1988). Models for longitudinal data: A generalized estimating equation approach. *Biometrics*, 1049–1060.

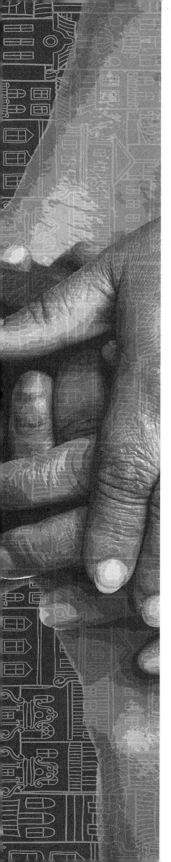

SECTION IV

Translation and Future Directions

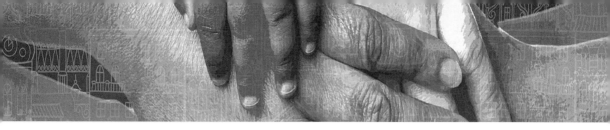

CHAPTER 14

Healthy Aging and Its Implications for Public Health: Social and Behavioral Interventions

Matthew Lee Smith, Marcia G. Ory, and **Thomas R. Prohaska**

ABSTRACT

Healthy aging is an achievable societal goal, especially as more is learned about the interacting influences of biological, behavioral, social, and environmental processes on health and functioning over the life course. While there are many definitions and synonyms for "healthy aging," this chapter adopts the broad public health conceptualization and associated solutions employed by the Centers for Disease Control and Prevention's Healthy Aging Research Network. In this context, the chapter introduces core concepts and principles associated with healthy aging research and practice, which are then followed by descriptions of known risk factors for aging populations and exemplars of healthful aging as related to behavioral and environmental influences on health. The chapter continues with an account of the evolution of aging research (from determinants to dissemination) and provides practical examples of translational research (as well as the foundational concepts and benefits of such research endeavors). It describes the "evidence-based movement" as a means to disseminate effective programs and explores pragmatic issues including program fidelity, scalability, and sustainability. The chapter concludes with recommended strategies to integrate clinical- and community-level interventions as well as policy considerations and future directions for the field.

▶ Introduction

Healthy aging is no longer a dream; rather, it is an achievable societal goal as more is learned about the interacting influences of biological, behavioral, social, and environmental processes on health and functioning over the life course (Satariano & Maus 2017a , Maus & Satariano 2017b). While many definitions and synonyms for "healthy aging" exist, this chapter adopts the broad public health conceptualization and solutions employed by the Centers for Disease Control and Prevention's (CDC's) Healthy Aging Research Network. It defines healthy aging as "the development and maintenance of optimal physical, mental, and social well-being in older adults. For healthy aging, we need safe physical environments and communities that support attitudes and behaviors leading to health and well-being, and effective use of health services and community programs to prevent or minimize the effects of acute and chronic disease" (Belza, Altpeter, Hooker, & Moni, 2014; CDC, 2011; Wilcox et al., 2013). This framework for viewing healthy aging reflects several generations of work and scholarship.

Nearly 70 years ago, the World Health Organization (WHO, 1946) moved health from a medical construct to a population health concept by defining health broadly as a "state of complete physical, mental, and social well-being and not merely the absence of disease or infirmity." Starting in the late 1970s, scholars began identifying the linkages between health and behavior, thereby defining the then-new field of behavioral medicine (Institute of Medicine [IOM], 1982). Notably, a systematic review of research publications based on the Alameda County Study documented the link between lifestyle and health outcomes among older adults (Housman & Dorman, 2005). This longitudinal study was one of the first to document the long-term consequences of excessive alcohol consumption, sedentary behavior, smoking, and other health risk behaviors on all-cause mortality, mobility, and disability among older adults (Belloc & Breslow, 1972). Findings from this longitudinal survey also linked education, gender, and ethnicity to mortality among older adults. It also documented that older adults with multiple risk factors (e.g., smoking, excessive alcohol use, and sedentary lifestyle) were at considerably greater risk for poor health outcomes. Further, in the 1980s and 1990s, scholars at the National Institute on Aging expanded these concepts to consider how health and behavior were intertwined with aging processes (Ory, Abeles, & Lipman, 1992).

Several core principles of the **social and behavioral** aspects on aging have been postulated that have implications for public health and aging **interventions**:

■ *The heterogeneity of the older population.* Despite lingering stereotypes of older people as either ill and dependent on others for their care—or healthy and wealthy—there is great variability in the health and functioning of older people, and often more variability among older adults than in any other life stage. This is not surprising considering the accumulated diversity in experiences and social, environmental, and behavioral exposures over the course of the lifespan.

■ *Aging as a life course phenomenon.* This perspective implies that people do not suddenly become old at a specific age; rather, they are the product of their combined lifetime experiences interacting with social, behavioral, and biomedical processes. There is no single chronological marker of old age; instead, each person ages from birth to death.

■ *Aging and the social context.* Aging is influenced by, and also influences, the macro and micro social contexts in which people grow older. While aging is universal, how an individual grows old will vary depending on whether one grows up in North America, Japan, or Western Europe versus less industrialized and less prosperous countries. Additionally, individuals born during the same period have some common defining experiences and represent unique age cohorts, such as those persons coming of age in the Great Depression, baby boomers, or more recently Millennials. This concept of cohort aging is in contrast to personal or individual aging.

■ *The potential for intervention.* The variability in aging across time and space underscores that the aging process is malleable and hence responsive to some degree of human intervention and control. This relationship is the root for the mantra of aging researchers: "It's never too late" to make changes that can influence an individual's life trajectory. Indeed, research demonstrating the mutability of chronic illness and disability provided the foundation for translating this research to practice and policy (Prohaska, Smith-Ray, & Glasgow, 2012).

PEARL 14-1 Aging and Negative Stereotypes

The core principles of the behavioral and social aspects of aging have implications for public health and aging interventions. The varied needs of a diverse aging population require differing solutions to improve health and well-being. The paradigm about the abilities of older adults must be changed to embrace the abilities of older adults and avoid negative stereotypes. Older adults are not incapable of change; rather, through appropriate evidence-based interventions, they can and will improve their functional abilities and overall quality of life.

In summary, aging-research attention has shifted from emphasizing length of life to stressing the quality of additional years (U.S. Department of Health and Human Services, 2000). While this change in emphasis seems obvious, it is important to note that living a longer life without quality (e.g., with medical complications, frequent hospitalizations, or reduced motor or cognitive functioning) is more draining on the affected individuals, their families, and society relative to those persons living more quality years with reduced morbidity and health-related ramification. Even so, the presence of disease is not the ultimate indicator of poorer quality health; an individual living with diabetes, for example, can have a well-managed disease and live multiple quality years post diagnosis. Indeed, concepts such as active life expectancy (Katz et al., 1983) and successful aging (Rowe & Kahn, 1987) have been widely used to emphasize the quality of life among older adults.

▶ Risk Factors

The Alameda County Study is probably the most cited large-scale population-based study of lifestyle factors associated with longevity (Belloc et al., 1972; Berkman & Breslow, 1983; Housman & Dorman, 2005). After following up with the 1965 cohort years later, investigators noted that five practices were generally associated with longer and healthier lives: avoiding smoking, exercising regularly, maintaining a healthy body weight, sleeping between seven and eight hours nightly, and limiting consumption of alcoholic drinks (Kaplan et al., 1987; Wingard, Berkman, & Brand, 1982). What was most revealing about the Alameda County Study was that these risk factors remained potent in later life, confirming the assertion that natural and planned changes can make a significant difference in individuals' health and functioning (Kaplan et al., 1987). This initial research led to many other community studies demonstrating that how and where one lives determine health and vitality above and beyond the effects of the genes with which a person was born (Rowe & Kahn, 1987, 2015). Once the initial risk factors were identified, subsequent investigations confirmed their relevance to different populations and settings (Abramson, Trejo, & Lai, 2002; Prohaska et al., 2006).

▶ Exemplars

We selected one behavioral and one environmental risk factor to highlight regarding what is currently known.

Physical Activity

Physical activity—a lifestyle behavior—is one of the most salient risk factors for health and longevity. Physical inactivity has been related to the onset and progression of most chronic conditions, including those of both a physical and mental health nature. The 2008 U.S. Department of Health and Human Services' *Physical Activity Guidelines for Americans* report provides scientific evidence for the importance of being physically active across the life course. Older adults do not "get a pass" from being physically active, but instead are encouraged to get at least 150 minutes each week of moderate-intensity physical activity such as brisk walking, as long as they have no limiting chronic conditions prohibiting physical activity (Nelson et al., 2007). Nevertheless, older adults are, on average, the least physically active of any age group.

Many reasons have been cited for this resistance to physical activity, including stereotypes held by older adults, their families, and even healthcare professionals that "exercise" is harmful for older adults or has fewer benefits for older adults, or that older adults are unwilling or unable to change their lifestyle habits (Ory, Hoffman, Hawkins, Sanner, & Mockenhaupt, 2003). The classic study of the fall-reduction benefits of weight training for frail older nursing home residents—many of whom were octogenarians or even nonagenarians—confirms the

importance of adopting a life course perspective in which appropriately designed and targeted interventions are seen as beneficial at most ages and disability levels (Fiatarone et al., 1994).

Currently, it is unknown exactly how much and which types of activity are best for adults, with special reference to older adults. The current guidelines set "minimum" standards, with the assumption that more is typically better. However, it is important to emphasize the public health message that some is better than none, and that the best strategy is to start slow and build up an individual's activity regimen. For both initiation and long-term maintenance, it is less important which activity is pursued (e.g., walking, gardening, or dancing) than whether it will be appealing to the older adult and feasible for engagement as part of routine daily behaviors.

The best physical activity interventions include a supportive environment for enhancing motivation for being physically active as well as opportunities to engage in physical activity/exercises in a supervised setting (King, 2001; Lewthwaite, 1990; McAuley & Blissmer, 2000). A growing consensus agrees that the essential elements needed for successful programs include attention to key behavioral change principles for initiating and maintaining physical activity (Cress et al., 2006, Cress et al., 2004), such as social support, self-efficacy, active choices, health contracts, regular performance feedback, and positive reinforcement.

Built and Natural Environment

Recent research emphasizes the importance of social determinants for understanding variants in health across populations and settings (Diaz Moore, Greenfield, & Scharlach, 2017). In particular, ZIP code (i.e., geographic location of residence) has been postulated as a key risk factor on par with other documented biological or behavioral risk factors, reflecting the importance of an individual's physical and social environment in determining health and well-being (Humpel, Owen & Leslie, 2002). Clearly, ZIP code may be a proxy for a complex set of inter-correlated social, economic, environmental, and resource factors within a specific geospatial area. In parallel fashion, there is now greater appreciation of the link between place and health—especially for older adults, for whom there often needs to be an accommodation between their changing physical capacities and the environmental demands (Diaz Moore, Greenfield, & Scharlach, 2017; Lawton, 1985). Some evidence indicates that older adults' functional capacity and environmental demands are associated with walking for exercise (Satariano et al., 2010) and that level of cognitive impairment is associated with the types of environments in which older adults walk for exercise (Prohaska et al., 2009). To move the field forward, a conceptual framework for investigation has been proposed that links environmental design features to behavior. which in turn impacts health outcomes (Ory, Lee, & Satariano, in press; Satariano, Ory, & Lee, 2012).

At the macro level, the "smart growth" movement has delineated specific principles that are associated with many population benefits (Durand, Andalib, Dunton, Wolch, & Pentz, 2011), including indirect impacts on lifestyle behaviors and population health outcomes. These principles include supporting mixed land uses; taking advantage of compact building design; creating a range of housing opportunities and choices; creating walkable neighborhoods; fostering distinct, attractive communities with a strong sense of pride; preserving open space, farmland, natural beauty, and critical environmental areas; strengthening and directing development toward existing communities; providing a variety of transportation choices; making development decisions predictable, fair, and cost-effective; and encouraging community and stakeholder collaboration in development decisions.

At the more micro or meso level, urban planners are identifying modifiable environmental design features that have been shown to influence neighborhood walkability and to be associated with more downstream indicators such as obesity and prevalence of lifestyle-related

PEARL 14-2 Partnership and Collaboration in Research

Extensive research has informed us about what works to improve the health of older adults—ranging from understanding the determinants of health and risk to understanding intervention effectiveness to embedding successful programs that can reach older adults in organizations and settings that serve the masses. Interventions can be disseminated throughout communities to enhance clinical, community, and policy influences. These influences must not be isolated in silos, but rather must be coordinated and integrated to yield anticipated outcomes and sustain programs capable of improving older adults' health. Partnership and collaboration are key to accomplishing this task.

conditions. These features include access to services; street connectivity, infrastructure, and safety for walking; aesthetics; traffic hazards; neighborhood; and crime. Safety has been found to be a major factor in walkability—whether it involves parents letting their children walk to school or older adults feeling comfortable about walking in their neighborhoods.

A recent study confirmed the strong association between neighborhood walkability and physical activity levels for middle-aged and older adults (Towne et al., 2016). Physical activity is also strongly associated with having a positive view of one's neighborhood in terms of both safety and cohesion. Interestingly, "perceptions of safety" are often as predictive—or even more predictive—of walking as objective environmental measures, and this is likely to be more so with older adults.

Several observations can be made about the findings from environmental studies. Despite the challenges of conducting research in this area, some universal lessons are emerging. Universal design elements are being touted as a best strategy for ensuring that both young and old live in environments that are supportive to being more physically active. A nonprofit organization,

8 80 Cities, aims to improve the quality of lives of people living in cities by creating safe environments for 8 year olds to 80 year olds. The "8 80 Cities" movement emphasizes that the environmental conditions that will enable a young child to be active will also likely make it easier for older adults to partake in more neighborhood-based physical activity (8 80 Cities, 2016).

While the number of environmental studies has certainly proliferated over the past two decades, most of these investigations have been based on cross-sectional designs and rely on "natural experiments" involving the creation of new activity-friendly communities—or more micro changes in the environment. Environmental research calls for different research paradigms given that it is not feasible to "assign" persons to different neighborhoods, and given that it is labor intensive and expensive to follow residents over time with precise measurement instruments more typical of those used in smaller, controlled studies. A recent article by Rosenberg and colleagues (2015) provided a number of novel strategies for conducting sedentary behavioral research among older adults, including randomized environmental interventions and environmental policy research.

▸ Research Evolution: From Determinants to Dissemination

Over the years, **aging research** has evolved from efforts to understand what works to promote health and healthful aging to the widespread dissemination of evidence-based programs to the organizations and individuals who need such services most. In terms of research and national funding, there has been a transition away from determinant studies that examine the contributors to health and illness and toward efficacy studies that utilize strictly controlled methods (e.g., randomized controlled trials) to identify the impact of interventions. Following these efficacy efforts, the field capitalized on the accumulating evidence from highly controlled randomized trials to translate and disseminate evidence-based interventions in community settings and support policies promoting the health of older adults. Ultimately, such broader translation of such effective interventions must be based on a clear understanding and adherence to the intervention's therapeutic elements and delivery mechanisms.

Once the benefits of interventions and their essential elements for success were understood, researchers began to focus on dissemination and implementation research, which emphasizes adapting strategies and methods to embed programs in those settings, organizations, and environments that are most likely to enhance the programs' effectiveness, promote their organizational adoption, increase their reach, and encourage their sustainability. This process is bidirectional in that, ultimately, findings from these dissemination and implementation efforts will be evaluated to inform subsequent research (from research to practice, and from practice to research). That is, research on determinants of dissemination is an iterative process that includes efforts to examine health determinants and illness as well as efficacy and effectiveness to better understand and refine interventions based on evidence of their impact in the context of evolving population demographics, participant demands, and community/clinical systems used to reach older adult participants (**FIGURE 14-1**).

▸ Guiding Questions for the Research Translation Process

In thinking about research translation, there is a continuum that spans from problem identification and risk factor correlation, to testing and

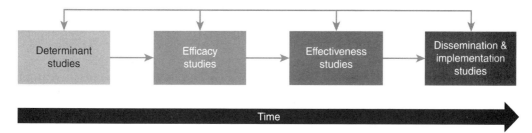

FIGURE 14-1 Research from determinants to dissemination.
Contributed by: Matthew Lee Smith.

creation of interventions, to dissemination and scalability, to sustainability of the intervention effort. From a public health perspective, four sequential and fundamental questions must be answered to understand the existing evidence base (Brownson, Fielding, & Maylahn, 2009; Prohaska et al., 2006):

1. What are the types and levels of lifestyle behaviors among diverse older populations that are related to the problem of interest? This question goes beyond incidence and prevalence of behavioral risk factors, including sub-questions to elucidate the context—for example, Which social and behavioral and environmental factors influence engagement in healthy lifestyles?
2. What are the health benefits and consequences of these lifestyle behaviors among diverse older populations?
3. Based on known linkages between health and behavior, and an understanding of behavior change principles, which interventions have been created and tested that have been proven to work, and what are the criteria used to evaluate their success?
4. Which factors are most effective in ensuring successful translation and broader dissemination of programs with demonstrated efficacy and effectiveness?

These are interrelated but different questions that require different information. For example, question 1 may identify that specific demographic groups of older adults have a greater prevalence of a specific risk factor—for example, older women might be found to be less physically active than men. Question 2 can be addressed with cross-sectional studies establishing an association between risk factors and health, and with longitudinal research that examines the natural history between the risk factors and the development of health consequences. A body of evidence from randomized clinical trials in which a random set

PEARL 14-3 Improvement versus New Programs

While many evidence-based programs for older adults exist, there are opportunities to translate the existing efforts to serve new older adult populations and serve them in new settings. There is no reason to "re-create the wheel" when improving the design of the "wheel" can accomplish the same goal as creating new programs. If an existing program does not adequately meet the needs of the population being served, then modifications to the content, format, or delivery modality should be encouraged to improve outcomes and diversify the menu of solutions to address older adults' health and well-being. However, these new, translated solutions must adhere to the intervention's essential elements to ensure the anticipated outcomes are achieved.

of individuals are exposed to health promotion behaviors (e.g., smoking cessation, exercise program) can help establish the causal association between the behavior and health outcomes. In question 3, the benefits of the behavior have been established and the issue becomes one of broader implementation. Question 4 focuses on dissemination and sustainability.

▶ The Evidence-Based Movement

In the United States, the **evidence-based movement** exists to promote, deliver, and embed evidence-based programs in communities (Boutaugh et al., 2014; Boutaugh & Lawrence, 2014). Each of these interventions was selected for grand-scale dissemination because of its documented effectiveness in randomized controlled trials. Each of these programs was subsequently translated for use in community settings, and is endorsed by the National Council on Aging (NCOA, 2016) as being within the highest tier of evidence. These programs address topics including, but are not limited to, chronic disease self-management, fall prevention,

physical activity, mental health, medication adherence, and caregiving. Many national stakeholders, including the NCOA, have supported the national dissemination of these programs, including the Administration for Community Living (ACL), Centers for Disease Control and Prevention, and Archstone Foundation (Ory & Smith, 2015). In addition to providing financial support for these interventions, a variety of networks have been instrumental in promoting and delivering them throughout the United States. For example, the Evidence-Based Leadership Council (EBLC) consists of program developers and selected community partners (Haynes et al., 2014); the FallsFree Initiative represents all active fall-prevention coalitions across the United States (Beattie, 2014; Schneider & Beattie, 2014); and the CDC's Healthy Aging Research Network comprises an impressive collection of aging scholars at institutions of higher learning and medical facilities (Belza et al., 2014). Because of these coordinated and synchronized efforts, these programs are now proliferating across the nation and widely available in community settings, being delivered through the aging services network in senior centers, residential facilities, faith-based organizations, and healthcare facilities, among others (**FIGURE 14-2**).

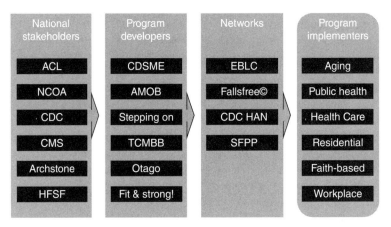

FIGURE 14-2 Evidence-based programs in communities in the United States.
Contributed by: Matthew Lee Smith.

► Fundamentals of Evidence-Based Programs

At the macro level, all evidence-based programs have two components: the therapeutic element and the delivery mechanism (Prohaska et al., 2012). Therapeutic element studies and delivery mechanism research have emerged and are gaining traction. Some researchers examine only variations in the delivery mechanism (e.g., which behavioral change strategies promote optimal adherence to the health practice). Others study only behavioral factors or only genetic factors. Still others suggest that a bio-psychosocial model is no longer sufficient; genetics and environment are now considered critical factors, but little research has been conducted that combined all of the various elements (the point of the NIA Symposium).

Building the Mechanisms in Silos

Personalized (precision) medicine has drawn attention to the concept of personalized risk factors, just as it has highlighted the possibility of precisely targeted health methods to prevent or delay disease and disability. We have only recently been successful in building the body of literature on the role of the environment in healthy aging. To date, however, much of this work has focused on environmental characteristics influencing walking, ways to prevent falls, and how work settings and home environments contribute to sedentary behavior.

The therapeutic elements of evidence-based programs focus on behavioral risk factors such as exercise, diet, stress reduction, smoking cessation, and medication management. The delivery mechanism for such programs is the means by which older adults are motivated to implement and maintain the appropriate health practices. One problem at this macro level is that researchers have often tended to focus on one component or the other, becoming specialized

in exercise or dietary behavior or in elements of the delivery mechanism, such as the examination of the role of environmental factors or social support on exercise. A consequence of this "silo approach" has been the formation of groups who examine only the amount of change in the health behavior needed to have a meaningful effect or only focused practice implementation. Likewise, knowledge on health practices has been built in silos. Some researchers investigate only social determinants, only environmental influences, only behavioral risk factors, or only the mechanisms of behavioral change. As noted earlier, this narrow focus has resulted in relatively few studies that have incorporated a comprehensive bio-psychosocial approach.

An Integrated Approach

Fortunately, the field has matured. Increasingly, the movement from research to practice has facilitated the transition to more multifaceted interventions addressing multiple risk factors in an environmental context. As a consequence, the field is developing an even more complex understanding of health promotion among older populations, with a focus on phenotypes and genetic contributions to health. Early indications are that personalized medicine or precision health might spur a trend toward a silo approach. However, this new approach to health also offers an opportunity to incorporate genetic personalized health into the broader discussion of the relative contributions of multiple influences on older adult health—that is, behavioral, environmental, genetic, and psychosocial factors. Possible questions in research devoted to this angle include the following: Why do some older adults experience better outcomes compared to others when exposed to the same level of health promotion? Under which circumstances are genetic, environmental, and behavioral factors more influential in determining the health of older adults.

The body of literature on behavioral risk factors and the impact of changing these behaviors has led a consensus on the level needed to obtain meaningful improvements in health for many of the health behaviors. For example, the CDC and the American College for Sports Medicine (ACSM) have recommended that older adults engage in aerobic exercise for 150 minutes per week at least at a moderate level and perform strength training two times per week. We now have a general understanding about the relative effect of most health-promotion behaviors on the health among older populations. We know that to accomplish behavior change and improve health and well-being, multilevel (i.e., clinical, community, and policy) approaches and multidisciplinary teams (e.g., public health, gerontology, social work, psychology, medicine, transportation) are necessary (**FIGURE 14-3**).

▶ More About Translation and Adaptation

Translation of interventions is necessary to disseminate the known benefits of evidence-based interventions to new populations and new

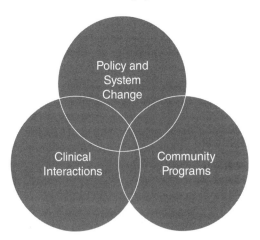

FIGURE 14-3 Multilevel approaches and multidisciplinary teams for behavior change and health and well-being improvement.

Contributed by: Matthew Lee Smith.

settings. Further, translation is a useful endeavor to expand the effectiveness of known interventions to address new societal problems, cover new content, or assess new treatments. The essential concept when translating an intervention is to make modifications to the content and format necessary to meet the new objectives while maintaining the essential elements from the original program necessary for success. Researchers must strike a balance between maintaining the effectiveness of the original intervention even as they advance knowledge and expand the intervention's utility and utilization. However, researchers must be cognizant that too much change will result in a total transformation of the intervention, thereby creating a new intervention that does not adhere to the original principles or contain the original essential elements. The intervention is deemed to be successfully translated if it is still capable of achieving the same outcomes as the original intervention while also yielding new information.

Translation, or intervention adaptation, is needed to develop programs that are responsive to the changing needs and demands of populations and settings. For example, the Chronic Disease Self-Management Program (CDSMP) has reached more than 252,000 participants in the United States, but it has not been successfully delivered in workplace settings (Smith et al., 2014). To address this issue, through a grant from the National Institutes of Health, a series of activities were initiated to translate the intervention to enhance the feasibility of its use in the workplace. By collecting data from various stakeholders, including program master trainers and employees working with chronic conditions, the program developers and interventionists were able to modify the program's format (i.e., to be more palatable to employers) and content (i.e., to be more applicable for working-age adults). The resulting intervention is being tested to determine its effectiveness in terms of known health outcomes and new indicators of worker performance (Smith et al., 2014).

Another example of translation will serve to illustrate how an intervention can be changed to reach new populations. Research with Hispanic older adults at the Texas–Mexico border is addressing the reality that motivating behavioral changes among these individuals requires more than simply delivering a program in Spanish. When translating an intervention for this population, it is important for researchers to keep the basic behavioral change strategies but adapt them to meet the target population's cultural and familial values and the issues that are important to the participants. The point is to engage in "precision health." The translated programs still have the therapeutic elements, but they are tailored to better align with the needs, beliefs, and values of the target population.

As this example shows, it is the match of the intervention with the population and settings that is needed to ensure program effectiveness. For example, falls interventions among older adults may focus on physical activity, balance training, and elimination of fall hazards in the home, yet new risk factors continue to be discovered. Most recently, cognitive distraction while walking has been suggested to be a mutable risk factor (Smith-Ray et al., 2013). A randomized trial based on a 10-week, computer-based cognitive training intervention was designed to reduce participants' level of being distracted. The findings showed a significant difference on measures predictive of falls, including balance and gait speed. The intervention was most effective among older adults with slower gait speed, which in turn suggests the potential of tailored and targeted or precision interventions among older adults with specific disabilities. Intervention programs should be tailored to the underlying causes of falls, which tend to be multidimensional rather than addressable through a single-strategy approach.

▶ Treatment Fidelity

Treatment fidelity refers to the degree that an intervention is delivered in the way it was originally intended. Stated differently,

treatment fidelity assesses the accuracy of any intervention's delivery in terms of the manuals, protocols, and models from which it was derived. In many grand-scale disseminations, the same program must be delivered multiple times to serve large numbers of participants (e.g., multiple workshops of 20 participants must be offered to reach 1000 people). Given this reality, it is important that each time the intervention is delivered, it is consistent with the interventions occurring before and after it, so as to ensure that all participants receive the same content and program benefits. In theory, fidelity is important to ensure the intervention outcomes observed are a result of the intervention model and its implementation. Interventions delivered with high fidelity have a greater chance of attaining the predetermined, anticipated outcomes. If there is a lack of fidelity, the ability to determine the effectiveness of the program is hindered, leaving researchers and practitioners wondering if the results were due to external factors (and if internal and external fidelity were compromised).

Program drift often occurs when an intervention is delivered over a period of time and/or in multiple settings. By definition, program drift consists of slight modifications, intentional or unintentional, that result in less than perfect replication and program delivery. Sometimes program drift can be a positive outcome, such as when the program developers attempt to scale up their dissemination efforts. For example, to embed A Matter of Balance (AMOB) into community organizations for grand-scale delivery, the original 8-week intervention (delivered once a week for 8 weeks) was also delivered in a 4-week version (delivered twice a week for 4 weeks). Although the essential elements of the intervention were maintained, this drift was essential for organizational adoption in some settings. At other times, program drift can be a negative outcome, as when a health professional facilitates a program and modifies the content because the professional believes he or she "knows better" or "knows more" than what the program manual contains. To avoid this risk, the developers of the Chronic Disease Self-Management Program (CDSMP) use nonprofessional lay leaders (e.g., those who are not nurses or physical therapists) to monitor drift and ensure consistent replication across time and space.

When delivering evidence-based programs, it is important to monitor fidelity, and most of these interventions were developed with a specific fidelity protocol in mind. The most common way of ensuring treatment fidelity is to host in-depth training of intervention facilitators and to require that they be certified (by meeting certain criteria) prior to offering the program in their community. Another common method of fidelity monitoring is to have other trained facilitators observe newly trained facilitators. This sort of review often occurs using fidelity instruments, which document adherence to the content delivered as well as the processes that must occur before, during, and after the program is delivered.

Fidelity is certainly an extremely important concept, because only through adherence can participants be sure to consistently receive the intended concepts and obtain the intended benefits. Nevertheless, fidelity monitoring can become cumbersome. For example, when too many items are being observed before, during, and after the program is delivered, this overly complicated review places an additional burden on the observers and may deter their participation in the monitoring process. Therefore, the processes used to monitor program fidelity must be carefully considered to match the intervention's delivery modality and to focus primarily on the essential elements for success. While fidelity checklists are often used to monitor programs, the mere nature and scope of certain interventions may require such checklists to become long and difficult to follow. As such, efforts have been made to refine and mainstream fidelity checklists so that they can be used more easily in the field across time and space (Ahn et al., 2015).

PEARL 14-4 Fidelity Monitoring of Programs

Fidelity monitoring is critical to ensure programs are delivered as intended. In turn, adequate training and observation efforts are needed to ensure programs can be delivered to older adults across time and space. The successes of a program can be attributed to the intervention (and not to some external set of factors) only if the program is delivered with adherence to program-specific manuals, processes, and content delivery (occurring before, during, and after the intervention). Assessing and monitoring program drift is essential to know what the program is, who it serves and benefits, and whether modifications or translational efforts are necessary.

▶ Scalability

As with any effective intervention, increasing the number of individuals served is essential to ensure aging-related programs meet their goals. When delivering interventions to older adults, then, the program's implementers must consider ways to maximize its reach. Further, given the specified budget, only a certain number of individuals can be served by a given intervention.

If the program's funding remains consistent, there are only a few ways that reach can be enhanced. The first consideration is to reduce or eliminate program content deemed to be unnecessary for program success while retaining only the intervention's essential elements. The second consideration is to change the target participant focus and the intent to reach the same number of individuals, while having each potential participant have certain demographic characteristics, have a specific health status, or reside within a geographic location. This process is often guided by outcome evaluation findings and helps to ensure that those persons who are likely to benefit most from the program will be enrolled, whereas others are not actively recruited into the program.

Ultimately, decisions about scalability based on a fixed budget are contingent upon the purpose of the delivery effort. Are the program's implementers attempting to obtain the same outcomes with more people? Are they looking to obtain stronger outcomes with fewer people? Are they attempting to get the same number of people, but have them look more similar in terms of health risk or demographics? Regardless of the answer to these questions, the decision to scale up the intervention should include strategies that do not compromise the integrity or effectiveness of the intervention.

▶ Sustainability

The sustainability of a program within a given community begins prior to its implementation. Sustainability planning is essential when determining target populations, community partners, and annual budgets. A multiyear plan should be considered. Community-based participatory research (CBPR), or action research, is a strong strategy that should be utilized when planning for initial program delivery and long-term sustainability. CBPR is a way of engaging community organizations, leaders, and stakeholders to better understand the context and climate of the environment in which a program will be introduced and delivered. Through these interactions and other forms of needs assessment, community and organizational priorities can be identified and collectively met by selecting appropriate interventions. If the intervention and its associated benefits align with the mission and ongoing services of an organization and the needs of a community, the program is more likely to be adopted and delivered faithfully over time.

Many strategies can be applied to enhance sustainability. One strategy is to identify an innovative partner who can help advance the intervention's delivery within a given community. For example, many programs that target older adults for participation may be delivered in senior centers or residential facilities (places where older adults typically live and congregate). At the same time, it has been seen that faith-based organizations, YMCAs, and even schools are useful partners for delivering programs to older adults. For example, given the changing demographics of U.S. society and the intergenerational nature of many homes, especially within the Hispanic and African American communities, engaging schools and school-aged children in interventions can, in turn, indirectly engage and recruit older adults.

Another strategy depends on leverage—that is, leveraging funds, target populations, and referrals. In a given community, many organizations are likely to offer health-related services and resources. Given that federal, state, and philanthropic funds are limited in the current economic environment, the level of competition for scarce funding has skyrocketed in recent years. Therefore, when introducing interventions into communities, a single organization's budget can go further when it is enhanced with partnerships than when it is subjected to additional competition. Because many organizations serve the same older adults in a given community, participants should not be fought over; rather, they should be shared and served collectively. Thus, one organization should offer a particular program (or set of services), then refer older adults to another organization that can provide additional, noncompeting services. In this scenario, older adults receive additional services and have better chances for optimized health, and each organization provides the service(s) most aligned with its mission and relies on its community partners to offer other services/resources, thereby avoiding wasting funds on duplicated services. Not every organization can offer every intervention, so collaboration is key to ensure maximization of benefits to intervention recipients.

PEARL 14-5 Partnership with Communities

To impact organizational or community-level outcomes, strategic efforts are needed to reach enough older adults to move the "health needle." These scalable efforts are better achieved through diverse partnerships that foster communication between clinical and community entities. Once plans to increase the volume of older adults served are developed, these partnerships can again be utilized to encourage sustainability of interventions in a community. Ethical considerations necessitate that program deliverers and decision makers be accountable for ensuring that these evidence-based services and resources do not go away once the funding ends. If efforts are not embedded into communities in a long-standing, ongoing capacity, the initial introduction of an intervention cannot be justified.

To further increase participation in interventions, it is important to bring programs to where the older adults reside and naturally congregate. Participants are less likely to attend the program, especially if it requires multiple sessions, if they must travel great distances to the program site.

▶ Integrating Community and Clinical Interventions

Many interventions for older adults are delivered in silos (i.e., independently based on funding source, discipline, or community setting). While we try to embed interventions in communities and environments, oftentimes organizations in different sectors are not aware of what is happening external to their own silos.

For example, falls-prevention programs include both clinical interventions and community-based interventions. The STEADI Toolkit is a clinical intervention that focuses on fall-related screening, treatment, and referral for older adults using an algorithm utilized by clinicians during regular physician visits (Stevens & Phelan, 2012). During a visit with their physician, older adults answer a series of questions and undergo several procedures that determine their fall-related risk. Based on those risk factors, additional tests are performed and referrals to specialists are made. Depending on patients' level of fall-related risk, they can also be referred to community-based falls-prevention programs.

Simultaneously, many community-based programs currently serve older adults that emphasize fall prevention (e.g., AMOB, Stepping On, Otago, Tai Chi). These interventions are often hosted in community settings such as senior centers, faith-based organizations, residential facilities, and libraries. Although clinicians are aware that these programs exist, they may not be fully aware of where or when these programs are offered in the community. For this reason, integrating clinical and community interventions can be challenging. There is a need for real-time interaction to ensure that older adults get the clinical screenings and treatments needed to assess their fall-related risk, while also getting the education, physical activity, and social support necessary to prevent falls in the community.

Although falls are used as an example here, this type of community–clinical interaction is necessary when thinking about interventions for disease management, medication management, physical activity, and other initiatives for older adults (**FIGURE 14-4**; **TABLE 14-1**). Many different strategies can be used to facilitate this type of real-time community–clinical integration.

For example, one solution is to create commonly used and managed calendars that show clinicians when and where community-based programs will be delivered in their area. Another approach is to provide clinicians with information about organizations offering these programs and the benefits of these interventions. Such materials can increase the clinicians' knowledge about these programs and foster

Community-clinical integration

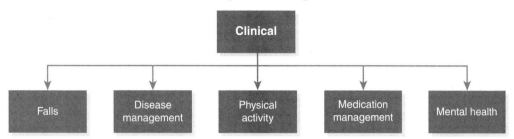

FIGURE 14-4 Community–clinical integration of interventions for disease management and other initiatives for older adults.

Contributed by: Matthew Lee Smith.

future referrals. Yet another solution is to create detailed referral forms that can be completed by clinicians and given to patients so they can provide program deliverers at community-based organizations with their health-related risks and recommendations for appropriate programs.

While it is important for clinicians to know about the community-based programs and refer accordingly, it is also important that patients tell their healthcare providers about programs in which they are participating. When patients share this information, clinicians are better prepared to contextualize their health-related risks, manage their progress, and make subsequent referrals, as necessary.

▶ Policy

A major concern in intervention science research is not whether we know what works, but rather whether we as a society can implement what is known to work. In health care, the long lag time between discovery and widespread dissemination of best clinical practices is well documented (Glasgow & Emmons, 2007; Glasgow, Lichtenstein, & Marcus, 2003). This delay is also evident for behavioral interventions. As one example, it took more than 20 years for CDSMP, which was first developed and tested in the 1990s as an effective program impacting many individual and healthcare outcomes, to be adopted by major federal agencies

and funding provided for its national dissemination (Boutagh et al., 2014). Similarly, principles of urban planning and environmental design for health have been known for decades, but the adoption of best practices at the community and home levels is more theoretical than the norm.

Several lessons from the past can be applied to speed up the transition from theory to practice. First is to design the "intervention" with the end user in mind. This means employing a community participatory approach in which key stakeholders are involved throughout the process—from discovery to implementation to dissemination to sustainability. It also means setting up the infrastructure to support program implementation and dissemination with fidelity. Second, a funding stream must be secured that can support the interventions after their initial testing or first phase of dissemination. This requires documenting the business case for evidence-based programs in general as well as for the specific programs of interest. Tools such as the health cost savings estimator (http://www.ebp-savings.info/) are now available to help communities understand the value of implementing programs in terms of savings to their high-cost healthcare programs (Ahn, Smith, Altpeter, Post, & Ory, 2015). For example, if only 5% of adults with chronic conditions enrolled in CDSMP, then approximately $3.3 billion in emergency room and hospitalization costs would be saved (Ahn et al., 2013).

TABLE 14-1 Selected Examples of the Highest-Level Disease Prevention Evidence-Based Programs for Seniors

Program Name	Goals	Audience	Duration	Delivered By	Website
Active Living Every Day (ALED)	Evoke behavior change by reducing barriers to physical activity	Adults interested in incorporating physical activity into their daily lives	12-week sessions	Trained facilitators (at least 1 per session)	www.ActiveLiving.info
A Matter of Balance (AMOB)	Reduce falls risk and fear of falling; improve falls efficacy and management; promote physical activity	Adults age 60 and older who are ambulatory and able to problem solve	8 sessions (meeting weekly or twice weekly), 2 hours per session	2 trained lay leaders	www.mainehealth.org/mob
Chronic Disease Self-Management (CDSMP) Program	Build self-confidence in clients to take part in maintaining their health and managing their chronic health conditions	Adults with chronic conditions	6 sessions, about 2 hours per session	2 trained lay leaders	http:// patienteducation. stanford.edu/ programs/cdsmp. html
Fit & Strong!	Manage lower-extremity osteoarthritis	Sedentary older adults with lower-extremity joint pain and stiffness; participants must be cleared by a physician to participate in exercise	8 weeks, 3 times per week, 90 minutes per session	Trained facilitator	www.fitandstrong.org
EnhanceFitness	Improve overall functional fitness and well-being	Sedentary older adults	Ongoing: 1-hour sessions, 3 times per week (group physical activity)	Certified fitness instructor	www. projectenhance. org/EnhanceFitness. aspx

(continues)

TABLE 14-1 Selected Examples of the Highest-Level Disease Prevention Evidence-Based Programs for Seniors *(continued)*

Program Name	Goals	Audience	Duration	Delivered By	Website
Otago Exercise Program	Increase strength, balance, and endurance	Community-dwelling frail older adults	4–5 home visits over 8 weeks; monthly phone calls for a year; optional follow-up visits (6, 9, and 12 months)	Physical therapist	http://www.med.unc.edu/aging/cgec/exercise-program
Program to Encourage Active, Rewarding Lives for Seniors (PEARLS)	Reduce symptoms of depression and improve health-related quality of life	Adults age 60 and older with minor depression or dysthymia and are receiving home-based social services	8 sessions, 50 minutes per session (occurs over 19 weeks)	Trained social services worker	www.pearlsprogram.org
Stepping On	Increase self-confidence in making decisions and changing behavior (e.g., exercise) to reduce falls	Community-residing, cognitively intact, older adults at risk for falling	7-week program, 2 hours per session; home or telephone visit; booster session after 3 months	1 trained leader; 1 peer leader	http://wihealthyaging.org/stepping-on
Tai Chi: Moving for Better Balance (TCMBB)	Improve balance, strength, and physical performance to prevent falls	Adults age 65 and older	24- to 26-week program, 3 classes per week, 1 hour per session	Qualified instructors	www.tjqmbb.org

Data from: National Council on Aging. Highest Tier Evidence-Based Health Promotion/Disease Prevention Programs. Available at: https://www.ncoa.org/resources/highest-tier-evidence-based-health-promotiondisease-prevention-programs/

The newest generation of funding for evidence-based programming from ACL requires upfront planning for sustainability. Creative models are being considered, such as seeking reimbursement from insurers or healthcare partners (Shubert et al., 2014). Given the growing numbers of older adults and the higher potential burden of care associated with this population, as a society we cannot afford to stand pat and bemoan the current situation; rather, we must look forward and forge creative partnerships and solutions.

▶ Conclusion and New Directions

The field of evidence-based interventions for seniors is evolving rapidly. Indeed, the seeds for its future directions are already being sowed.

Programmatic Efforts

Lists of recommended evidence-based programs based on the best behavioral and social behavior change principles have been developed. A direction that seems to be emerging from this work is consideration for bundling the different programs to better reinforce and sustain programmatic gains (Towne et al., 2015). For example, an older individual might enroll in CDSMP or AMOB, but at the end of the workshop, be encouraged to join a hands-on exercise program such as Enhance-Fitness. Right now, we know very little about how different programs fit together, and what the best sequencing might be, and for whom. This is a practical area for future inquiry.

Revisiting Research Paradigms

Researchers have spent decades developing the "best" intervention strategies and now have a vast portfolio of evidence-based practices. According to Larry Green, "If we want more evidence-based practice, we need more practice-based evidence." This means going back to

community-based or clinical settings and seeing "what works," and then standardizing best practices so they can be broadly implemented outside of the original setting and population. An example of this approach is the Texercise Program (Riley, 2014), a governor-endorsed physical activity program that had wide coverage but was not being delivered in a consistent manner. Efforts have since been made to develop a standard procedure ("manualize") for the intervention's implementation, create uniform training and facilitator protocols, and test the new Texercise Select Program for effectiveness (Ory, Smith, Howell, et al., 2015; Ory, Smith, Jiang, et al., 2015; Smith et al., 2015). As mentioned previously in the translation and fidelity portions of this chapter, standardizing an intervention produces many benefits by ensuring consistency regarding content delivery, activity participation, and intervention dose. Such consistency enables the program's implementers to identify the "borders" of their interventions and to more successfully replicate the program over time and space and link intervention processes to outcomes.

Dissemination of New Advances in Science

Dissemination by program developers used to be defined in terms of published literature and reports to funding agencies—a factor that may have been one cause of the long delays in translating research into practice. Researchers are now recognizing the importance of bringing their findings back to community stakeholders and seeking advice on the best ways to accomplish scalability and sustainability. Toward this end, researchers are developing policy briefs and holding feedback sessions to formulate next steps after the initial program efficacy has been demonstrated. Further, researchers should select dissemination channels for research and practice findings that reach those audiences who can best use the information. An example of this could be the publication of findings in credible online, open-access journals that make articles available in a timely manner and do not require subscription fees (often associated with academic institutions).

The Role of Technology

There is growing interest in how technology can support behavioral and social interventions—or serve as an actual intervention for screening, diagnosis, treatment, or environmental modification. For example, mHealth tools are being used to help with initial assessments of behavior and social supports, to support behavioral adherence through reminders, and to make and track referrals (Dahlke et al., 2015). Similarly, mTools are being used to engage and motivate older adults to be more physically active and mentally alert (Satariano, Scharlach, & Lindeman, 2014).

There have also been significant advances in the use of technology for making homes safer, enabling older adults to live independently longer (Magnusson, Hanson, & Borg, 2014). For example, the use of video game technology (e.g., Kinect motion-sensing input devices) has enabled clinicians and agencies to monitor fall occurrences in the home and program officials to improve intervention engagement remotely (e.g., assessing the accuracy of Tai Chi poses in online delivery).

Further, the integration of technology into existing program and community initiatives facilitates community–clinical connectivity (as previously stated) and can allow for the collection of uniform data from patients. For example, the CDC has partnered with Epic to integrate the STEADI Toolkit as a standard module in its electronic medical records (http://www.cdc.gov/steadi). Further, technology has enabled electronic training for the STEADI Toolkit and continuing education credits to be earned for clinicians and allied health professionals (e.g., nurses, physical therapists, occupational therapists, health educators) who complete such training.

Intergenerational Emphases

Consistent with considerations of aging as a life course phenomenon, there is growing recognition of the interdependence of generations. This perspective is reflected in universal design principles for housing and community spaces. It is also reflected in programmatic activities where caregivers of all ages are invited to participate in evidence-based practices, and in the growing number of intervention strategies designed to ease stress among intergenerational caregivers. To this end, efforts have been made to account for generational shifts in evidence-based programming, with programs that traditionally have targeted older adults being translated to meet the needs of middle-aged and older adults. For example, the previously mentioned translation of CDSMP for use in the workplace (Smith et al., 2014) is intended to bring about immediate health- and work-related benefits to participants, but it is also intended to prevent negative health- and work-related ramifications associated with unmanaged conditions as these employees transition into older adulthood.

References

8 80 Cities. (2016). Available at: http://880cities.org

Abramson, T. A., Trejo, L., & Lai, D. W. (2002). Culture and mental health: Providing appropriate services for a diverse older population. *Generations*, *26*(1), 21.

Ahn, S., Basu, R., Smith, M. L., Jiang, L., Lorig, K., Whitelaw, N., & Ory, M. G. (2013). The impact of chronic disease self-management programs: Healthcare savings through a community-based intervention. *BMC Public Health*, *13*, 1141. doi:10.1186/1471-2458-13-1141

Ahn, S., Smith, M. L., Altpeter, M., Belza, B., Post, L., & Ory, M. G. (2014). Methods for streamlining intervention fidelity checklists: An example from the chronic disease self-management program. *Frontiers in Public Health*, *2*, 139–146.

Ahn, S., Smith, M. L., Altpeter, M., Post, L., & Ory, M. G. (2015). Healthcare cost savings estimator tool for chronic disease self-management program: A new tool for program administrators and decision makers. *Frontiers in Public Health*, *3*, 197–208.

Beattie, B. L. (2014). Working toward a multi-program strategy in fall prevention. *Frontiers in Public Health*, *2*, 62–63.

Belloc, N. B., & Breslow, L. (1972). Relationship of physical health status and health practices. *Preventive medicine, 1*(3),409-421. doi:http://dx.doi.org/10.1016/0091-7435(72)90014-X

Belloc, B., Breslow, L., & Hochstim, J. R. (1972). Measurement of physical health in a general population survey. *American Journal of Epidemiology, 92*(5), 328–336.

Belza, B., Altpeter, M., Hooker, S. P., & Moni, G. (2014). The CDC Healthy Aging Research Network: Advancing science toward action and policy for the evidence-based health promotion movement. *Frontiers in Public Health, 2,* 50–52.

Berkman, L. F., & Breslow, L. (1983). Health and ways of living: The Alameda County study. New York, NY: Oxford University Press.

Boutaugh, M. L., Jenkins, S. M., Kulinski, K. P., Lorig, K. L., Ory, M. G., & Smith, M. L. (2014). Closing the disparity: The work of the Administration on Aging. *Generations, 38*(4), 107–118.

Boutaugh, M. L., & Lawrence, L. J. (2014). Fostering healthy aging through evidence-based prevention programs: Perspectives from the administration for community living/administration on aging. *Frontiers in Public Health, 2,* 18–20.

Brownson, R. C., Fielding, J. E., & Maylahn, C. M. (2009). Evidence-based public health: A fundamental concept for public health practice. *Annual Review of Public Health, 30,* 175–201.

Centers for Disease Control and Prevention (CDC). (2011). *Healthy Aging Research Network: Putting collective wisdom to work for older Americans.* Atlanta, GA: National Center for Chronic Disease Prevention and Health Promotion, Division of Adult and Community Health.

Cress, E., Buchner, D., Prohaska, T., Rimmer, J., Brown, M., Macera, C., DePietro, L. & Chodzko-Zajko, W. (2004). Physical activity programs and behavior counseling in older adult populations, *Medicine & Science in Sports & Exercise, 36*(11), 1997–2003.

Cress, M. E., Buchner, D. M., Prohaska, T., Rimmer, J., Brown, M., Macera, C.,... Chodzko-Zajko, W. (2006). Best practices for physical activity programs and behavior counseling in older adult populations. *European Review of Aging and Physical Activity, 3*(1), 34–42.

Dahlke, D. V., Fair, K., Hong, Y. A., Beaudoin, C. E., Pulczinski, J., & Ory, M. G. (2015). Apps seeking theories: Results of a study on the use of health behavior change theories in cancer survivorship mobile apps. *JMIR mHealth and uHealth, 3*(1), e31.

Diaz Moore, K., Greenfield, E. A., & Scharlach, A. (2017). Healthy aging and its implications for public health: Healthy communities. In W. Satariano & M. Maus (Eds.), *Aging, place, and health: A global perspective.* Burlington, MA: Jones & Bartlett Learning.

Durand, C. P., Andalib, M., Dunton, G. F., Wolch, J., & Pentz, M. A. (2011). A systematic review of built environment factors related to physical activity and obesity risk: Implications for smart growth urban planning. *Obesity Reviews, 12*(5), e173–e182.

Fiatarone, M. A., O'Neill, E. F., Ryan, N. D., Clements, K. M., Solares, G. R., Nelson, M. E.,... Evans, W. J. (1994). Exercise training and nutritional supplementation for physical frailty in very elderly people. *New England Journal of Medicine, 330*(25), 1769–1775.

Glasgow, R. E., & Emmons, K. M. (2007). How can we increase translation of research into practice? Types of evidence needed. *Annual Reviews of Public Health, 28,* 413–433.

Glasgow, R. E., Lichtenstein, E., & Marcus, A. C. (2003). Why don't we see more translation of health promotion research to practice? Rethinking the efficacy-to-effectiveness transition? *American Journal of Public Health, 93*(8), 1261–1267.

Haynes, M., Hughes, S., Lorig, K., Simmons, J., Snyder, S. J., Steinman, L.,... Pelaez, M. B. (2014). Evidence-Based Leadership Council: A national collaborative. *Frontiers in Public Health, 2,* 59–61.

Housman, J., & Dorman, S. (2005). The Alameda County Study: A systematic, chronological review. *Journal of Health Education, 36*(5), 302–308.

Humpel, N., Owen, N., & Leslie, E. (2002). Environmental factors associated with adults' participation in physical activity: A review. *American Journal of Preventive Medicine, 22*(3), 188–199.

Institute of Medicine (IOM). (1982). *Health and behavior: Frontiers of research in the behavioral sciences.* Hamburg, D. A, Elliott, G. R., & Parron, D. L. (Eds.). Washington, DC: National Academy Press.

Kaplan, G., Seeman, T., Cohen, R., Knudsen, L., & Guralnik, J. (1987). Mortality among the elderly in the Alameda County Study: Behavioral and demographic risk factors. *American Journal of Public Health, 77*(3), 307–312.

Katz, S., Branch, L. G., Branson, M. H., Papsidero, J. A., Beck, J. C., & Greer, D. S. (1983). Active life expectancy. *New England Journal of Medicine, 309*(20), 1218–1224.

King, A. C. (2001). Interventions to promote physical activity by older adults. *Journals of Gerontology, Series A: Biological Sciences and Medical Sciences, 56*(suppl 2), 36–46.

Lawton, M. P. (1985). The elderly in context perspectives from environmental psychology and gerontology. *Environment and Behavior, 17,* 501–519.

Lewthwaite, R. (1990). Motivational considerations in physical activity involvement. *Physical Therapy, 70*(12), 808–819.

Magnusson, L., Hanson, E., & Borg, M. (2004). A literature review study of information and communication technology as a support for frail older people living at home and their family carers. *Technology and Disability, 16*(4), 223–235.

Maus, M., & Satariano, W. (2017b). Aging, health, and the environment: An ecological model. In W. Satariano & M. Maus (Eds.), *Aging, place, and health: A global perspective*. Burlington, MA: Jones & Bartlett Learning.

McAuley, E., & Blissmer, B. (2000). Self-efficacy determinants and consequences of physical activity. *Exercise and Sport Sciences Reviews*, *28*(2), 85-88.

National Council on Aging. (2016). Key components of evidence-based programming. Available at: https://www.ncoa.org/resources/highest-tier-evidence-based-health-promotiondisease-prevention-programs/

Nelson, M. E., Rejeski, W. J., Blair, S. N., Duncan, P. W., Judge, J. O., King, A. C.,... Castaneda-Sceppa, C. (2007). Physical activity and public health in older adults: Recommendation from the American College of Sports Medicine and the American Heart Association. *Circulation*, *116*(9), 1094.

Ory, M. G., Abeles, R. P. E., & Lipman, P. D. E. (1992). *Aging, health, and behavior*. Newbury Park, CA: Sage Publications.

Ory, M., Hoffman, M. K., Hawkins, M., Sanner, B., & Mockenhaupt, R. (2003). Challenging aging stereotypes: Strategies for creating a more active society. *American Journal of Preventive Medicine*, *25*(3S2), 164-171.

Ory, M. G., Lee, C., & Satariano, W. A. (In press). Health and the built environment: Enhancing healthy aging through environmental intervention. In C. Browning & S. Thomas (Eds.), *Interdisciplinary perspectives of healthy ageing: Improving the quality of life for older persons*. New York, NY: Springer.

Ory, M. G., & Smith, M. L. (Eds.). (2015). *Evidence-based programming for older adults*. Lausanne, Switzerland: Frontiers Media. doi:10.3389/978-2-88919-585-5

Ory, M. G., Smith, M. L., Howell, D., Zollinger, A., Quinn, C., Swierc, S. M., & Stevens, A. B. (2015). The conversion of a practice-based lifestyle enhancement program into a formalized, testable program: From Texercise Classic to Texercise Select. *Frontiers in Public Health—Public Health Education and Promotion*. doi:10.3389/fpubh.2014.00291

Ory, M. G., Smith, M. L., Jiang, L., Howell, D., Chen, S., Pulczinski, J. C., & Stevens, A. B. (2015). Texercise effectiveness: Impacts on physical functioning and quality of life. *Journal of Aging and Physical Activity*, *23*(4), 622-629. doi:10.1123/japa.2014-0072

Prohaska, T., Belansky, E., Belza, B., Buchner, D., Marshall, V., McTigue, K.,... Wilcox, S. (2006). Physical activity, public health, and aging: Critical issues and research priorities. *Journals of Gerontology, Series B: Psychological Sciences and Social Sciences*, *61*(5), S267-S273.

Prohaska, T., Eisenstein, A., Satariano, W., Bayles, C., Kurtovich, E., Kealey, M., & Ivey, S. (2009). Walking and the preservation of cognitive function in older populations. *Gerontologist*, *49*(suppl 1), S86-S93.

Prohaska, T., Smith-Ray, R., & Glasgow, R. (2012). Translation, dissemination and implementation issues. In T. Prohaska, L. Anderson, & R. Binstock (Eds.), *Public health for an aging society* (pp. 161-180). Baltimore, MD: Johns Hopkins University Press.

Riley, H. (2014). Texercise: The evolution of a health promotion program. *Frontiers in Public Health*, *2*, 45-46.

Rosenberg, D. E., Gell, N. M., Jones, S. M., Renz, A., Kerr, J., Gardiner, P. A., & Arterburn, D. (2015). The feasibility of reducing sitting time in overweight and obese older adults. *Health Education & Behavior*, 1090198115577378.

Rowe, J. W., & Kahn, R. L. (1987). Human aging: Usual and successful. *Science*, *237*(4811), 143-149.

Rowe, J. W., & Kahn, R. L. (2015). Successful aging 2.0: Conceptual expansions for the 21st century. *Journals of Gerontology, Series B: Psychological Sciences and Social Sciences*, *70*(4), 593-596.

Satariano, W., Ivey, S., Kurtovich, E., Keley, M., Hubberd, A., Bayles, C.,... Prohaska, T. (2010). Lower body function, neighborhoods and walking in an older population. *American Journal of Preventive Medicine*, *38*(4), 419-428.

Satariano, W., & Maus, M. (2017a). Global aging of the population: The significance of an epidemiological perspective.. In W. Satariano & M. Maus (Eds.), *Aging, place, and health: A global perspective*. Burlington, MA: Jones & Bartlett Learning.

Satariano, W. A., Ory, M. G., & Lee, C. (2012). Planned and built environments: Interactions with aging. In T. R. Prohaska, L. A. Anderson, & R. H. Binstock (Eds.), *Public health in an aging society*, 327–352. Baltimore, MD: Johns Hopkins Press.

Satariano, W. A., Scharlach, A. E., & Lindeman, D. (2014). Aging, place, and technology: Toward improving access and wellness in older populations. *Journal of Aging and Health*, *26*(8), 1373-1389.

Schneider, E. C., & Beattie, B. L. (2014). Building the older adult fall prevention movement: Steps and lessons learned. *Frontiers in Public Health*, *2*, 64-69.

Shubert, T. E., Smith, M. L., Ory, M. G., Clarke, C. B., Bomberger, S. A., Roberts, E., & Busby-Whitehead, J. (2014). Translation of the Otago Exercise Program for adoption and implementation in the United States. *Frontiers in Public Health*, *2*, 224-235.

Smith, M. L., Ory, M. G., Jiang, L., Howell, D., Chen, S., Pulczinski, J. C., Swierc, S. M., & Stevens, A. B. (2015). Texercise Select effectiveness: An examination of physical activity and nutrition outcomes. *Translational Behavioral Medicine: Practice, Policy and Research*, *5*(4), 433-442. doi:10.1007/s13142-014-0299-3

Smith, M. L., Wilson, M. G., DeJoy, D. M., Padilla, H., Zuercher, H., Corso, P.,... Ory, M. G. (2014). Chronic Disease Self-Management Program in the workplace: Opportunities for health improvement. *Frontiers in Public Health*, *2*, 166-171.

Smith-Ray, R., Hughes, S., Prohaska, T., Little, D., Jurivich, D., & Hedeker, D. (2013). Impact of cognitive training on balance and gate in older adults. *Journals of Gerontology, Series B: Psychological Sciences and Social Sciences, 70*(3), 357-366.

Stevens, J. A., & Phelan, E. A. (2012). Development of STEADI: A fall prevention resource for health care providers. *Health Promotion Practice*, 15248399 12463576.

Towne, S. D. Jr., Smith, M. L., Ahn, S., Altpeter, M., Belza, B., Kulinski, K. P., & Ory, M. G. (2015). National dissemination of multiple evidence-based disease prevention programs: Reach to vulnerable older adults. *Frontiers in Public Health, 2*, 156. doi: 10.3389/fpubh.2014.00156

Towne, S. D. Jr., Won, J., Lee, S., Ory, M. G., Forjuoh, S. N., Wang, S., & Lee, C. (2016). Using Walk Score and neighborhood perceptions to assess walking among middle-aged and older adults. *Journal of Community Health*, 1-12.

U.S. Department of Health and Human Services. (2000). *Healthy people 2010*. Washington, DC: Author.

U.S. Department of Health and Human Services. (2008). *Physical activity guidelines for Americans*. Washington, DC: Author.

Wilcox, S., Altpeter, M., Anderson, L. A., Belza, B., Bryant, L., Jones, D. L.,… Satariano, W. A. (2013). The Healthy Aging Research Network: Resources for building capacity for public health and aging practice. *American Journal of Health Promotion, 28*(1), 2-6.

Wingard. D. B. L., Berkman, L. F., & Brand, R. J. (1982). A multivariate analysis of health-related practices: A nine-year mortality follow-up of the Alameda County Study. *American Journal of Epidemiology, 116*(5), 765–775. PMID: 7148802

World Health Organization (WHO). (1946). Preamble to the Constitution of the World Health Organization as adopted by the International Health Conference, New York, 19-22 June, 1946; signed on 22 July 1946 by the representatives of 61 States (Official Records of the World Health Organization, no. 2, p. 100) and entered into force on 7 April 1948.

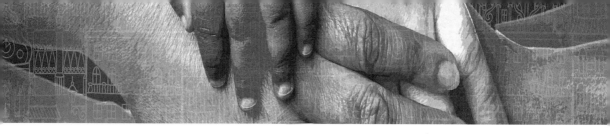

CHAPTER 15

Healthy Aging and Its Implications for Public Health: Healthy Communities

Keith Diaz Moore, Emily A. Greenfield, and **Andrew Scharlach**

ABSTRACT

This chapter explores how healthy aging is influenced by the communities in which we live. It does so by viewing the concept of healthy aging from a lifespan development perspective and by viewing communities as places. There are six developmentally salient attributes that person–place transactions should enable: continuity, compensation, control, connection, contribution, and challenge/comfort. The chapter draws upon the ecological framework of place to assert that place comprises the people, the physical setting, and the program (the socially shared expectations that inform action and then shape appraisals of those actions). These concepts are explored in relation to various place-based initiatives, including both those that are "setting oriented" (visitability, complete streets, age-friendly community initiatives) and those that are "support oriented" (naturally occurring retirement community [NORC] supportive service programs, villages). Healthy places are considered to be those milieus of people, programs, and physical settings that facilitate the six developmentally salient attributes of person–place transactions.

KEYWORDS

healthy places	visitability	naturally occurring retirement
age-friendly	universal design	community (NORC)
community initiatives	villages	environmental gerontology

Image: Hands © Shutterstock, Inc./Dewald Kirsten; Buildings © Shutterstock, Inc./Bariskina.

▶ Introduction

"Healthy aging" is a popular, yet nebulous phrase. Schulz and Heckhausen (1996) position healthy aging within a life course perspective, emphasizing outcomes such as a decrease in morbidity and an increase in life expectancy. The European Union's Health Ageing Project (2006, p. 16) defines healthy aging somewhat differently, as "the process of optimising opportunities for physical, social, and mental health to enable older people to take an active part in society without discrimination and to enjoy an independent and good quality of life." In both cases, healthy aging is viewed as a process, although the anticipated outcomes are different.

This chapter explores the interplay of place with healthy aging. In so doing, we will focus on the following objectives:

■ Examine healthy aging as a lifelong pursuit, with a focus on domains of human development that are particularly salient to the latter part of the life course

■ Discuss places as ecological phenomena that have special significance for the potential of healthy aging

■ Describe how healthy aging involves an ongoing, dynamic negotiation of place involving the process of adaptation

■ Consider existing and potential place-based initiatives that may further facilitate healthy aging

Healthy aging can be situated according to an **environmental gerontology** perspective. Golant's (2011) theory of residential normalcy argues that older adults engage in the processes of assimilation and accommodation so as to maintain themselves within appropriate zones of "residential normalcy," or person–environment congruence. Assimilation and accommodation are concepts identified by Piaget (1932), who conceived of psychological development as a process of active and intentional engagement with external reality. For Golant, assimilation refers to individuals'

efforts to alter their environments—for example, through home modification or relocation—so as to preserve their internal cognitive structures. Accommodation refers to internally focused strategies such as altering one's aspirations or changing comparison standards (e.g., "others have it worse"). Personal and physical resources as well as opportunity structures may then impact the efficacy of such strategies. For instance, personal wealth and disposable income not only shape the range of assimilative efforts an individual can consider adopting, but also influence how the person may perceive and value such interventions. This process is related to the concept of opportunity structures, which suggest that the opportunity for anyone to achieve particular goals requires certain necessary conditions that vary depending on social networks and membership (Silverstein & Bengston, 1997).

The notion that zones of person–environment fit are connected to optimal functioning was advanced by Lawton and Nahemow (1973) as they presented the cornerstone of environmental gerontology, the ecological model of aging. Building upon the work of Wohlwill (1966), these authors identified that optimization does not occur at a specific point, but rather within a zone stretching both positively and negatively from what they term the "adaptation level," reflecting interactions between the person and his or her environment. Lawton and Nahemow's theory rests on the notion that people seek to maintain homeostasis: Sometimes this may mean a need for restoration, and at other times it may mean a need for challenge. Ultimately, this model might be considered to give rise to Golant's (2011) identification of residential normalcy, which encompasses a zone of comfort (less environmental pressure) and a zone of mastery (greater pressure) as two key dimensions of person–environment fit.

Both the ecological model of aging and the theory of residential normalcy acknowledge that the negotiation between the person and the environment also needs to consider that the needs, desires, abilities, and resources involved in the person–environment transaction change over time and in regard to social situations. However, neither of these theoretical conceptualizations fully integrates these critical issues. As Lawton (1989, p. 57) wrote, "the language of process, temporal state, and development must be supplied by those more gifted than I." What follows is an effort to more fully articulate and integrate such concerns.

▸ Human Development and the Negotiation of Person–Environment Fit

Scharlach and his colleagues (e.g., Scharlach & Diaz Moore, 2016; Scharlach & Lehning, 2015) have expanded the concept of person–environment fit by incorporating principles from lifespan developmental theory. They identify six constructs as developmentally salient attributes of person–environment transactions in later life: (1) continuity; (2) compensation; (3) control; (4) connection; (5) contribution; and (6) [the previously mentioned] challenge/comfort. We now examine in greater detail the developmental salience of each of these six attributes.

Continuity

Maintaining continuity with regard to self-identity can be challenging in later life when confronting developmental transitions that may potentially disconnect a person from what previously gave his or her life meaning (Hazan, 2011). An example of such a change is retirement in a society that ties identity with work. Atchley's (1989) continuity theory holds that older adults adapt using psychological strategies tied to their past experiences of themselves and their social world. Adaptive efforts are therefore negotiated within the context of their perceived past, their individual

preferences, and their social identity. Maintaining lifelong interests and activities that support one's continued sense of self can become more challenging in later life, not only as a result of age-related reductions in functional ability, but also because environments are not always well designed to enhance the functioning of older community members. For instance, to preserve a relatively stable self-construct, individuals may modify their activities, their aspirations, and even their constructions of reality (e.g., Herzog & Markus, 1999).

Compensation

Compensation refers to the application of alternative methods to achieve goals when circumstances make prior methods less usable. This concept comes from Paul and Margaret Baltes' selective optimization with compensation lifespan developmental model (Baltes & Baltes, 1990). Compensation efforts can be facilitated by resources within the individual's local environment, such as assistance with tasks that can no longer be performed independently, assistive devices, ambient assistive technologies (e.g., "smart home" apps), environmental modifications, or other sources of support. Compensation can also involve behavioral changes, including developing new abilities or finding alternative means of achieving goals, as well as adjustments in aspirations and social reference standards to reflect changing circumstances (Romo et al., 2013). Compensation in later life has been found to have a positive effect on various indicators of healthy aging such as emotional well-being and satisfaction (Freund, 2008).

Control

Whereas compensation focuses on the need for support, control focuses on the actual and perceived ability to effect changes in oneself and one's environment so as to achieve one's aims. Control theory posits that individuals will actively strive to modify their environments and themselves in an effort to maximize goal achievement and minimize distress (Schulz & Heckhausen, 1996). Two types of control are suggested to exist: primary control and secondary control (Heckhausen, Wrosch, & Schulz, 2010). Primary control, which targets the external world, involves actively attempting to manipulate the physical or social environment with the aim of attaining one's goals. Secondary control involves internal psychological processes, such as adoption of more attainable goals, strategic social comparisons, less-demanding comparisons with one's earlier self, and self-protective causal attributions (Heckhausen et al., 2010). Research findings suggest that secondary control processes tend to increase throughout life, whereas primary control peaks in mid-life and declines thereafter, perhaps in response to the lack of adequate external options for resolving complex age-related challenges (Heckhausen et al., 2010). When adopting a life course perspective, it is important to note that actions taken earlier in life in preparation for later life (e.g., health promotion, financial planning, skill acquisition, investing in long-term relationships) are associated with better quality of life years later (Kahana, Kelley-Moore, & Kahana, 2012; Prenda & Lachman, 2001).

Connection

Older adults generally strive to remain socially engaged as they grow older, even in the face of substantial personal and contextual barriers. Carstensen's (1993) socioemotional selectivity theory (SST) emphasizes that meaningful interpersonal relationships assume increased importance when people view themselves as being closer to the end of their life, especially when those relationships reinforce a positive sense of self. A person's time horizon—that is, the period of life believed to be remaining—shapes the investment of that individual's time and energy so as to maximize positive interactions with familiar interpersonal contacts

(Scheibe & Carstensen, 2010). Maintaining meaningful social relationships can become more challenging in later life as a result of factors such as health problems, disabling conditions, and interpersonal communication (Weir, Meisner, & Baker, 2010); depletion of social networks due to death, illness, and retirement; ageist and disablist norms that contribute to social isolation by fostering feelings of inadequacy and invisibility; and unsupportive physical environments that limit mobility and restrict access to community participation.

Contribution

Classic lifespan developmental theory identifies generativity—which can be broadly defined as caring for the well-being and welfare of others—as a hallmark feature of adult development (Erikson, 1963). Building from this idea, scholars have posited that generative concern increases with age because of both societal expectations and intrinsic desires (McAdams & de St. Aubin, 1992). Empirical evidence suggests that concern for younger generations among older adults is especially strong when older adults sense their own lifetimes as limited (Maxfield et al., 2014). Moreover, there has been growing attention within gerontology on how environmental contexts—including social and organizational policies—can facilitate or constrain outlets for older adults' prosocial behaviors (Morrow-Howell, Gonzales, Matz-Costa, & Greenfield, 2015). Research has found that prosocial behaviors in later life can yield benefits for the individuals who engage in them, especially when motivated by an other-oriented (rather than self-oriented) perspective (e.g., Brown & Brown, 2014; Konrath, Fuhrel-Forbis, Lou, & Brown, 2012). Particularly for older adults who are at risk for poorer well-being, perhaps because of health problems or widowhood, prosocial behaviors can provide positive psychosocial outcomes, such as a renewed sense of meaning and purpose (Greenfield & Marks, 2004).

Public health initiatives serving older adults would be greatly enhanced if they pursued issues from a lifespan perspective and focused on promoting the six developmentally salient attributes of person–place transactions: continuity, compensation, control, connection, contribution, and challenge/comfort.

Challenge/Comfort

The ecological model of aging is predicated on the concept of adaptation and its related desired outcome of homeostasis (Lawton & Nahemow, 1973). In short, there are times when a person needs some challenge to return to maximum potential, while at other times the individual may have been under stress and requires some comfort. Within the biology of aging, the concept of challenge is expressed within hormesis theory (Rattan, 2008), which suggests that organisms, from the cellular level to social organizations, require ongoing challenges if they are to grow and flourish. This challenge is subject to a "Goldilocks principle," however: Hormesis describes a process in which exposure to a "low dose" of an intervention, which is typically damaging at higher doses and intensities, induces an adaptive beneficial effect. Through a process of stress conditioning, successful encounters with manageable challenges can foster positive compensatory responses that strengthen the organism's ability to adapt constructively when faced subsequently with more intense situations.

On the flip side, after experiencing stress, the body may require restoration—that is, comfort—to again achieve homeostasis. In gerontology, we see this concept illustrated in the progressively lowered stress threshold (PLST) model (Hall & Buckwalter, 1987); it suggests that, as people experience the daily stress associated with dementia, their intrinsic capacity or threshold is progressively

compromised. Interventions have been proposed to alter the trajectory toward anxiety and ultimately dysfunctional behavior that are comforting in nature. Building upon the PLST model, Diaz Moore (2007) suggests that attention restoration theory (Kaplan, 1995) is relevant to designing environments for people with dementia. Specifically, this theory suggests that environments should have four characteristics—being away (different from the stress-inducing environment), fascination (capturing attention), extent (depth and richness to maintain fascination), and compatibility (fit between environment and one's purposes)—if they are to restore expended directed attentional capacity. In reality, physical and social environments seldom provide the optimal levels of stimulation and growth appropriate for aging bodies and minds, but instead may potentially induce excess dependency and learned helplessness. As an example, disuse, rather than actual disease, appears to be a greater contributor to cardiovascular vulnerability, musculoskeletal fragility, and premature frailty in later life (Bortz, 2009).

▶ The Ecological Framework of Place

From a life course perspective, the six previously mentioned attributes are central to the process of healthy aging. We view that process as involving a constant dynamic negotiation of the person with place over the life course. We use the term "place" advisedly, as far too often discussions of aging and environment focus solely on either the physical environment or the social environment, but miss the important interdependency between them. As Proshansky and colleagues (1983) identified, there is no physical environment that is not also a social environment, and vice versa. Thus we agree with Wahl and Lang (2004, pp. 17-18), who suggest that place should be viewed as encompassing three premises: (1) "behavior is embedded" in places, which "combine both a physical-spatial as well as social-cultural dimension"; (2) places are "socially constructed... socially shaped" physical environments; and (3) "places are dynamic and show both change and stability over time, as people age."

Aspects of place that are likely to influence healthy aging can be further identified through the ecological framework of place (EFP) heuristic (Diaz Moore, 2014). The EFP defines a place as "a milieu involving people ('place participants'), the physical setting, and the program of the place, all catalyzed by situated human activity and fully acknowledging that all four may change over time" (p. 184). We briefly describe each of these components in the following subsections.

People

People may be conceptualized at multiple levels of aggregation (individual, group, organizational, cultural) and encompass not only objective characteristics (e.g., various measured competences such as independent activities of daily living) but also experiential modalities (e.g., motivation, perception, cognition, affect [Weisman, Chaudhury, & Diaz Moore, 2000]). Importantly, regardless of the level of aggregation employed, the EFP views people as expressing agency (c.f. List & Petit, 2011), an underlying assumption of the model.

Physical Setting

As with people, we must consider not only the objective characteristics of the physical setting, but also what Moos (1980) refers to as the "personality of the place." The objective characteristics of the physical setting include objective sensory (e.g., olfactory) and spatial (e.g., degree of enclosure) properties as well as the systems that constitute the physical setting (e.g., roads, sidewalks, lawn, utility infrastructure). However, we also develop perceptual-cognitive assessments of the intentions of the setting that often become anthropomorphized

in terms such as "friendly" or "hostile." Importantly, the EFP notes that any given physical setting exists within a system of other settings, which may be conceptualized at different scales (proximate, building/site, neighborhood/community, and settlement). This facilitates potential consideration of what Bronfenbrenner (2009) terms the mesosystem, or the relationships between these scales.

Program

The concept of the "program" of place is perhaps the most difficult to understand, yet we argue it is a powerful construct in understanding the negotiation of aging and place. Specifically, the program refers to the typically unspoken, socially shared expectations associated with a place that informs action and then shapes the subsequent interpretation of the resulting transaction. In this way, program captures the influence of culture, which Rubinstein and de Medeiros (2003) suggest has two roles in regard to place: (1) as an originating frame of reference colored by assumptions about space, language, narration, and expectations of self and others; and (2) as a mediating, or interpretive, lens for ongoing transactions, shaped by an individual's past experiences, social status, and the like.

The program may best be recognized in a situation where its precepts are violated. As an example, surprise parties are most effective when they occur at a time and place when the program suggests something else is to take place. Participants get excited by the notion of engaging in something otherwise taboo, and the celebrant is surprised only because the program—that is, the socially shared expectations—was violated. Programs are essential to understand, as their fundamental purpose is to further the intention of the place. People may or may not share that intention (e.g., the surprise party), and it is not uncommon for the physical setting to constrain the intentions of the program. How else do we explain the great occurrence of remodeling or rearranging furniture?

What the EFP adds to the conversation on healthy aging is a conceptualization suggesting that the dynamic process of person-environment fit actually should be viewed as the dynamic negotiation of place experience involving an individual with all three aspects of place: people, physical setting, and program. At its heart, the process of healthy aging for individuals would involve the negotiation of their own intentionality with that of the places they experience. Building upon the European Union's definition of healthy aging, **healthy places** might then be defined as those milieus of people, programs, and physical settings that facilitate opportunities for optimal physical, social, and mental health. A developmental perspective would suggest that those health outcomes rely on individuals' engagement with these milieus, particularly for the purposes of continuity, compensation, control, connection, contribution, and challenge/comfort. In other words, healthy places might be considered to be those milieus of people, program, and physical settings that facilitate continuity, compensation, control, connection, contribution, and challenge/comfort.

Examples of Place-Based Initiatives to Promote Healthy Aging

We now turn our attention to several prominent models that explicitly focus on modifying aspects of people's immediate social and physical environments to enhance healthy aging, which is perceived as a person–place process. We first discuss visitability and complete streets as two initiatives that focus on the "physical setting" dimension of place. We then turn our attention to **age-friendly community initiatives** with a focus on the "people" dimension of place. Finally, we provide an overview of villages and naturally occurring retirement community supportive service programs, which represent initiatives that focus on the "program" aspect of place.

Visitability

The concept of **visitability** is defined by Pynoos and colleagues (2010, p. 332) as "a small set of basic accessibility features that enable older adults and persons with disabilities to access the main level of family homes." As such, visitability may be viewed as a subset of the interventions necessary to overcome mobility barriers and thereby promote "optimal mobility."

Four public health burdens are associated with mobility disability: reduced access to goods and services, increased sedentary behavior, social isolation, and older adults' potentially compromised ability to contribute to their communities (Satariano et al., 2012). While all four are critical detriments to healthy aging, the term "visitability" makes it clear that the emphasis for these interventions is promoting social engagement. Declines in social engagement place individuals at increased risk of dementia (Fratiglioni, Paillard-Borg, & Winblad, 2004), cardiovascular disease (Barth, Schneider, & von Känel, 2010), heightened allostatic load as demonstrated by heightened inflammatory and metabolic responses (Grant, Hammer, & Steptoe, 2009; Uchino, 2006), lowered quality of life and health-related quality of life (Hawton et al., 2011; Rantakokko et al., 2015), and increased risk of mortality (Holt-Lundstad, Smith, Baker, Harris, & Stephenson, 2015). Current evidence indicates that the heightened risk for mortality from a lack of social relationships is greater than that from obesity (Flegal, Kit, Orpana, & Graubard, 2013). With an elderly population, we do need to distinguish between social withdrawal (an active choice made by the person) and true social isolation (which involves a sense of distress) (Kim & Clarke, 2015). In fact, a number of researchers suggest that efforts should be directed not so much toward treating social isolation but rather toward preventing it (e.g.,

Dickens, Richards, Greaves, & Campbell, 2011; Nicholson, 2012).

Visitability emphasizes the implementation of a few core accessibility features in residential environments, including a zero-step entrance (an entrance threshold where the accessible floor height is the same as the exterior grade), 32-inch clear doorways, and at least a half bath on the accessible floor with maneuvering space for a walker or wheelchair (and preferably a three-fourths bath) (Maisel, Smith, & Steinfeld, 2008). This concept is based on the assumption that these essential interventions allow individuals experiencing increasing physical limitations to extend the period of time and the range of disability during which they may still age-in-place. In terms of spatial organization, visitability assumes that the kitchen is on the accessible floor of the dwelling, as is a space that might be turned into a sleeping area. Remodeling costs associated with such alterations are significant, however, which is why visitability advocates continue to push for such common-sense guidelines to be implemented in new construction (Concrete Change, 2016).

Visitability has its roots in the paradigm shift that has occurred in the disability movement—from viewing disability as a medical condition, to viewing functionality as a result of the negotiation between persons and their environment, in relation to the goal-oriented action they seek to engage (World Health Organization [WHO], 2001). This profound shift emphasizes the centrality of the physical environment in determining functionality. Thus, someone with a broken right leg and using crutches is temporarily disabled and may be "mobility disabled" in terms of the inability to drive, at heightened risk of falls (e.g., using stairs), and having difficulty using facilities such as bathrooms.

Currently, only a very narrow range of the suggestions found in the accessibility literature address visitability concerns. Accessibility, from a design perspective, aims for environments to provide an assortment of design interventions,

products, and information that support long-term use by individuals with mobility limitations (Maisel et al., 2008). As such, Iwarsson and Ståhl (2003, p. 61) suggest that "accessibility is the encounter between the person's or group's functional capacity and the design and demands of the physical environment." This definition led to the development of the Housing Enabler instrument (Iwarsson, 1999; Iwarsson & Slaug, 2010), which involves a checklist for functional capacity (personal component) and a checklist for environmental barriers (environmental component), followed by an analysis relating the two to determine person–environment fit. The Housing Enabler provides a robust methodology for developing highly personalized interventions for those persons with participatory restrictions due to physical limitations. This tool has recently been translated and tested for the U.S. context (Lien, Steggell, Slaug, & Iwarsson, 2015) and suggests exciting possibilities for advancement in this area.

Another possible advance would come with the adoption of a "**universal design**" approach, which Steinfeld and Maisel (2012, p. 29) define as "a process that enables and empowers a diverse population by improving human performance, health and wellness, and social participation." Such a process-focused change suggests the need to retrain architects, designers, and occupational and recreational therapists to focus on design and intervention decisions designed to promote a more inclusive society. One step in this direction is the Lifetime Homes (2015) concept found in the United Kingdom, which suggests 16 design criteria for promoting accessibility rooted in five overarching principles: inclusivity, accessibility, adaptability, sustainability, and good value.

The intent of improved accessibility in residential environments is to provide a minimum baseline for the provisions in the physical setting that may enable extended duration of aging-in-place for older adults. If we view functional capacity as having a bell curve in society, the aim for accessibility is to minimize participatory restriction due to environmental barriers for a wider range of individuals along that curve. How far along the tails of the population might an intervention extend? Universal design pushes this concept further by asking how far along the tails might environments be designed to enable the performance, health, and participation of all. In so doing, universal design provides a challenge to the "program"—our socially shared norms—regarding our housing stock, the people whom we are housing, and perhaps even why we are housing them.

From a developmental perspective, "visitable" environments serve a compensatory function to support the longest possible duration of optimal mobility. The design interventions discussed previously allow residents to maintain continuity by more easily navigating access to and from their dwellings, and facilitating continuance of familiar and meaningful behavior patterns either in or out of the house, including maintaining socializing patterns and social relationships. Visitability should also extend the amount of time an individual can continue to reside in the home, as it provides a more adaptive spatial organization that can maintain a person in his or her zones of mastery and comfort longer within the same dwelling.

Complete Streets

A complete street is "a road that is designed to be safe for drivers; bicyclists; transit vehicles and users; and pedestrians of all ages and abilities" (LaPlante & McCann, 2008, p. 24). The complete street movement began with the formation, inside Smart Growth America, of the National Complete Streets Coalition in 2004. This organization recognized that, for the most part, transportation engineering has defined the problem of the street as an automobile-oriented problem. Complete streets emphasize the context-appropriate consideration of all modes of transportation in street design (**FIGURE 15-1**). According to Smart Growth America (2016), "a complete street may include: sidewalks, bike lanes (or wide paved shoulders), special bus lanes, comfortable and accessible public transportation stops, frequent and safe crossing opportunities, median islands, accessible pedestrian signals, curb extensions, narrower travel lanes, roundabouts, and more."

Even if an older adult has a residence that is fully accessible, it is quite possible, given the development patterns of the past half-century, that the residence might be located in a neighborhood that in various ways still limits accessibility to amenities, goods, and services. Many residential developments have been created that forego sidewalks on one or both sides of the street, limit connectivity of walking and biking paths through the creation of winding streets and cul-de-sacs, and provide limited access points to, and most importantly across, arterials filled with fast-moving traffic—in other words, the traditional suburban development pattern.

While complete streets, like visitability, are related to optimal mobility for older adults, they also address three of the four public health

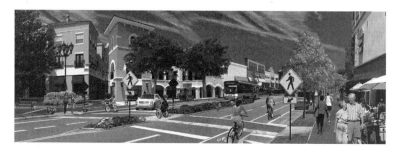

FIGURE 15-1 Example of a Complete Street approach to street design.

burdens associated with mobility limitations: social engagement, access, and physical activity. The issues of social isolation were discussed earlier in this chapter. Typical suburban street design limits access to resources such as groceries and health care, resulting in negative health outcomes (Glass et al., 2003). Sedentary behavior has been linked to increased risk of mortality (Katzmarzyk, Church, Craig, & Bouchard, 2009), cardiovascular disease (Manson et al., 2003), and metabolic syndrome (Gao, Nelson, & Tucker, 2007). Lack of physical activity in older individuals can also lead to loss of musculoskeletal strength and an increase in obesity (DiPetro, 2001; Frank, Kerr, Rosenberg, & King, 2010). In a preliminary study, Watts and colleagues (2015) have found that neighborhoods exhibiting greater connectivity (e.g., high intersection densities providing more potential routes for walking) are associated with better cognitive function, both at baseline and two years later.

One of the premises of complete streets is that such design elements make a neighborhood more connected and accessible by multimodal mobility options, particularly walking. Walking most frequently occurs in one's own neighborhood (Eyler, Brownson, Bacak, & Housemann, 2003) and is highly influenced by characteristics of the physical environment (Van Cauwenberg et al., 2011). Walking for exercise and transportation purposes is associated with a number of neighborhood characteristics, including availability of sidewalks, accessibility of desirable destinations, aesthetic attributes, and perceptions of safety from traffic or crime (Owen, Humpel, Leslie, Bauman, & Sallis, 2004). Satariano and colleagues (2012) add that transportation or utilitarian walking integrated into everyday life is most likely to occur in mixed-use neighborhoods that have short block lengths, include frequent intersections, and are perceived to be free from crime, heavy traffic, and other threats.

At the heart of the complete streets concept are efforts to increase the safety and accessibility associated with multimodal travel. Many of its core design suggestions are illustrated simply by considering pedestrian crossings. From a complete streets perspective, pedestrian crossings are enhanced by the following features:

- Narrower lanes
- Roadway reconfigurations
- Sidewalk bulb-outs that also shorten the travel distance across the street
- Continental-style crosswalk painting ("zebra striping")
- Pedestrian-actuated crosswalk signs
- Longer walk signals (LaPlante & McCann, 2008)

The transportation logic for changes to lane configuration stem from research suggesting that 10-foot driving lanes are equally as safe and tend to slow traffic in comparison to 12-foot driving lanes (National Cooperative Highway Research Program, 2007), and that four-lane roads are more efficient when they are transformed into one lane in each direction and a center turn lane (which then provides additional space that can be reclaimed for bulb-outs, bus stops, and the like on each side of the road). Where multiple lanes in each direction are necessary, the provision of a median pedestrian island ought to be considered. Sidewalk bulb-outs often go hand-in-hand with parallel parking, in that those bulb-outs do double duty by shortening the travel distance across the street for pedestrians and simultaneously providing a modicum of protection to parked cars from cars turning corners. Where blocks are long, mid-block pedestrian crossings should be considered.

While complete streets offer multiple suggestions for facilitating optimal mobility through the design of the physical setting, this concept fundamentally challenges the program that our society has chosen to engineer in the past. For nearly a century, transportation engineering has focused on issues of speed and convenience, resulting in an automobile-oriented hierarchy. This design was predicated on low fuel prices, affordability of cars, and heavy subsidization of such travel through road and highway improvement projects (e.g., the Federal Highway Bill). As energy and automobile prices have risen over time, however, the threshold for low-income families to enter the automobile world and then maintain such mobility has been set increasingly higher. Slowly changing settlement patterns to more mixed-use developments, higher-density urbanization, and growing health and environmental concerns associated with an automobile-centric society are changing consumer preferences and behavior (Van Dender & Clever, 2013). Likewise, our aging society is influencing these patterns, as automobile travel decreases in older populations (Van Dender & Clever, 2013). Increasingly, a green transportation hierarchy is being advocated that not only favors multimodality, but also sets priorities to put pedestrians first, followed by bicycles, public transportation, service and freight vehicles, taxis, carpools, and finally single-occupant vehicles (Litman, 2011).

Complete streets address the full range of developmentally salient attributes and, therefore, should receive much greater consideration in the planning of new neighborhoods for the lifespan. At its core, the complete streets concept focuses on providing mobility choices and access to all citizens, thereby furthering participation in the community. With such design choices, older adults are more likely to achieve a sense of continuity and connection without being thwarted by mobility limitations. Complete streets provide the connective tissue for older adults to civic institutions. By providing choices (auto, transit, bike, walking), they also promote personal control, thereby enhancing individuals' sense of empowerment. As such, complete streets support the developmentally salient attributes of continuity, connection, and control.

Age-Friendly Community Initiatives

Age-friendly community initiatives (AFCIs) represent an important approach for modifying the "people" dimension of local communities to create healthy places for older adults. The World Health Organization popularized the term "age-friendly" upon initiating its Age-Friendly Cities and Communities program in 2006, which now spans nearly 300 localities across 33 countries (WHO, 2015). This network is charged with identifying, addressing, and creating opportunities for healthy aging, specifically by facilitating "collaborative thinking and coordination across sectors" to make sustainable and effective improvements to localities' built and social environments (Beard & Warth, 2013, p. xvii).

The very idea of age-friendly communities emerged, in part, from a healthy aging perspective. According to Buffel and Phillipson (2016), the WHO launched its age-friendly network in response to earlier policy initiatives on active aging. Active aging was intended to address older adults' participation in "meaningful pursuits that contribute to the well-being of the individual concerned"—including activities within family, the paid labor force, and society at large (Walker, 2002, p. 124). Fitting with this perspective, the WHO framework for age-friendliness emphasizes the importance of both social and physical environments that promote older adults' active inclusion in their residential communities (Moulaert, Boudiny, & Paris, 2016). **TABLE 15-1** summarizes features of age-friendly communities, as identified by WHO.

Beyond the WHO network, the understanding of exactly what AFCIs constitute continues to evolve. Integrating findings from prior scholarship, Greenfield and colleagues (2015) defined AFCIs broadly as "deliberate and distinct efforts across stakeholders from multiple sectors within a defined and typically local geographic area to make social and/or physical environments more conducive to older adults' health, well-being, and ability to age in place and in the community" (p. 192). Others, however, have defined AFCIs somewhat differently. Golant (2015), for example, has situated AFCIs as part of local government and leadership, akin

TABLE 15-1 Indicators of Age-Friendliness According to the World Health Organization Framework

Dimension	Examples
Outdoor space and buildings	Safe and well-maintained outdoor seating is available, especially near transit, parks, and other public spaces; buildings are accessible. Public toilets are clean, accessible, and well maintained.
Transportation	Public transportation is affordable, reliable, and frequent, and reaches important destinations, such as health and commercial centers. Supports are available for older adults who drive, such as refresher driving courses and accessible and affordable parking.
Housing	A range of affordable and safe housing options with key services are available for all older people. Older adults' housing is integrated within the broader community.
Social participation	Older people have access to a range of affordable and engaging community events and activities. Organizations conduct specialized outreach to socially isolated older adults.
Respect and social inclusion	Older adults are included in community decision making, including those who are economically disadvantaged. Service staff are courteous and helpful to older adults.
Civic participation and employment	A variety of options are available for older adults to volunteer and engage in paid work. Training is available for older workers and volunteers.
Communication and information	There is a communication system that reaches every resident. Access to the Internet is available in public places at no or little cost.
Community and health services	Health and social services are co-located, coordinated as much as possible, and easily accessible. Service professionals have skills and knowledge in the area of aging.

Reprinted from World Health Organization. Global Age-Friendly Cities: A Guide, Copyright 2007. Available at: http://apps.who.int/iris/bitstream/10665/43755/1/9789241547307_eng.pdf.

to regulatory environments, public programs, and competent private and public leaders. Ball and Lawler (2014) more recently called for AFCIs to be considered more than just stand-alone programs or pilot efforts within a particular place, with program developers focusing on instigating collective systems so as to make their effects more long-lasting, comprehensive, and far-reaching.

Although what an AFCI involves is likely to differ from one community to the next, AFCIs oftentimes take form as a collaborative or coalition involving multiple organizations, sectors, and private citizens—including older adults themselves. These initiatives typically include a planning stage, during which stakeholders work in partnership to assess needs and assets within a local area to prioritize actions for improving a locality for the benefit of current and future cohorts of older residents. Based on this information, many AFCIs work on strategically and collaboratively supporting changes at the community level to make the locality more supportive of older residents. Examples of such changes include making intersections safer for pedestrians of all mobility levels, advocating for decisions by local zoning boards to promote the development of new and affordable senior housing, supporting the introduction of a farmer's market where people of all ages can access fresh produce, and improving sidewalks for safer mobility (Caro & Fitzgerald, 2015). In this sense, AFCIs can be considered catalysts for systematically improving features of a locality to benefit residents over the entirety of their lives.

AFCIs have been championed largely by private philanthropy (Scharlach, 2012) and, in some cases, by local government (e.g., Goldman, Owusu, Smith, Martens, & Lynch, 2016). In the United States, for the most part, national support has been limited to small pilot programs and web-based technical assistance, such as through AARP (http://www.aarp.org) and Grantmakers in Aging (http://giaging .org). Greenfield and colleagues (2015) identified four major challenges to the expansion of AFCIs in the United States: (1) the entrenched focus of national aging policy on funding services for individuals (as opposed to funding for communities as a whole); (2) challenges around engaging people outside of the field of aging to become invested in AFCIs; (3) fragmentation across networks that have promoted AFCIs, thereby reducing their potential collective impact; and (4) the overall lack of rigorous research evidence concerning the impact of AFCIs on valued outcomes among older adults. Nevertheless, the ideas that are central to AFCIs—including strategically

convening diverse stakeholders within a locality, engaging older adults as advocates and informants, and creating systems-level changes at a local level—continue to capture the attention of gerontologists and society as a whole (e.g., Eisenberg, 2015).

▶ Support-Oriented Initiatives

Although age does not determine the need for assistance, age-related vulnerabilities—especially in the context of communities developed for younger and more able-bodied persons—increase the importance of programs offering supportive services in later life. Such supports can include assistance with both basic and instrumental tasks of daily living, such as driving, grocery shopping, cooking, and safely ambulating around one's home and neighborhood. They also can foster more expressive opportunities, such as maintaining social connections, engaging in lifelong learning, and being civically engaged. Supportive services can be offered by paid providers—such as nursing aides or private drivers—as well as by unpaid family members, friends, neighbors, and community volunteers.

In the United States, programs and policies for supportive services for older adults largely have focused on funding particular types of organizations to provide specific types of assistance to specific subgroups of individuals. For example, many of the programs offered through the U.S. federal Older Americans Act focus on certain types of services, such as home-delivered meals, information and referrals, or chronic disease self-management programs (Niles-Yokum & Wagner, 2016). Medicaid—as the largest source of funding for services provided within people's homes and communities—is reserved for people with very low incomes and those with significant levels of functional impairment (O'Keeffe et al., 2010).

New models to enhance supports for all older adults within local communities have emerged, in part as a response to limitations of these longer-standing public programs. Two prominent examples are **naturally occurring retirement community (NORC)** supportive service programs and "village" organizations. NORCs are a demographic phenomenon in which a critical mass of older adults is concentrated within a geographic area or housing development that was not planned as senior housing (Hunt & Ross, 1990). The classic NORC is an apartment building that, due to its proximity to services and amenities (e.g., pharmacies and grocery stores), access to social groups, and "the surrounding neighborhood and its characteristics" (Hunt & Gunter-Hunt, 1986, p. 13; Kahana, Bhatta, Lovegreen, Kahana, & Midlarsky, 2013), attracts and retains older adults as residents. Thus, NORCs as geographic phenomena further the attributes of control and challenge/comfort. Others have identified neighborhood-based NORCs—which often include single-family residences that house both an aging-in-place population (e.g., "empty nesters") and in-migrating older residents—as well as rural NORCs whose populations often become age-concentrated due to out-migration of younger adults and families.

The geographic phenomenon of NORCs has led to the development of NORC supportive service programs. These programs are designed to be implemented in NORCs to support older residents' healthy aging as they age in place. NORC programs are typically developed within long-standing, nonprofit, community-based organizations in partnership with a range of other stakeholders, such as housing managers, faith-based organizations, neighborhood associations, voluntary groups, and older adults themselves (Greenfield, Scharlach, Graham, Lehning, & Davitt, 2012). As a "community-level intervention" (Bedney, Goldberg, & Josephson, 2010, p. 304), NORC programs are not designed just to provide supportive services, but rather seek to enhance both formal and informal networks of place-based supports through activities such

> ### PEARL 15-2 Complementary Approaches to Support Healthy Aging
>
> Complete streets, visitability, age-friendly community initiatives, villages, and NORC programs are complementary place-based approaches to make localities more supportive of healthy aging. They are likely to be most effective at the population level when implemented in parallel with each other.

as relationship building, assessing community needs, and coordinating services.

Villages are membership organizations that provide older adults in a particular neighborhood with a range of nonprofessional services, such as transportation, housekeeping, and companionship, as well as referrals to existing community services (McDonough & Davitt, 2011). This model was developed in 2002 by a group of older adults residing in the Beacon Hill neighborhood of Boston (McWhinney-Morse, 2009), as an alternative to having to move to retirement or assisted living communities (Beacon Hill Village, 2011). Older adults pay membership dues to gain access to an array of supportive services. These services are hyperlocal by definition, as villages are governed by the older adult membership, and their members often volunteer to provide services for other members. As such, villages are a potential neighborhood-based mechanism to promote the empowerment of older adults. Most are free-standing grassroots efforts of varying scales, with some serving fewer than 20 members, and others having more than 500 members. Despite this variation, most existing villages share five characteristics: They are (1) self-governing, (2) geographically defined, (3) membership organizations, that (4) provide or arrange for services, (5) with the goal of helping their members to age in place (Scharlach, Lehning, & Graham, 2010).

Villages and NORC programs both aim to enhance the health, well-being, and quality of life of older adults as they age in place within their communities. Similar to traditional supportive service organizations, these place-based supportive service initiatives seek, in part, to link individuals with resources that can better meet their potential supportive service needs, such as making referrals to vetted service providers. However, unlike traditional service entities, villages and NORC programs also seek to promote older adults' community contributions as well as their connections to others within their local communities (Greenfield et al., 2012). These models work toward these aims by, for example, providing opportunities for older adults to serve on organizational governance bodies, encouraging older adults to participate in community-wide social events, and facilitating opportunities for them to provide support to each other. Both NORC programs and villages are designed to offer these benefits based on their specialized knowledge of their local community; they are charged with deeply understanding local norms and conditions so as to optimize their service offerings specifically in the context of their localities.

While NORC programs and villages are similar in their goals and overall categories of activities, prior research has identified several key differences between them. First, NORC programs are typically developed as part of a larger multi-service organization, such as a family service organization that serves a variety of age groups and addresses a variety of social issues. Villages, in contrast, typically emerge as free-standing organizations that develop their own status as private nonprofit organizations (Greenfield, Scharlach, Lehning, Davitt, & Graham, 2013). NORC programs also are more likely to receive funding from government grants and contracts, especially in New York, where state and city government have designated public funding specifically for NORC programs (Greenfield et al., 2012). In contrast, villages' funding model emphasizes annual membership dues, whereby older residents themselves pay an annual fee that gives them access to the organizations' services and activities (Scharlach et al., 2010). Finally, NORC

programs and villages differ somewhat in the predominant types of services that they offer. Although both typically offer a central telephone number that members can use to request services and social-recreational activities, villages are more likely to offer assistance that can be provided by volunteers, such as transportation assistance and help with minor home repairs. With their larger numbers of paid staff, on average, NORC programs are more likely to offer skilled services, such as professional care coordination, benefits counseling, and preventive health services (Greenfield et al., 2013).

Despite these differences, villages and NORC programs reflect enthusiasm for place-based supportive service initiatives for older adults. Villages, in particular, have proliferated rapidly over the past 15 years, beginning with a single village in 2002 and numbering more than 180 villages by the end of 2015 (Village to Village, 2015). This growth suggests the relevance of local, grassroots, and consumer-driven responses to long-standing limitations in aging services. It also indicates the need for place-based initiatives that not only address long-term services and supports (e.g., providing help with activities of daily living) or wellness (e.g., providing opportunities for social, physical, and civic activity), but also more deeply foster healthy aging through coordinated approaches that take advantage of the efficiencies and synergies within a single organizational entity.

It should be noted that programs similar to the Village model exist in a number of other countries, including the Netherlands, Australia, Sweden, and Israel. Israel's government-sponsored Supportive Community Program, for example, combines an emergency call service, home repairs, friendly visiting, and social activities, developed and coordinated by retired community residents and provided by neighborhood volunteers. Evaluations of the Supportive Community Program have shown high levels of satisfaction, with 70% of members surveyed reporting increased sense of security, 33% reporting decreased burden on adult children, and 25% reporting an increased ability to age-in-place (Berg-Warman & Brodsky, 2006).

Studies to evaluate the extent to which NORC programs and villages achieve their intended outcomes among older individuals are in their nascence. The largest evaluation studies to date have used survey research methods to examine perceived benefits according to participants. For example, a study based on a convenience sample of NORC program participants across the United States found that the overwhelming majority of respondents agreed that the NORC program helped them to socialize more, increased their knowledge of community services, and contributed to their confidence in their ability to age in place (Bedney, Schimmel, Goldberg, Kotler-Berkowitz, & Bursztyn, 2007). Similarly, in a study of village members in California, the vast majority of participants reported that the village enhanced their ability to age in place; moreover, perceived benefits were generally greater among people who more regularly utilized the village's programs and services (Graham, Scharlach, & Price Wolf, 2014). A more recent study based on data from village members in California found that older adults' confidence in their ability to age in place, social support, and intentions to stay put increased, on average, over the first year of membership in a village (Graham, Scharlach, & Kurtovich, 2016). These findings, in combination with a growing body of conceptual scholarship that articulates the underlying program models for NORC programs and villages (Greenfield, 2016; Greenfield et al., 2013), are important steps toward the design and implementation of increasingly rigorous outcomes studies.

▶ Conclusion and Future Directions

Through the discussion of place-based initiatives to promote healthy aging—as well as conceptual models emphasizing physical setting, people, and programs—this chapter has highlighted strategic and potentially scalable efforts to optimize environments for healthy aging. By orienting attention to theoretical frameworks on persons and places, as well as place-based practice approaches, we hope to generate new insights for research, policy, and practice on healthy aging.

The presentation of insights from lifespan developmental theory—alongside environmental gerontological theory on dimensions of place—indicates the importance of initiatives to make physical settings, people, and programs more conducive to continuity, compensation, control, connection, contribution, and challenge/comfort. We believe that innovation occurs when shared intentionality is present, and the articulation of these six fundamental attributes helps bring focus to the overall core intentions that place-based initiatives to promote healthy aging ought to seek to foster. Continuity involves the preservation of the self-construct in the face of internal or external threats. Compensation involves behavioral and/or socio-psychological adaptation to challenges. Control encompasses perceived self-efficacy and its preservation. Having meaningful interpersonal relationships and experiencing generativity in various social spheres are captured by the notions of connection and contribution, respectively. Finally, stimulation and growth in various functional domains are enabled by periods of challenge and periods of comfort.

The ecological framework of place perspective is especially valuable for elucidating multiple components of place and determining how they matter for individual outcomes. In particular, the EFP reframes person-environment fit from an interaction between person and environment to a dynamic that explicitly considers the powerful effect of the sociocultural milieu. In so doing, it challenges the "user needs" approach to design for older adults, which has typified architectural design for the past four decades. While user needs are certainly important, the EFP posits that those needs exist within a set of socio-normative understandings—a program—that sets the expectations and assumptions regarding older adults and their social relationship partners. This position, in turn, suggests that place-based approaches need to not only respond to user needs, but also negotiate cultural norms and assumptions. Thus, places can be—and ought to be—powerful agents of social change.

Our discussion has also highlighted the integrative negotiation of aging as involving not just the program, physical setting, and people, but also the interpenetrating nature of the negotiation among all three of these elements. Mobility is a case in point. While the key components of the complete streets concept clearly may enhance older adults' potential for mobility, the underlying precepts of the program emphasize that to be even more inclusive to those with functional limitations, supportive services—ranging from assistive technologies (e.g., walkers) to community volunteers—should be offered to provide another layer of inclusion. At the same time, the theoretical perspectives in this chapter suggest that each individual reacts differently to environmental conditions. For example, some people might see the availability of supports in their community as symbols of dependence, whereas others might view them as enablers of independence (for further discussion, see Abramson, 2015), thereby influencing individuals' use of these supports and potentially their healthy aging.

It is highly unlikely than any single place-based initiative will promote healthy aging for all people and in all ways. Thus, communities that adopt a variety of approaches that address complementary aspects of physical settings,

people, and programs are more likely to profoundly affect healthy aging at a population level than communities that implement just one initiative. For example, both visitability and complete streets, as setting-oriented initiatives, are likely to support developmental needs, such as continuity and connection, especially for older adults with mobility limitations. Conversely, NORC programs and villages have real strengths in terms of their ability to support connection, contribution, and control, particularly for people who lack other sources of support. Age-friendly community initiatives have the potential to serve as people-powered catalysts to integrate these various interventions and ensure that they systematically build upon each other for the purposes of improving population health.

In the spirit of the Kurt Lewin quote that "there is nothing so practical as good theory," the theoretical perspective offered here links lifespan development theory with both environmental and geographical gerontology through their emphases on the concept of place. We believe that the field of public health may be served well by the theories offered within both domains and that these theories have much to offer in terms of shaping meaningful research, policy, and practice for our aging society. In terms of research recommendations, the discussion highlights the importance of employing longitudinal, multimethod, multilevel approaches to understand healthy aging from a public health perspective. The people, program, and physical setting components of place-based interventions in aging need to be measured over time.

In addition to theoretically guided and longitudinal research, research is needed on the diffusion of place-based approaches across diverse communities. For example, what are the key factors that lead to a locality's adoption of a complete streets policy? Do age-friendly community initiatives support the integration of other place-based strategies, such as visitability being part of a municipality's master plans? How can greater partnerships among public health, architecture, and gerontology facilitate principles in practice, such as universal design?

PEARL 15-3 Healthy Places and Shared Expectations

Healthy places need to consider not only the needs of the person and the characteristics of the setting, but also the ways in which our goals, actions, and subsequent appraisals are informed by socioculturally shared expectations (the program of the place).

How can public health help extend the advance of interprofessional education in the health sciences to a broader range of fields, including design, public policy, and geography?

All too often, the aging of our society is labeled the "silver tsunami," implying that it is a huge, unstoppable wave that will leave destruction in its wake. Through the dialogue in this chapter, we have highlighted the exciting new possibilities of this demographic reality and noted how place-based theories and initiatives in aging provide insights for moving policy, practice, and research forward. In the end, our aging population presents both challenges and opportunities that have the potential to drive change toward healthier, more age-inclusive communities that can benefit people across the entirety of their lives. We believe that integrating conceptual frameworks on person-and-place in later life to enhance place-based initiatives in aging can help to more fully achieve this potential.

References

Abramson, C. (2015). *The end game: How inequality shapes our final years.* New York, NY: Oxford University Press.

Atchley, R. C. (1989). A continuity theory of normal aging. *Gerontologist, 29*(2), 183-190.

Ball, M. S., & Lawler, K. (2014). Changing practice and policy to move to scale: A framework for age-friendly communities across the United States. *Journal of Aging & Social Policy, 26(1-2),* 19-32.

Baltes, P. B., & Baltes, M. M. (1990). Psychological perspectives on successful aging: The model of selective optimization with compensation. *Successful Aging: Perspectives from the Behavioral Sciences, 1,* 1-34.

Barth, J., Schneider, S. & von Känel, R. (2010). Lack of social support in the etiology and the prognosis of coronary heart disease: A systematic review and meta-analysis. *Psychosomatic Medicine, 72*(3), 229-238.

Beard, J. R., & Warth, L. (2013). Building an age-friendly world, one city at a time. *Aging Today, 34*(3), 7.

Beacon Hill Village. (2011). Available at: http://www.beaconhillvillage.org

Bedney, B. J., Goldberg, R. B., & Josephson, K. (2010). Aging in place in naturally occurring retirement communities: Transforming aging through supportive service programs. *Journal of Housing for the Elderly, 24,* 304-321.

Bedney, B. J., Schimmel, D., Goldberg, R., Kotler-Berkowitz, L., & Bursztyn, D. (2007). Rethinking aging in place: Exploring the impact of NORC supportive service programs on older adult participants. Available at: https://fedweb-assets.s3.amazonaws.com/fed-74/2/Rethinking%2520Aging%2520in%2520Place.pdf

Berg-Warman, A., & Brodsky, J. (2006). The supportive community: A new concept for enhancing the quality of life of elderly living in the community. *Journal of aging and social policy,* 18(2), 69–83.

Bortz, W. (2009). Understanding frailty. *Journals of Gerontology, Series A: Biological Sciences and Medical Sciences, 162,* 1–2.

Bronfenbrenner, U. (2009). *The ecology of human development: Experiments by nature and design.* Cambridge, MA: Harvard University Press.

Brown, R. M., & Brown, S. L. (2014). Informal caregiving: A reappraisal of effects on caregivers. *Social Issues and Policy Review, 8,* 74–102. doi:10.1111/sipr.12002

Buffel, T., & Phillipson, C. (2016). Can global cities be "age-friendly cities"? Urban development and ageing populations. *Cities, 55,* 94-100.

Caro, F. G., & Fitzgerald, K. G. (Eds.). (2015). *International perspectives on age-friendly cities.* London, UK: Routledge.

Carstensen, L. L. (1993). Motivation for social contact across the life span: A theory of socioemotional selectivity. *Nebraska Symposium on Motivation, 40,* 209-254.

Concrete Change. (2016). Visitability: Basic access in every new house. Available at: http://www.concretechange.org/

Diaz Moore, K. (2007). Restorative dementia gardens: Exploring how design may ameliorate attention fatigue. *Journal of Housing for the Elderly, 21*(1-2), 73-88.

Diaz Moore, K. (2014). An ecological framework of place: Situating environmental gerontology within a life course perspective. *International Journal of Aging and Human Development, 79*(3), 183-209.

Dickens, A. P., Richards, S. H., Greaves, C. J., & Campbell, J. L. (2011). Interventions targeting social isolation in older people: A systematic review. *BMC Public Health, 11*(1), 647.

DiPietro, L. (2006). Physical activity in aging: Changes in patterns and their relationship to health and function. *Journals of Gerontology, Series A, 56*(2), 13–22.

Eisenberg, R. (2015). Why are there so age-friendly cities? Available at: http://www.forbes.com/sites/nextavenue/2015/08/12/why-are-there-so-few-age-friendly-cities/#134fef6991fd

Erikson, E. (1963). *Childhood and society.* New York, NY: W. W. Norton & Company.

European Union's Health Ageing Project. (2006). Healthy ageing: A challenge for Europe. Available at: http://www.healthyageing.eu/sites/www.healthyageing.eu/files/resources/Healthy%20Ageing%20-%20A%20Challenge%20for%20Europe.pdf

Eyler, A. A., Brownson, R. C., Bacak, S. J., & Housemann, R. A. (2003). The epidemiology of walking for physical activity in the United States. *Medicine and Science in Sports and Exercise, 35*(9), 1529-1536.

Flegal, K. M., Kit, B. K., Orpana, H., & Graubard, B. I. (2013). Association of all-cause mortality with overweight and obesity using standard body mass index categories: A systematic review and meta-analysis. *Journal of the American Medical Association, 309*(1), 71-82.

Frank, L., Kerr, J., Rosenberg, D., & King, A. (2010). Healthy aging and where you live: Community design relationships with physical activity and body weight in older Americans. *Journal of Physical Activity and Health, 7*(suppl 1), S82–S90.

Fratiglioni, L., Paillard-Borg, S., & Winblad, B. (2004). An active and socially integrated lifestyle in late life might protect against dementia. *Lancet Neurology, 3*(6), 343–353.

Freund, A. M. (2008). Successful aging as management of resources: The role of selection, optimization, and compensation. *Research in Human Development, 5*(2), 94-106.

Gao, X., Nelson, M., & Tucker K. (2007). Television viewing is associated with prevalence of metabolic syndrome in Hispanic elders. *Diabetes Care, 30*, 694–700.

Glass, T., Balfour, J. (2003). Neighborhoods, aging, and functional limitations. In I. Kawachi & L. F. Berkman (Eds.), *Neighborhoods and health* (pp. 303–334). New York, NY: Oxford University Press.

Golant, S. M. (2011). The quest for residential normalcy by older adults: Relocation but one pathway. *Journal of Aging Studies, 25*(3), 193-205.

Golant, S. M. (2015). *Aging in the right place.* Baltimore, MD: Health Professions Press.

Goldman, L., Owusu, S., Smith, C., Martens, D., & Lynch, M. (2016). Age-friendly New York City: A case study. In T. Moulaert & S. Garon, *Age-friendly cities and communities in international comparison* (pp. 171-190). New York, NY: Springer.

Graham, C. L., Scharlach, A. E., & Kurtovich, E. (2016). Do villages promote aging in place? Manuscript submitted for publication.

Graham, C. L., Scharlach, A. E., & Price Wolf, J. (2014). The impact of the "village" model on health, well-being, service access, and social engagement of older adults. *Health Education & Behavior, 41*(1 suppl), 91S-97S. doi:10.1177/1090198114532290

Grant, N., Hamer, M., & Steptoe, A. (2009). Social isolation and stress-related cardiovascular, lipid, and cortisol responses. *Annals of Behavioral Medicine, 37*(1), 29–37.

Greenfield, E. A. (2012). Using ecological frameworks to advance a field of research, practice, and policy on aging-in-place initiatives. *Gerontologist, 52*(1), 1–12.

Greenfield, E. A. (2016). Support from neighbors and aging in place: Can NORC programs make a difference? *Gerontologist, 56*(4), 651-659. doi:10.1093/geront/gnu162

Greenfield, E. A., & Marks, N. F. (2004). Formal volunteering as a protective factor for older adults' psychological well-being. *Journals of Gerontology: Social Sciences, 59*(5), S258-S264. doi:10.1093/geronb/59.5.S258

Greenfield, E. A., Oberlink, M., Scharlach, A. E., Neal, M. B., & Stafford, P. B. (2015). Age-friendly community initiatives: Conceptual issues and key questions. *Gerontologist, 55*(2), 191-198.

Greenfield, E. A., Scharlach, A., Graham, C., Lehning, A. J., & Davitt, J. K. (2012). An overview of NORC programs in New York: Findings from a 2012 national survey. Available at: http://agingandcommunity.org/publications

Greenfield, E. A., Scharlach, A. E., Lehning, A. J., Davitt, J. K., & Graham, C. L. (2013). A tale of two community initiatives for promoting aging in place: Similarities and differences in the national implementation of NORC programs and villages. *Gerontologist*, gnt035.

Hall, G., & Buckwalter, K. (1987). Progressively lowered stress threshold: A conceptual model for care of adults with Alzheimer's disease. *Archives of Psychiatric Nursing, 1*, 399–406.

Hawton, A., Green, C., Dickens, A. P., Richards, S. H., Taylor, R. S., Edwards, R.,… Campbell, J. L. (2011). The impact of social isolation on the health status and health-related quality of life of older people. *Quality of Life Research, 20*(1), 57-67.

Hazan, H. (2011). Gerontological autism: Terms of accountability in the cultural study of the category of the Fourth Age. *Ageing and Society, 31*(7), 1125-1140.

Heckhausen, J., Wrosch, C., & Schulz, R. (2010). A motivational theory of life-span development. *Psychological Review, 117*(1), 32.

Herzog, A. R., & Markus, H. R. (1999). The self-concept in life span and aging research. In V. L. Bengtson, & K. W. Schaie (Eds.), *Handbook of theories of aging* (pp. 227–252). New York, NY: Springer.

Holt-Lunstad, J., Smith, T. B., Baker, M., Harris, T., & Stephenson, D. (2015). Loneliness and social isolation as risk factors for mortality: A meta-analytic review. *Perspectives on Psychological Science, 10*(2), 227-237.

Hunt, M. E., & Gunter-Hunt, G. (1986). Naturally occurring retirement communities. *Journal of Housing for the Elderly, 3*(3-4), 3-22.

Hunt, M. E., & Ross, L. E. (1990). Naturally occurring retirement communities: A multi-attribute examination of desirability factors. *Gerontologist, 30*(5), 667-674.

Iwarsson, S. (1999). The Housing Enabler: An objective tool for assessing accessibility. *British Journal of Occupational Therapy, 62*(11), 491-497.

Iwarsson, S., & Slaug, B. (2010). *Housing Enabler: A method for rating/screening and analysing accessibility problems in housing. Manual for the complete instrument and screening tool.* Lund, Sweden: Veten & Skapen HB & Slaug Data Management.

Iwarsson, S., & Ståhl, A. (2003). Accessibility, usability and universal design-positioning and definition of concepts describing person-environment relationships. *Disability & Rehabilitation, 25*(2), 57-66.

Kahana, E., Bhatta, T., Lovegreen, L. D., Kahana, B., & Midlarsky, E. (2013). Altruism, helping, and volunteering pathways to well-being in late life. *Journal of Aging and Health, 25*(1), 159-187.

Kahana, E., Kelley-Moore, J., & Kahana, B. (2012). Proactive aging: A longitudinal study of stress, resources, agency, and well-being in late life. *Aging & Mental Health, 16*(4), 438-451.

Kaplan, S. (1995). The restorative benefits of nature: Toward an integrative framework. *Journal of Environmental Psychology, 15*(3), 169-182.

Katzmarzyk, P. T., Church, T. S., Craig, C. L., & Bouchard, C. (2009). Sitting time and mortality from all causes, cardiovascular disease, and cancer. *Medicine and Science in Sports and Exercise, 41*(5), 998-1005.

Kim, M., & Clarke, P. (2015). Urban social and built environments and trajectories of decline in social engagement in vulnerable elders findings from Detroit's Medicaid home and community-based waiver population. *Research on Aging, 37*(4), 413-435.

Konrath, S., Fuhrel-Forbis, A., Lou, A., & Brown, S. (2012). Motives for volunteering are associated with mortality risk in older adults. *Health Psychology, 31*(1), 87-96.

LaPlante, J., & McCann, B. (2008). Complete streets: We can get there from here. *ITE Journal, 78*(5), 24.

Lawton, M. P. (1989). Behavior-relevant ecological factors. In K. Schaie & K. Schooler (Eds.), *Social structure and aging: Psychological processes* (pp. 57-78). Hillsdale, NJ: LEA Publishers.

Lawton, M. P., & Nahemow, L. (1973). Ecology and the aging process. In C. Eisdorfer & M. P. Lawton (Eds.), *The psychology of adult development and aging* (pp. 619-674). Washington, DC: American Psychological Association.

Lien, L. L., Steggell, C. D., Slaug, B., & Iwarsson, S. (2015). Assessment and analysis of housing accessibility: Adapting the environmental component of the Housing Enabler to United States applications. *Journal of Housing and the Built Environment*, 1-16.

Lifetime Homes. (2015). Available at: http://www.lifetimehomes.org.uk/

List, C., & Pettit, P. (2011). *Group agency: The possibility, design, and status of corporate agents.* Oxford, UK: Oxford University Press.

Litman, T. (2011). Introduction to multi-modal transportation planning: Principles and practices. Available at: http://www.vtpi.org/multimodal_planning.pdf

Maisel, J., Smith, E., & Steinfeld, E. (2008). *Increasing home access: Designing for visitability.* Washington, DC: AARP Public Policy Institute.

Manson, J. E., Hsia, J., Johnson, K. C., Rossouw, J. E., Assaf, A. R., Lasser, N. L.,… Strickland, O. L. (2003). Estrogen plus progestin and the risk of coronary heart disease. *New England Journal of Medicine, 349*(6), 523-534.

Maxfield, M., Greenberg, J., Pyszczynski, T., Weise, D. R., Kosloff, S., Soenke, M.,… Blatter, J. (2014). Increases in generative concern among older adults following reminders of mortality. *International Journal of Aging and Human Development, 79*(1), 1-21.

McAdams, D. P., & de St. Aubin, E. (1992). A theory of generativity and its assessment through self-report, behavioral acts, and narrative themes in autobiography. *Journal of Personality and Social Psychology, 62*, 1003-1015.

McDonough, K. E., & Davitt, J. K. (2011). It takes a village: Community practice, social work, and aging-in-place. *Journal of Gerontological Social Work, 54*(5), 528-541.

McWhinney-Morse, S. (2009). Beacon Hill Village. *Generations, 33*(2), 85-86.

Moos, R. H. (1980). *The social climate scales: An overview.* Palo Alto, CA: Consulting Psychologists Press.

Morrrow-Howell, N., Gonzales, E., Matz-Costa, C., & Greenfield, E. A. (2015). *Increasing productive aging in later life* (Grand Challenges for Social Work Initiative Working Paper No. 8). Cleveland, OH: American Academy of Social Work and Social Welfare. Available at: http://aaswsw.org/wp-content/uploads/2015/12/WP8-with-cover.pdf

Moulaert, T., Boudiny, K., & Paris, M. (2015). *Active and healthy ageing: Blended models and common challenges in supporting age-friendly cities and communities.* New York, NY: Springer.

National Cooperative Highway Research Program. (2007). *Project 3-27: Preliminary report: Urban and suburban lane widths.* Kansas City, MO: Midwest Research Institute.

Nicholson, N. R. (2012). A review of social isolation: An important but under assessed condition in older adults. *Journal of Primary Prevention, 33*(2-3), 137-152.

Niles-Yokum, K., & Wagner, D. (2015). *The aging networks: A guide to programs and services.* New York, NY: Springer.

O'Keefe, J., Saucier, P., Jackson, B., Cooper, R., McKenney, E., Crisp, S., & Moseley, C. (2010). Understanding Medicaid home and community services: A primer, 2010 edition. Available at: https://aspe.hhs.gov/understanding-medicaid-home-and-community-services-primer-2010-edition

Owen, N., Humpel, N., Leslie, E., Bauman, A., & Sallis, J. F. (2004). Understanding environmental influences on walking: Review and research agenda. *American Journal of Preventive Medicine, 27*(1), 67-76.

Piaget, J. (1932). *The moral development of the child.* London, UK: Kegan Paul.

Prenda, K. M., & Lachman, M. E. (2001). Planning for the future: A life management strategy for increasing control and life satisfaction in adulthood. *Psychology and Aging, 16*(2), 206.

Proshansky, H. M., Fabian, A. K., & Kaminoff, R. (1983). Place-identity: Physical world socialization of the self. *Journal of Environmental Psychology, 3*(1), 57-83.

Pynoos, J., Steinman, B. A., & Nguyen, A. Q. (2010). Environmental assessment and modification as fall-prevention strategies for older adults. *Clinics in Geriatric Medicine, 26*(4), 633-644.

Rantakokko, M., Portegijs, E., Viljanen, A., Iwarsson, S., Kauppinen, M., & Rantanen, T. (2015). Changes in life-space mobility and quality of life among community-dwelling older people: A 2-year follow-up study. *Quality of Life Research,* 1-9.

Rattan, S. I. (2008). Hormesis in aging. *Ageing Research Reviews, 7*(1), 63-78.

Romo, R. D., Wallhagen, M. I., Yourman, L., Yeung, C. C., Eng, C., Micco, G.,... Smith, A. K. (2013). Perceptions of successful aging among diverse elders with late-life disability. *Gerontologist, 53*(6), 939-949.

Rubinstein, R. L., & de Medeiros, K. (2003). Aging in context: Socio-physical environments. *Annual Review of Gerontology and Geriatrics, 23,* 59.

Satariano, W. A., Guralnik, J. M., Jackson, R. J., Marottoli, R. A., Phelan, E. A., & Prohaska, T. R. (2012). Mobility and aging: New directions for public health action. *American Journal of Public Health, 102*(8), 1508-1515.

Scharlach, A. (2012). Creating aging-friendly communities in the United States. *Ageing International, 37,* 25-38. doi:10.1007/s12126-011-9140-1

Scharlach, A., & Diaz Moore, K. (2016). Aging-in-place. In V. Bengston & R. Settersten (Eds.), *Handbook of the theories of aging* (3rd ed.). New York, NY: Springer.

Scharlach, A., & Lehning, A. (2015). *Creating aging-friendly communities.* Oxford, UK: Oxford University Press.

Scharlach, A. E., Lehning, A. J., & Graham, C. (2010, October). Proliferation of the "village" model: Neighborhood associations for aging in place. *Gerontologist, 50,* 256-257.

Scheibe, S., & Carstensen, L. L. (2010). Emotional aging: Recent findings and future trends. *Journals of Gerontology, Series B: Psychological Sciences and Social Sciences, 132.*

Schulz, R., & Heckhausen, J. (1996). A life span model of successful aging. *American Psychologist, 51*(7), 702.

Silverstein, M., & Bengston, V. (2007). Intergenerational solidarity and the structure of adult child-parent relationships in American families. *American Journal of Sociology, 103,* 429-460. doi:10.1086/231213

Smart Growth America. (2016). National Complete Streets Coalition. Available at: https://smartgrowthamerica.org/program/national-complete-streets-coalition/

Steinfeld, E., & Maisel, J. (2012). *Universal design: Creating inclusive environments.* New York, NY: John Wiley & Sons.

Uchino, B. (2006). Social support and health: A review of physiological processes potentially underlying links to disease outcomes. *Journal of Behavioral Medicine, 29*(4), 377-387.

Van Cauwenberg, J., De Bourdeaudhuij, I., De Meester, F., Van Dyck, D., Salmon, J., Clarys, P., & Deforche, B. (2011). Relationship between the physical environment and physical activity in older adults: A systematic review. *Health & Place, 17*(2), 458-469.

Van Dender, K., & Clever, M. (2013). Recent trends in car usage in advanced economies: Slower growth ahead? Available at: http://www.itf-oecd.org/sites/default/files/docs/dp201309.pdf

Village to Village. (2015). Available at: http://www.vtvnetwork.org/

Wahl, H. W., & Lang, F. R. (2004). Aging in context across the adult life course: Integrating physical and social environmental research perspectives. *Annual Review of Gerontology and Geriatrics, 23,* 1-33.

Walker, A. (2002). A strategy for active ageing. *International Social Security Review, 55*(1), 121-139.

Watts, A., Ferdous, F., Diaz Moore, K., & Burns, J. M. (2015). Neighborhood integration and connectivity predict cognitive performance and decline. *Gerontology and Geriatric Medicine, 1,* 2333721415599141.

Weir, P. L., Meisner, B. A., & Baker, J. (2010). Successful aging across the years: Does one model fit everyone? *Journal of Health Psychology, 15*(5), 680-687.

Weisman, G. D., Chaudhury, H., & Diaz Moore, K. (2000). Theory and practice of place: Toward an integrative model. *The Many Dimensions of Aging,* 3-21.

Wohlwill, J. F. (1966). The physical environment: A problem for a psychology of stimulation. *Journal of Social Issues, 22*(4), 29-38.

World Health Organization (WHO). (2001). *International classification of functioning, disability and health: ICF.* Geneva, Switzerland: Author.

World Health Organization (WHO). (2015). Age-friendly world. Available at: https://extranet.who.int/agefriendlyworld/

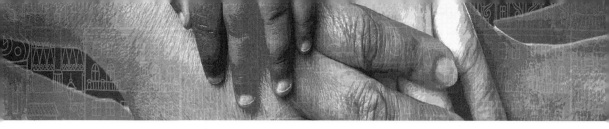

CHAPTER 16

Aging and Public Health: New Directions

Marlon Maus and **William A. Satariano**

ABSTRACT

This chapter summarizes some possible future directions in the epidemiology of aging as identified through a collaborative effort by the contributing authors of this text. Five themes emerged that may assist readers in identifying areas for further research and practice in the epidemiology of aging: a life course perspective on the epidemiology of aging, the natural/built environment, technology, new conceptual models, and international studies. Although not by any means exhaustive or all-inclusive, these themes help provide a roadmap for the initiation of future endeavors.

KEYWORDS

epidemiology of aging   future directions   aging research

▶ Introduction

"It's tough to make predictions, especially about the future."

—Danish proverb

When we were planning this text, we realized that one of the most important functions that it could serve was to assist readers in identifying areas where further research and practice in the **epidemiology of aging** are needed. The World Health Organization's (WHO's)

World Report on Aging and Health states that "comprehensive public-health action on aging is urgently needed. Although there are major knowledge gaps, we have sufficient evidence to act now…" (WHO, 2015).

It is precisely to recognize and enumerate those gaps that we asked the contributors to this volume to identify what they considered to be **future directions** in their area of **aging research**. In other words, what is likely to be done in the future? What should be done? In the chapters of this text, we have attempted to identify some common themes. Each senior author also had the opportunity to comment on our final list. While the resulting list of themes certainly is not completely comprehensive, we believe it reflects many of the key points made by the authors. Of course, for your own consideration of future directions, we recommend that you study the future directions (last) section of each chapter as well as the Pearls features. In the end, each of these future directions seeks to better understand the etiology of healthy aging and develop better strategies to enhance healthy aging among a diverse population of older adults.

We began this text with a consideration of the Epidemiologic Transition Theory (ETT). There is general agreement that ETT provides a useful context (really, a grand vision) for a consideration of demographic patterns of global aging. Most important, this theory provides a framework for describing and explaining the global diversity of aging—for example, the populations of the developing world who are aging are "older" than the populations of the developing world. This diversity is associated with both economic and social factors.

Despite the significance of ETT for achieving an understanding of global aging, there have been a number of recommendations to enrich the theory. Specifically, recommendations have been made to examine aging diversity within developed and developing countries. Some evidence suggests that there is not a single aging process at work within each country, but rather multiple processes. It is also recommended that the effects of economic factors

and the implications of migration patterns, including the movement of refugees, be given greater attention so as to identify factors that may help clarify demographic patterns of aging. Other recommendations include a consideration of the life course and the natural and built environments.

We believe that the ecological model continues to serves as a useful template—that is, as a guide for continuing needed research in the future. Although various definitions of the ecological model have been proposed, in this text we define it as a model that assumes "patterns of health and well-being are due to a dynamic interplay of biological, social, economic, and environmental factors that play out over the life course of individuals, families, neighborhoods, and communities." The ecological model provides a multidisciplinary, multilevel framework. Although this model has been in place for some time, only recently has a new generation of work been undertaken to conduct the research specified by the model. In particular, there is a growing body of research on the life course and human-environmental interactions, two of the important themes made apparent by reviewing the chapters in this volume.

▶ Themes

Five themes emerged that may assist the readers identify areas for further research and practice in the epidemiology of aging. This list is by no means exhaustive, and the choices on it reflect the interests and expertise of the contributing panel. The themes are not mutually exclusive, and there are elements that either overlap with or could have been placed in other categories. The five themes are:

- Life course perspective
- Natural and built environments
- Technology
- Conceptual models
- International studies

Life Course Perspective

There is a growing recognition that the heterogeneity of life expectancy and health outcomes cannot be completely understood without an understanding of the life course. A growing body of evidence indicates that we cannot fully understand the late chapters of life without understanding the early years, including the period of conception. By studying the life course, it becomes possible to understand periods of susceptibility and periods of resiliency and, therefore, to better understand the heterogeneity of life expectancy and health outcomes. A life course is also critical for understanding how these patterns, in turn, vary by race, socioeconomic status, and region. As noted earlier in this text, "Continued research on age-specific changes or the transmission of epigenetic marks to future generations will be important for understanding the determinants of aging and trajectories of age-related morbidities." In a recommendation that has special relevance to ETT, it is seen as necessary to "examine biodemography studies that characterize functionality over the life course and examine age- and/or sex-specific processes critical to our understanding of how morbidity emerges and evolves in a population as it ages." A life course approach of this kind is also critical for understanding the etiology of frailty. Rather than using a cross-sectional approach to focus on one dysregulated system at a time, a temporal approach is able to examine the extent and timing of "multisystem dysregulation" and "implementation of frailty assessment in clinical settings."

Furthermore, health in late life reflects not only contemporaneous conditions, but also the biological forces and lifestyle factors that shape an individual's development from the earliest stage to maturity. This reality also motivates the use of a life course perspective.

One area that should be addressed by future studies is how sexual dimorphism contributes to differences in contextual susceptibility to stressors or their differential health effects at the population level. Differences in social standing or economic status may at least partially account for apparent gender differences in exposures and health outcomes. For this reason, it is important that future research consider the socioeconomic partitioning of health outcomes across the life course and its relation to sex differences in health and well-being.

Finally, there are many biomarkers, effect modifications, interactions, additive effects, and selection biases, among others, that remain undiscovered as yet. These factors need to be addressed in the general older population. Of course, people with specific conditions and disabilities are also growing old, and they should not be forgotten in studies either.

Natural and Built Environment

There is a growing interest in examining how climatic change and other environmental events affect social, economic, and political aspects of everyday life. Research to date indicates that older adults are most vulnerable to the ill effects of heat waves, floods, and major storms. It is clear that global warming will have negative influences on aging populations, in that older people are especially vulnerable to heat waves and other climatic events (Finch et al., 2014). Given the anticipated increase in these events' incidence, it is important to develop better strategies of adaptation to reduce the risks faced by a growing older population.

More detailed and sophisticated research is also needed on the effects of the built environment (e.g., residential housing patterns, density, and transportation patterns), on health behavior (e.g., walking and access to goods and services), and on health outcomes. Although a number of chapters in this text argue for the importance of research on the built environment, the most developed research to date has focused on mobility and falls. From the time that the disability model—really a variant of an ecological model—was developed, researchers have recognized that mobility (e.g., walking or driving) can be either enhanced or impeded by environmental factors. Today, there is a need to determine the independent and joint effects of environmental factors on different mobility outcomes. Research on falls is especially noteworthy. Indeed, falls research may serve as a model for better understanding the health effects of environmental factors. Elsewhere in this text, it is recommended that falls research should focus on the intersection of the "location, activity, and consequences of falling, [as] the specific fall outcomes may vary by older adults' health outcomes and behavioral phenotype." In addition, it is not enough to classify environments by location; rather, they must be categorized based on by the activities pursued there and the time spent in those activities.

Technology

The recent achievements in informatics technology and mobile computing have created both multiple challenges and extraordinary opportunities for the field of the epidemiology of aging. Mobile devices can improve social interactions, allow family members and friends to be socially connected in real time regardless of physical distances, and reduce the social isolation that is all too common in older age. At the same time, they may potentially increase the time spent on sedentary activities and reduce physical activity, especially the outdoor activities that are critical to maintaining physical and mental health in older age.

Technology can be thought of in two ways. First, technology can be defined as various devices, such as electronic medical records, walking aids, and environmental sensors (Lindeman, 2012). Although a growing number of technological devices are being produced to make life easier for older adults, relatively little systematic research has been conducted to determine whether specific devices are effective, especially among diverse populations of older people (Maus, Lindeman, & Satariano, 2016). Likewise, little

research has sought to examine factors associated with access to technological devices, regardless of how effective those devices are (Satariano, Scharlach, & Lindeman, 2014). In addition, with the development of new transportation systems (e.g., self-driving cars, new forms of passenger transport), there is a need to examine their effects on the everyday lives of older people.

Second, technology can be thought of as innovative systems through which to better conduct aging research. Mobile devices, including wearable gadgets, may open up new opportunities for continuously collecting personal data on health, mobility, lifestyles, falls/injury events, and ecological moments. The use of natural-language processing makes it possible to turn older adults' electronic medical records into individual-level longitudinal quantitative databases on fall history or other health-related events, and risk factors can be processed and made available in nearly real time.

Technology related to mobility and transportation holds great promise as a means to address the increased risk for adverse events and injuries among older individuals, their increasing fragility, and the sequelae of certain diseases, functional impairments, and use of medications that may limit the safe use of different transportation modes such as driving, walking, cycling, or riding in vehicles. In the future, we will need to determine the effects of the increasing range of interventions that become available to enhance the health and function of older transportation users, as well as to make their vehicles and environments safer and more accommodating, on a broader range of outcomes and in different groups of individuals. Globally, there is a need to understand the changes that are occurring in middle- and lower-income countries with respect to older drivers and transportation users, the particular challenges these countries face in implementing programs, and the "best practices" in terms of possible solutions to these challenges.

New-technology development will need to ensure that the needs of older individuals are considered when these technologies are developed and tested, and that older individuals have sufficient access to beneficial technologies and are appropriately trained in their use. Some examples from the transportation realm include in-vehicle technologies, driverless cars, and ride services.

There is also growing interest in how technology might potentially support behavioral and social interventions—or serve as an actual intervention for screening, diagnosis, treatment, or environmental modification. Some examples include the use of mHealth tools to help with initial assessments of behavior and social supports, support behavioral adherence through reminders, or make and track referrals (Dahlke et al., 2015). Similarly, mTools are being used to engage and motivate older adults to be more physically active and mentally alert (Satariano et al., 2014).

Other important technological areas that are rapidly developing include the use of technology for making homes safer, thereby enabling older adults to live independently longer (Magnusson, Hanson, & Borg, 2004). Examples include monitoring for fall occurrences in the home, uniform data collection from patients in existing programs and community initiatives by facilitating community-clinical connectivity, and electronic training for the STEADI Toolkit and continuing education credits for such training for clinicians and allied health professionals.

Conceptual Models

More sophisticated conceptual models are needed that will better capture patterns of health, functioning, and life expectancy over the life course. Research on comorbidity and multimorbidity illustrates the utility of looking beyond categorical conditions (e.g., heart disease or diabetes) given that older people are likely to have more than one condition. While the early work in this area has typically focused on the number of multiple morbidities found among older adults, more recent research has sought to understand "clusters" of multimorbidities—that is, particular combinations of conditions. A new generation of studies will require common definitions and standard measurement and methodological protocols to examine these issues. This approach also may be useful to examine clusters of health-promoting behaviors. That is, rather than examining just physical activity or diet or tobacco exposure, new insights may be obtained by examining the patterns or clusters of health behaviors. Research in this area, in turn, may lead to more innovative and efficient health promotion programs.

To speed the design and development of effective frailty surveillance and intervention strategies, and to translate those strategies into the routine clinical management of frail older adults, researchers need to refine and standardize measurements of frailty. It is also necessary to advance three other major areas: (1) design of integrative approaches for etiologic research, (2) development of methodologies to evaluate interventions targeting multisystem dysregulation, and (3) implementation of frailty assessment in clinical settings.

To date, most of the studies conducted in this area so far have two major limitations. First, most have been cross-sectional and correlative, which means that they could not identify causal relationships. Second, the underlying individual-level aging-related physiologic changes have not been well characterized. The individual trajectories, therefore, may be better predictors of frailty than simply a snapshot of a biomediator's level at one point of time (Xue, Beamer, Chaves, Guralnik, & Fried, 2010; Xue, Guralnik, Beamer, Fried, & Chaves, 2015; Xue, Walston, Fried, & Beamer, 2011).

To test hypotheses related to multisystem decline with aging, we will need multisystem data collected prospectively over the lifespan. Collecting such data in humans is a labor-intensive and costly endeavor, but animal models with diverse genetic backgrounds may serve as alternatives for the study of complex disease risks and aging. An example is the rat model of low versus high intrinsic aerobic exercise capacity developed by researchers at the University of Michigan (Koch & Britton, 2001; Xue et al., 2016).

Clinical translation of frailty research will require the use of new approaches and models. Some areas to be addressed include the adaptation of theory-based operational definitions, such as the PFP, which include performance-based measures that are not standard in clinical practice. In addition, short self-report frailty questionnaires may not accurately identify frail patients. Other questions include whether frailty assessment should be standardized for all clinical care settings, or if it should be tailored to each application. There is also a need to develop specific treatment options for frailty that are tailored to a given clinical population. The current incorporation of frailty into clinical settings is largely based on observational findings; clinical trials evidence is needed. Future studies are also needed to independently validate frailty measures in different specialties, so as to better understand the feasibility and predictive ability of frailty for risk stratification of treatments and procedures. Finally, the identification of clinical and laboratory biomarkers to diagnose frailty and to guide the development and targeting of preventive strategies should be explored (Walston et al., 2006).

International Studies

If we are to truly understand global patterns of aging, it will be necessary to conduct more international studies. To make global comparisons of data, however, researchers working in this area will need to identify a common set of important questions and a common methodology for carrying out such investigations. It is also important to realize that some studies will require international comparisons among a subset of nations. For example, with the rapid introduction of the automobile and other forms of mass transit, it will be important to determine the extent to which such technological innovations either enhance or impede mobility and other behavioral outcomes in populations (e.g., Mexico, China, and India).

To facilitate future international research that furthers the agenda on human aging, greater collaboration will be needed among various partners, including academia and research institutions, international organizations (e.g., United Nations, World Health Organization, International Labor Organization), and international donors and charities (e.g., Bill and Melinda Gates Foundation, nongovernmental associations such as Help Age). A paramount concern is the need to mobilize local resources to encourage local health professionals and older adults to take part in the research and knowledge translation activities so as to produce locally relevant research.

International researchers should jointly formulate and examine hypotheses that explore how the economic and social contexts influence physical functioning and mental health of older populations. Organizing international workshops to design conceptual frameworks that integrate biological, economic, psychological, and social aspects of aging and facilitating consortia to fund such research projects in specific regions are two examples of these collaborations.

Finally, greater efforts should be devoted to pooling international population-based data to make those data available to interested researchers. One example of this kind of activity is the Gateway to Global Aging Data (https://g2aging.org/index.php?section=homepage), a platform for population survey data on aging from around the world. This platform provides a digital library of searchable survey items that opens up the possibility for finding comparable questions across surveys. Most of the countries contributing data to this data set are high-income countries, but there are also data from middle-income countries such as Mexico, Indonesia, Costa Rica, and India. Another platform worth mentioning is Maelstrom Research (https://www.maelstrom-research.org/), which brings together an international team of epidemiologists, statisticians, and computer scientists to propose data-harmonization tools and data-sharing models. The ultimate goal is facilitation of collaborative epidemiological research, through the application of the principles of "team science."

The following examples suggest the kinds of potential research projects that are feasible to conduct through international collaborations:

- Examination of pathways through which diseases result in disability, using identical conceptual frameworks in different contexts.
- Establishment of evidence-based links between universal healthcare accessibility, universal old-age pensions, and opportunities for active aging by cross-country analyses, similar to what has been done in the SHARE study within European countries (Borsch-Supan et al., 2013).
- Collection of new data when it is necessary to test new and innovative hypotheses in response to new challenges that populations face, such as studying the impact of climate change (e.g., nutritional changes imposed on older adults due to climate change; mortality related to heat waves in poor countries), emerging infectious diseases (e.g., chikungunya, dengue fever, and Zika in Latin America), and financial fraud by banks and financial institutions geared toward older adults' lifelong savings.
- Evaluation of the impacts of social and economic interventions within both local and wider contexts on the health of older populations. For example, one might study the health benefits associated with improvements in social cohesion and personal safety as well as with decreased crime rates in neighborhoods.
- Evaluation of the rapid changes in the structure of modern societies and their potential effects on the health status of older adults. Recent decades have witnessed events such as urbanization and migration that involve a large proportion of the population as well as very fast-paced changes in social constructs and values that have happened within the lifespan of a single generation. Today's older adults were brought up with different family values, more conservative gender roles, and fewer uses of technologies in their daily life compared to younger generations. Although these social changes have happened all over the world, the degree of changes varies across countries. Exploration of the health attributes of these social changes is another international research opportunity.

▶ Conclusion

If Moore's law were to be applied to the exponential increase in the body of information about the aging of the world's population, we could foresee the need to identify significant areas where our research efforts would be best directed. The ultimate goal is not just to continue expanding our knowledge of the subject, but rather to encourage the translation of this knowledge and aging research into practice and policy so as to improve the chances that people will age in a healthy manner. We hope that this summary chapter on future directions will contribute in some measure toward this crucial goal.

References

Borsch-Supan, A., Brandt, M., Hunkler, C., Kneip, T., Korbmacher, J., Malter, F.,... Zuber, S. (2013). Data resource profile: The Survey of Health, Aging and Retirement in Europe (SHARE). *International Journal of Epidemiology*, dyt088.

Dahlke, D. V., Fair, K., Hong, Y. A., Beaudoin, C. E., Pulczinski, J., & Ory, M. G. (2015). Apps seeking theories: Results of a study on the use of health behavior change theories in cancer survivorship mobile apps. *JMIR mHealth and uHealth*, 3(1), e31.

Finch, C. E., Beltrán-Sánchez, H., & Crimmins, E. M. (2013). Uneven futures of human lifespans: Reckonings from Gompertz mortality rates, climate change, and air pollution. *Gerontology*, *60*(2), 183–188.

Koch, L. G., & Britton, S. L. (2001). Artificial selection for intrinsic aerobic endurance running capacity in rats. *Physiological Genomics*, *5*(1), 45–52.

Lindeman, D. (2012). Technology and aging. In T. R. Prohaska, L. A. Anderson, & R. H. Binstock (Eds.), *Public health for an aging society* (p. 253). Baltimore, MD: The Johns Hopkins University Press.

Magnusson, L., Hanson, E., & Borg, M. (2004). A literature review study of information and communication technology as a support for frail older people living at home and their family carers. *Technology and Disability*, *16*(4), 223–235.

Maus, M., Lindeman, D. A., & Satariano, W. A. (2016). Wayfinding, mobility, and technology for an aging society. In R. H. Hunter, A. L. Anderson, & L. B. Belza (Eds.), *Community wayfinding: Pathways to understanding* (pp. 153–167). Cham, Switzerland: Springer International.

Satariano, W. A., Scharlach, A. E., & Lindeman, D. (2014). Aging, place, and technology: Toward improving access and wellness in older populations. *Journal of Aging and Health*, *26*(8), 1373–1389. doi:10.1177/0898264314543470

Walston, J., Hadley, E. C., Ferrucci, L., Guralnik, J. M., Newman, A. B., Studenski, S. A.,… Fried, L. P. (2006). Research agenda for frailty in older adults: Toward a better understanding of physiology and etiology: Summary from the American Geriatrics Society/National Institute on Aging Research Conference on Frailty in Older Adults. *Journal of the American Geriatrics Society*, *54*(6), 991–1001.

World Health Organization (WHO). (2015). *World report on aging and health*. Luxembourg: Author.

Xue, Q. L., Beamer, B. A., Chaves, P. H., Guralnik, J. M., & Fried, L. P. (2010). Heterogeneity in rate of decline in grip, hip, and knee strength and the risk of all-cause mortality: The Women's Health and Aging Study II. *Journal of the American Geriatrics Society*, *58*(11), 2076–2084.

Xue, Q.-L., Guralnik, J. M., Beamer, B. A., Fried, L. P., & Chaves, P. H. (2015). Monitoring 6-month trajectory of grip strength improves the prediction of long-term change in grip strength in disabled older women. *Journals of Gerontology, Series A: Biological Sciences and Medical Sciences*, *70*(3), 365–371.

Xue, Q.-L., Walston, J. D., Fried, L. P., & Beamer, B. A. (2011). Prediction of risk of falling, physical disability, and frailty by rate of decline in grip strength: The Women's Health and Aging Study. *Archives of Internal Medicine*, *171*(12), 1119–1121.

Xue, Q.-L., Yang, H., Li, H.-F., Abadir, P. M., Burks, T. N., Koch, L. G.,… Walston, J. D. (2016). Rapamycin increases grip strength and attenuates age-related decline in maximal running distance in old low capacity runner rats. *Aging*, *8*(4), 769–776.

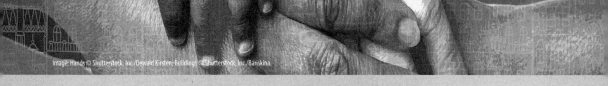

Index

Page numbers followed by 'f' and 't' refer to figures and tables respectively.